IRON METABOLISM

AN INTERNATIONAL SYMPOSIUM

SPONSORED BY

CIBA

AIX-EN-PROVENCE, 1st-5th JULY, 1963

CHAIRMEN

J.-C. DREYFUS AND G. SCHAPIRA

PARIS

EDITED BY

F. GROSS

WITH THE ASSISTANCE OF

S. R. NAEGELI AND H. D. PHILPS

BASLE

WITH 234 FIGURES

SPRINGER-VERLAG

BERLIN · GÖTTINGEN · HEIDELBERG

1964

Softcover reprint of the hardcover 1st edition 1964

Library of Congress Catalog Card Number 64—17311

ISBN 978-3-642-87154-2 ISBN 978-3-642-87152-8 (eBook)
DOI 10.1007/ 978-3-642-87152-8

Title No. 1226

Preface

International Symposia sponsored by CIBA Basle have been held once a year since 1959 in various European countries. In contrast to the many scientific meetings organised by the CIBA FOUNDATION either at its headquarters in London or occasionally abroad, the subjects dealt with at these International Symposia have concerned problems more directly related to CIBA's own research work in the pharmaceutical field. The various topics covered up to the present reflect the far-reaching interests and the widespread activities that a pharmaceutical enterprise develops in quite diverse fields of chemical, biological, and medical research, and to which the basic approach is an increasingly important prerequisite for the development of a new and useful therapeutic agent.

Iron metabolism came into the sphere of interest in connection with CIBA's research on antibiotics and related natural products containing iron, substances which act in their metal-free form as strong and specific chelating agents. Of course, these observations, interesting though they are, would not in themselves have justified a symposium. It seemed, however, useful to examine the new results from a wider perspective and to attempt to relate them to present-day knowledge of iron metabolism in general — its physiology, its pathology, and therapeutic aspects.

The success of a scientific symposium depends on the conception of the programme and the selection of the participants. Dr. J.-C. DREYFUS and Dr. G. SCHAPIRA, who kindly took over the burden of organising the meeting, achieved both these aims and had the satisfaction that almost all the specialists asked to participate accepted the invitation. They were also responsible for the selection of Aix-en-Provence as a meeting place, where the beautiful surroundings beneath the blue sky of Provence provided an ideal atmosphere not only for scientific discussions, but also for relaxation and diversion. Special thanks are also due to Dr. P. SAGAUT who was responsible for the local arrangements.

An international meeting which gathers people from various parts of the world inevitably poses a linguistic problem. We are particularly grateful to the chairmen and their compatriots who — albeit in the heart of their own country — accepted the inconvenience of speaking a foreign language. Although one perfect and impressive example of the beauty of the French language was given, there was a general agreement to communicate in English, which is now accepted as the most useful means of understanding at international conferences of this kind. When, however, we were confronted with the problem of the difference between English and American spelling, we chose a compromise solution, adhering to the American usage for the papers by American speakers and to British spelling for the other papers and for the record of the discussions.

That it was possible to edit the proceedings of the symposium without much delay was due to the willing co-operation of all participants, to the efforts of the publishers and their staff, and to the help of various people in our office. The editor is deeply indebted to all who have contributed to the preparation of this volume, including especially Dr. R. Deguillaume who translated the summaries into French, Dr. Wiltrud Hatzinger who prepared the index, and Miss B. Pfeifer who typed part of the discussions during the meeting. Thanks are given to Springer-Verlag, who again on this occasion did everything possible to ensure publication by the date we had taken as our target.

Basle, November 1963 *F. G.*

Contents

Iron deficiency

Iron overload

Therapeutics

Participants in the Symposium

ALBAHARY, C.	Centre Hospitalier de Saint-Denis, Saint-Denis, Seine (France)
BEARN, A. G..	The Rockefeller Institute for Medical Research, New York, N.Y. (U.S.A.)
BEUTLER, E..	Department of Medicine, City of Hope Medical Center, Duarte, Calif. (U.S.A.)
BICKEL, H.	Forschungslaboratorien der CIBA Aktiengesellschaft, Basel (Switzerland)
BOTHWELL, T. H. . .	Department of Medicine, University of Witwatersrand, Johannesburg (South Africa)
BOYE NIELSEN, J. . .	Medicinsk Afdeling A, Rigshospitalet, København (Denmark)
BRICK, I. B.	Department of Medicine, Georgetown University School of Medicine and Hospital, Washington, D.C. (U.S.A.)
CALLENDER, SHEILA T.	The Nuffield Department of Clinical Medicine, The Radcliffe Infirmary, Oxford (Great Britain)
CAROLI, J..	Hôpital Saint-Antoine, Paris (France)
CHATTERJEA, J. B. . .	Department of Haematology, Calcutta School of Tropical Medicine, Calcutta (India)
CLETON, F. J.	Instituut voor Radiopathologie en Stralenbescherming, Academisch Ziekenhuis, Leiden (The Netherlands)
DREYFUS, B..	Hôpital Saint-Antoine, Paris (France)
DREYFUS, J.-C. . . .	Laboratoire de Recherches de Biochimie Médicale, Hôpital des Enfants-Malades, Paris (France)
EICHHORN, G. L.. . .	Baltimore City Hospitals, Baltimore, Md. (U.S.A.)
FIGUEROA, W. G.. . .	Department of Medicine, University of California, Los Angeles, Calif. (U.S.A.)
FINCH, C. A..	Department of Medicine, University of Washington, Seattle, Wash. (U.S.A.)
FRICK, P.	Medizinische Universitätsklinik, Kantonsspital Zürich, Zürich (Switzerland)
GAJDOS, A.	Clinique Médicale de l'Hôtel-Dieu, Paris (France)
GROSS, F.	Forschungslaboratorien der CIBA Aktiengesellschaft, Basel (Switzerland)

HALLBERG, L. . . . . Medicinska kliniken II, Göteborgs Universitet, Göteborg (Sweden)

HARRISON, PAULINE M. Department of Biochemistry, University of Sheffield, Sheffield (Great Britain)

HEILMEYER, L. . . . Medizinische Universitätsklinik, Freiburg im Breisgau (Germany)

IMHOF, P. . . . . . . Forschungslaboratorien der CIBA Aktiengesellschaft, Basel (Switzerland)

KATZ, J. H. . . . . . Radioisotope Service, Veterans Administration Hospital, Boston, Mass. (U.S.A.)

KEBERLE, H. . . . . Forschungslaboratorien der CIBA Aktiengesellschaft, Basel (Switzerland)

KRUH, J. . . . . . . Laboratoire de Recherches de Biochimie Médicale, Hôpital des Enfants-Malades, Paris (France)

LABIE, DOMINIQUE . . Laboratoire de Recherches de Biochimie Médicale, Hôpital des Enfants-Malades, Paris (France)

LONDON, I. M.. . . . Department of Medicine, Albert Einstein College of Medicine, New York, N.Y. (U.S.A.)

MOESCHLIN, S.. . . . Medizinische Klinik, Bürgerspital, Solothurn (Switzerland)

MOORE, C. V. . . . . Department of Medicine, Washington University School of Medicine, St. Louis, Missouri (U.S.A.)

MORGAN, E. H. . . . Department of Physiology, University of Western Australia, Nedlands (Australia)

MOURIQUAND, C. . . . Laboratoire d'Histologie, Faculté de Médecine et de Pharmacie, Grenoble (France)

NAJEAN, Y. . . . . . Institut de Recherches de la Faculté de Médecine, Hôpital Saint-Louis, Paris (France)

OLMER, J.. . . . . . Clinique Médicale Thérapeutique, Hôpital de la Conception, Marseille (France)

PETERS, G. . . . . . Forschungslaboratorien der CIBA Aktiengesellschaft, Basel (Switzerland)

POLLYCOVE, M. . . . University of California School of Medicine, San Francisco, Calif. (U.S.A.)

PRELOG, V. . . . . . Laboratorium für organische Chemie, Eidgenössische Technische Hochschule, Zürich (Switzerland)

RITTENBERG, D. . . . Department of Biochemistry, College of Physicians and Surgeons of Columbia University, New York, N.Y. (U.S.A.)

ROSA, J. . . . . . . Laboratoire de Recherches de Biochimie Médicale, Hôpital des Enfants-Malades, Paris (France)

SAADI, R. . . . . . . Laboratoire de Recherches de Biochimie Médicale, Hôpital des Enfants-Malades, Paris (France)

SALERA, U. . . . . . Clinica Medica, Università di Roma, Roma (Italy)

SCHÄFER, K. H. . . . Universitäts-Kinderklinik, Hamburg-Eppendorf (Germany)

SCHAPIRA, G. . . . . Laboratoire de Recherches de Biochimie Médicale, Hôpital des Enfants-Malades, Paris (France)

SCHUBERT, J. . . . . Facultad de Ciencias Exactas y Naturales, Universidad de Buenos Aires, Buenos Aires (Argentina)

SCHWARZMANN, V. . . Laboratoire de Recherches d'Enzymologie Clinique et Expérimentale, Hôpital Saint-Antoine, Paris (France)

SHERLOCK, SHEILA . . Department of Medicine, The Royal Free Hospital, London (Great Britain)

STURGEON, P. . . . . National Research Laboratory, The American National Red Cross, Los Angeles, Calif. (U.S.A.)

TRIPOD, J.. . . . . . Forschungslaboratorien der CIBA Aktiengesellschaft, Basel (Switzerland)

TUBIANA, M.. . . . . Institut Gustave-Roussy, Centre Clinique et Thérapeutique, Villejuif, Seine (France)

UNDRITZ, E.. . . . . Pharmakologisches Laboratorium, Sandoz A.G., Basel (Switzerland)

VANNOTTI, A. . . . . Clinique Médicale Universitaire, Hôpital Cantonal, Lausanne (Switzerland)

VENTURA, S.. . . . . Clinica Medica, Università di Perugia, Perugia (Italy)

VERLOOP, M. C. . . . Haematologisch Laboratorium, Geneeskundige Universiteitskliniek, Utrecht (The Netherlands)

VISCHER, E. . . . . . Forschungslaboratorien der CIBA Aktiengesellschaft, Basel (Switzerland)

WITTS, L. J.. . . . . The Nuffield Department of Clinical Medicine, The Radcliffe Infirmary, Oxford (Great Britain)

WÖHLER, F. . . . . . Medizinische Universitätsklinik, Freiburg im Breisgau (Germany)

YOSHIKAWA, H. . . . Department of Physiological Chemistry and Nutrition, Faculty of Medicine, University of Tokyo, Tokyo (Japan)

ZÄHNER, H. . . . . . Institut für Spezielle Botanik, Eidgenössische Technische Hochschule, Zürich (Switzerland)

Iron metabolism, past, present, and future

Introduction

By

G. Schapira

Briefly, the purpose of this Symposium is to discuss the subject of iron from the biological and medical aspect, both in the light of present-day knowledge and with a view to future developments.

By way of introduction, let us first take a glance at the history of iron.

The Ancients believed that iron was of heavenly origin. The Greeks, in fact, referred to it as *sideros* — a word which indicates its connotation with the stars — and one of the oldest names for iron was *anbar*, meaning sky and fire.

Iron was prized by the Greeks and the Romans as a gift from Mars, the warrior god, and some meteorites may indeed well have proved a gift to them.

Having been used in the making of tools as far back as the Iron Age, this metal was eventually to find its way into the physician's armamentarium. We have now reached what might be described as the biochemical era of iron — an era in which we are gaining a deeper insight into the role played by iron as a trace element in the physiology and pathology of the living organism.

From the time of Sydenham in the 17th century to the early 20th century, the history of iron in relation to medicine was closely interlinked with that of chlorosis, although, despite the efforts of Blaud, the effect exerted by iron in this connection was long to remain controversial.

Today our medical knowledge of iron and its properties is far greater. Nevertheless, as Bothwell has pointed out: "Current practices in iron therapy can give the physicians little cause for pride. Although a great variety of preparations are being promoted at the present time, their so-called advantages have no foundation in fact and, for the most part, depend on some special gimmick to attract the physician's or patient's eye".

In some cases, treatment in the form of injections of an iron preparation is undoubtedly justified. But the decision whether or not to use such a preparation may well be a difficult one — as, for example, in the case of the iron-dextran complex, Imferon.

An article bearing the arresting title "Carcinogenic risks of iron dextran" (Editorial) describes experiments on rats and mice in which repeated injections of massive doses of Imferon at the same site resulted in the development of a local sarcoma in a high percentage of the animals (HADDOW and HORNING). On the other hand, it must be conceded that, under the appropriate experimental conditions, given the right species and the right strain of animal, many harmless substances — even ordinary glucose and fructose — can be made to induce malignant tumours. Are we therefore to ban the use of such substances for the treatment of patients?

The answer to this question depends firstly on the magnitude of the risk involved. In this instance, the risk is very slight, because nobody has yet reported a case in which cancer has developed in man under such conditions.

The second consideration is whether the risk, be it great or small, is justified by the patient's condition. This point is often lost sight of, but we shall no doubt have an opportunity of discussing it in the course of this Symposium.

It was in 1713 that LEMMERY and GEOFFROY first demonstrated the presence of iron in tissues. Various types of haemin iron were subsequently described, but the very fact that the molecules contained such small amounts of iron frequently gave rise to controversies and misinterpretations.

In LIEBIG's "Tierchemie", published in 1843, there is a chapter entitled "The Theory of Respiration", in which combustion in the animal body is related to the presence of iron. LIEBIG believed that combustion took place in the blood, where the haemoglobin iron oxidised the biological substrates: "The blood corpuscles contain an iron compound; no other component of which the various parts of the body consist contains iron".

Working on LIEBIG's theory of respiration, HOPPE-SEYLER succeeded in crystallising haemoglobin in 1867. The discovery by MCMUNN that not only the red cells, but all cells contained haem was challenged by LEVY, an associate of HOPPE-SEYLER, and the influence of HOPPE-SEYLER was such that MCMUNN remained silent.

Non-haemin iron was not in fact described until the present century. It was FONTES and THIVOLLE who, in 1925, first demonstrated that plasma iron was different from haemoglobin iron; two years later, BARKAN observed that iron was bound to plasma protein. HOLMBERG and LAURELL discovered the iron-binding properties of plasma, and SURGENOR (with KOECHLIN and STRONG) isolated siderophilin; finally, twelve years previously, LAUFBERGER had isolated ferritin.

There are still iron compounds which have not been identified. If 3 out of 4 g. are contained in the haemoglobin, there remains in the muscles (excluding myoglobin) 0.5 g. of non-haemin iron, which, as we observed many years ago, is a complex (Table 1).

Table 1. *Iron in the human body (in g.)*

Haemoglobin	3.00
Cytochromes, catalase, siderophilin	0.01
Ferritin + haemosiderin	0.70
Muscular iron:	
myoglobin	0.15
non-haemin iron	0.50

Some of the iron is easily extractable, but some is not, and the pattern of extractability may change in pathological states (Fig. 1). The biochemical nature of this iron-containing complex, however, is still something of a mystery and cannot be explained in terms of the ferro-flavo-proteins which have been described since.

Two discoveries by CLAUDE BERNARD contributed towards an understanding of the function of iron in the animal organism, viz. the effect of hydrogen cyanide and of carbon monoxide on chemical reactions in the cell. "*En faisant respirer de l'acide prussique à un animal, on voit que son sang veineux devient rutilant. Quelquefois, le lendemain de la mort on retrouve encore la même coloration dans le sang du cœur. Bien que la quantité de l'acide respirée soit extrêmement minime, le chien est très malade. Si d'ici quelques instants il ne succombe pas rapidement, il reviendra à une santé parfaite.*"

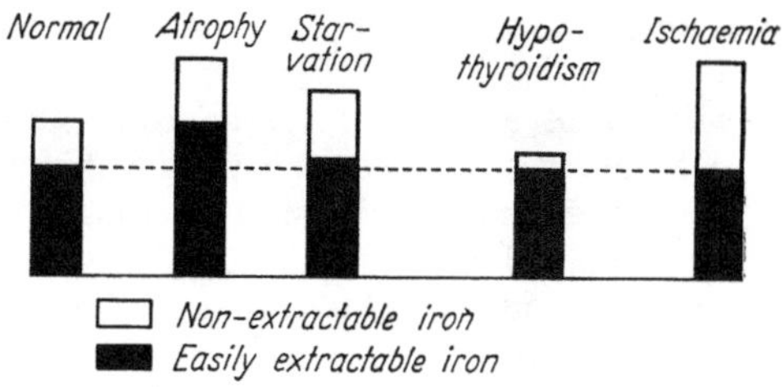

Fig. 1. Non-haemin iron from muscle in normal and pathological conditions

Since a small amount of cellular substance can deal with large amounts of substrate, aerobic respiration, anaerobic glycolysis, carbon dioxide, and nitrate assimilation are catalytic processes, and since a small amount of cyanide will inhibit the metabolism of much substrate, cyanide inhibition is therefore an anticatalytic process, and enzymes involved in this metabolism must have catalytically active groups which are chemically alike. This was one of the principles underlying the investigations of biochemical processes carried out by OTTO WARBURG.

In studies of this type, use was also made of carbon monoxide, which exerts its poisonous effect by acting on haemoglobin. CLAUDE BERNARD therefore concluded: "*On voit par ces résultats que l'oxyde de carbone déplace l'oxygène du sang.*" The action exerted by light on carbonyl haemoglobin was studied by HALDANE and LORRAINE SMITH, who likewise discovered that carbon monoxide compounds underwent photochemical dissociation. The fact that an enzymatic reaction could be reversed by carbon monoxide indicated that the reacting group of the enzyme was a heavy metal. Since the carbon monoxide inhibitor was sensitive to light, this meant that the heavy metal was iron.

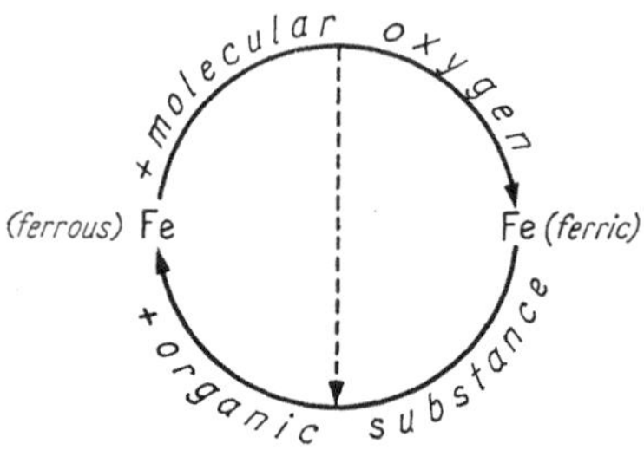

Fig. 2. Oxidoreduction of iron in a metabolic chain (From O. WARBURG)

A chemical model of what was supposed to be a process of auto-oxidation was provided by cysteine in solution, which is oxidised to cystine when left to stand in the air (Fig. 2). "*Bei der Darstellung des Cysteins, Reduktion des Cystins mit Zink und Salzsäure, ist eine Verunreinigung mit Eisen schwer zu vermeiden*", said WARBURG, but when the cysteine was purified and pure buffer solution and quartz vessels were used, auto-oxidation no longer occurred. The oxidation of cysteine, which is inhibited by cyanide, was not in fact attributable to auto-oxidation, but was an example of oxygen transport by a heavy metal.

"Molecular oxygen which is used up by the respiration of aerobic cells never reacts directly with the biological substrates, but always and exclusively with divalent iron combined in a complex. Iron of a higher valency is thereby formed, and this is reduced back again to the divalent state by organic substances. Thus, in so far as the iron is concerned, the original state is regained" (WARBURG). A valency change therefore takes place in a complex iron compound by which the oxygen required for cell respiration is transported; in other words, iron is the oxygen-transporting part of the respiratory enzyme.

In 1937, an entirely new light was shed on the physiology of iron by MCCANCE, who observed that the parenteral injection of iron was not followed by any increase in faecal excretion of the metal.

With regard to the physiological difference in the iron balances of males and females, this phenomenon, although better understood today, was already noted many years ago, as mentioned by UNDRITZ in his work "Significance and Beauty of Colours in Haematology". Men are in fact darker than women. However, as MOORE pointed out in his Harvey Lecture, the most exciting chapter in the story of iron concerns the movement of iron into and out of the cells — rather than into and out of the body — and the functions fulfilled by iron within the cell. It is particularly these aspects of the problem which are at present being studied and which we shall be discussing today and tomorrow. We are, in fact, now on the brink of a new era in medicine: the molecular age.

There are two principal pigments encountered in living matter: one is the green pigment, chlorophyll, and the other is the red pigment, haemin. Both are porphyrin compounds. It is interesting to speculate how these pigments evolved and what metabolic pathways their evolution followed.

Is it likely that, after the many different stages of evolution which gave rise to haem, the properties of oxidation were suddenly created? Might it not be reasonable to postulate, as GRANICK did, that the function of oxidation was so fundamental that it must have been part of the first protoplasm arising from an inorganic origin? The coelacanths *Latimeria chalumnae* are known to have remained morphologically unchanged for hundreds of millions of years; if their biochemistry is also unchanged, their iron enzymes are perhaps as old as life itself.

The properties of haem are those of the iron atom. We can discuss the ability of a simple, hydrated ferric ion to break down hydrogen peroxide, yielding water and oxygen, or to act as a peroxidase. "Simple aqueous ferric ion has a catalytic activity expressed by the number 10^{-5}. If, however, we surround that iron ion with a suitable organic grouping, it turns out that the catalytic ability of that iron has been enhanced by a factor of 1,000 (Fig. 3). If we build the haem into a still more complex structure with a protein around it, we can increase the catalytic ability by several more powers of 10" (CALVIN).

This raises the question as to how this can come about in a natural, evolutionary manner. The answer given by CALVIN is that the process occurs by "autocatalysis and self-selection. There is a sequence of reactions, leading from the compounds which were randoms synthesised by radiation (succinic acid and glycine) to the porphyrins (Fig. 4). The sequence of reactions involves simple condensation, followed by decarboxylation and another condensation (a double condensation really), followed by a series of oxi-

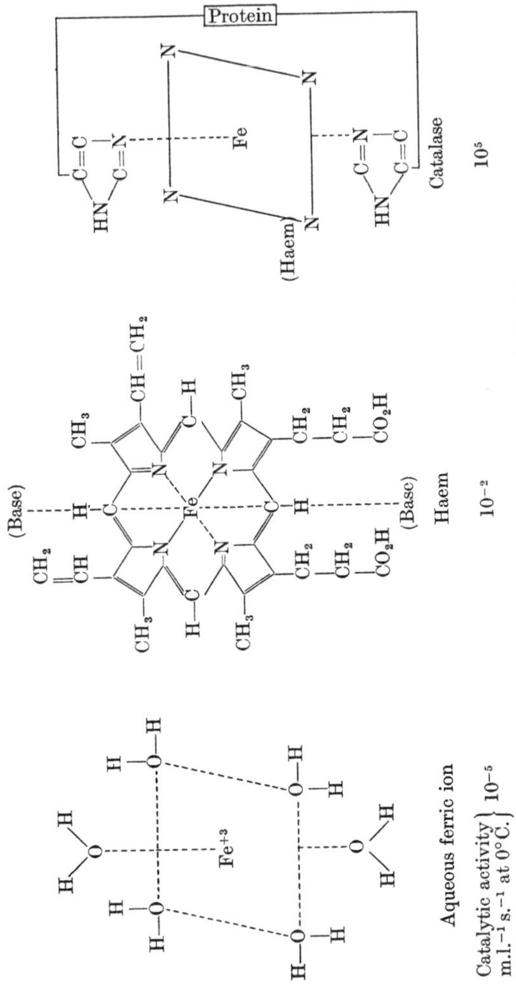

Fig. 3. Catalytic properties of iron (from M. Calvin)

dation steps, leading finally to the tetrapyrrole. If any of these steps is catalysed by iron and if the iron porphyrin structures turn out to be better catalysts for any of these steps than the bare iron

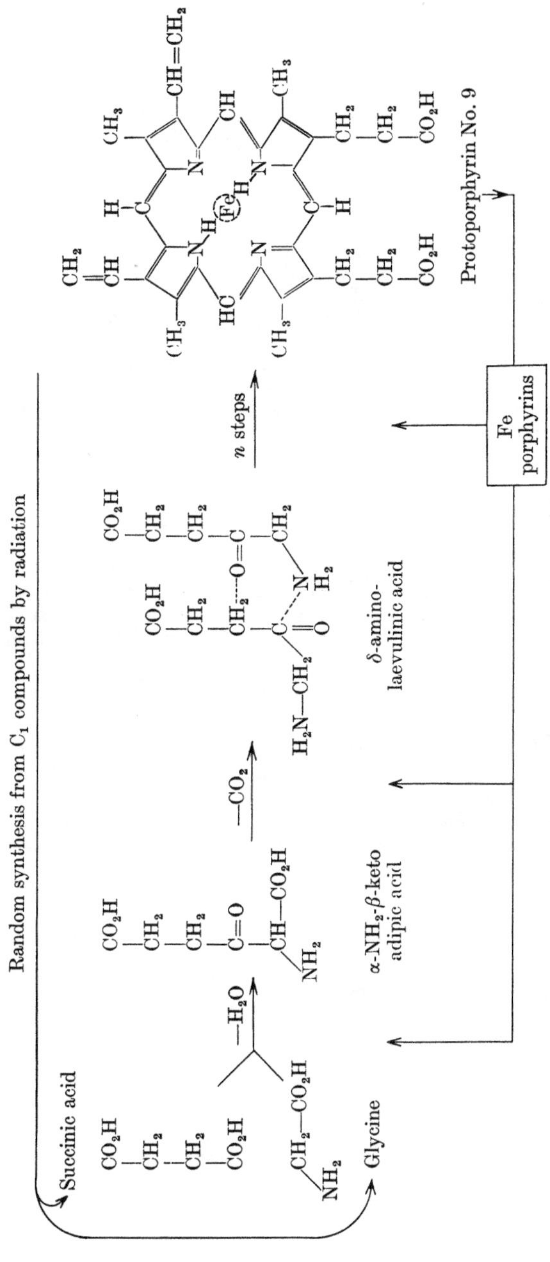

Fig. 4. Possible points for catalytic activities of iron (from M. CALVIN)

itself, you can see that once this process begins (as it would have begun here by random synthesis and condensation), an autoselection of this sequence would enhance the transformation of the succinic acid and glycine into delta-aminolevulinic acid and finally into the porphyrin". And then you know all about the origin of life!

References

BARKAN, G.: Zschr. physiol. Chem. (G.) **170**, 194 (1927). — BERNARD, C.: Leçons sur les effets des substances toxiques. Paris, 1887. — BEUTLER, E., V. F. FAIRBANKS, and J. L. FAHEY: Clinical Disorders of Iron Metabolism. Grune & Stratton, New York/London, 1962. — BLAUD, P.: Rev. méd. franç. étrang. **45**, 337 (1832). — BOTHWELL, T. H., and C. A. FINCH: In: Iron Metabolism. Little, Brown & Co., Boston/Toronto, 1962, p. 339. — CALVIN, M.: Advances Biol. Med. Phys. (U.S.A.) 8, 322 (1962). — DREYFUS, J.-C., and G. SCHAPIRA: Le fer. Biochimie, Physiologie, Pathologie. Expansion Scient. Franç., Paris, 1958. — *Editorial*: Brit. Med. J. **1960**/I, 788 (see also HADDOW and HORNING). — FONTES, G., and L. THIVOLLE: Compt. rend. Soc. biol. (Fr.) **93**, 687 (1925). — GRANICK, S.: Amer. Naturalist **87**, 65 (1953). — HADDOW, A., and E. S. HORNING: J. Nat. Cancer Inst. (U.S.A.) **24**, 109 (1960). — HALDANE, J., and J. L. SMITH: J. Physiol. (G.B.) **20**, 497 (1896). — HOLMBERG, C. G., and C. B. LAURELL: Acta physiol. Scand. **10**, 307 (1945). — HOPPE-SEYLER, F.: Zschr. physiol. Chem. (G.) **14**, 106 (1890). — LAUFBERGER, V.: Bull. Soc. chim. biol. (Fr.) **19**, 1575 (1937). — LEMERY, N., and E. GEOFFROY: In: CHRISTIAN, H. A.: Med. Libr. Hist. J. (U.S.A.) **1**, 176 (1903). — LEVY, L.: Zschr. physiol. Chem. (G.) **13**, 309 (1889). — LIEBIG, J.: Tierchemie, quoted by WARBURG. — MCCANCE, R. A., and E. M. WIDDOWSON: Lancet (G.B.) **1937**/II, 680. — MCMUNN, C. A.: Philos. Transact. Roy. Soc. London **177**, 267 (1886). — MOORE, C. V.: Harvey Lect. (U.S.A.) **55**, 67 (1961). — SURGENOR, D. M., B. A. KOECHLIN, and L. E. STRONG: J. Clin. Invest. (U.S.A.) **28**, 73 (1949). — SYDENHAM, T.: In: CHRISTIAN, H. A.: The Works of Thomas Sydenham. Allard, London, 1850. — UNDRITZ, E.: Signification et beauté des couleurs en hématologie, la science du sang. "Palette", Sandoz Ltd., Basle, No. **11**, 10—20 (1962). — WARBURG, O.: Heavy metal prosthetic groups and enzyme action. Clarendon Press, Oxford, 1949, pp. 27, 46, 63.

Biochemistry of iron

The function of iron in biochemistry

By

G. L. Eichhorn

A perusal of the various titles encompassed by this Symposium suggests that its primary concern is not with the *function* of iron in biochemistry, but rather with the *concentrations* of iron in biochemical systems. The biochemistry that is most immediately pertinent in such a context involves to a large extent molecules in which the iron really has no function at all.

The function of these molecules is, in fact, to transport the iron to the sites in which *it* has a function, or else to store the iron until the need for its function arises.

There is, nevertheless, a compelling reason for a consideration of function at the beginning of such a conference. There exist, of course, thermodynamic and kinetic relationships between the iron-storage and transport molecules and the substances that contain functioning iron. Therefore any acceleration or inhibition of the activity of the functional molecules will affect the concentration of iron in the storage and transport molecules. The former constitute the *raison d'être* of the latter, and consequently it is pointless to attempt to discuss the latter without an understanding of the molecules in which iron fulfils its biochemical role.

Attributes of iron useful in biochemical processes

Iron is the most versatile of all biochemically active metals and can be found associated with a large variety of biological molecules of many sizes and shapes. For this reason, a discussion of the function of iron in biochemistry is practically illustrative of the many different ways in which metallic ions generally participate in biological reactions. There is, in fact, no function served by iron that is not also served by another metal in a different system. The greater importance of iron is perhaps an accident of evolution.

The characteristics of iron which make it useful in biological systems are the following:

(1) Like other metallic ions, iron in solution represents a concentration of positive charge. This charge can distort molecular dipoles

in such a manner that covalent bonds are weakened and made more susceptible to cleavage. Another valuable result of this charge is that it can bring two molecules into close contact so that interaction may readily occur.

(2) The covalent bonds emanating from the iron atom are directed toward the six corners of an octahedron. This feature serves to orient molecules that interact while bound to the iron, and thus influences the stereochemistry of the reaction.

(3) Iron has two stable oxidation states and several more unstable oxidation states in aqueous solution, and the redox potential between these varies widely, depending upon the nature of the ligands. For this reason, iron complexes are useful in electron-transfer reactions.

(4) Both iron (II) and iron (III) can exhibit two different electronic configurations, which vary in the number of unpaired electrons. As a result, iron forms complexes of varying stabilities, again depending upon the ligands. This property of iron causes small changes in the ligands to effect large changes in the character of the iron, making possible a variety of reactions of apparently similar iron complexes.

The versatility of iron in the exercise of a variety of activities is exemplified by the hemoproteins, a group of iron compounds in which the coordination sphere around the iron is remarkably similar.

The hemoproteins

In all of these compounds, four of the six coordination positions around the iron are occupied by the nitrogen atoms of a porphyrin,

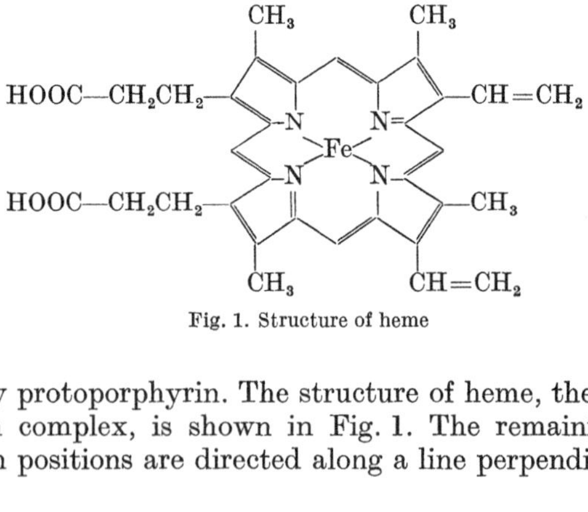

Fig. 1. Structure of heme

frequently protoporphyrin. The structure of heme, the iron protoporphyrin complex, is shown in Fig. 1. The remaining two coordination positions are directed along a line perpendicular to the plane of the porphyrin, and, in hemoproteins, they may be taken up by either two donor groups on the protein, as in cytochrome C, or only one such group and a small molecule (as in hemoglobin, catalase, and peroxidase).

The functions of the hemoproteins include the binding of molecular oxygen in hemoglobin, the transfer of electrons as in the cytochromes, and the cleavage of the peroxide structure, as in catalase and peroxidase. The ability of the iron atom bound to the porphyrin structure to engage in such a diversity of tasks is intimately related to the electronic configuration of iron, which can be most usefully considered from the point of view of the ligand field theory (*12*, *24*).

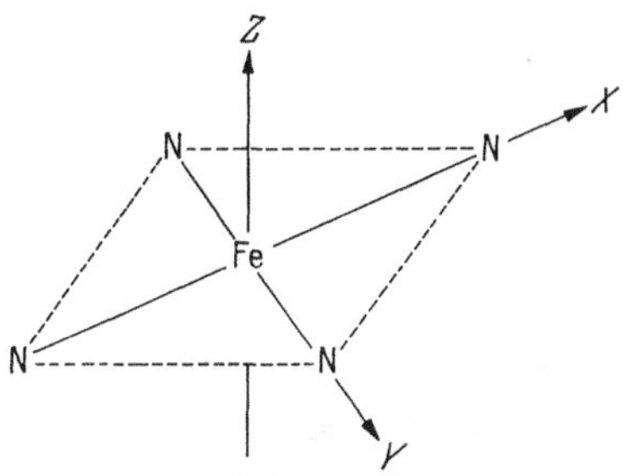

Fig. 2. Stereochemistry of iron

The iron atom in a hemoprotein can be considered as the focal point of a Cartesian coordinate system, with the porphyrin in the xy plane and the iron to nitrogen bonds in the heme pointing in the x and y directions (*6*, *7*). The fifth and sixth coordination positions of the iron will then point in the z direction, as is shown in Fig. 2.

The chemical properties of iron in either the $+2$ or the $+3$ oxidation state are determined primarily by the electrons in the $3d$ shell. This shell contains five orbitals, each of which is capable of accommodating two electrons of opposite spin, so that a total of ten electrons can be placed into a completed shell. In iron, the shell is not completed, having only six electrons in iron (II) and five in iron (III). The five orbitals into which these electrons are placed differ in the directional properties of the electrons, as shown in Fig. 3, in which the directional electron intensity is indicated schematically for three of the five orbitals. The electrons in Fig. 3 have been placed in the same coordinate system as the iron atom in Fig. 2. The significance of the diagrams in Fig. 3 is that the length of a line drawn from any point on the solid line in each drawing to the center is proportional to the electron density in the direction of the line. (Thus, the $d_{x^2-y^2}$ electron has maximal electron density in the x and y directions and zero electron density along a line bisecting the angle $x-\mathrm{Fe}-y$ in the xy plane, and zero electron density in the z direction.)

It can be seen from Fig. 3 that the electrons in the d_{z^2} and the $d_{x^2-y^2}$ orbitals point in the direction of the ligands, and therefore these electrons will repel the electrons on the ligands. The electrons in the d_{xy} orbital, on the other hand, have zero electron density in the direction of the ligands, and therefore there will be very little repulsion between a d_{xy} electron and the ligand electrons. The two additional orbitals, d_{xz} and d_{yz}, have not been shown, since their shapes are identical to the shape of the d_{xy} orbital,

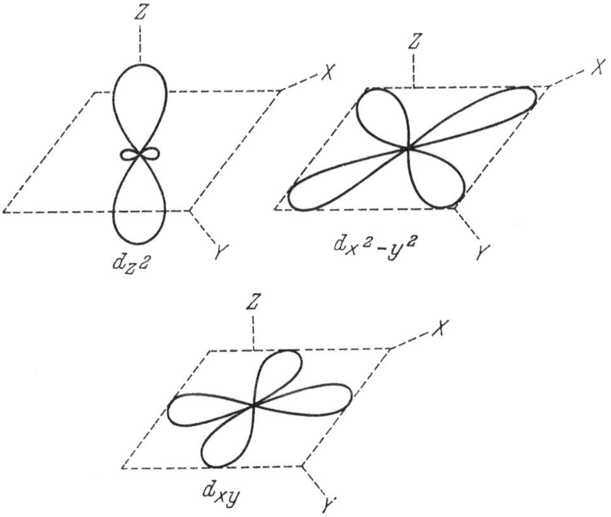

Fig. 3. Directional properties of *d*-orbitals

except that they are in different planes, as indicated by the subscripts. It is apparent that the d_{xz} and d_{yz} orbitals also exert very little repulsion against the electrons on the ligands.

Of the five orbitals available to the iron electrons, two of them, d_{z^2} and $d_{x^2-y^2}$, will therefore have a higher energy than the other three, d_{xy}, d_{xz}, and d_{yz}. It is therefore to be anticipated that the electrons will tend to fill the lower energy orbitals before any of them go into the higher energy orbitals. There is, however, another effect which counteracts the ligand-repulsion phenomenon. According to HUND's rule, two electrons in the same orbital repel each other, so that all orbitals tend to be singly occupied before any of them are filled by two electrons.

The conflict between HUND's rule and the ligand-repulsion phenomenon is responsible for the two different electronic configurations which both iron (II) and iron (III) can exhibit. If the ligands are held strongly enough, the repulsion between ligand electrons and the higher energy orbitals is large enough to overcome the HUND repulsion between electrons in the same orbital, and a *strong* field complex results. If, on the other hand, the ligand repulsion is weaker than the HUND effect, a weak field complex is produced instead. The electronic structures of the strong and weak field complexes of iron (II) and iron (III) are shown in Table 1 (which also includes structures for iron (IV) and (V) for later

Table 1. *Electronic configurations of iron*

	Fe(II)		Fe(III)	
	Weak	Strong	Weak	Strong
d_{z^2}	×	—	×	—
$d_{x^2-y^2}$	×	—	×	—
d_{xy}	×	××	×	×
d_{xz}	×	××	×	××
d_{yz}	××	××	×	××

	Fe(IV)		Fe(V)	
	Weak	Strong	Weak	Strong
d_{z^2}	—	—	—	—
$d_{x^2-y^2}$	×	—	—	—
d_{xy}	×	×	×	×
d_{xz}	×	×	×	×
d_{yz}	×	××	×	×

reference). It can be seen from the table that iron (II) has four unpaired electrons in a weak field complex and none in a strong field complex. Iron (III) has five and one unpaired electrons in weak and strong field complexes, respectively. A determination of the magnetic moment therefore provides a simple experimental means by which to determine the electronic configuration.

Thus it becomes possible to correlate the functions of the hemoproteins with the electronic configuration of the iron in these molecules.

Strong field hemoproteins

The purpose of the various hemoproteins that make up the cytochrome system is to transfer an electron (*16*) stepwise from molecular oxygen to other electron-carriers of lower potential. Cytochrome C is by far the most thoroughly investigated and best understood of the group. Its magnetic moment corresponds to one unpaired electron in its oxidized form, and it is diamagnetic in its reduced form (*13*). Cytochrome C is therefore a strong field complex. In order to carry out its electron-transfer mission, the molecule remains intact, and no change occurs in the coordination sphere around the iron. The requirement for the structure of cytochrome C is, in fact, that the addition and subtraction of an electron can take place with no effect upon the remainder of the molecule. The resulting constancy in the environment of the iron atom is achieved through the tight binding of a strong field complex. Thus, the electron transfer agent, requiring stability, has the electron configuration that confers the greatest amount of stability.

Little is known about the passage of electrons from one cytochrome molecule to another. It has been recently suggested that the imidazole rings bound to the iron could serve as passageways for electrons between the iron atoms (*21*).

Hemoproteins which alternate between weak and strong fields

The structural requirements of hemoglobin, catalase, and peroxidase are, in a sense, opposite to those of cytochrome C. In these molecules, only five of the coordination bonds to the iron are permanent, while the sixth coordination position is reserved for the substrates in peroxidase and catalase, and for oxygen in hemoglobin. All of these molecules are weak field complexes in the absence of substrate (or oxygen), when the sixth position is occupied by water, and they become strong field complexes when peroxide or oxygen are attached. As we shall see, these changes in electronic configuration are perfectly suited to the functional processes of the hemoproteins during which they occur.

The function of peroxidase is to break down peroxide molecules (*3*), which become attached to the sixth coordination position, in the presence of reducing agents (whose oxidation may be the ultimate purpose of the reaction in some instances). In the absence of substrate, peroxidase has a magnetic moment corresponding to five unpaired electrons (*19*); it is thus a weak field iron (III) complex. During the course of the reaction with hydrogen peroxide, there are formed two complexes containing iron in formal oxidation states of +5 and +4 (*2*, *8*, *20*). George's formulation (*8*) of the reaction sequence is represented schematically as follows:

(1) $$\text{—Fe}^{\text{III}}\text{—OH}_2 + \text{H}_2\text{O}_2 \rightarrow \text{—Fe}^{\text{V}} :: \ddot{\underset{\cdot\cdot}{\text{O}}} : \overset{\text{H}}{\ddot{\underset{\cdot\cdot}{\text{O}}}} : \text{H}$$

peroxidase complex I

(2) 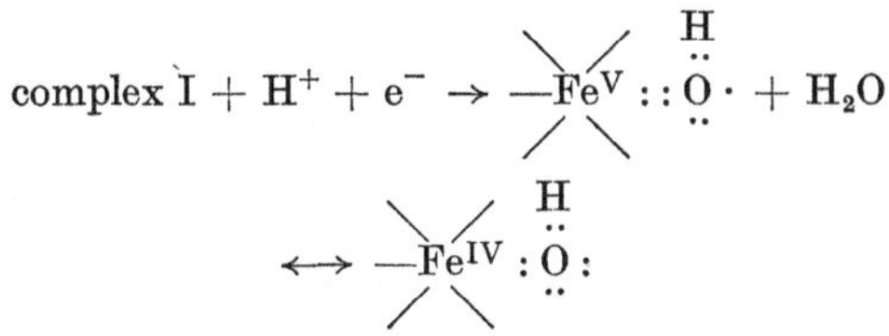

complex II

(3) 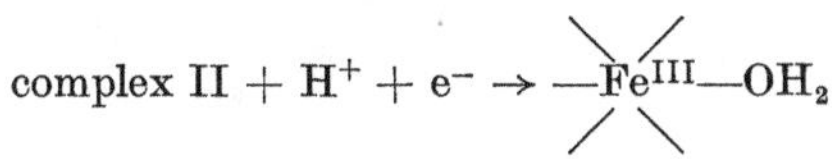

peroxidase

The electrons in the equations, of course, come from the reducing agents. Complex I has three unpaired electrons, which would be characteristic of iron (V) in either a weak or strong field complex, but complex II has only two unpaired electrons, the correct number for a strong field iron (IV) complex (*20*) (Table 1). The weak field hydrated peroxidase molecule readily gives up water in exchange for H_2O_2, which is bound sufficiently more tightly than water to give rise to a strong field complex. This complex is, however, unstable in the presence of reducing agents, which replenish the iron with electrons while breaking down the H_2O_2 molecule in the process.

Thus, the relatively weak peroxidase-water complex is readily converted into the relatively strong peroxidase-peroxide complex, which reverts to the former in the presence of the reducing agent. Catalase apparently works very similarly to peroxidase, except that another molecule of H_2O_2 can act as the reducing agent.

The function of hemoglobin is to transport molecular oxygen. In analogy with the interpretation of the electron configurations in peroxidase, it may be anticipated that the hydrated form of hemoglobin is a weak field complex which is then readily converted to oxyhemoglobin, which should be a strong field complex. Such is indeed the case; as the classical magnetic susceptibility studies of Pauling and Coryell have shown, hemoglobin containing iron (II) has four unpaired electrons, and oxyhemoglobin has none (*14*).

To sum up, then, hemoglobin, peroxidase, and catalase have an interesting property in common inasmuch as all these molecules are weak field complexes in the aquo form and turn into strong field complexes when they are bound to oxygen or peroxide. This change in electron configuration can provide the driving force for the substitution of water by the oxygen and peroxide molecules. To remove these molecules from the iron atom, the peroxide must be decomposed or the oxygen molecule removed by mass-action effects. Cytochrome C, on the other hand, requires structural stability during electron transfer and remains a strong field complex at all times.

Non-heme iron in biological catalysis

Even though a large proportion of the activity of iron in biochemical systems is carried out while the iron is bound to a porphyrin, there are many other biologically active iron compounds in which the iron is bound in some other fashion. It is quite possible that eventually the proportion of non-heme-bound functional iron compounds to the heme compounds will turn out to be much greater than is now suspected, since the stability of the iron-porphyrin attachment makes it so much easier to isolate the hemoproteins with the iron still in its place than it is to isolate other compounds in which the iron is much less strongly held, without detaching the iron from the molecules.

The aconitase reaction

Among the non-heme iron catalyzed reactions that have received relatively careful study is the aconitase reaction (*4*), which catalyzes the interconversion of citric, isocitric, and aconitic acids.

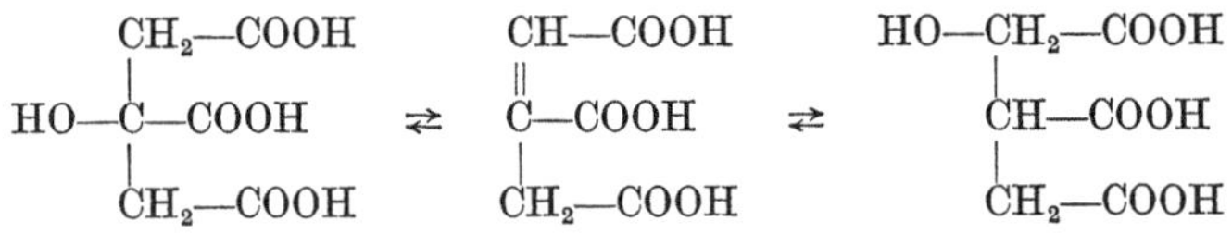

Citric acid Aconitic acid Isocitric acid

Little is known about the nature of the binding of the iron (II) to the enzyme, but evidence has been obtained that this reaction proceeds through carbonium ion intermediates (*17*), as is shown in Fig. 4. This mechanism illustrates, first of all, the importance of the positive charge on the iron in bringing about these conversions. In the iron (II) citrate complex (c) the iron withdraws electrons from the hydroxyl group, weakening the bond holding that group to the citrate molecule and resulting eventually in the formation of carbonium ion (a). The same effect in the iron (II) isocitrate complex (d) produces carbonium ion (b). In the iron (II) aconitate complex (e), the coordination position held by the hydroxyl groups in (c) and (d) is occupied, presumably, by a water molecule, and the electron-withdrawing effect of the iron would then release a proton from the water molecule. This proton can move to the carbon atom at either end of the double bond, resulting in the formation of one or the other of carbonium ions (A) or (B).

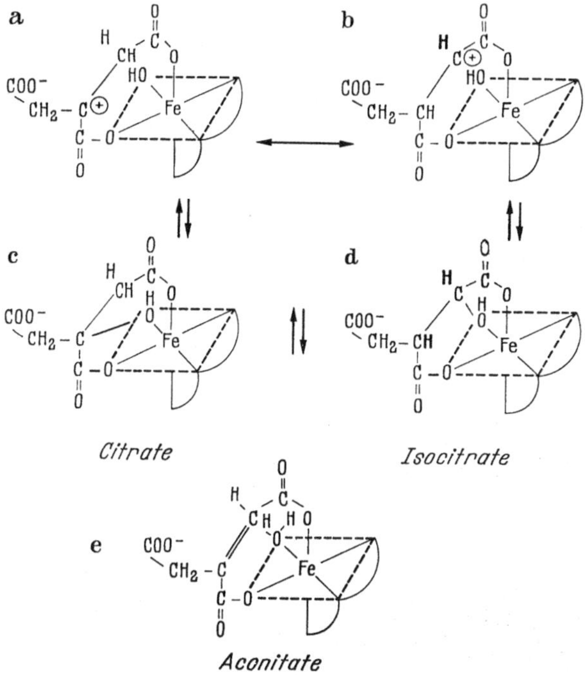

Fig. 4. Mechanism of aconitase reaction [SPEYER and DICKMAN (*17*)]

This mechanism also illustrates the influence of the stereochemistry of iron upon a reaction which it mediates (*5*). Five different molecular species are depicted in Fig. 4, yet none of them differs in the ligand attachment to the iron. Thus, the iron atom serves to maintain the proper spatial relationship between the hydroxyl group and the carbonium ions. This constancy in the coordination sphere of the iron should greatly accelerate the rate of the interconversions.

Phenolytic oxygenases

The last decade has witnessed the discovery of a variety of different enzymes which catalyze the cleavage of the aromatic ring of phenolic compounds in the presence of molecular oxygen (*10*). All of these enzymes require iron for their activity, even though the presence of iron in the native enzymes has not been demonstrated in all cases. These enzymes are exemplified by pyrocatechase, which splits the carbon-carbon bond of catechol into *cis, cis*-muconic acid (*9*):

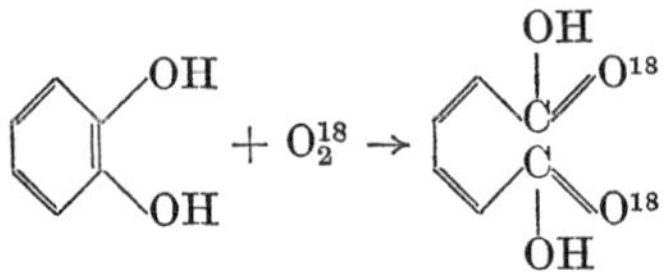

As shown in the equation, experiments with oxygen-18 revealed that both atoms of the molecular oxygen are found in the muconic acid at the conclusion of the reaction. Mehler (*10*) has proposed a mechanism for the action of these oxygenases in which the iron atom serves as a carrier of molecular oxygen in much the same way as in hemoglobin. His proposal is illustrated for pyrocatechase in Fig. 5. The atoms of the oxygen molecule are aligned with the

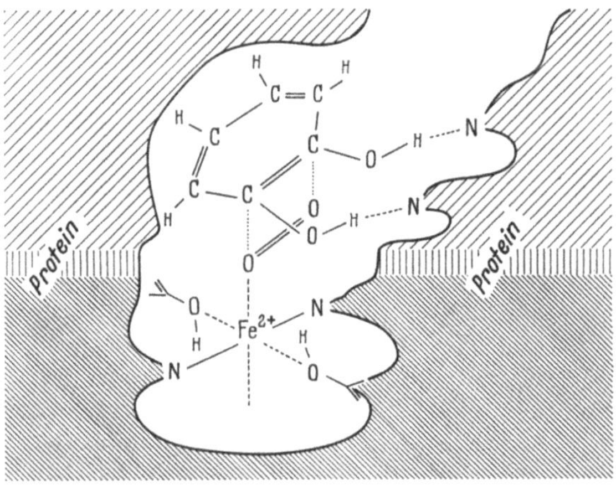

Fig. 5. Mechanism of pyrocatechase reaction [Mehler (*10*)], by permission of Academic Press, New York

appropriate carbon atoms in pyrocatechol. As a consequence of its coordination with iron, the oxygen atom directly bound to iron is relatively electron-deficient, compared with the oxygen atom further removed from the iron. Possibly the initial step in the degradation of the catechol is the movement of electrons from the double bond toward the positive dipole oxygen, thus creating a carbon-oxygen bond and an electron-deficient carbon atom. The latter can remove this deficiency by the formation of a second carbon-oxygen bond. Cleavage of the oxygen-oxygen bond and electron rearrangement would lead to the final product.

Ferredoxin

It would be negligent to conclude a discussion of iron function at the present time without at least a cursory reference to the recent investigations on ferredoxin. This enzyme, first discovered by SAN PIETRO and LANG (*15*), has been shown to be essential for a number of different electron transfer reactions (*11*, *22*). One of the most interesting of these is involved in the role of ferredoxin in the separation of the light and dark reactions of photosynthesis (*23*). It was shown that ferredoxin is reduced by a chloroplast pigment in light and re-oxidized by T.P.N. in the dark. The redox potential of ferredoxin is $-.432$ volts, making it one of the most readily oxidizable known biological electron-carriers (*18*).

Unfortunately, present knowledge makes it useless to attempt an analysis of how the iron operates in this molecule. There is no doubt that the iron is important; each molecule of ferredoxin, of molecular weight approximating 12,000, contains ten atoms of iron (*18*). One of the most curious aspects of the ferredoxin structure is that the release of iron by the action of acid is accompanied by the release of sulfide, and the iron and sulfide are produced in equivalent amounts (*1*). It would seem that much more information is required before these phenomena can be interpreted.

Conclusion

I have confined this discussion to the functional iron compounds only partly because I wished to conform to the title of my talk. The more important reason is that the iron-transport and storage molecules will be thoroughly covered by Drs. HARRISON and BEARN. For the same reason, I have not mentioned any of the iron-containing growth factors and their antagonists in micro-organisms, since Dr. PRELOG will be dealing with these substances in his paper. Perhaps the iron in some of these latter substances is functional, and we shall know before the morning is over.

Summary

The characteristics of coordinated iron that make it useful in biochemistry are its charge, its existence in a number of oxidation states, its stereochemistry, and its ability to attain different electronic configurations.

The hemoproteins have been placed in two categories. The first includes the cytochromes, which transfer electrons without change in molecular structure. These molecules are strong field complexes in both oxidation states. The second includes hemoglobin, which transports molecular oxygen, and catalase and peroxidase, which cleave the peroxide structure. These molecules are weak field complexes in their aquo forms and strong field complexes when bound to molecular oxygen or hydrogen peroxide.

The aconitase reaction illustrates the importance of the stereochemistry of iron during the course of an enzymatic process. The phenolytic oxygenases demonstrate the ability of non-heme iron to transfer molecular oxygen to phenolic compounds that undergo ring cleavage as a result. Recent studies on ferredoxin are briefly taken into consideration.

Zusammenfassung

Die Eigenschaften, die komplexgebundenes Eisen zu einem zweckmäßigen Bestandteil biochemisch aktiver Verbindungen machen, sind seine Ladung, seine Stereochemie, sowie die Tatsache, daß es in verschiedenen Oxydationszuständen vorliegt, und daß es fähig ist, verschiedene elektronische Konfigurationen einzunehmen.

Die Haemoproteine lassen sich in zwei Gruppen einteilen. Die erste enthält die Zytochrome, die Elektronen übertragen, ohne dabei ihre molekulare Struktur zu verändern. Diese Moleküle stellen in beiden Oxydationszuständen Komplexe mit starkem Ligandenfeld dar. Zur zweiten zählen Haemoglobin, das molekularen Sauerstoff transportiert, sowie Katalase und Peroxydase, die die Peroxydstruktur spalten. Diese Moleküle sind in ihrer Hydratform Komplexe mit schwachem Ligandenfeld, dagegen solche mit starkem Ligandenfeld, wenn sie an molekularen Sauerstoff oder Wasserstoffperoxyd gebunden sind.

Die Akonitase-Reaktion ist ein Beispiel für die Bedeutung der Stereochemie von Eisen im Verlaufe eines enzymatischen Prozesses. Mit Hilfe der phenolytischen Oxygenasen, für deren Wirkung die Anwesenheit von Eisen notwendig ist, läßt sich zeigen, daß nicht an Haem gebundenes Eisen die Fähigkeit besitzt, molekularen Sauerstoff auf phenolytische Verbindungen zu übertragen, deren Ring dadurch gespalten wird. Neue Untersuchungen über Ferredoxin werden kurz erwähnt.

Résumé

Les propriétés du fer qui donnent à un composé qui le contient une activité biochimique sont: sa charge électrique, sa structure stéréochimique, son existence sous différents états d'oxydation ainsi que sous différentes configurations électroniques.

Les hémoprotéines peuvent être classées en deux groupes. Le premier comprend les cytochromes, qui transportent les électrons sans modification de leur structure moléculaire. Ces molécules sont des complexes avec champ de ligands fort dans leurs deux états d'oxydation. Au deuxième groupe appartiennent l'hémoglobine, qui transporte l'oxygène moléculaire, ainsi que les catalases et les peroxydases, qui scindent la structure des peroxydes. Ces molécules sont des complexes avec champ de ligands faible sous leur forme hydratée et des complexes avec champ de ligands fort quand elles sont liées à de l'oxygène moléculaire ou à de l'eau oxygénée.

La réaction de l'aconitase est un exemple de l'importance de la stéréochimie du fer au cours d'un processus enzymatique. A l'aide des oxygénases phénolytiques, dont l'action exige la présence de fer, on peut montrer que le fer non lié à l'hème est capable de transporter de l'oxygène moléculaire sur les composés phénoliques, dont l'anneau se trouve ainsi brisé. Des recherches récentes sur la ferrédoxine sont brièvement mentionnées.

References

1. Buchanan, B., W. Lovenberg, and J. C. Rabinowitz: Proc. Nat. Acad. Sc. U.S.A. **49**, 345 (1963). — 2. Chance, B.: Arch. Biochem. Biophysics (U.S.A.) **37**, 235 (1952). — 3. Chance, B.: In: The Enzymes, 1st ed. Ed. by J. B. Sumner and K. Myrbäck, Vol. I. Academic Press, New York, 1951, p. 440. — 4. Dickman, S. R., and A. A. Cloutier: J. Biol. Chem. (U.S.A.) **188**, 379 (1951). — 5. Eichhorn, G. L.: Advances Chem. (U.S.A.) **37**, 37 (1963). — 6. Eichhorn, G. L.: Fed. Proc. (U.S.A.) **20**, Suppl. 10, 40 (1961). — 7. Eichhorn, G. L.: In: Metal Binding in Medicine. Ed. by M. J. Seven and L. A. Johnson. Lippincott, Philadelphia, 1960. p. 19. — 8. George, P.: Biochem. J. (G.B.) **54**, 267 (1953). — 9. Hayaishi, O., M. Katagiri, and S. Rothberg: J. Amer. Chem. Soc. **77**, 5450 (1955). — 10. Mehler, A. H.: In: Oxygenases. Ed. by O. Hayaishi. Academic Press, New York, 1962, p. 87. — 11. Mortensen, L. E., R. C. Valentine, and J. E. Carnahan: Biochem. Biophys. Res. Comm. (U.S.A.) **7**, 448 (1962). — 12. Orgel, L. E.: An Introduction to Transition-Metal Chemistry. Ligand Field Theory. John Wiley & Sons, New York, 1960, 180 pp. — 13. Paul, K. G.: In: The Enzymes, 2nd ed. Ed. by P. D. Boyer, H. Lardy, and K. Myrbäck, Vol. III. Academic Press, New York, 1960, p. 303. — 14. Pauling, L., and C. D. Coryell: Proc. Nat. Acad. Sc. U.S.A. **22**, 210 (1936). — 15. San Pietro, A., and H. N. Lang: J. Biol. Chem. (U.S.A.) **231**, 211 (1958). — 16. Slater, E. C.: In: Metals and Enzyme Activity. Ed. by E. M. Crook. University Press, Cambridge, 1958, p. 76. — 17. Speyer, J. R., and S. R. Dickman: J. Biol. Chem. (U.S.A.) **220**, 193 (1956). — 18. Tagawa, K., and D. I. Arnon: Nature (G.B.) **195**, 537 (1962). — 19. Theorell, H.: Ark. Kemi. Mineral. Geol. (Sweden) **16** A, No. 3 (1942). — 20. Theorell, H., A. Ehrenberg, and B. Chance: Arch. Biochem. Biophysics (U.S.A.) **37**, 237 (1952). — 21. Urry, D. W., and H. Eyring: Proc. Nat. Acad. Sc. U.S.A. **49**, 253 (1963). — 22. Valentine, R. C., R. L. Jackson, and R. S. Wolfe: Biochem. Biophys. Res. Comm. (U.S.A.) **7**, 453 (1962). — 23. Whatley, F. R., K. Tagawa, and D. I. Arnon: Proc. Nat. Acad. Sc. U.S.A. **49**, 266 (1963). — 24. Williams, R. J. P.: Chem. Rev. (U.S.A.) **56**, 299 (1955).

Discussion

LONDON: Dr. EICHHORN, you made the important point that the electronic configuration of the iron helps to determine the biological function of the various haem proteins. I wonder therefore whether you would care to consider what is known, or what you could predict, with respect to the intimate chemical configuration of the iron and of its linkage to the specific proteins.

EICHHORN: I don't really think I can answer your question, but perhaps one can say that a primary consideration in the determination of the different electronic structures that I have indicated is the nature of the sixth ligand. If it can form a π-bond, as peroxide or molecular oxygen, then there is an opportunity for strengthening of the coordination. Of course, in cytochrome C there is not even the opportunity of forming such a bond, because the protein occupies both the fifth and the sixth coordination position. So the only generalisation I can really make on the basis of known haemoprotein structures is that strong field complexes appear to result whenever the protein is bound in two places, or else when the protein is bound in only one place and a π-bonding group occupies the sixth coordination position. But as regards the specific groups on the protein that are required for strong field bonding, there is little that can be said on this point, except, perhaps, that groups such as imidazole groups would be favourable.

SCHUBERT: As you know, copper is associated with iron in the cytochromes. I was wondering if you would care to comment on the cooperative effects between iron and copper.

EICHHORN: I don't feel very competent to discuss the cooperative effects between iron and copper. However, I should perhaps point out that in a recent paper by URRY and EYRING[1] they propose a mechanism for the electron movements from one cytochrome to another through the conjugated double-bond system of imidazole rings.

RITTENBERG: I have often thought that the function of the various complexes of iron in the organism is to keep the iron in solution. At pH 7, Fe^{+++} is quite insoluble. The function of the porphyrin complexes is to combine with four sites of the octahedral configuration of iron. The four sites lie in one plane and prevent the other two sites lying on each side of the plane from being complexed by a simple amino acid. I wonder whether the importance of the protein in a metallic protein lies in its contribution not only to specificity but also to solubilisation of the metal. The figures which were quoted on the catalase-like activity of iron are somewhat misleading, because a pH was chosen at which inorganic iron is quite inactive. If you could keep iron in solution at a higher pH, it would have a very respectable activity.

EICHHORN: You have made a very important point there. I think that generally one function of the proteins in enzymes is to make the biological actions more specific. Metallic ions are notoriously non-specific, and in order to prevent them from doing things that they shouldn't do, the proteins are

[1] URRY, D. W., and H. EYRING: Proc. Nat. Acad. Sc. U.S.A. **49**, 253 (1963).

essential. You pointed out one way in which the haemoprotein structure prevents some undesirable things from happening by preventing chelation.

SCHUBERT: As far as keeping the iron in solution is concerned, I should just like to mention that there exists what is called a mononuclear barrier. This means that the normal concentration of "free" iron in the blood is so low that the iron would exist in the form of soluble mononuclear complexes, as discussed in my paper (p. 482). For Fe^{+++} the critical concentration below which it exists in a mononuclear state, even in the absence of complexing agents other than OH^-, is roughly 10^{-4} M. The normal concentration of iron in the blood, excluding that bound in haemoglobin, is so low that the other protein and non-protein iron-binding constituents serve functions other than to keep iron from precipitating.

EICHHORN: Nevertheless, there seem to be biological mechanisms that prevent the iron from existing in the ionic form throughout the whole physiological process.

SCHUBERT: It is always in a complex state.

Incorporation of iron in the haem moiety of chromoproteins

By

H. Yoshikawa and Y. Yoneyama

The biosynthesis of haem in the immature or nucleated erythrocyte has been studied extensively by Shemin, Neuberger, Rimington, and Granick, with the result that the mechanism of porphyrin synthesis is now known. The final step in the biosynthetic chain involves the incorporation of an iron atom into the porphyrin ring. In recent years, evidence has accumulated to support – although admittedly not to prove – the view that protoporphyrin is the direct precursor of haem and that the insertion of iron into protoporphyrin is enzymatically catalysed.

Localisation of iron-inserting activity

The mechanism of this reaction was investigated initially by studying the incorporation of radioactive iron *in vitro* into the haem of bone-marrow cells (Kasuga, Konno, and Sakai, 1954), reticulocytes (Walsh, Thomas, Chow, Fluharty, and Finch, 1949), and avian erythrocytes (Jensen, Ashenbrucker, Cartwright, and Wintrobe, 1953). Granick (1954) observed the reaction in chicken-erythrocyte extract by determining the disappearance of protoporphyrin and the appearance of Fe^{59}-haem. Konno (1954) fractionated the homogenate of bone-marrow cells by the method of differential centrifugation and claimed that the activity exists in the nuclear fraction. Recent investigations suggest, however, that haem biosynthesis is effected mainly in mitochondria which are closely attached to the nuclei of erythroblasts and avian erythrocytes (Sano, 1958).

Haem synthesis is not confined to bone-marrow cells and erythrocytes. Every aerobic cell has haemoproteins for respiration and synthesises their prosthetic group *in situ*. For instance, yeast cells take up inorganic iron from a culture medium to form haem during growth (Yoshikawa, 1937). Theorell, Béznak, Bonnichsen, Paul, and Åkeson (1951) investigated the incorporation of isotopic iron into various haemoproteins of tissues *in vivo* and suggested that they were independently synthesised in the cells. In our laboratory, MINAKAMI, YONEYAMA, and YOSHIKAWA (1958) observed the incorporation of Fe^{59} into haem in homogenates of rat liver, as well as of other organs, and they also found that the activity was located in the liver mitochondria – a finding which was confirmed by NISHIDA and LABBE (1959).

Solubilisation of the active principle

Treatment of insoluble materials with surface-active agents brings about solubilisation of the active principle. Tween 20 was employed for the insoluble particles of duck erythrocytes by KRUEGER, MELNICK, and KLEIN (1956), and sodium cholate for the particulate fraction of chicken haemolysate by KAGAWA, MINIKAMI, YONEYAMA, and URATA (1957). The active principle was also prepared in soluble form from a liver-mitochondria fraction by treating with sodium cholate (MINAKAMI, YONEYAMA, and YOSHIKAWA, 1958; MINAKAMI, 1958) or with Tween 20 (LABBE, 1959). Upon fractionation of the cholate extract of mitochondria with ammonium sulphate, the major part of the enzyme activity was found in the 50–75% saturated fraction (MINAKAMI, 1958). Similar fractionation was carried out by NEVÉ (1961), who found the active principle in the 50–60% saturated fraction of a bicarbonate-Tween 40 extract of chicken erythrocytes.

The active preparations from different sources have a number of properties in common. The active principle is heat-labile and temperature-dependent, and has a pH optimum and substrate specificity. These properties are compatible with the enzymic nature of this biochemical reaction. Anaerobic conditions favour the insertion of iron into protoporphyrin (GRANICK, 1954; KRUEGER, MELNIK, and KLEIN, 1956), and the presence of reducing substances enhances the enzymic reaction (GOLDBERG, 1959; KAGAWA, MINAKAMI, and YONEYAMA, 1959). The activity is inhibited by p-chloromercuribenzoate and other sulphydryl-binding reagents (KAGAWA, MINAKAMI, and YONEYAMA, 1959; LABBE and HUBBARD, 1960). The inhibitory effect of lead has been repeatedly discussed in relation to the disturbances of porphyrin metabolism occurring in lead poisoning.

Haemoglobin-free enzyme preparation

We managed to prepare the enzyme in a form free from haemoglobin (MINAKAMI, KAGAWA, SUGITA, YONEYAMA, and YOSHIKAWA, 1959). Thoroughly washed duck-erythrocyte stroma was extracted with sodium cholate, and the extract was chromatographed on Amberlite IRC 50 to separate the iron-inserting enzyme from the haemoglobin. In later experiments, a larger amount of the enzyme was prepared in the following manner (YONEYAMA, OHYAMA, SUGITA, and YOSHIKAWA, 1962). Duck erythrocytes were washed with cold isotonic KCl and haemolysed by the addition of water. The haemolysate was centrifuged at 8,000 × G. for 10 minutes. The precipitate was re-suspended in a large volume of water, and the suspension was made isotonic by the addition of hypertonic KCl and centrifuged. The washing process was repeated several times until the supernatant had become colourless. The pale yellow precipitate was extracted with an equal volume of cholate-Tris buffer (pH 7.4) solution for 15 hours at 4° C. The mixture was centrifuged at 8,000 × G. for 15 minutes. The clear supernatant was used as the enzyme. Mercapto-ethanol was added to stabilise the enzyme, which was an SH enzyme. If necessary, further fractionation was carried out by ammonium sulphate saturation.

The enzyme activity was assayed by measuring the Fe^{59} incorporation into haem or by determining the decrease in protoporphyrin (DRESEL and FALK, 1956).

Table 1. *Specific activity of each fraction during purification*

1 ml. of each fraction was incubated with 0.2 μmol of $FeCl_3$, 0.2 μmol of protoporphyrin, 4 μmols of cysteine, and 200 μmols of Tris buffer (pH 8.0) in a final volume of 3.3 ml. for 30 min. at 37° C. S represents haemolysate supernatant, 0.2 ml. of which was added in place of 0.2 ml. buffer solution.

Fraction	Total activity (c.p.m./mg.)	Protein (mg./ml.)	Specific activity (c.p.m./mg.)	Yield (%)
Haemolysate	6,520	204	32	100
Cholate extract	4,700	1.06	4,560	
Cholate extract + S	5,110		4,860	48
$(NH_4)_2SO_4$ fraction				
0—28% saturation	82	0.98	84	
28—50% saturation	1,248	0.56	2,230	
28—50% saturation + S	3,835		6,850	14
50—75% saturation	121	0.43	280	

The result of a typical fractionation is shown in Table 1. At purified stages of the enzyme, maximum activity is attained by the addition of haemolysate supernatant, which is inactive by itself, as observed previously by us (MINAKAMI, YONEYAMA, and YOSHIKAWA, 1960) and by others (SCHWARTZ, HILL, CARTWRIGHT, and WINTROBE, 1959). This will be discussed later.

Properties of the enzyme

Spectral change during the course of the reaction is shown in Fig. 1. The increase in transmission at 409 mμ (protoporphyrin) and its decrease at 424 mμ (haem) are clearly demonstrated. The reaction proceeds almost linearly with time for at least 30 minutes.

The temperature-dependency of the activity shows a maximum at 37° C., and practically no reaction occurs at 0° C. The activity is almost completely destroyed by heating the preparation

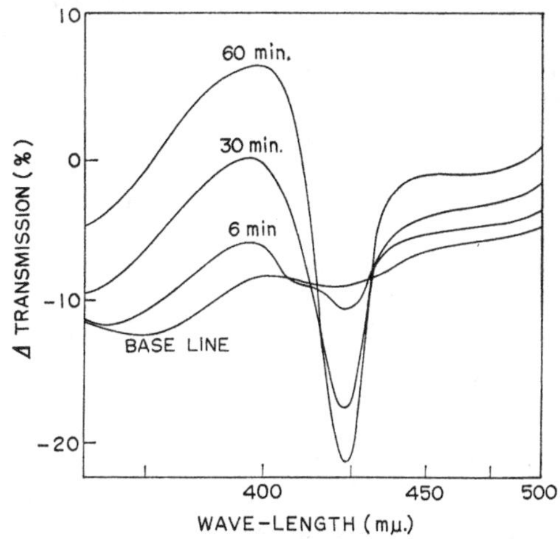

Fig. 1. Spectra representing differences between reaction mixtures with and without active enzyme preparation at different time intervals

to 56° C. for 30 minutes. The optimum pH lies at 8.2. This value differs considerably from that reported previously by KAGAWA, MINAKAMI, and YONEYAMA (1959), who obtained the greatest activity at pH 7.2 with a crude preparation. A similar difference in pH optimum has been reported for liver iron-inserting enzyme. The value is 8.2 for the soluble form (LABBE and HUBBARD, 1960), as compared with 7.4 for the particulate form (NISHIDA and LABBE, 1959).

The Michaelis constant for ferrous iron is $8 \cdot 10^{-5}$ *M* and that for protoporphyrin is $7 \cdot 10^{-6}$ *M*.

The reaction product

The removal of haemoglobin from the enzyme preparation enabled us to investigate the nature of the reaction product and to observe its stoichiometric formation from iron and protoporphyrin. KLEIN (1959) demonstrated the net synthesis of haem in crude enzyme preparations, but precise measurement of the synthesis was hampered by large amounts of preformed haemoglobin and haemoprotein in the preparation.

The haem which is produced from iron and protoporphyrin in our enzyme system is protohaem. This has been proved by the absorption spectra of haematin in the ethyl-acetate extract of the reaction mixture and its pyridine haemochromogen, and by paper chromatography run in acetic acid in water-saturated toluene.

Formation of haem is negligible when the incubation is carried out without the addition of protoporphyrin. No haem synthesis is observed from δ-aminolaevulinic acid. This indicates that the preparation is free from the enzyme system involved in the synthesis of protoporphyrin from δ-aminolaevulinic acid.

When deutero-, meso-, or haematoporphyrin is added to the reaction mixture instead of protoporphyrin, corresponding haems are produced (Table 2). The products were identified by determining the absorption spectra of pyridine haemochromogens. On the

Table 2. *Substrate specificity of porphyrins and α-peak of pyridine haemochromogens from the haems produced*

Substrate	Fe^{59} incorporation into haem (% protoporphyrin)	α-peak of pyridine haemochromogen (mμ)	
		Product	Authentic
δ-Aminolaevulinic acid	0	—	—
Protoporphyrin	100	556	557
Mesoporphyrin	87	546	547
Haematoporphyrin.	179	550	548
Deuteroporphyrin	270	544	545
Coproporphyrin	0		
Uroporphyrin	0		

other hand, uroporphyrin with 8 carboxylic groups and coproporphyrin with 4 carboxylic groups cannot serve as substrate for the enzyme. Thus, the enzyme has a specificity towards porphyrins with 2 carboxylic groups. These findings are in accord with the results obtained by GOLDBERG, ASHENBRUCKER, CARTWRIGHT, and WINTROBE (1956) in experiments with chicken haemolysate, and by LABBE and HUBBARD (1961) in experiments with liver-mitochondria extract.

Metal specificity has been studied by comparing the coordination of Fe^{59}, Co^{60}, and Zn^{65}. Of these metals, only iron is incorporated at a fast rate. Because the reaction mixture contains an excess of cysteine, added ferric iron must be reduced to ferrous iron and then inserted into the protoporphyrin. No radioactivity is found in the cobalt-porphyrin complex which has been added as the carrier. This is in striking contrast with the results obtained by LABBE and HUBBARD (1961) in the case of liver-mitochondria enzyme, where cobalt was inserted into protoporphyrin as fast as ferrous iron. These substrate specificities strongly suggest that the active principle involved in iron insertion is enzymic in nature.

The stoichiometry of the reaction has been established by measuring simultaneously the amount of haem formed and the decrease in iron and protoporphyrin, as shown in Table 3. This result indicates that side reactions, such as destruction of haem and protoporphyrin, do not occur in this reaction system.

Table 3. *Stoichiometry of haem formation*

The mixture contained 2 ml. of enzyme solution, 400 μmols of Tris buffer (pH 8.0), 0.126 μmol of protoporphyrin, 0.355 μmol of iron, and 6 μmols of cysteine in a total volume of 5 ml. Incubation was at 37° C.

Substrates and product	0 min. (μmol)	30 min. (μmol)	Difference (μmol)
Protoporphyrin	0.126	0.077	—0.049
Iron	0.355	0.305	—0.050
Haem	0.014	0.064	+0.050

Nature of the initial product and formation of haemoglobin

Our earlier study revealed that, if the cholate extract of duck-erythrocyte stroma was freed from haemoglobin by ion-exchange resin chromatography, the main product of the reaction from iron and porphyrin was not haemoglobin, as determined with the aid of Fe^{59} (MINAKAMI, KAGAWA, SUGITA, YONEYAMA, and YOSHIKAWA, 1959). The radioactive haem produced by the enzyme remained adsorbed at the upper portion of the Amberlite IRC 50 column when 0.1 *M* phosphate buffer (pH 7.4) was run through, whereas haemoglobin was eluted by the same treatment. Free haem, which is essentially insoluble in a neutral pH, behaved similarly on the column. If a supernatant from duck-erythrocyte haemolysate was added to the reaction system, haem synthesis was remarkably potentiated, and the main product was duck haemoglobin, whereas, if the supernatant was from horse haemolysate, most of the labelled haem belonged to horse haemoglobin (MINAKAMI, YONEYAMA, and YOSHIKAWA, 1960).

These findings led us to the conclusion that the haem synthesised by this enzyme combines with a specific acceptor in the haemolysate to form the respective haemoglobin. This acceptor in the supernatant resembled haemoglobin in ammonium sulphate fractionation, but clearly differed from it in ion-exchange resin chromatography. It was thought that the acceptor may have been free globin, although no direct evidence for this assumption was obtainable. The existence of free globin in duck erythrocytes was also suggested by the fact that the ratio of specific activities of carbon atoms from 2-C^{14}-glycine in haem and globin was always more than unity and decreased as the incubation was prolonged (SUGITA, 1959).

SCHWARTZ, HILL, CARTWRIGHT, and WINTROBE (1959) similarly showed that the addition of an inactive supernatant from a chicken-erythrocyte haemolysate to their enzyme preparation resulted in a marked increase in activity. However, they could not identify the non-haemoglobin intermediate.

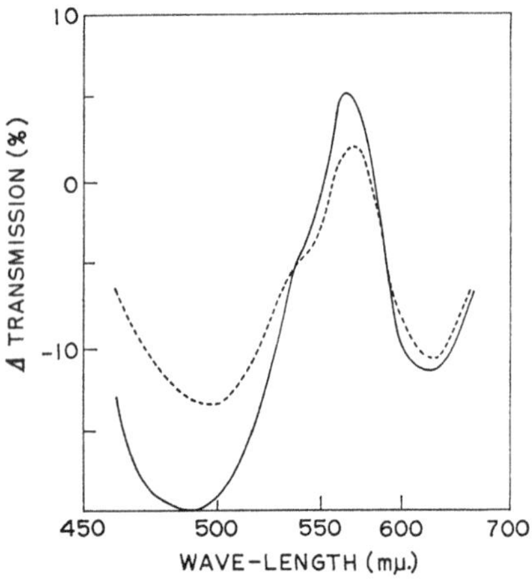

Fig. 2. Spectra representing the difference between the oxidised and reduced forms of the reaction product (——) and haemalbumin (···)

Recently, we succeeded in characterising the initial product of the reaction with the haemoglobin-free preparation (YONEYAMA, OHYAMA, SUGITA, and YOSHIKAWA, 1962). At the end of incubation, the reaction was stopped by chilling and the solution divided into two portions, one of which was aerated and the other reduced with dithionite. The spectrum representing the difference between the oxidised and reduced forms of the product is shown in Fig. 2.

The spectrum of haemalbumin is also shown in the same figure for reference. There is a striking similarity between the spectra. It will be seen from Fig. 3 that the spectrum obtained with haemoglobin, as described below, is entirely different from these spectra. Using radioactive iron as the tracer, the haem produced was subjected to ion-exchange chromatography. A part of the labelled haem was eluted from the column of CG-50 by NaCl-sodium citrate solution, and the rest was attached to the resin and only eluted by NaOH. The former was probably the haem bound to iron-inserting enzyme and the latter free haem (YONEYAMA, OHYAMA, SUGITA, and YOSHIKAWA, in press).

These findings confirm our former observation that the initial product yielded from iron and protoporphyrin by the enzymic reaction is not haemoglobin but protohaem, which is loosely combined with non-globin protein (presumably the enzyme protein).

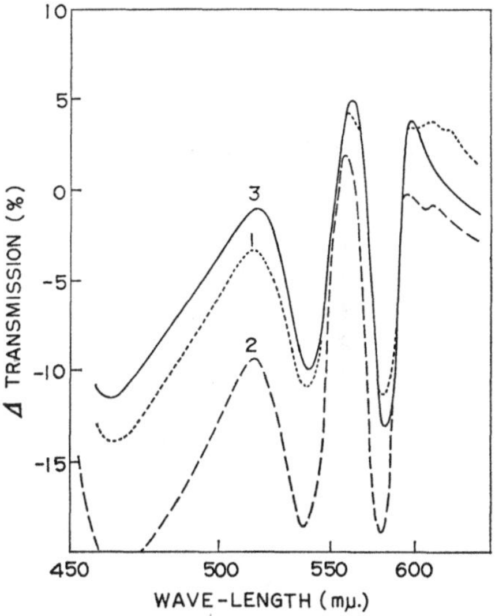

Fig. 3. Spectra representing differences between oxygenated and de-oxygenated forms of haemoglobin. 1. Incubation mixture (globin was added at the beginning). 2. Incubation mixture (globin was added after the incubation). 3. Haemoglobin

Haemoglobin synthesis from iron, protoporphyrin, and globin

With our enzyme preparation we also investigated the *in vitro* formation of haemoglobin from iron, protoporphyrin, and globin (SUGITA, YONEYAMA, and OHYAMA, 1962). The mixture containing ferric chloride, protoporphyrin, globin, cysteine, and the enzyme in Tris buffer (pH 8.0) was incubated in a Thunberg tube at 37° C. for one hour under nitrogen. The subsequent procedure for obtaining the spectrum representing the difference between oxygenated and de-oxygenated forms of the product was the same as described above. Another experiment was carried out in the same way, except that globin was added to the mixture after incubating and chilling the tube, and the mixture was allowed to stand at 4° C. The spectra in the two experiments were essentially the same as that of haemoglobin shown in Fig. 3.

A similar experiment, in which apomyoglobin was used instead of globin, resulted in the formation of myoglobin, which was distinguished from haemoglobin as CO compound spectrophotometrically (OHYAMA, YONEYAMA, and YOSHIKAWA, 1962).

These findings support the view that the insertion of iron into porphyrin occurs enzymatically to form haem and that the haem is accepted by globin.

SCHWARTZ, GOUDSMIT, HILL, CARTWRIGHT, and WINTROBE (1961) reported stimulation of haem synthesis by the addition of globin to their enzyme preparation to form haemoglobin. We could not, however, confirm their observation. It appeared rather as if globin exerted some inhibitory effect (YONEYAMA, OHYAMA, SUGITA, and YOSHIKAWA, in press). No sign of denaturation was present in our globin preparations, but we cannot exclude the possibility that a slight change in molecular structure may have been the cause of our failure to observe any stimulating effect of globin upon haem synthesis. Indeed, globin was so unstable in the reaction mixture that it tended to flocculate during incubation. Apomyoglobin, which is more stable than globin, gave the same results. It is suggested that the globin in the haemolysates exists in a stabilised form and draws the enzyme reaction in the direction of haem synthesis as haemoglobin is formed.

Role of phospholipid

All attempts to obtain the enzyme in soluble form without the aid of surface-active agents have failed. It seems highly probable that the enzyme is of a lipoprotein nature and only solubilised by detergents which act primarily on lipid-protein interfaces. This view is supported by the fact that the enzyme activity of the particulate preparation, as well as of the cholate extract, is impaired when phospholipase of Naja-naja snake venom is added.

In addition, we found that the re-combination of aqueous extract from acetone powder and phospholipid from acetone extract of duck-erythrocyte stroma resulted in a marked increase in haem synthesis. This prompted us to investigate further the role of lipid in this reaction (YONEYAMA, IRISAWA, TANAKA, and KASUGA, 1963).

Acetone powder was prepared in the conventional manner from thoroughly washed stroma. It retained most of its enzyme activity, as was shown by an assay performed on its cholate extract. The dry powder was extracted with 0.2 *M* Tris buffer (pH 8.0) at 4° C. and centrifuged. The clear or slightly opalescent supernatant was separated for assay of the enzyme. Lipid was extracted from the stroma with chloroform-methanol (1:1), and the extract was washed with water. The lipid, in a chloroform layer, was applied on a silica column. At first, chloroform was run through the column to elute the simple lipid, followed by methanol to elute the phospholipid. The latter effluent was mixed with an adequate amount of water, and methanol was driven off *in vacuo* to obtain an emulsion of phospholipid.

The enzyme activity was determined by Fe^{59} incorporation into haem with and without addition of the phospholipid emulsion

Table 4. *The effect of phospholipid on synthesis of haem from iron and protoporphyrin*

Tris buffer extract from the acetone powder of duck-erythrocyte stroma was used as the enzyme. The mixtures contained the enzyme, protoporphyrin, and phospholipid as indicated, and 0.05 μmol of $FeCl_3$ labelled with Fe^{59}, 2 μmols of cysteine, and 0.5 ml. of 0.2 *M* Tris buffer (pH 8.0) in a final volume of 2.0 ml. Incubations were for 30 min. at 37° C. under nitrogen.

	Enzyme (ml.)	Phospholipid (mg.)	Protoporphyrin (μmol)	Fe^{59} incorporation (%)
I	0.5	0	0.025	0.32
II	0.5	2.0	0.025	1.23
III	0	2.0	0.025	0.14
IV	0	0	0.025	0

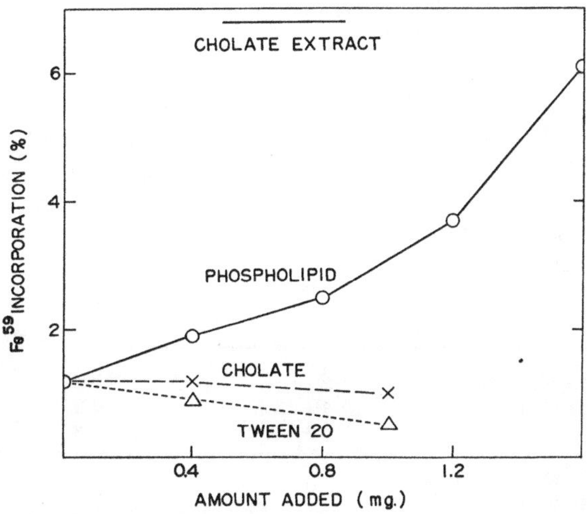

Fig. 4. Influence of phospholipid, cholate, and Tween 20 on haem synthesis

to the reaction mixture. As shown in Table 4, when the enzyme activity was assayed without the addition of phospholipid, little haem synthesis occurred. However, the addition of phospholipid resulted in a considerable increase in the reaction. Phospholipid alone did not catalyse the insertion of iron into protoporphyrin.

To study the effect of the phospholipid concentration, various amounts of phospholipid were added to the enzyme solution and the activity was assayed. Iron incorporation increased along with the phospholipid concentration, as shown in Fig. 4. It was possible, however, that the increase in haem synthesis might have been due to solubilisation of protoporphyrin in the presence of phospholipid; but this was ruled out by the fact that surface-active substances such as Tween 20 and cholate did not accelerate the reaction (Fig. 4).

Particulate-bound protoporphyrin

When duck haemolysate was incubated with δ-aminolaevulinic acid, the greater part of the protoporphyrin synthesised was found in the stroma in a form which it was not possible to wash out with isotonic KCl solution. On the other hand, uroporphyrin, coproporphyrin, and haemoglobin were readily removed from the stroma by the washing.

Homogenate of the stroma with bound protoporphyrin was incubated with iron and C^{14}-protoporphyrin which had been

Table 5. *Incorporation of free C^{14}-protoporphyrin in the presence and absence of bound protoporphyrin*

The reaction mixture contained 2 ml. of stroma homogenate, 8 μmols of cysteine, 0.4 μmol of $FeCl_3$, 400 μmols of Tris buffer (pH 8.0), 44 μmols of free C^{14}-protoporphyrin, and 4 mg. of sodium cholate. The amount of bound protoporphyrin was 61 μmols per 2 ml. of the homogenate. Incubation was at 37° C. The amount of haem which was supposed to originate from free protoporphyrin was calculated from the radioactivity in haem.

	Time (min.)	Protoporphyrin (μmol)	Haem	
			Total (μmol)	From free protoporphyrin (μmol)
Homogenate with bound protoporphyrin	20	—14.3	15.2	0.3
	40	—30.5	29.9	2.7
	60	—37.3	35.8	3.1
Homogenate without bound protoporphyrin	60	—	7.9	5.5

prepared enzymatically in accordance with the method described by KAWAI, SUGITA, and YONEYAMA (1961). The results shown in Table 5 indicate that the particulate-bound protoporphyrin is preferentially converted to haem without prior exchange with added free protoporphyrin. More haem was formed in the homogenate with bound protoporphyrin than in the homogenate without it, and free protoporphyrin was not incorporated into haem to any great extent (SUGITA, 1962).

Synthesised stroma-bound protoporphyrin was extracted by a chloroform-methanol mixture (1:1), together with lipid, and fractionated by the use of a silica column. Protoporphyrin was not eluted by chloroform, and methanol therefore had to be employed to elute the pigment (YONEYAMA, IRISAWA, TANAKA, and KASUGA, 1963). Since free protoporphyrin is known to be eluted from the column by chloroform, the stroma-bound protoporphyrin must be extracted in combination with phospholipid.

ERIKSEN (1955) reported that protoporphyrin in the reticulocytes consisted of two fractions which differ from each other in respect to their solubility in acetone, and he suggested that bound protoporphyrin, presumably the protoporphyrin-globin complex, was probably the immediate precursor of haemoglobin. It is known that globin combines with protoporphyrin, as shown by HILL and HOLDEN (1926). If the stroma-bound porphyrin in SUGITA's experiments had been the protoporphyrin-globin complex, it should have been washed out from the stroma by KCl solution as readily as haemoglobin.

Our results suggest that the phospholipid portion of the particulate iron-inserting enzyme may act as the binding site of protoporphyrin for the incorporation of iron, and that the haem thus formed is transferred to globin which has been synthesised by the microsomes. That protoporphyrin has a strong affinity for phospholipid is presumptive evidence in favour of this mechanism. Further purification of the enzyme and subsequent kinetic studies will be necessary if the mechanism of these reactions is to be successfully elucidated.

Summary

The enzyme responsible for the synthesis of haem from iron and protoporphyrin was studied.

The enzyme was prepared from duck erythrocytes in haemoglobin-free form. It had a broad specificity towards porphyrins with 2 carboxylic acids, producing corresponding haems. On the other hand, porphyrins with 4 and 8 carboxylic groups showed no reaction of this kind. Metal-specificity studies further showed that ferrous iron was the most efficient of the metals tested.

The absorption spectrum of the reaction mixture after incubation closely resembled that of haemalbumin. If the enzymic synthesis of haem took place in the presence of globin, most of the haem produced was found in the form of haemoglobin. Apomyoglobin was also utilised in this system to form myoglobin.

The aqueous extract from dry acetone powder of duck-erythrocyte stroma showed only weak enzyme activity, but the addition of phospholipid obtained from stroma led to a remarkable potentiation of the reaction.

It was observed that stroma-bound protoporphyrin synthesised by avian erythrocytes was utilised for haem formation in preference to free porphyrin. Our results suggest that the iron-inserting enzyme is a lipoprotein and that the haem which is synthesised by the enzyme is accepted by globin to form haemoglobin.

Zusammenfassung

Es wurde das Ferment untersucht, das verantwortlich für die Synthese von Haem aus Protoporphyrin und Eisen ist.

Das Ferment wurde aus Enten-Erythrozyten dargestellt, und zwar frei von Haemoglobin. Es besitzt eine breite Spezifität gegenüber Porphyrinen mit 2 Carboxylgruppen, die entsprechendes Haem produzieren. Andererseits zeigen Porphyrine mit 4 oder 8 Carboxylgruppen keine entsprechende Reaktion. Untersuchungen über die Spezifität des metallischen Anteils zeigten außerdem, daß Ferroeisen das wirksamste der geprüften Metalle ist.

Das Absorptionsspektrum des Reaktionsgemisches nach der Inkubation glich weitgehend demjenigen von Haemalbumin. Erfolgte die enzymatische Synthese von Haem in Gegenwart von Globin, so fand sich der größte Teil des gebildeten Haems in Form von Haemoglobin. Im gleichen System wurde Apomyoglobin verwendet, um Myoglobin zu bilden.

Wäßriger Extrakt von Azeton-Trockenpulver des Stromas von Enten-Erythrozyten zeigte nur eine geringgradige enzymatische Aktivität, jedoch verstärkte die Zugabe von Phospholipid aus dem Stroma die Reaktion beträchtlich.

Es fand sich, daß an Stroma gebundenes Protoporphyrin, synthetisiert durch Vogel-Erythrozyten, für die Haembildung dem freien Porphyrin vorgezogen wurde. Unsere Befunde machen es wahrscheinlich, daß das Eisen einbauende Ferment ein Lipoprotein ist, und daß Haem, welches durch das Enzym synthetisiert wird, durch Globin aufgenommen wird, um Haemoglobin zu bilden.

Résumé

L'enzyme responsable de la synthèse de l'hème à partir du fer et de la protoporphyrine a été étudié.

Il a été préparé, sous une forme ne contenant pas d'hémoglobine, à partir d'hématies de canard. Il possède une grande spécificité à l'égard des porphyrines contenant 2 groupes carboxyliques dans la formation des hèmes correspondants. D'autre part, avec les porphyrines contenant 4 ou 8 groupes carboxyliques on n'observe aucune réaction de ce genre. Des études sur la spécificité du métal ont de plus montré que le fer bivalent est le plus actif de tous les métaux étudiés.

Le spectre d'absorption du mélange en réaction après incubation ressemble de très près à celui de l'hémalbumine. Si la synthèse enzymatique de l'hème se fait en présence de globine, la plus grande partie de l'hème produit se trouve sous forme d'hémoglobine. L'apomyoglobine a aussi été utilisée dans ce système pour former de la myoglobine.

L'extrait aqueux obtenu à partir d'une poudre de stroma d'hématies de canard séché à l'acétone s'est montré d'une activité enzymatique faible, mais qui s'est remarquablement renforcée après adjonction de phospholipide provenant du stroma.

On a observé que la porphyrine liée au stroma synthétisée par les hématies d'oiseau est utilisée pour la formation de l'hème de préférence à la porphyrine libre. Nos résultats suggèrent que l'enzyme permettant l'insertion du fer dans la porphyrine est une lipoprotéine, et que l'hème synthétisé par cet enzyme est accepté par la globine pour former l'hémoglobine.

References

DRESEL, E. I. B., and J. E. FALK: Biochem. J. (G. B.) **63**, 72 (1956). — GOLDBERG, A.: Brit. J. Haemat. **5**, 150 (1959). — GOLDBERG, A., H. ASHENBRUCKER, G. E. CARTWRIGHT, and M. M. WINTROBE: Blood (U.S.A.) **11**, 821 (1956). — GRANICK, S.: Fed. Proc. (U.S.A.) **13**, 319 (1954). — HILL, R., and H. F. HOLDEN: Biochem. J. (G.B.) **20**, 1326 (1926). — JENSEN, W. N., H. ASHENBRUCKER, G. E. CARTWRIGHT, and M. M. WINTROBE: J. Laborat. Clin. Med. (U.S.A.) **42**, 833 (1953). — KAGAWA, Y., S. MINAKAMI, and Y. YONEYAMA: J. Biochem. (Japan) **46**, 711 (1959). — KAGAWA, Y., S. MINAKAMI, Y. YONEYAMA, and G. URATA: J. Jap. Biochem. Soc. **29**, 611 (1957). — KASUGA, S., K. KONNO, and Y. SAKAI: J. Jap. Biochem. Soc. **26**, 282 (1954). — KAWAI, Y., Y. SUGITA, and Y. YONEYAMA: J. Biochem. (Japan) **49**, 89 (1961). — KLEIN, J. R.: Proc. Soc. Exper. Biol. Med. (U.S.A.) **101**, 6 (1959). — KONNO, K.: J. Jap. Biochem. Soc. **26**, 260 (1954). — KRUEGER, R. C., I. MELNICK, and J. R. KLEIN: Arch. Biochem. Biophysics (U.S.A.) **64**, 302 (1956). — LABBE, R. F.: Biochim. biophysica acta (Neths) **31**, 589 (1959). — LABBE, R. F., and N. HUBBARD: Biochim. biophysica acta (Neths) **41**, 185 (1960). — LABBE, R. F., and N. HUBBARD: Fed. Proc. (U.S.A.) **20**, 376 (1961). — MINAKAMI, S.: J. Biochem. (Japan) **45**, 833 (1958). — MINAKAMI, S., Y. KAGAWA, Y. SUGITA, Y. YONEYAMA, and H. YOSHIKAWA: Biochim. biophysica acta (Neths) **35**, 569 (1959). — MINAKAMI, S., Y. YONEYAMA, and H. YOSHIKAWA: Biochim. biophysica acta (Neths) **28**, 447 (1958). — MINAKAMI, S., Y. YONEYAMA, and H. YOSHIKAWA: J. Biochem. (Japan) **47**, 269 (1960). — NEVÉ, R. A.: Haematin Enzymes. Pergamon Press, Oxford, 1961, p. 207. — NISHIDA, G., and R. F. LABBE: Biochim. biophysica acta (Neths) **31**, 519 (1959). — OHYAMA, H., Y. SUGITA, Y. YONEYAMA, and H. YOSHIKAWA: Biochim. biophysica acta (Neths) **47**, 413 (1961). — OHYAMA, H., Y. YONEYAMA, and H. YOSHIKAWA: Biochim. biophysica acta (Neths) **63**, 535 (1962). — SANO, S.: Acta haemat. Japon. **21**, 337 (1958). — SCHWARTZ, H. C., R. GOUDSMIT, R. L. HILL, G. E. CARTWRIGHT, and M. M. WINTROBE: J. Clin. Invest. (U.S.A.) **40**, 188 (1961). — SCHWARTZ, H. C., R. L. HILL, G. E. CARTWRIGHT, and M. M. WINTROBE: Biochim. biophysica acta (Neths) **36**, 567 (1959). — SUGITA, Y.: J. Jap. Biochem. Soc. **31**, 318 (1959). — SUGITA, Y.: J. Biochem. (Japan) **51**, 436 (1962). — SUGITA, Y., Y. YONEYAMA, and H. OHYAMA: J. Biochem. (Japan) **51**, 450 (1962). — THEORELL, H., M. BÉZNAK, R. BONNICHSEN, K. G. PAUL, and A. ÅKESON: Acta chem. Scand. **5**, 445 (1951). — WALSH, R. J., E. D. THOMAS, S. K. CHOW, R. G. FLUHARTY, and C. A. FINCH: Science (U.S.A.) **110**, 396 (1949). — YONEYAMA, Y., K. IRISAWA, S. TANAKA, and S. KASUGA: paper presented at the 15th Symposium on Enzyme Chemistry, Osaka, Japan, 1963. — YONEYAMA, Y., H. OHYAMA, Y. SUGITA, and H. YOSHIKAWA: Biochim. biophysica acta (Neths) **62**, 261 (1962). — YONEYAMA, Y., H. OHYAMA, Y. SUGITA, and H. YOSHIKAWA: Biochim. biophysica acta (Neths) (in press). — YOSHIKAWA, H.: J. Biochem. (Japan) **25**, 627 (1937).

Discussion

GAJDOS: Do you think that the effect of lead on haem synthesis is a real inhibitory effect? In our own experiments, the results were somewhat disturbing. In *in vitro* experiments, an inhibitory effect was observed, as it has been by others. In order to investigate the problem *in vivo* we poisoned rabbits with lead and then studied a haem synthetase preparation obtained from the red cells by the method of GOLDBERG[1]. This preparation, incubated with protoporphyrin and radioactive iron, showed a very high enzyme activity. This was unexpected, for lead in the blood is accumulated exclusively in the red blood cells. Thus, we have the feeling that the *in vitro* inhibition by lead is artificial and may be explained by the protein-precipitating effect of lead. Now, in lead-poisoned animals, haem synthesis is actually diminished. We think that one of the reasons for this is the enhancing effect of lead on iron accumulation in the stroma of the red cells. This was shown by JANDL[2], and we could entirely confirm his findings.

YOSHIKAWA: I don't know whether lead acts as a real inhibitor of enzyme activity or whether it just denaturates the enzyme protein. It may be nonspecific, because copper and mercury also exert an inhibitory effect upon the enzyme. High enzyme activity in the erythrocytes obtained from lead-poisoned animals can be explained by stippled cells in the blood, as pointed out by SANO[3] in Kyoto.

NAJEAN: Does the inserting enzyme show the same activity with bivalent iron or with trivalent iron?

YOSHIKAWA: I did not use ferrous iron. Usually we add cysteine to the reaction mixture for incubation. Without the addition of cysteine or other reducing substances the enzyme activity is pretty low. Ferric iron must be reduced to ferrous iron by these substances.

NAJEAN: Did you try to separate your final product from haemoglobin by sephadex chromatography?

YOSHIKAWA: No, I didn't.

KRUH: When we incubate a cell-free system of reticulocytes, i.e. ribosomes and a soluble fraction, we get a synthesis of haemoglobin, and in this condition haem is probably not synthesised[4]. So we believe that the system could have a pool of haem which would combine with globin as soon as globin is synthesised.

YOSHIKAWA: That's right. I think that probably haem is synthesised in the mitochondrial system and globin formed by a microsomal system, whereupon the newly formed globin draws the haem out of the mitochondria in some way. But this is just a hypothesis.

MOESCHLIN: I was very interested to learn that the complex of protoporphyrin may be attached to a lipid porphyrin complex. From the toxi-

---

[1] GOLDBERG, A.: Brit. J. Haemat. **5**, 150 (1959).
[2] JANDL, J. H., et al.: J. Clin. Invest. (U.S.A.) **38**, 161 (1959).
[3] SANO, S.: Acta haemat. Japon. **21**, 157 (1958).
[4] KRUH, J., J. ROSA, J.-C. DREYFUS, and G. SCHAPIRA: Biochim. biophysica acta (U.S.A.) **49**, 509 (1961).

cological point of view this might explain the action of benzene and nitrobenzene and also that of the benzene derivative chloramphenicol. Have you studied the possible inhibitory effect of these compounds on synthesis in your experiments? I think it would be very interesting to do this, because clinically we find that the formation of haemoglobin is arrested at the protoporphyrin level. So it might be just this lipid complex which is responsible for the effect of the toxic action of these lipid solvents.

I would also like to ask Dr. GAJDOS a question. If I understand you correctly, you do not think that a toxic enzyme blockade occurs at the level preceding the protoporphyrins. The first thing we find clinically is the very high excretion of delta-aminolaevulinic acid. How do you explain this in relation to your theory?

GAJDOS: It is very difficult to explain the *accumulation* of porphyrins and porphyrin precursors during lead poisoning. The *in vitro* experiments always show *inhibition* of porphyrin synthesis. Perhaps our present investigations will shed some fresh light on this problem. We have isolated mitochondria from the hepatic cells of lead-poisoned rabbits and studied the kinetics of aminolaevulinic acid synthesis by this preparation. We found an approximately twofold increase in aminolaevulinic acid synthesis as compared with mitochondria isolated from normal rabbit livers. It seems therefore that lead poisoning enhances the first step of porphyrin biosynthesis. But this enhancement, which still needs confirmation, is far less important than that which GRANICK[1] has recently observed in mitochondrial preparations obtained from animals with experimental porphyria.

YOSHIKAWA: Dr. MOESCHLIN's suggestion is a valuable one. I should like to study inhibition by the lipid solvents afterwards.

LONDON: Earlier work has indicated that the vinyl groups are essential for the incorporation of iron into the porphyrin ring. Now your work seems to suggest that they are certainly not essential.

YOSHIKAWA: That is correct. Vinyl groups are not essential, but the presence of two carboxylic groups is essential.

LONDON: This is an important point, because it would represent a significant departure from what has hitherto been accepted as fact. The second question I would like to ask Dr. YOSHIKAWA relates to the enzyme which he has been purifying from either bone marrow or duck erythrocytes. Duck erythrocytes normally contain a large fraction of reticulocytes. Have you found the enzyme in mature mammalian erythrocytes?

YOSHIKAWA: No; mature mammalian erythrocytes do not contain it.

LONDON: Do you believe, then, that the source of the enzyme is the mitochondria?

YOSHIKAWA: I think so. But mitochondria of avian erythrocytes are not easily separated from the nuclei. So I cannot say definitely that the enzyme is confined to the mitochondria.

LONDON: In mammalian reticulocytes you would have cells with mitochondria but without nuclei.

YOSHIKAWA: We have unpublished experimental data showing that rabbit reticulocyte particles incorporate iron into haem.

---

[1] GRANICK, S., and G. URATA: J. Biol. Chem. (U.S.A.) **238**, 821 (1963).

Ferritin and haemosiderin

By

PAULINE M. HARRISON

I. The nature of ferritin and haemosiderin

Storage iron occurs in two physically different forms known as ferritin and haemosiderin. These are present in various organs, especially in the liver, spleen, and red bone marrow. The levels of ferritin and haemosiderin are increased during rapid breakdown of haemoglobin (GRANICK, 1946a), and tracer experiments confirm that haemoglobin iron can be transferred to haemosiderin and ferritin (HAHN et al., 1943). Ferritin and haemosiderin are also formed in response to the administration of large amounts of various iron compounds (GRANICK and HAHN, 1944; GRANICK, 1946; KUFF and DALTON, 1957; RICHTER, 1957, 1959a; BESSIS and BRETON-GORIUS, 1959; MUIR and GOLDBERG, 1961; THERAYOTHIN and CROSBY, 1962), the relative amounts of iron appearing in the ferritin and haemosiderin fractions depending on a number of factors (SHODEN et al., 1953; SHODEN and STURGEON, 1958, 1959).

Ferritin is a water-soluble crystalline protein, consisting of a well-defined and constant protein moiety, known as apoferritin (GRANICK and MICHAELIS, 1943), and micelles of a colloidal hydrated iron oxide ("iron hydroxide")-phosphate complex, the amount of which is variable. Ferritin isolated from horse spleen contains 17–23% of its dry weight as iron (GRANICK, 1943); smaller amounts have been reported for other species (SHODEN and STURGEON, 1960). The micelles have a characteristic and relatively constant magnetic susceptibility corresponding to a magnetic moment of 3.8 Bohr magnetons (MICHAELIS et al., 1943). As was first shown by FARRANT (1954) and has since been confirmed by other workers, the iron micelles are situated inside the protein shell. The size of the micelles is therefore limited by the space inside the protein; as seen in the electron microscope it is 55–60 Å, the protein shell having an external diameter of 94–110 Å (FARRANT, 1954; KUFF and DALTON, 1957; LABAW and WYCKOFF,

1957). In the electron microscope, the micelles quite frequently appear to be composed of subunits about 27–30 Å in diameter, a view of the molecule in which four subunits can be seen generally being regarded as characteristic of ferritin. In wet ferritin crystals, rather larger molecular dimensions have been found by X-ray diffraction; the micelles have a diameter of about 74 Å and the protein shell an external diameter of about 122Å (HARRISON, 1960, 1963). Similar dimensions have been found by low-angle X-ray scattering in solution (J. W. ANDEREGG, private communication). The function of the protein may be to "protect" the micelles and render them soluble.

Haemosiderin is a rather ill-defined and variable entity. Microscopically visible, iron-rich granules can be isolated, the spleen of old horses in which the granules have accumulated being a good source (GRANICK, 1946a). The composition of haemosiderin granules is very variable. The percentage of iron reported varies from 8 to 45% (COOK, 1929; ASHER, 1933; GRANICK, 1942; RICHTER, 1959b; WÖHLER, 1960; SHODEN and STURGEON, 1960). Protein and other organic constituents are also present. The variability in composition probably depends in part on the source of the haemosiderin granules and in part on the isolation procedure. Haemosiderin iron, like that of ferritin, is present in the form of a colloidal "iron hydroxide" complex, some phosphate also being present. It has a magnetic moment similar to that of ferritin, although its magnitude is rather more variable (MICHAELIS et al., 1943; SHODEN and STURGEON, 1960).

Massive iron-rich deposits have also been observed in a variety of cells by electron microscopy (e.g. BESSIS and BRETON-GORIUS, 1957a and b; RICHTER, 1957; REGER et al., 1961). These deposits occur in the cytoplasm and sometimes in the nuclei (NISSIM, 1953; RICHTER, 1961a; LADDA, 1962). They are often surrounded by membranes. Sometimes the deposits occur inside mitochondria. Many of them may be composed, wholly or largely, of ferritin, and in some of them a regular lattice structure similar to that of crystalline ferritin has been observed (BESSIS and BRETON-GORIUS, 1957, 1959; RICHTER, 1958). In others, the iron-containing particles appear to differ from those of ferritin: they are more variable in size and lack the characteristic appearance of ferritin micelles (RICHTER, 1957). These observations have led to the following definition of haemosiderin by RICHTER (1959a):

"Haemosiderin is a substance occurring in the form of intra- or extracellular deposits that (1) are visible in the light microscope as brown granules, (2) contain trivalent iron as demonstrated by histochemical tests such as Perls' test, and (3) often contain variable amounts of ferritin as revealed by electron microscopy."

The presence of ferritin or of apoferritin has also been reported in isolated haemosiderin granules (McKAY and FINEBERG, 1958; RICHTER, 1959b; WÖHLER, 1960). WÖHLER (1960) has pointed to similarities in the amino-acid composition of the protein components of haemosiderin and ferritin from horse spleen, but the similarities are less marked than those between apoferritins from different species (see Table 1), which suggests that other proteins are present. McKAY and FINEBERG (1958) have reported the presence of at least two other proteins in horse-spleen haemosiderin.

In an attempt to differentiate haemosiderin from ferritin SHODEN and STURGEON (1961) recommend that the term "haemosiderin" be applied only to the water-insoluble material obtained after the extraction of ferritin. Electron micrographs of such granules show aggregates of electron-dense particles, but neither

Table 1. *Amino-acid compositions of*
AHI = apohaemosiderin I, AF = apoferritin. Figures in columns 2—6 = g. residues/molecule, mol. wt. 480,000. Figures in columns

Amino acid	AHI[1] (1960)	Horse AF[2] (1950)	Horse AF[1] (1960)	Horse AF[3] (1962)
Glutamic acid	22.50	15.1	18.08	15.6
Aspartic acid .	4.15	5.9	7.13	10.4
Lysine . . .	8.25	6.8	6.79	5.2
Arginine. . .	7.84	8.2	7.61	6.95
Histidine . .	1.90	4.2	2.15	3.71
Tyrosine. . .	1.28	4.5	3.07	4.53
Phenylalanine	1.86	5.4	3.26	5.40
Tryptophan .	1.82	1.1	1.20	0.82
Leucine . . .	11.26	16.5	19.12	13.4, 14.7
Isoleucine . .		1.2		1.84, 2.17
Valine. . . .	1.64	3.6	3.86	3.57
Alanine . . .	8.72	1.5	6.70	5.15
Glycine . . .	6.54	2.6	4.88	2.98
Serine	7.29	—	4.54	3.85, 3.26
Threonine . .	4.38	3.7	3.65	2.95
Proline . . .	2.62	1.3	2.26	1.67, 1.13
$^1/_2$-Cystine . .	2.05	1.4	1.86	1.02
Methionine. .	4.79	1.7	3.02	1.83, 2.02

[1] Analyses by paper chromatography (WÖHLER, 1960).
[2] Analysis mainly by microbiological methods (MAZUR et al., 1950).
[3] Analysis mainly by methods of MOORE and STEIN, and MOORE, SPACKMAN, and STEIN (HARRISON et al., 1962). Figures are averages of those for two different preparations except where these differ significantly, in which case the results are given separately. Recovery 94%.

ferritin crystals nor the "tetrad" appearance of ferritin micelles. They suggest the following description of a haemosiderin granule (or at least one from the rabbit-liver parenchymal cell):

(1) that it is a relatively amorphous condensation of electron-dense particles into an essentially protein-free aggregate;

(2) that it consists mainly of ferric hydroxide;

(3) that it originates in liver-cell vacuoles through a process of degradation of the protein matrix of ferritin.

As SHODEN and STURGEON pointed out, there may be intermediate stages between water-soluble ferritin and "haemosiderin" as defined by them. The granules isolated from human liver [RICHTER (1959b)] by differential centrifugation may be such an intermediate stage. Soluble ferritin should have been removed from these granules during the extraction procedure. Precipitin tests on aqueous extracts of the granules showed only traces of apoferritin. Nevertheless, ferritin micelles and apoferritin mole-

apoferritin and "apohaemosiderin I"

amino-acid residues/100 g. protein. Figures in columns 7—8 = number of 9—10 = number of residues/subunit, mol. wt. 24,000

Guinea-pig AF[4] (1962)	Horse AF[3] (1962)	Guinea-pig AF[4] (1962)	Horse AF[3] (1962)	Guinea-pig AF[4] (1962)
16.92	577	629	29	31.4
12.21	435	509	21.8	25.4
6.72	195	209	9.7	12.6
7.81	213	240	10.6	12.0
5.21	118, 129	182	5.9, 6.5	9.1
5.49	134	161	6.7	8.1
5.10	175	166	8.8	8.4
1.92	21 ± 1	49.4	1.05	2.5
13.93	570, 620	596	28.6, 31	29.8
2.35	78, 92	99.8	3.8, 4.6	5.0
3.77	173	183	8.7	9.1
5.18	348	349	17.4	17.4
3.23	250	271	12.5	13.6
3.65	212, 180	201	10.6, 9.0	10.1
3.37	140	160	7.0	8.0
1.82	72, 56	90	3.6, 2.8	4.5
0.61	48 ± 2	28.6	2.4	1.4
1.98	67, 74	72.5	3.4, 3.7	3.6

[4] Analysis by method of MOORE, SPACKMAN, and STEIN (FRIEDBERG, 1960). Recovery 101%. The molecular weight and subunit molecular weight found for horse apoferritin (see text) have been assumed for guinea-pig apoferritin.

cules were seen in electron micrographs. Evidently, although insoluble, some of the apoferritin had retained its hollow shell form[1]. However, the very high iron content of these granules, reported to be up to 45% (this would correspond to 77% FeOOH), is much higher than the probable maximum iron content of ferritin molecules discussed below (26%). This suggests that, if the iron micelles of these granules had been derived from ferritin, much of the apoferritin must have been degraded.

II. The structure and properties of ferritin

The occurrence, isolation, and some properties of ferritin

Ferritin is well known to occur in a number of mammals (MICHAELIS, 1943). Ferritin or ferritin-like molecules have also been reported in the marine elasmobranch, *Scyllium canicula* (TECCE, 1952), in the lugworm, *Arenicola marina* (ROCHE et al., 1951), and in plants (HYDE et al., 1962). Horse ferritin has been most widely studied.

The usual isolation procedure for ferritin from horse spleen (LAUFBERGER, 1937; GRANICK, 1942) depends on its comparative stability towards heat. It can be separated from denatured proteins after heating an aqueous extract of minced spleen to 80° C. It is purified by precipitation with ammonium sulphate and crystallisation with cadmium sulphate. Some insoluble material separates during the purification procedure. We have confirmed that this is denatured ferritin.

Apoferritin, the iron-free protein, is obtained when ferritin ferric iron is reduced to the ferrous state. Reduction can be achieved by "biological" reducing agents, such as cysteine, glutathione, and ascorbic acid (BIELIG and BAYER, 1955a; MAZUR, BAEZ, and SHORR, 1955), but experimental evidence suggests (GREEN and MAZUR, 1957) that reduction of ferritin iron in the liver involves xanthine oxidase. In the laboratory, the iron can be removed most conveniently by reduction with dithionite (GRANICK and MICHAELIS, 1943; BEHRENS and TAUBERT, 1952). Apoferritin crystallises from cadmium sulphate as colourless octahedral crystals isomorphous with those of ferritin.

---

[1] We have made a similar observation in another connection (HOFMANN and HARRISON, 1963). We have found that it is possible to render apoferritin insoluble and "denatured" by freezing an aqueous solution to —15° C. Nevertheless, as shown by X-ray diffraction, the insoluble material has retained a configuration similar to that of the native protein.

For many years the inorganic component of ferritin was believed to be attached to the surface of the protein (GRANICK, 1951). MAZUR and SHORR (1950) showed, however, that ferritin and apoferritin have the same electrophoretic mobility and that horse-ferritin antibody precipitates the same amounts of ferritin and apoferritin nitrogen. Electron micrographs of ferritin obtained by FARRANT (1954) first clearly demonstrated that the micelles are situated inside a shell of protein. Nevertheless, their presence affects the behaviour of the molecules in a number of ways. Thus, a concentrated solution of ferritin, heated to about 65° C., forms a granular precipitate, which redissolves on cooling (GRANICK, 1942). Apoferritin does not behave in this way. Even at lower temperatures, ferritin shows some tendency to aggregate. In the ultracentrifuge, ferritin solutions are found to be inhomogeneous (ROTHEN, 1944). The schlieren pattern shows a sharp peak with a sedimentation coefficient corresponding to that of apoferritin (s^0_{20}, $w = 17.65$) and a broad diffuse one with an average sedimentation coefficient about 65 s. On ROTHEN's calculations this would correspond roughly to an average molecular weight twice that expected for ferritin.

The presence of iron also affects the ease of precipitation with ammonium sulphate, and this property can be used to fractionate ferritin, the iron-rich fractions coming down first (MAZUR et al., 1950; PHILIPPOT and DE BORNIER, 1959). MAZUR has also fractionated ferritin by centrifugation.

We have made a preliminary examination of ferritin fractions in the ultracentrifuge. Unfractionated ferritin contains about 20–25% of apoferritin (ROTHEN, 1944). In low-iron fractions, the relative amount of apoferritin is increased and the sedimentation coefficient of the diffuse fast peak is decreased. VAN BRUGGEN (1962) has estimated the numbers of full, empty, and partially full molecules in various fractions as seen in the electron microscope. The percentage of the latter remained constant, while the proportion of empty molecules increased in the low-iron fractions.

Ferritin has recently been separated into three or four components by starch-gel electrophoresis (KOPP et al., 1963). These authors found that apoferritin gives a single band (band 1). Bands 2 and 3 are evidently associated with iron-rich components, since they are enriched by repeated fractional precipitation at very low ammonium sulphate concentrations. In the ultracentrifuge, the authors found that enrichment with components 2 and 3 increased the sedimentation coefficient. They consider that bands 2 and 3 are not associated with dimers and trimers or polymers produced in the isolation procedure, since they are also given by crude extracts of ferritin. This does not, however, rule out the possibility that the latter contained molecular aggregates, although the presence of large amounts of iron in the molecule could be associated with conformational changes.

Molecular weight and chemical composition of apoferritin

Apoferritin from horse spleen is relatively homogeneous, with a reproducible nitrogen content (16.1–16.3%) and sedimentation coefficient $s^0_{20,w} = 17.6$, although its extinction at 280 mμ is somewhat variable ($E^{1\,mg./ml.}_{1\,cm.} = 0.860$ to 0.970) (HOFMANN and HARRISON, 1963), probably owing to the presence of traces of yellow contaminants (see GRANICK and MICHAELIS, 1954). A somewhat higher extinction, at 280 mμ ($E^{1\,mg./ml.}_{1\,cm.} = 1.01$), has been reported for guinea-pig apoferritin (FRIEDBERG, 1962).

The molecular weight of horse apoferritin has been determined as 465,000 by sedimentation-diffusion (ROTHEN, 1944) and 480,000 by X-ray diffraction and crystal-density measurements (HARRISON, 1963). A smaller value, 340,500, has been obtained from osmotic-pressure measurements (DE BORNIER, 1957).

The amino-acid composition has been determined for apoferritin from horse spleen (MAZUR, LITT, and SHORR, 1950; WÖHLER, 1960; HARRISON, HOFMANN, and MAINWARING, 1962) and from guinea-pig liver (FRIEDBERG, 1962). The results are given in Table 1. If the more recent results are compared for the two species, it is found that the amino-acid compositions are in general very similar, although there are some interesting differences (some allowance must be made for the differences in recovery of amino acids in the analyses: 94% for horse and 101% for guinea-pig apoferritin). The numbers of acidic residues are nearly the same, but guinea-pig apoferritin contains rather more basic residues and has an isoelectric point (4.8) which is slightly higher than that of horse apoferritin (4.4). Guinea-pig apoferritin contains about twice as much tryptophan and about half as much cysteine-plus-cystine as horse apoferritin.

The composition of the micelles and the molecular weight of ferritin

The exact nature of the colloidal iron complex in the micelles is still uncertain. The 1.0–1.5% of ferritin phosphorus, present as phosphate, is associated with the micelles. It occurs both on the surface and in the inside, and the composition $(FeOOH)_8 \cdot (FeO{:}PO_3H_2)$ has been suggested (MICHAELIS, CORYELL, and GRANICK,

1943; GRANICK and HAHN, 1944). Ferritin fractions with different iron contents have the same Fe:P ratio (MAZUR, LITT, and SHORR, 1950), confirming that the phosphorus is an integral part of the micelles. The analytical figures in the literature are not very numerous, but I have collected the results of twelve analyses for horse, rabbit, and human ferritin, where iron and nitrogen are given as percentages of the dry weight, and, taking the nitrogen content of the protein to be 16.1% (GRANICK and MICHAELIS, 1943), I have calculated the percentage weights of protein and micelles. The percentage of iron in the latter can thus be obtained. The figures vary from 46% to 104%, but most are between 50% and 70%, the average being 59% (excluding the value 104%). The theoretical percentages of iron in the following are: $(FeOOH)_8 \cdot (FeO:OPO_3H_2)$, 57%; Fe_2O_3, 70%; $Fe_2O_3 \cdot H_2O$, 63%; and $Fe_2O_3 \cdot 3H_2O$, 52%. The variations in the experimental values may be due to variations in the extent of drying of the specimen before analysis, to experimental error, or to variations in the composition of the micelles.

The highest Fe:N ratio determined for iron-rich ferritin fractions is 2.5 (MAZUR, LITT, and SHORR, 1950; PHILLIPPOT and DE BORNIER, 1959). Assuming 16.1% N in the protein and 59% Fe in the micelles, the molecules would contain 24% of their weight as Fe and 40.6% of their weight as micelles. If the protein component has a weight of 480,000, then the molecular weight of this fraction would be 808,000. KLEINWACHTER (1961) states that the fraction with Fe:N equal to 2.5 contains 27.7% Fe. This value must be too high, since it would imply that 88.5% of the micelle is Fe. I have determined the molecular weight of an iron-rich fraction to be 800,000 by X-ray diffraction and crystal-density measurements, but I have not obtained analytical data for these crystals. As a result of an electron-microscope study of ferritin fractions, VAN BRUGGEN (1962) concluded that ferritin molecules completely filled with iron would have an Fe:N ratio of 2.9. On the assumptions given above, the molecular weight of full ferritin molecules would then be 860,000. They would contain 26% of iron, or 4,000 iron atoms, and the micelles would account for 44% of the molecular weight.

Chemical evidence for subunits in apoferritin

X-ray crystallographic studies (HARRISON, 1959) suggested that apoferritin contained subunits. Chemical evidence summarised below shows that there are about twenty identical peptide chains in horse apoferritin.

Horse apoferritin contains 21 tryptophan residues, and this must be the maximum number of identical chains (HARRISON, HOFMANN, and MAINWARING, 1962). N-terminal amino groups are absent, but there are 19.7 $\pm$ 5% acetyl residues/mole apoferritin, and N-acetyl serine has been detected in enzymic digests (W. I. P. MAINWARING, personal communication). MAINWARING has also isolated about 19 moles of arginine from the C-terminal end of horse apoferritin using carboxypeptidase B, the C-terminal sequence being leucyl-lysyl-arginine. The number of peptides found in "fingerprints" of tryptic digests is also consistent with twenty identical peptide chains (HARRISON and HOFMANN, 1962).

The degradation of apoferritin into subunits

Ferritin is relatively resistant to denaturation at high pH, even above 12, and at high concentrations of urea except at high pH (MAZUR et al., 1950). In acid, ferritin iron goes into solution and the protein forms insoluble aggregates (BÉNÉZECH and DE BORNIER, 1955).

We have found (HOFMANN and HARRISON, 1963) that *native* apoferritin is not degraded into subunits by 8M urea or by 1% sodium dodecyl sulphate. Up to about 50% degradation to a 2.1s component occurs after prolonged incubation at pH 12.6, the process apparently having an all-or-none character. If ferritin is treated with 1N NaOH for 10 minutes (MICHAELIS et al., 1943) or with concentrations down to 0.2N NaOH for longer periods (DE BORNIER, 1956), the iron micelles are released. A preliminary examination suggests that under these conditions the protein is completely degraded.

Complete degradation under mild conditions can be achieved if apoferritin is first dehydrated by alcohol precipitation, or freeze-drying, and then dissolved in sodium dodecyl sulphate, with which it forms a complex having a sedimentation coefficient of 2.5s. The weight of protein in the complex is 25,000–27,000, corresponding to 18–19 subunits per molecule. MAINWARING has recently found that apoferritin splits into subunits having a molecular weight of 25,000 if the positive charges on the lysine residues are replaced by negative ones by succinylation (KLOTZ et al., 1962).

The quaternary structure of apoferritin

A model for the quaternary structure of apoferritin, which is in agreement with recent X-ray diffraction evidence (HARRISON, 1963) and with the results discussed above, consists of twenty subunits, each composed of a single peptide chain and situated at the twenty vertices of a pentagonal dodecahedron. A model of such an arrangement is shown in Fig. 1. In the proposed structure, each subunit is centred at a radius of 49–50 Å, and the centres of neighbouring subunits are 35 Å apart. In the actual molecule, the subunits cannot all be structurally equivalent.

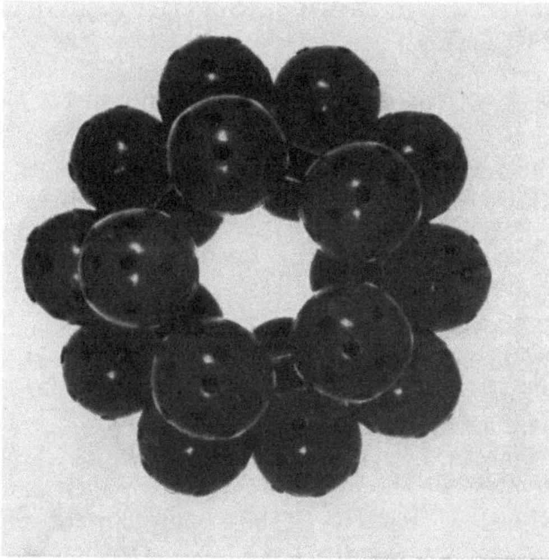

Fig. 1. Model of proposed quaternary structure of apoferritin — twenty subunits at the vertices of a pentagonal dodecahedron — viewed perpendicular to a pentagon face. Each ball represents a single peptide chain. In the actual molecule, the subunits would be in contact with one another. They would not be expected to be exactly spherical.

The properties and functions of ferritin in relation to its structure

In the preceding sections, I have discussed the chemical composition of the ferritin molecule, its size and shape, and the basic architecture of the protein shell. It is now pertinent to ask a number of questions. How are ferritin molecules formed *in vivo* and how are they broken down? What is the structure of the micelles? How are the protein subunits held together? How are the micelles attached to the protein? In what ways are the physiological functions of the molecules related to their chemical composition and structure?

Ferritin synthesis

The administration of iron compounds leads to an increase in the amounts of ferritin formed in various types of cell *in vivo.*

Ferritin synthesis can also be activated in tissue cultures of HeLa cells by the addition of small amounts of ferrous sulphate to the medium (RICHTER, 1961). Tracer experiments of FINEBERG and GREENBERG (1955) have demonstrated that an increase in the level of iron leads to the *de novo* synthesis of apoferritin and that the iron enters the completed protein shell. MAZUR and GREEN (1959) also report that Fe^{59} is taken up most rapidly by apoferritin-rich fractions of ferritin. An *in vitro* incorporation of iron into apoferritin can occur if the latter is incubated at pH 7.4 in the presence of *ferrous* ammonium sulphate which is allowed to oxidise slowly in the air (BIELIG and BAYER, 1955b). Experiments of LOEWUS and FINEBERG (1957) suggest that *in vivo* the iron must also be in the ferrous state before it is taken up by apoferritin. Thus, it appears that both the uptake and release of iron by ferritin are by way of Fe^{++}. GRANICK (1946b) has suggested that in the mucosal cells Fe^{++} is in equilibrium with ferritin Fe^{+++} and that this equilibrium plays a part in the regulation of iron absorption. Evidence has been obtained for the presence of a small amount of ferrous iron associated with ferritin (MAZUR et al., 1955), and this may be responsible for its vasodepressor and antidiuretic effects under certain conditions (MAZUR, 1956).

An examination of the model in Fig. 1 shows that the protein subunits are situated at the corners of the pentagonal faces, the centres of which are empty. If the subunits were spherical, this central space would measure 24 Å across. Density measurements, however, indicate that the subunits must be mere space-fillers rather than spheres, and the central space is probably considerably smaller than this. "Negative staining" methods (RICHTER, 1959c; VAN BRUGGEN, 1962) show that the channels through which the reagents pass must be at least 8.5 Å across. They are certainly large enough for Fe^{++} and PO_4''' ions to pass through, and the oxidation to Fe^{+++} and the formation of the micelles may take place inside the protein shell. Once formed, the colloidal complex may be held inside the protein by chemical links or simply because the particles are too large to pass through the inter-subunit spaces. Alternatively, the protein may act as a sieve. The ferric hydroxide, which forms as the Fe^{++} is oxidised, starts to eliminate water and form polymers. Possibly only those polymers which are formed in the initial stages are small enough to enter the protein shell. Inside the shell, they may condense further and also form links with groups in the inner surface of the protein. Preliminary observations made by J. W. ANDEREGG (personal communication) on ferritin fractions having a very low iron content suggest that the first iron to enter the shell is bound at a radius of about 40 Å. This is just the radius of the centre of the pentagonal faces.

"Synthetic ferritin" made by the method of BIELIG and BAYER is not identical with native material. In the electron microscope, completely filled molecules are absent, about half the molecules being partly full (VAN BRUGGEN, 1963). I have also found that the X-ray diffraction patterns differ from those of native ferritin. These differences may be due to the absence of phosphate.

The structure of the micelles

From the foregoing discussion it may be concluded that the structure of the micelles is determined by that of the protein. Various structures have been proposed to account for the appearance of the micelles in electron micrographs. These include four subunits at the vertices of a square (FARRANT, 1954) or of a tetrahedron (RICHTER, 1959a) or six subunits at the vertices of an octahedron (MUIR, 1960; BESSIS and BRETON-GORIUS, 1960) or of a trilateral prism (VAN BRUGGEN, WIEBENGA, and GRUBER, 1960). In some photographs, however, particularly ones taken very close to true focus (H. E. HUXLEY, private communication), the micelles seem to be rather uniform in density and to have a polyhedral appearance. In some views they seem to be roughly square in outline, in others pentagonal. If the protein consists of twenty subunits at the apices of a pentagonal dodecahedron, and the micelles fill the available space in the inside, then their shape would be expected to approximate to that of a solid icosahedron. X-ray diffraction photographs of wet ferritin-apoferritin mixed crystals (HARRISON, 1963) suggest that the micelles are roughly spherical, but probably actually polyhedral objects, about 74 Å in diameter. The details of their shape are not yet clear, however.

The stability of ferritin molecules: inter-subunit and protein-micelle linkages

Native ferritin and apoferritin are rather stable molecules, as shown by their resistance to denaturation and degradation. Nevertheless, the fact that freeze-dried apoferritin can be degraded by detergent shows that the subunits are not held together by S-S bridges or other covalent bonds. Van der Waals and electrostatic interactions and hydrogen bonds (for example, between tyrosyl and carboxyl groups) may all play a part in holding the subunits together. The presence of water appears to be necessary for the maintenance of the native configuration. Shrinkage occurs on drying, the molecular diameter decreasing from 122 Å (wet) to 112 Å (air-dried) and then to about 100 Å (vacuum-dried). After thorough dehydration the protein can readily be split into subunits.

Ferritin is somewhat more resistant to denaturation and enzymatic hydrolysis than apoferritin. This may be due to the binding of the protein to the micelles. MAZUR and GREEN (1959) have suggested that there is a mercaptide linkage between protein sulphydryl groups and Fe^{+++}, since the number of reactive SH groups is greater in low-iron fractions. We have confirmed this finding. In horse ferritin, the number of reactive SH groups increases from about 1 per subunit in iron-rich fractions to about 1.5 per subunit in apoferritin-rich fractions (and to about 2 per subunit on denaturation). This correlation, however, does not necessarily imply a direct linkage; the increased iron content might have made some of the SH groups inaccessible. A study of guinea-pig ferritin would be of interest in this connection, since the total number of "half-cystine" residues is rather less than in horse ferritin.

The uptake and release of iron by the intact protein shell has been discussed above. The protein itself can also be broken down in the tissues, since apoferritin does not accumulate when the iron is released (GRANICK, 1951). Ferritin micelles may be converted to "haemosiderin" by partial or complete breakdown of the protein, probably by the action of proteolytic enzymes (cathepsins have been reported to attack native ferritin [RENDL, 1954]). GRANICK (1951) has suggested that ferritin may be considered not only as a storage form of iron, but also as one of the reserve storage proteins.

Summary

Ferritin and haemosiderin are the two forms in which iron is stored in the body. Ferritin is a relatively well-defined water-soluble crystalline protein, although its iron content is variable. It consists of a protein shell surrounding a "ferric hydroxide"-phosphate complex. The size of the inorganic component is delimited by the space available inside the protein, so that, as seen in the electron microscope, the electron-dense core has a constant diameter of about 55 Å, while the external diameter of the protein shell is about 105 Å. In the native state, these dimensions are about 74 Å and 122 Å, respectively. The ferric hydroxide accounts for up to about 40—44% of the weight of the ferritin molecule.

Haemosiderin is granular and insoluble in water. The granules may contain as much as 58—77% of their weight as ferric hydroxide, the size and shape of which is variable. Haemosiderin granules also contain protein — and the presence of apoferritin has been reported — as well as non-protein organic components and phosphorus. Haemosiderin may be largely a breakdown product of ferritin.

Although stored as Fe^{+++}, the uptake and release of ferritin iron appears to be in the ferrous form. The *in vivo* synthesis of apoferritin occurs in response to ferrous iron, and the iron enters the completed protein shell. An *in vitro* "synthetic ferritin" can be formed when ferrous ammonium sulphate is oxidised by atmospheric oxygen in the presence of apoferritin. Ferritin iron can be released *in vitro* by reducing agents such as dithionite. At low pH, ferritin iron goes into solution and the denatured protein is precipitated. At high pH, the iron micelles are precipitated and the protein remains in solution, although no longer in its native form.

Some of the properties of ferritin outlined above may be explained in terms of the structure of its molecules. Horse-spleen apoferritin has a molecular weight of about 480,000 and consists of twenty peptide chains. X-ray diffraction evidence suggests that the chains are situated at the twenty vertices of a pentagonal dodecahedron. Ferrous ions could pass through the spaces between subunits at the centres of the pentagonal faces. The structure of the ferric hydroxide micelles would be expected to be complementary to that of the protein. The protein subunits are hard to separate, although they are not held together by covalent bonds. At high pH, the structure falls apart and the micelles are released. Apoferritin can also be degraded if first dehydrated. The amino-acid composition has been determined for apoferritin from horse spleen and from guinea-pig liver. There are a number of significant differences.

Zusammenfassung

Ferritin und Haemosiderin sind die beiden Formen, in denen Eisen im Organismus gespeichert wird. Ferritin ist ein verhältnismäßig gut definiertes wasserlösliches, kristallines Eiweiß, dessen Eisengehalt variiert. Es besteht aus einer Eiweißhülle, die einen Ferrihydroxyd-phosphat Komplex umgibt. Die Größe des anorganischen Anteils des Moleküls ist durch den vorhandenen Raum innerhalb des Proteins begrenzt. Mit Hilfe des Elektronenmikroskopes ist nachweisbar, daß der elektronendichte Kern einen konstanten Durchmesser von ungefähr 55 Å besitzt, während der äußere Durchmesser der Proteinhülle etwa 105 Å beträgt. Im Nativzustand liegen diese Durchmesser bei etwa 74 Å bzw. 122 Å. Ferrihydroxyd hat einen Anteil bis zu 40—44% am Gewicht des Ferritinmoleküls.

Haemosiderin liegt in Form von Granula vor und ist unlöslich in Wasser. Die Granula, deren Größe und Gestalt variieren, können bis zu 58—77% Ferrihydroxyd enthalten. Daneben bestehen die Haemosiderin-Granula aus Eiweiß — auch Apoferritin soll darin vorkommen — sowie aus anderen organischen Bestandteilen und Phosphor. Haemosiderin stellt zum großen Teil ein Abbauprodukt von Ferritin dar.

Obgleich als Ferrieisen abgelagert, scheint die Aufnahme und Abgabe von Ferritineisen in der Ferroform zu erfolgen. Die *in vivo* Synthese von Apoferritin erfolgt als Reaktion auf Ferroeisen, wobei das Eisen in die vollständige Proteinhülle eingebaut wird. Ein „synthetisches Ferritin" kann *in vitro* gebildet werden, wenn Ferroammoniumsulfat durch atmosphärischen Sauerstoff in Gegenwart von Apoferritin oxydiert wird. Ferritineisen kann *in vitro* durch reduzierende Substanzen wie Dithionit freigesetzt werden. Bei niedrigem pH geht Ferritineisen in Lösung, und das denaturierte Eiweiß fällt aus. Bei hohem pH werden die eisenhaltigen Micellen präzipitiert, während das Eiweiß in Lösung bleibt, allerdings nicht in seiner ursprünglichen Form.

Einige der angegebenen Eigenschaften von Ferritin lassen sich auf Grund seiner Molekülstruktur erklären. Aus Pferdemilz isoliertes Apoferritin hat ein Molekulargewicht von etwa 480'000 und besteht aus zwanzig Peptidketten. Röntgenspektrographische Untersuchungen sprechen dafür, daß die Ketten an den zwanzig Ecken eines pentagonalen Dodecaeders sitzen. Ferroionen könnten durch die Abstände zwischen den Untereinheiten an den Zentren der fünf Flächen gehen. Die Struktur der Ferrihydroxyd-Micellen dürfte komplementär zu der des Proteins sein. Die Untereinheiten des Eiweißes sind nur schwer voneinander abzutrennen, obgleich sie nicht durch kovalente Bindungen zusammengehalten werden. Bei hohem pH fällt die Struktur auseinander, und die Micellen werden freigesetzt. Apoferritin kann auch abgebaut werden, wenn es zuerst dehydriert wird. Der Aminosäuregehalt für Apoferritin aus Pferdemilz und aus Meerschweinchenleber wurde bestimmt. Dabei ergeben sich wesentliche Unterschiede.

Résumé

La ferritine et l'hémosidérine sont les deux formes sous lesquelles le fer est stocké dans l'organisme. La ferritine est une protéine relativement bien définie, cristalline, soluble dans l'eau, mais dont la teneur en fer est variable. Elle se compose d'une enveloppe protéique entourant un complexe d'hydroxyde de fer phosphaté. La dimension de la partie inorganique de la molécule est limitée par l'espace disponible à l'intérieur de la protéine. Le microscope électronique montre que le noyau imperméable aux électrons a un diamètre constant d'environ 55 Å, tandis que le diamètre extérieur de la couche protéique est d'environ 105 Å. A l'état naissant, ces deux diamètres sont respectivement d'environ 74Å et 122Å. L'oxyde ferrique participe pour 40 à 44% au poids de la molécule de ferritine.

L'hémosidérine se présente sous forme granulaire et est insoluble dans l'eau. Les granules, de dimension et de forme variables, peuvent contenir jusqu'à 58 à 77% d'oxyde ferrique. Par ailleurs, ces granules d'hémosidérine contiennent des protéines — de l'apoferritine s'y trouverait également — ainsi que d'autres constituants organiques et phosphorés. L'hémosidérine pourrait éventuellement être un produit de dégradation de la ferritine.

Bien que le fer soit stocké sous forme trivalente, la ferritine semble fixer et céder son fer sous forme bivalente. La synthèse de l'apoferritine *in vivo* s'effectue selon une réaction où le fer intervient sous forme bivalente et par laquelle le fer est fixé dans l'enveloppe protéique globale. On peut préparer *in vitro* une «ferritine synthétique» en oxydant du sulfate d'ammoniaque ferreux par l'oxygène de l'atmosphère en présence d'apoferritine. Le fer de la ferritine peut être libéré *in vitro* par des substances réductrices comme le $Na_2S_2O_4$ (dithionate de soude). A des pH peu élevés, le fer de la ferritine passe en solution, et la protéine dénaturée précipite. A des pH élevés, les micelles contenant du fer précipitent, tandis que la protéine reste en solution, mais sous une forme autre que sa forme primitive.

Quelques-unes des propriétés mentionnées de la ferritine peuvent s'expliquer par sa structure moléculaire. L'apoferritine isolée de la rate de cheval a un poids moléculaire de 480.000 environ et se compose de vingt chaînes peptidiques. L'étude du spectre de diffraction aux rayons X semble montrer que ces chaînes sont fixées aux vingt sommets d'un dodécaèdre pentagonal. Les ions ferreux pourraient traverser l'espace compris entre les chaînes peptidiques aux centres des cinq faces. La structure des micelles d'oxyde ferrique devrait être complémentaire de celle de la protéine. Les chaînes peptidiques de la protéine ne se laissent que difficilement séparer, bien qu'elles ne soient pas fixées par des liaisons covalentes. Aux pH élevés, la structure est désorganisée, et les micelles sont libérées. Après déshydratation, l'apoferritine peut aussi être dégradée. La composition en acides aminés de l'apoferritine de la rate de cheval ainsi que celle du foie de cobaye ont été déterminées. Des différences notables ont été trouvées.

Acknowledgement

The author would like to thank the Medical Research Council, London, for their personal research grant.

References

Asher, T.: Hoppe-Seyler's Zschr. physiol. Chem. (G). **220**, 97 (1933). — Behrens, M., and M. Taubert: Hoppe-Seyler's Zschr. physiol. Chem. (G.) **290**, 156 (1952). — Bénézech, C., and B. M. de Bornier: Compt. rend. Soc. biol. (Fr.) **149**, 774 (1955). — Bessis, M., and J. Breton-Gorius: Compt. rend. Acad. sc. (Fr.) **244**, 2846 (1957a). — Bessis, M., and J. Breton-Gorius: Compt. rend. Acad. sc. (Fr.) **245**, 1271 (1957b). — Bessis, M., and J. Breton-Gorius: J. Biophys. Biochem. Cytol. (U.S.A.) **6**, 231, 237 (1959). — Bessis, M., and J. Breton-Gorius: Compt. rend. Acad. sc. (Fr.) **250**, 1360 (1960). — Bielig, H. J., and E. Bayer: Naturwissenschaften (G.) **42**, 466 (1955a). — Bielig, H. J., and E. Bayer: Naturwissenschaften (G.) **42**, 125 (1955b). — de Bornier, B. M.: Compt. rend. Soc. biol. (Fr.) **150**, 1595 (1956). — de Bornier, B. M.: Bull. Soc. chim. biol. (Fr.) **39**, 1067 (1957). — van Bruggen, E. F. J.: Ph. D. Thesis, Groningen (1962). — van Bruggen, E. F. J., E. H. Wiebenga, and M. Gruber: J. Mol. Biol. (G.B.) **2**, 81 (1960). — Cook, S. F.: J. Biol. Chem. (U.S.A.) **82**, 595 (1929). — Farrant, J. L.: Biochim. biophysica acta (U.S.A.) **13**, 569 (1954). — Fineberg, R. A., and D. M. Greenberg: J. Biol. Chem. (U.S.A.) **214**, 97, 107 (1955). — Friedberg, F.: Canad. J. Biochem. **40**, 983 (1962). — Gabrio, B. W., and K. Solomon: Proc. Soc. Exper. Biol. Med. (U.S.A.) **75**, 124 (1950). — Granick, S.: J. Biol. Chem. (U.S.A.) **146**, 451 (1942). — Granick, S.: Chem. Rev. (U.S.A.) **38**, 379 (1946a). — Granick, S.: J. Biol. Chem. (U.S.A.) **164**, 737 (1946b). — Granick, S.: Physiol. Rev. (U.S.A.) **31**, 489 (1951). — Granick, S., and P. F. Hahn: J. Biol. Chem. (U.S.A.) **155**, 661 (1944). — Granick, S., and L. Michaelis: J. Biol. Chem. (U.S.A.) **147**, 91 (1943). — Hahn, P. F., S. Granick, W. F. Bale, and L. Michaelis: J. Biol. Chem. (U.S.A.) **150**, 407 (1943). — Harrison, P. M.: J. Mol. Biol. (G.B.) **1**, 69 (1959). — Harrison, P. M.,: Acta cryst. (Den.) **13**, 1060 (1960). — Harrison, P. M.: J. Mol. Biol. (G.B.) **6**, 404 (1963). — Harrison, P. M., and T. Hofmann: J. Mol. Biol. (G.B.) **4**, 239 (1962). — Harrison, P. M., T. Hofmann, and W. I. P. Mainwaring: J. Mol. Biol. (G.B.) **4**, 251 (1962). — Hofmann, T., and P. M. Harrison: J. Mol. Biol. (G.B.) **6**, 256 (1963). — Hyde, B. B., A. J. Hodge, and M. L. Birnstiel: Fifth International Congress for Electron Microscopy, Vol. 2. Academic Press, New York, 1962, p. T-1. — Kleinwachter, V.: Chem. listy (Czech.) **55**, 234 (1961). — Klotz, I. M., and S. Keresztes-Nagy: Nature (G.B.) **195**, 900 (1962). — Kopp, R., A. Vogt, and G. Maass: Nature (G.B.) **198**, 892 (1963). — Kuff, E. L., and A. J. Dalton: J. Ultrastruct. Res. (U.S.A.) **1**, 62 (1957). — Labaw, L. W., and R. W. G. Wyckoff: Biochim. biophysica acta (U.S.A.) **25**, 263 (1957). — Laufberger, V.: Bull. Soc. chim. biol. (Fr.) **19**, 1575 (1937). — Loewus,

M. W., and R. A. FINEBERG: Biochim. biophysica acta (U.S.A.) **26**, 441 (1957). — MAZUR, A.: In: Essays in Biochemistry. John Wiley & Sons, New York, 1956, p. 198. — MAZUR, A., S. BAEZ, and E. SHORR: J. Biol. Chem. (U.S.A.) **213**, 147 (1955). — MAZUR, A., and S. GREEN: In: Sulfur in Proteins. Academic Press, New York and London, 1959, p. 189. — MAZUR, A., J. LITT, and E. SHORR: J. Biol. Chem. (U.S.A.) **187**, 473 (1950). — MAZUR, A., and E. SHORR: J. Biol. Chem. (U.S.A.) **182**, 607 (1950). — MCKAY, R. H., and R. A. FINEBERG: Fed. Proc. (U.S.A.) **17**, 272 (1958). — MICHAELIS, L.: Advanc. Protein Chem. (U.S.A.) **3**, 53 (1947). — MICHAELIS, L., C. D. CORYELL, and S. GRANICK: J. Biol. Chem. (U.S.A.) **148**, 463 (1943). — MUIR, A. R.: Quart. J. Exper. Physiol. (G.B.) **45**, 192 (1960). — MUIR, A. R., and L. GOLDBERG: J. Path. Bact. (G.B.) **82**, 471 (1961). — NISSIM, J. A.: J. Path. Bact. (G.B.) **66**, 185 (1953). — PHILIPPOT, J., and B. M. DE BORNIER: Bull. Soc. chim. biol. (Fr.) **41**, 119 (1959). — REGER, J. F., M. P. HUTT, and H. B. NENSTEIN: J. Ultrastruct. Res. (U.S.A.) **5**, 28 (1961). — RENDI, R.: Boll. Soc. ital. biol. sper. **30**, 508 (1954). — RICHTER, G. W.: J. Exper. Med. (U.S.A.) **106**, 203 (1957). — RICHTER, G. W.: J. Biophys. Biochem. Cytol. (U.S.A.) **4**, 55 (1958). — RICHTER, G. W.: J. Exper. Med. (U.S.A.) **109**, 197 (1959a). — RICHTER, G. W.: Amer. J. Path, **35**, 690 (1959b). — RICHTER, G. W.: J. Biophys. Biochem. Cytol. (U.S.A.) **6**, 531 (1959c). — RICHTER, G. W.: J. Biophys. Biochem. Cytol. (U.S.A.) **9**, 263 (1961a). — RICHTER, G. W.: Nature (G.B.) **190**, 413 (1961b). — ROCHE, J., M. BESSIS, and J. BRETON-GORIUS: Compt. rend. Acad. sc. (Fr.) **252**, 3886 (1961). — ROTHEN, A.: J. Biol. Chem. (U.S.A.) **182**, 607 (1944). — SHODEN, A., B. W. GABRIO, and C. A. FINCH: J. Biol. Chem. (U.S.A.) **204**, 823 (1953). — SHODEN, A., and P. STURGEON: Amer. J. Path. **34**, 1139 (1958). — SHODEN, A., and P. STURGEON: Acta haemat. (Switz.) **22**, 140 (1959). — SHODEN, A., and P. STURGEON: Acta haemat. (Switz.) **23**, 376 (1960). — SHODEN, A., and P. STURGEON: Nature (G.B.) **189**, 846 (1961). — TECCE, G.: Nature (G.B.) **170**, 75 (1952). — THERAYOTHIN, P., and W. H. CROSBY: J. Clin. Invest. (U.S.A.) **41**, 1206 (1962). — WÖHLER, F.: Acta haemat. (Switz.) **23**, 342 (1960).

Discussion

SAADI: We have done a little work on the same subject in Dr. SCHAPIRA's laboratory[1]. We were simply interested in comparing the ferritin of various normal subjects with that of patients suffering from haemochromatosis; for this purpose, we began by trying to find out how the ferritin was composed and whether we could draw any comparisons between ferritin from healthy subjects and from the patients. Dr. DREYFUS suggested that we should attempt to determine whether this protein of very high molecular weight is made up of subunits and whether it could thus easily be split by trypsin, resulting in various peptides which might be demonstrated by chromatography using the method of INGRAM[2]. When we carried out our experiments, we invariably found in horse ferritin (and in apoferritin, too) something like between 15 and 17 peptides — which suggested that we were not dealing with a single polypeptide chain. Then, as you have shown in your paper, Dr. HARRISON, we found that there was only one peptide with tryptophan. Thus, these results indicate that there cannot be more than between 15 and 20 peptides in the molecule; the subunit we found was therefore approximately the same as that which you found with a molecular weight of between 15,000 and 20,000.

I did not quite understand what you said about the difference between apoferritin and ferritin in starch-gel electrophoresis. I don't think that your findings in this connection were the same as ours.

HARRISON: The work that I was referring to was not ours, but that of KOPP, VOGT, and MAASS, recently published in Nature[3]. They obtained three, or sometimes four, bands with ferritin on starch-gel electrophoresis, but, as I understood it, they obtained only one band with apoferritin.

SAADI: This doesn't fit in with our findings at all. When we did starch-gel electrophoresis with ferritin from various species (horse, rat, healthy humans, diseased humans) there were always three bands, both in the case of apoferritin and ferritin. We tried to separate these bands from one another by cutting the starch gel, after which we eluted the ferritin by electrodialysis, concentrated it, and put it back again into the starch gel; but regardless of where we took the ferritin from, i.e. from the major band or from the others, we always found the two or three bands again after carrying out the procedures that I described; this led us to suppose — although I am not sure of it, since I am not a physical chemist — that there must presumably be some sort of equilibrium between ferritin in several states of molecular aggregation, particularly in view of the fact that the pores of the starch gel separate molecules of the same charge but of different size.

BEARN: I may have missed this, Dr. HARRISON, but can you re-associate the subunits?

---

[1] SAADI, R., G. SCHAPIRA, and J.-C. DREYFUS: Bull. Soc. chim. biol. (Fr.) **43**, 409 (1961).
SAADI, R.: Rev. franç. étud. clin. biol. **7**, 408 (1962).
[2] INGRAM, V. M.: Biochim. biophysica acta (U.S.A.) **28**, 539 (1959).
[3] KOPP, R., A. VOGT, and G. MAASS: Nature (G.B.) **198**, 892 (1963).

Harrison: We have not obtained complete re-association to apoferritin molecules, but this is a very interesting question and requires further study. Our results are only preliminary ones.

Granick[1] showed that ferritin micelles are precipitated at a pH of about 13. Under these conditions it seems that the protein subunits are separated. If the "ferric hydroxide" precipitate is spun off and the pH reduced to about 10, we have found — in one experiment — that the subunits re-aggregate to some extent, but we have not so far obtained a component with a sedimentation coefficient corresponding to that of apoferritin.

Bearn: Do the subunits bind iron?

Harrison: Not as far as I know.

Beutler: Are the subunits all identical or are there several different types, as seems to be the case with the haemoglobins and with the lactic dehydrogenases? In other words, are there several different types of amino-acid chain involved in the structure of ferritin? My other question is: if iron is really essential for the synthesis of apoferritin one would expect it to be very difficult to find iron-free apoferritin under physiological circumstances. Yet apoferritin can be extracted from tissues. I wonder how good the evidence is that iron is indeed necessary for *in vivo* apoferritin synthesis.

Harrison: Our results suggest that the subunits are *chemically* identical. Possibly there might be small differences, but for the moment we think that the subunits are all the same. But it is an interesting point that *structurally* the subunits cannot all be equivalent to one another, i.e. if there are twenty subunits, one at each vertex of a pentagonal dodecahedron. In the simple model built from spheres, the subunits are all equivalent and each has a threefold axis of symmetry passing through its centre. A polypeptide chain, however, is asymmetric and cannot have a threefold rotation axis. If twenty polypeptide chains are placed at each of the twenty vertices of a pentagonal dodecahedron, it is not possible to arrange them in such a way that they are all structurally equivalent. Two groups of ten subunits in which each member of a group has the same structural environment are possible. One might expect these structural differences to give rise to differences in the reactivity of otherwise equivalent residues. For example, there are twenty tryptophan residues, one for each subunit. Possibly one half of these residues might react differently from the other half. So far we have not found any such differences, but again this work is in a very preliminary state.

With regard to your question as to whether or not iron is *necessary*, its presence certainly seems to stimulate apoferritin synthesis. Perhaps someone else could say more about this.

Wöhler: We have found that there is always a small quantity of apoferritin in the cells, and we therefore think that iron is not necessary for the synthesis of apoferritin in the cells.

Gajdos: Is all the iron inside the protein moiety, or is some of it located at the surface? And if so, is there a difference in the electronic configuration of the two iron fractions? According to Mazur[2], 2% of the iron is on the

---

[1] Michaelis, L., C. D. Coryell, and S. Granick: J. Biol. Chem. (U.S.A.) **148**, 463 (1943).

[2] Mazur, A., S. Baez, and E. Schorr: J. Biol. Chem. (U.S.A.) **213**, 147 (1955).

surface, and this iron would be in the ferrous state, while the iron inside the apoferritin would be in the ferric state.

HARRISON: As far as we know, the iron in the micelles in the centre of the ferritin molecule is all in the ferric state. MAZUR's work, however, suggested that there was a small amount of iron — about 0.2% by weight — which was in the ferrous state. He thought that this iron was on or near the surface of the molecule.

EICHHORN: I wonder if it is possible to see anything of the structure of the ferric hydroxide micelle by X-rays, or is it completely amorphous?

HARRISON: The internal structure of the micelles is not a very regular one; X-ray diffraction patterns of ferritin and apoferritin at high angles look pretty similar. If the micelles are precipitated by NaOH, the precipitate gives two or three broad diffuse X-ray diffraction lines, from which it is not possible to say very much about the atomic arrangement. At low angles ferritin and also ferritin-apoferritin mixed crystals give diffraction patterns which clearly depend on the large-scale shape of the micelles. At present, however, this shape is not yet clear.

KRUH: Do you know if iron increases the amount of apoferritin by inducing a net biosynthesis of the protein, or has it a minor effect, for instance by binding together apoferritin subunits?

HARRISON: It appears to increase the biosynthesis of apoferritin.

KRUH: From amino acids?

HARRISON: Yes.

NAJEAN: Do you know if the ferritin of the erythroblast and of the reticulo-endothelial cell is the same as regards its capacity to take up and release iron?

HARRISON: No, I don't know.

Some observations on transferrin

By

A. G. Bearn and W. C. Parker

The observation by Barkan in 1927 (*2*) that serum iron was non-dialyzable at physiological pH marked the beginning of a trail of chemical and physiological research which led to the crystallization in 1952 (*14*) of transferrin, a serum protein with the specific properties of binding and transporting iron. In the last decade, the physiological aspects of iron transport have been greatly illuminated by the work of several investigators, but problems still exist. In particular, such detailed studies as have been undertaken on the structure of transferrin have barely scratched the surface of this problem.

Many of the chemical properties of transferrin are well established and need no extensive review. It will be recalled that transferrin is a glycoprotein with an approximate molecular weight of 83,000 (*1*, *11*). This estimate is rather lower than the earlier estimates which assigned transferrin a molecular weight of 90,000 (*14*). Under appropriate conditions, two atoms of iron can be bound, by ionic bonds, to each molecule of transferrin. Although the evidence is not conclusive, it has been suggested (*8*) that tyrosine and histidine are the sites on the transferrin molecule to which the ferric ion is bound. Transferrin occurs in human plasma in a concentration of 200–350 mg. %. Each g. of transferrin can bind about 1.25 mg. of iron, the total iron-binding capacity being approximately 200–400 μg. per 100 ml. of plasma. Transferrin is usually only one-third saturated with iron.

Until 1957, it had been assumed that transferrin represented a single molecular species, and indeed, as we have seen, a number of reassuring physical constants were assigned to it. In 1957, Smithies, using the recently developed starch-gel electrophoretic technique, disclosed two bands in the beta-globulin region (*25*). The following year, an additional beta-globulin band was observed with a mobility different from the two previously noted (*26*). It was subsequently shown that the beta-globulin bands bound radioactive iron and thus represented serum transferrin (*6*). The transferrins which migrated faster than normal transferrin were called transferrin B, and those migrating slower transferrin D, normal transferrin being designated transferrin C. Family studies demonstrated that these bands were genetically determined according to a simple co-dominant allelic system. Our interest in transferrin stemmed from the initial observations that genetic variants of transferrin occurred among normal healthy populations. In particular we were interested in the nature and extent of this particular genetic biochemical polymorphism, and in discovering whether and to what extent it existed in different species, and whether it would be possible to demonstrate physiological differences between normal and mutant transferrins. Progress has been slow, but a number of facts have come to light.

Genetic variation

As of now, there are 15 distinct electrophoretic species of normal transferrin. Seven migrate faster than normal transferrin and seven migrate slower. Fig. 1 illustrates the relative mobilities of the variants. Two aspects deserve particular emphasis. The wide geographic distribution of the populations in which the variants have been found and their relative frequency. Transferrins B_{Lae}, B_0, B_1, B_{1-2}, B_3, D_0, D_4, (D_{0-1}), $D_{Montreal}$, D_2, and D_3 have been reported only in isolated cases, and their occurrence can be plausibly ascribed to mutation pressure (*16*, *17*, *19*, *20*). However,

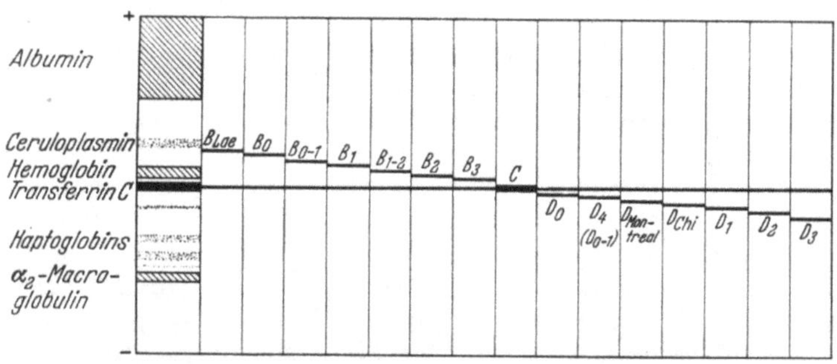

Fig. 1. Diagrammatic representation of known genetic variants of human transferrin

transferrins B_2, B_{0-1}, D_1, and D_{Chi} occur with a calculated gene frequency of 0.005, 0.04, 0.06, and 0.03, respectively, and with a heterozygous frequency corresponding to 1%, 8%, 12%, and 6% (*17*). The frequency of these four alleles is such as to make it extremely unlikely that they could be maintained by recurrent mutation, and one must therefore invoke the principle of balanced polymorphism. Strength to this hypothesis is lent by the occurrence of a unique transferrin in a particular population. Thus, B_2 occurs in Caucasian populations, B_{0-1} among Navajo Indians, D_1 among Negroes, and D_{Chi} among Chinese (Table 1). Indeed, the latter variant was specifically looked for when transferrin D_1, the variant commonly found among Negro populations, was reported to occur among Swedish Lapps and Chinese. *A priori*, this finding

Table 1. *Common transferrin variants in several populations*

	B_2	D_1	B_{0-1}	D_{Chi}
White	1%	0	0	0
Negro.	0	12%	0	0
Navajo Indian .	0	0	8%	0
Chinese	0	0	0	6%

was unexpected. These populations had not been subjected to similar environmental influences and would not be expected to have selected an identical genetic variant. Improvement in the technique of electrophoresis in the starch-gel system permitted the resolution of two bands in the D_1 region that had previously been unseparated. It is of interest that thus far the transferrin variant among the Lapps cannot be distinguished from D_{Chi} (*13*). In certain characteristics, the Lapps are similar to some Asiatic populations (high Fy^A and NS blood-group gene frequencies and very low *cde* Rh chromosome frequency). Thus, the presence in the Lapps of a transferrin indistinguishable from D_{Chi} lends support to the contention that the Lapps belong to the so-called Mongoloid race.

Outside Africa, the D_1 transferrin has been found among Australian aborigines, natives of New Guinea, Fiji, and New Caledonia, and Central and South American Indians. Although the appearance of D_1 transferrin among American Indians can be reasonably ascribed to Negro miscegenation, the finding of transferrin D_1 in Australian aborigines and Melanesian populations is less easy to understand. It is conceivable that improved resolution of the starch-gel technique may detect additional heterogeneity in the transferrin D_1 region.

No clear-cut physiological differences between normal and mutant transferrins have been demonstrated, and conjectures must remain very speculative. One unproved possibility concerns the uptake and release of iron from the transferrin molecule. The slower, more positively charged transferrins might favor the removal of iron from the tissues, whereas the faster, more negatively charged transferrins might favor the deposition of iron (*16*). The apparent failure to demonstrate a marked selective advantage should not be taken as evidence that none exists. If the system is balanced, the advantage is precisely equal to the gene frequency, and thus could be extremely difficult to detect.

Primate transferrin

The elaborate polymorphism observed in man is also found in several other mammalian species and will be only briefly summarized. Eight molecular species of transferrin have been observed in rhesus monkeys and four in chimpanzees (*17*). Unlike the situation found in man, the frequency of the various alleles is high and suggests a long-standing stable polymorphic system. All the variants found among rhesus monkeys migrate more rapidly than human transferrin, whereas all the chimpanzee variants migrate more slowly.

Isolation of transferrin

To determine whether there were any marked differences between normal and mutant transferrin, transferrin C, B_2, D_1, and D_3 were isolated by column chromatography and by starch-block electrophoresis and submitted to ultracentrifugation and quantitative amino-acid analysis (*18*). To compare normal transferrin with monkey transferrin, transferrin from a cynomolgus monkey was also prepared. A comparison of the amino-acid analyses is depicted in Table 2. It can be seen that no significant differences

Table 2. *Amino-acid composition of human and primate transferrins*
Residues per molecule of molecular weight 90,000

	Human (C, B_2, D_1)	Cynomolgus		Human (C, B_2, D_1)	Cynomolgus
Lysine	58	54	Alanine	59	65
Histidine	19	19	Half-cystine	40	39
Ammonia	62	64	Valine	49	54
Arginine	28	26	Methionine	10	11
Aspartate	82	83	Isoleucine	15	14
Threonine	32	34	Leucine	60	60
Serine	42	52	Tyrosine	26	27
Glutamate	63	65	Phenylalanine	28	30
Proline	36	36	Tryptophan	7	7
Glycine	51	49	Glucosamine	10	6

Half-cystine and methionine determined by performic-acid oxidation.
Tryptophan determined by alkaline hydrolysis in starch-barium hydroxide.

were detected among the four transferrins analysed. However, compared to normal transferrin, transferrin from the cynomolgus monkey contained 20% more serine and 40% less glucosamine. When human and cynomolgus-monkey transferrin were tested by the double diffusion method of OUCHTERLONY, against human transferrin, it could be shown that the monkey transferrin had relatively fewer antigenic sites on the molecule (Fig. 2).

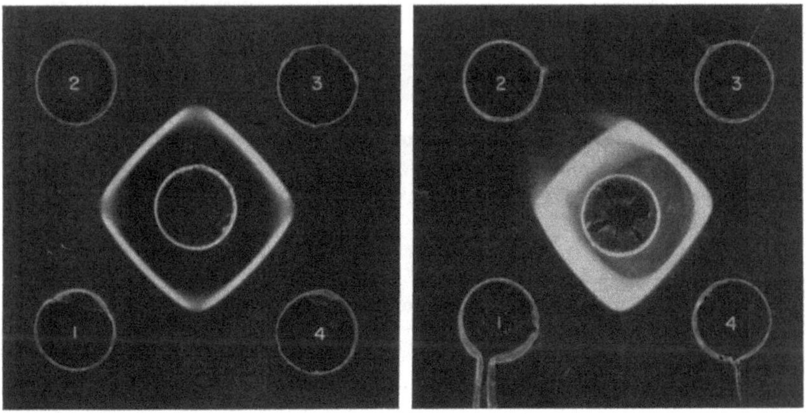

a b

Fig. 2. Immunological comparison (OUCHTERLONY method) of human and cynomolgus-monkey transferrin. (a) 1: Neuraminidase-treated transferrin C; 2: Transferrin C; 3: Transferrin B_2; 4: Transferrin C. (b) 1: Transferrin C; 2: Cynomolgus transferrin; 3: Transferrin D_1; 4: Transferrin B_{0-4}. Center wells: Anti-human transferrin serum [from PARKER and BEARN (*18*), by permission of The Journal of Experimental Medicine]

Attempts to separate transferrin into more than one polypeptide chain have proved unsuccessful. Since chemical analysis, by two separate methods, reveals only a single N-terminal residue of valine (*18*), the transferrin molecule may be regarded as being composed of a single polypeptide chain. The amino-acid composition of transferrin suggests that, if trypsin can be considered to hydrolyze lysine and arginine bonds selectively, the determination of the structural differences between normal and mutant transferrins could, theoretically, require the separation and sequencing of as many as 90–95 peptides. This formidable task lies ahead.

Multiple transferrins

Normal sera. In 1960, HARRIS (*7*), as well as BOYER and YOUNG (*3*), reported that autoradiographs obtained after separation of normal serum by starch-gel electrophoresis revealed a faint band migrating more slowly than the principal transferrin C band. In some sera, we have observed an additional slow component; and under conditions of high voltage a discrete faint component, migrating more rapidly than normal transferrin C, has been seen (*19*). This faint radioactive band has its counterpart as a protein band in the amidoschwarz stain. These "shadow" bands are not restricted to normal human sera, since they are well developed in the sera obtained from chimpanzees and rhesus monkeys.

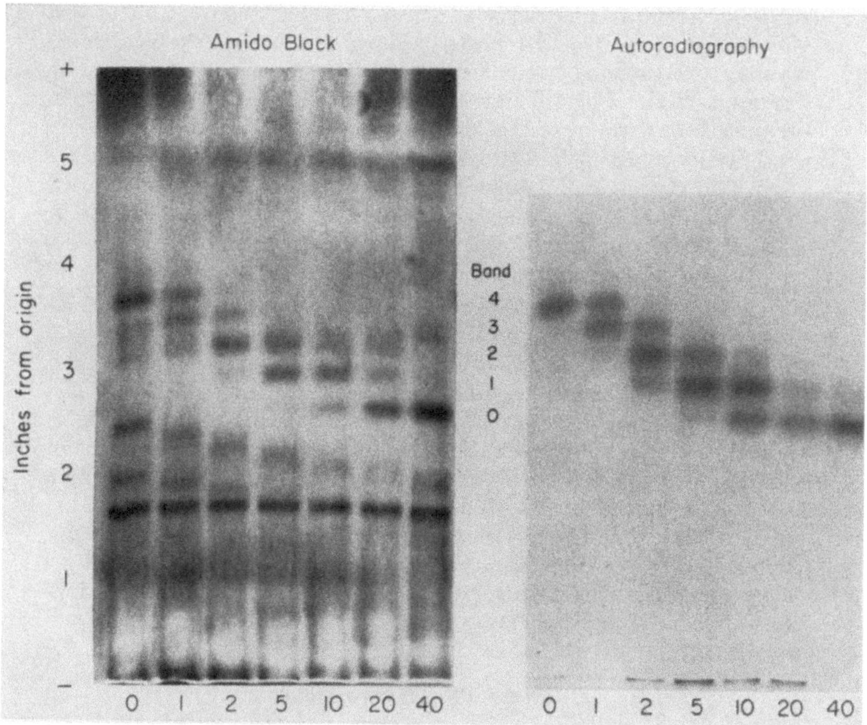

Fig. 3. Effect of neuraminidase on human serum. Left: starch-gel block; right: autoradiography [from PARKER and BEARN (*18*), by permission of The Journal of Experimental Medicine]

Effect of neuraminidase. Incubation of normal transferrin with neuraminidase results in a characteristic stepwise pattern of four slower migrating bands spaced at equal intervals (*15*). The number and intensity of the slowly migrating bands depend upon the concentration of neuraminidase employed. Prolonged incubation with excess neuraminidase leads to the appearance of all the transferrin in the slowest migrating band (Fig. 3). It is well established that neuraminidase has the specific property of hydrolyzing the glycosidic bond between sialic acid and protein. Thus, these experiments indicate that normal transferrin contains four sialic-acid residues per molecule; following incubation with neuraminidase, sialic acid is progressively removed. Each of the slowly migrating bands represents transferrin molecules with one less sialic-acid residue than the band migrating immediately ahead. The slowest band thus represents transferrin with all the sialic acid removed. This explanation is confirmed by comparative studies on the sialic-acid content of normal transferrin and transferrin incubated with neuraminidase. Chemical analyses indicate that normal transferrin contains four sialic-acid residues per molecule and that these are essentially completely removed by the enzyme. Similar experiments in which rhesus, chimpanzee, and cattle transferrin are incubated with neuraminidase disclose two additional slow-moving bands, suggesting that in these species transferrin contains only two sialic-acid residues per molecule.

It is of interest to note that purified conalbumin from egg white also contains a heterogeneous population of molecules which bind iron (*27*). Hen transferrin and conalbumin have a similar amino-acid composition and are immunologically indistinguishable. Experiments recently performed by PARKER indicate that the heterogeneity observed in conalbumin following starch-gel electrophoresis may be related to complexes with borate ion (*21*). Single or multiple bands can be obtained, depending on the concentration of the borate ion. The ultracentrifugal pattern of conalbumin is not dependent upon the number of bands seen during starch-gel electrophoresis, indicating that aggregation of conalbumin does not appear to occur under conditions where multiple bands were observed.

Transferrin in cord blood

A recent and rather surprising observation has been the multiplicity of transferrins occurring in normal cord sera that bind iron. In all sera examined (over 300), the cord blood showed a pattern that consisted of one fairly strong radioactive band, corresponding in position to normal transferrin C, and four faint slower bands of equal intensity. These faint bands have usually completely disappeared 12 weeks after birth. Superficially, the slower bands appeared to correspond in mobility to those seen when normal transferrin is incubated with neuraminidase. However, careful comparative studies of the stepwise pattern obtained on incubating normal adult transferrin, and the appearance of cord serum without the addition of neuraminidase, indicated that the minor components in cord serum migrated slightly more rapidly than the components observed in neuraminidase-treated adult serum. These experiments suggest that the minor bands in cord serum, in comparison to normal adult serum, lack more than just sialic acid. This is compatible with recent observations (*10*, *12*, *23*, *24*) which suggest that the carbohydrate prosthetic groups of proteins are prefabricated as units, usually containing sialic acid, hexose, and N-acetyl hexosamine, which are linked to the protein molecule by aspartic or glutamic acid. It appears, therefore, possible that the fetus may be relatively deficient in an enzyme system responsible for incorporating the prefabricated carbohydrate prosthetic groups into the transferrin molecule. Thus, at birth, although the majority of the transferrin molecules have their full complement of four carbohydrate prosthetic groups, some molecules have only three, two, or one prosthetic groups attached. The precise structure of the carbohydrate group in a transferrin is uncertain. It has recently been proposed that the carbohydrate moiety of normal human transferrin consists of four chains, each containing two residues of hexosamine, two of galactose, one of mannose, and one of sialic acid (*10*, *24*).

Cerebrospinal fluid

Starch-gel electrophoresis and immuno-electrophoresis of normal cerebrospinal fluid (C.S.F.) disclose two distinct proteins which have the electrophoretic and immunological characteristics of transferrin. In the starch-gel pattern, these proteins are two discrete bands of approximately equal intensity. One band migrates in the position of normal transferrin, and the second band migrates in the approximate position assumed by transferrin from which all the sialic acid has been removed. However, careful comparative studies reveal that the slow-moving band in C.S.F. is slightly faster than the bands observed in neuraminidase-treated normal serum and suggest that the more slowly migrating components lack the carbohydrate prosthetic group rather than just sialic acid. Earlier studies had indicated (*4*, *22*) that immuno-electrophoretic studies on C.S.F. revealed a double bow precipitate with antigenic properties similar to transferrin. Following incubation with neuraminidase, the fast-moving component in the C.S.F. becomes reduced in mobility and coincides with the slow-moving component. On the basis of these experiments, the authors concluded that the slow-moving transferrin lacked sialic acid (*22*).

Several explanations can be suggested for the curious double pattern of transferrin in C.S.F., but none seems entirely satisfactory. The central problem that confronts us is why there should be, in C.S.F., two populations of transferrin molecules, in approximately equal concentrations, one with the full complement of carbohydrate prosthetic groups and the other with no carbohydrate prosthetic groups.

The occurrence of the enzyme neuraminidase in C.S.F. (for which there is no compelling evidence) could not easily explain the findings obtained. The pattern observed in C.S.F. cannot be simulated by incubation studies with neuraminidase. Since the characteristic stepwise pattern is not obtained, it is necessary to postulate that the sialic acid on approximately half the transferrin molecules was inaccessible to the enzyme. Moreover, as already pointed out, the slow component migrates slightly faster than normal human transferrin stripped of sialic acid. Thus, neuraminidase in the C.S.F. would not account for the observations, and another hydrolytic enzyme such as glucosamidase or galactosidase must be postulated. The possibility that transferrin is made within the central nervous system appears unlikely. If, however, synthesis of transferrin without carbohydrate side-chains were to occur within the central nervous system the findings observed would be, to some extent, explicable. The evidence for synthesis of serum proteins, with the possible exception of gamma-globulin (*5*), within the central nervous system is slim and cannot be entertained too seriously.

Hereditary absence of transferrin

Apart from case reports in which a decreased plasma transferrin was observed just before death, there has been only one case reported in the literature where a deficiency of transferrin could reasonably be ascribed to genetical causes (*9*). The affected child suffered from a severe refractory hypochromic microcytic anemia, first diagnosed at the age of $3^1/_2$ months. The half-life of intravenously injected Fe^{59} was 5 minutes, compared to a normal value of approximately 50–150 minutes. An absence of transferrin was demonstrated immunologically. The most puzzling aspect of this case was the ability of sulfhydryl compounds to cause the appearance of a material which reacted with anti-transferrin antiserum. Paper electrophoresis following the addition of radioactive iron to the serum disclosed a peak of activity in the globulin region. The limited family data are compatible with an autosomal recessive disorder, since the child's parents were reported to have reduced levels of transferrin.

Summary

Genetic variations in the plasma proteins are now well recognized, but few proteins so far studied demonstrate the degree of variation exhibited by transferrin. A total of 15 variants have now been identified, which can be distinguished from normal transferrin by their electrophoretic mobility. Four of these variants exist in certain populations at a frequency which cannot plausibly be maintained by recurrent mutations, and the concept of balanced polymorphisms must therefore be introduced. The most rapidly moving transferrin has been found in a native of Lae, New Guinea, and the slowest in an American Negro. Quantitative amino-acid analyses of isolated and purified transferrin do not enable one to distinguish between the genetic variants thus far examined. The ultracentrifugal properties of the transferrin variants appear similar. Finger-printing of a protein with a molecular weight of 90,000, comprising approximately 90 tryptic peptides (based on the number of arginine and lysine residues), poses certain technical problems. Transferrin isolated from the cynomolgus monkey reveals both amino-acid and immunological differences from human transferrin. Two species of transferrin exist in the normal cerebrospinal fluid. These transferrins appear to differ in the carbohydrate prosthetic groups attached to the protein. Transferrin in normal cord serum exists as a series of five distinctly separable electrophoretic components. The four minor components have disappeared at the end of the first few weeks of life. Experiments in which the multiple bands in cord serum are compared with the series of bands obtained when adult serum transferrin is incubated with neuraminidase suggest that the newborn infant is deficient in an enzyme system necessary for the addition of carbohydrate prosthetic groups to the transferrin molecule.

Zusammenfassung

Genetische Abweichungen einzelner Plasmaproteine sind heute gut bekannt, aber wenige der bisher untersuchten Proteine zeigen so weitgehende Veränderungen wie Transferrin. Insgesamt sind bisher 15 Modifikationen identifiziert, die sich vom normalen Transferrin durch ihre verschiedene Wanderung bei der Elektrophorese auszeichnen. Vier dieser Varianten kommen bei verschiedenen Bevölkerungsgruppen mit einer Häufigkeit vor, die nicht durch wiederholte Mutationen zu erklären ist, so daß es berechtigt ist, einen ausgeglichenen Polymorphismus anzunehmen. Das am schnellsten wandernde Transferrin fand sich bei einem Eingeborenen von Lae, Neuguinea, das langsamste bei einem amerikanischen Neger. Quantitative Aminosäurebestimmungen von isoliertem und gereinigtem Transferrin haben keine Unterschiede bei den bisher untersuchten genetischen Varianten ergeben. Untersuchungen mit der Ultrazentrifuge zeigten ähnliche Eigenschaften der Transferrin-Varianten. „Finger printing" eines Proteins mit einem Molekulargewicht von 90'000, das ungefähr 90 tryptische Peptide enthält (bezogen auf die Zahl der Arginin- und Lysinreste), bietet gewisse technische Schwierigkeiten. Transferrin, das vom Cynomolgus-Affen isoliert wurde, unterscheidet sich sowohl in den Aminosäuren als auch immunologisch von menschlichem Transferrin. Zwei Arten von Transferrin liegen im normalen Liquor cerebrospinalis vor. Diese Transferrine scheinen sich in den prosthetischen Kohlenhydratgruppen zu unterscheiden, die mit dem Eiweiß verbunden sind. Im normalen Nabelschnurserum liegt Transferrin als eine Gruppe von fünf deutlich voneinander trennbaren elektrophoretischen Bestandteilen vor. Die vier Nebenkomponenten verschwinden am Ende der ersten Lebenswochen. Versuche, bei denen die einzelnen im Nabelschnurserum festgestellten Fraktionen mit den verschiedenen Banden verglichen werden, die bei Inkubation von Transferrin aus dem Serum Erwachsener mit Neuraminidase auftreten, sprechen dafür, daß bei Neugeborenen ein Enzymsystem fehlt, das für die Bindung der prosthetischen Kohlenhydratgruppen an das Transferrinmolekül notwendig ist.

Résumé

L'existence de variations génétiques dans les protéines plasmatiques est maintenant bien établie, mais parmi les protéines étudiées jusqu'à présent peu présentent le haut degré de variabilité de la transferrine. Quinze variantes au total ont été maintenant reconnues, qui peuvent être distinguées de la transferrine normale par leur rapidité de migration à l'électrophorèse. Quatre de ces variantes existent dans certaines populations à une fréquence qui ne peut raisonnablement pas s'expliquer par des mutations récurrentes et qui introduit la conception d'un polymorphisme équilibré. La transferrine migrant le plus rapidement a été trouvée chez un sujet originaire de Lae en Nouvelle Guinée, et la plus lente chez un noir américain. L'analyse quantitative des amino-acides de la transferrine isolée et purifiée ne permet pas de distinguer les variantes génétiques examinées jusqu'à présent. Les propriétés des variantes de la transferrine à l'ultracentrifugation sont identiques. Le «finger printing» d'une protéine d'un poids moléculaire de 90.000, comprenant environ 90 peptides obtenus par digestion tryptique (basé sur le nombre de résidus arginine et lysine) pose certains problèmes techniques. La transferrine isolée du singe Cynomolgus montre des différences à la fois dans son immunologie et dans ses amino-acides avec la transferrine humaine. Deux espèces de transferrine existent dans le liquide céphalo-rachidien normal. Ces transferrines semblent différer par les groupes prosthétiques hydro-carbonés fixés à la protéine. Dans le sérum normal prélevé du cordon ombilical, la transferrine existe sous forme d'une série de cinq composants nettement séparables par l'électrophorèse. Les quatre composants les moins importants disparaissent à la fin des premières semaines de la vie. Des expériences comparant les multiples fractions obtenues avec du sérum de cordon ombilicale, et la série de fractions obtenues avec de la transferrine de sérum d'adulte incubé avec de la neuraminidase sont en faveur d'une déficience chez le nouveau-né d'un système enzymatique nécessaire à la fixation du groupe prosthétique hydrocarboné sur la molécule de transferrine.

References

1. ALLERTON, S. E.: Doctoral Thesis, Division of Medical Sciences, Harvard University, U.S.A. (1962). — 2. BARKAN, G.: Zschr. physiol. Chem. (G.) **216**, 1 (1927). — 3. BOYER, S. H., and W. J. YOUNG: Nature (G.B.) **187**, 1035 (1960). — 4. BURTIN, P.: Clin. chim. acta (Neths) **4**, 72 (1959). — 5. FRICK, E., and L. SCHEID-SEYDEL: Klin. Wschr. (G). **36**, 837 (1958). — 6. GIBLETT, E. R., C. G. HICKMAN, and O. SMITHIES: Nature (G.B.) **183**, 1589 (1959). — 7. HARRIS, H., D. C. PENNINGTON, and E. B. ROBSON: Biochem. J. (G.B.) **74**, 44P (1960). — 8. HAZEN, E. E. Jr.: Doctoral Thesis, Division of Medical Sciences, Harvard University, U.S.A. (1963). — 9. HEILMEYER, L., W. KELLER, O. VIVELL, W. KEIDERLING, K. BERKE, F. WÖHLER, and H. E. SCHULTZE: Dtsch. med. Wschr. **86**, 1745 (1961). — 10. JAMIESON,

G. C.: Fed. Proc. (U.S.A.) **22**, 5338 (1963). — 11. JANDL, J., and J. H. KATZ: J. Clin. Invest. (U.S.A.) **42**, 314 (1963). — 12. JOURDIAN, G. W., F. SHIMUZU, and S. ROSEMAN: Fed. Proc. (U.S.A.) **20**, 161 (1961). — 13. KIRK, R. L., W. C. PARKER, and A. G. BEARN: To be published. — 14. KOECHLIN, B. A.: J. Amer. Chem. Soc. **74**, 2649 (1952). — 15. PARKER, W. C., and A. G. BEARN: Science (U.S.A.) **133**, 1014 (1961 a). — 16. PARKER, W. C., and A. G. BEARN: Science (U.S.A.) **134**, 106 (1961 b). — 17. PARKER, W. C., and A. G. BEARN: Ann. Human Genet. (G.B.) **25**, 227 (1961 c). — 18. PARKER, W. C., and A. G. BEARN: J. Exper. Med. (U.S.A.) **115**, 83 (1962). — 19. PARKER, W. C., and A. G. BEARN: Nature (G.B.) **196**, 477 (1962). — 20. PARKER, W. C., and A. G. BEARN: Science (U.S.A.) **137**, 854 (1962). — 21. PARKER, W. C.: Doctoral Thesis, The Rockefeller Institute, U.S.A. (1963). — 22. PETTE, D., and I. STUP: Klin. Wschr. (G.) **38**, 109 (1960). — 23. ROSEVEAR, J. W., and E. SMITH: J. Biol. Chem. (U.S.A.) **236**, 425 (1961). — 24. SCHULTZE, H. E., R. SCHMIDTBERGER, and H. HAUPT: Biochem. J. (G.B.) **329**, 490 (1958). — 25. SMITHIES, O.: Nature (G.B.) **180**, 1482 (1957). — 26. SMITHIES, O.: Nature (G.B.) **181**, 1203 (1958). — 27. WILLIAMS, J.: Biochem. J. (G.B.) **83**, 355 (1962).

Discussion

KATZ: How long do you wait after you have added the radioactive iron to the serum before you begin the electrophoresis?

BEARN: We run it almost immediately.

KATZ: Just one note of caution about this. I believe it takes a considerably longer period of time to complete binding than is generally assumed, particularly when the saturation of the serum transferrin is already high. The unbound Fe^{59} may adhere to various other proteins in a non-specific fashion. When one sees minor components in the autoradiograph this is a possible explanation. So one should wait at least 12 hours after addition of Fe^{59} to the serum in order to ensure complete and specific transferrin binding.

BEARN: We, too, have been concerned about this problem. However, we have not found any particular difference between patterns obtained when we wait 24 hours after adding Fe^{59} and when we run it immediately. To save time we do not routinely wait 24 hours.

CHATTERJEA: Did you have in your large series any instance of absence of transferrin in the serum?

BEARN: No, we did not. But Dr. HEILMEYER will be discussing this problem tomorrow.

VENTURA: Do the variants of transferrin have a different affinity for iron and do the normal variants of transferrin undergo modifications under pathological conditions, including especially those affecting haemopoietic tissue? If so, this may explain the abnormal behaviour of plasma radio-iron clearance which we sometimes see in anaemic diseases.

BEARN: The evidence, as far as it goes, is that there is no difference in binding between normal and variant transferrin. No correlation between variant transferrins and the disease has yet been disclosed.

MOESCHLIN: I have been very impressed by Dr. BEARN's new findings from the genetic point of view. Are there any correlations between the pathological haemoglobins and the different transferrin types? If abnormal transferrins are linked in some way with pathological haemoglobins this would offer very interesting possibilities in connection with racial studies and also as regards forensic studies relating to paternity suits.

KRUH: How do you visualise the variations in the transferrin molecule at the genetic level? Do you think there was once a mistake in the replication of D.N.A. in a non-essential locus — a mistake which became hereditary?

SAADI: I should like to know whether you have tried to see if there is any difference in the binding of iron by transferrin as such and by transferrin which has been treated by sialidase (transferrin devoid of sialic acid).

BEARN: I'm afraid we have not got any precise quantitative data on that. Qualitatively it appears the same.

Iron-containing compounds in micro-organisms

By

V. Prelog

Introduction. In the last 15 years, several iron-containing metabolites, characterised by a broad absorption band at 420 to 440 mμ, have been isolated from cultures of micro-organisms; these substances have been called "siderochromes" (*1*, *2*). Many siderochromes show strong biological activity even at very high dilution. Some of them display marked antibiotic activity, and these have been assigned the name "sideromycins". However, most of the siderochromes that have been isolated act as bacterial growth-factors and are known as "sideramines". Only a few siderochromes have been found to be biologically inactive. All the sideramines and sideromycins that have so far been isolated are listed in Table 1.

Table 1. Sideramines and sideromycins isolated to date

Siderochromes		
Sideramines		Sideromycins
Ferrichrome	Ferrioxamine A	Grisein
Coprogen	Ferrioxamine B	Albomycin
Terregens factor	Ferrioxamine C	
	Ferrioxamine D_1	Ferrimycin A_1
	Ferrioxamine D_2	Ferrimycin A_2
	Ferrioxamine E	Ferrimycin B
	Ferrioxamine F	ETH 22765
	Ferrioxamine G	
	Ferrichrysin	LA 5352
	Ferricrocin	LA 5937
	Ferrirhodin	
	Ferrirubin	

History. The first sideromycin to be discovered was grisein, described in 1947 by Reynolds, Schatz, and Waksman (*3*). The antibiotic albomycin, subsequently isolated by Gause and Brazhnikova (*4*), is identical with, or at least closely related to, grisein. In 1952, several sideramines were reported almost simultaneously:

ferrichrome by NEILANDS (*5*), coprogen by HESSELTINE and co-workers (*6*), and the terregens factor by LOCHHEAD and co-workers (*7*). As the outcome of a cooperative investigation undertaken by the Research Laboratories of CIBA Limited, Basle, by the Department for Special Botany of the Swiss Federal Institute of Technology in Zurich, and by the Organic Chemistry Laboratory of the same institute, the isolation of ferrimycin and of the ferrioxamine group of substances from Actinomyces cultures was announced in 1960 (*1, 8, 9*). The antagonism between the sideromycins and sideramines, discovered by ZÄHNER, HÜTTER, and BACHMANN (*10*), played an essential role in the exploration of this new group of compounds. The constitution of most of the ferrioxamines was soon established (*11–13*) and confirmed by partial and total syntheses (*14*). Meanwhile, NEILANDS and EMERY (*15*) had made important contributions to the determination of the constitution of the siderochromes from fungi—ferrichrome and ferrichrome A. Another interesting series of sideramines was isolated by KELLER-SCHIERLEIN (*16*) from fungi and their constitutions established. More recently, important advances have been made towards the determination of the constitutions of ferrimycin A(*17*) and δ-albomycin (*18, 19*), compounds which are apparently closely related in their chemistry to the sideramines. All the siderochromes that have so far been mentioned are iron (III) complexes of organic trihydroxamic acids, i.e. compounds which contain three –CO–NOH– residues.

One naturally occurring free trihydroxamic acid is the nocardamine, a metabolite of a Nocardia species, described in 1951 (*20*); its correct constitution was, however, only recognised later in the course of investigations on the ferrioxamines. The iron (III) complex of nocardamine was found to be identical with ferrioxamine E.

It should also be mentioned in this connection that the existence of a growth-factor for *Mycobacterium johnei* (*21*), chemically related to the sideramines, was already discovered as long ago as 1913. This factor, mycobactin, whose constitution was established in 1954 by SNOW and co-workers (*22, 23*), is a dihydroxamic acid and forms a stable iron (III) complex, which does not, however, act as an antagonist against sideromycins.

Occurrence. Siderochromes may be found in cultures of many micro-organisms. Certain strains are exceptional in that they produce considerable amounts of the corresponding iron-free trihydroxamic acids – desferri-siderochromes. So far, Streptomyces, Penicillium, Aspergillus, and Paecilomyces have been thoroughly studied as sources of siderochromes and desferri-siderochromes. The occurrence of siderochromes in higher plants and animals has not yet been established with certainty.

In the preparation of sideramines, advantage may be taken of the fact that many micro-organisms produce large amounts (up to 1 g. per litre of liquid culture) of desferri-siderochromes when grown on iron-deficient media. The siderochromes are then obtained by the addition of iron (III) salts (*24*).

Isolation and identification. The best procedures for the isolation of siderochromes are those which were developed for the isolation of cobalamines. Extraction with phenol-chloroform mixtures has proved particularly useful. By this means one usually obtains mixtures of related siderochromes, which can be separated, identified, and isolated by chromatography, by electrophoresis, or by counter-current distribution. Depending on their chemical constitutions, the compounds may be basic, neutral, acid, or amphoteric. The iron (III) ion can be removed from the siderochromes as iron (III) chloride by shaking with ether in hydrochloric acid solution, as insoluble iron (III) oxinate by addition of 8-hydroxyquinoline to a neutral solution, or as iron (III) hydroxide by making the solution strongly alkaline. Siderochromes with full biological activity can be recovered by the addition of iron (III) to the colourless desferri-siderochromes thus obtained. For chemical investigations it is advantageous to remove the iron right at the start, since otherwise the iron (III) ions may, under certain conditions, react with the organic degradation products to produce unwanted artefacts.

Constitution. The constitutions that have been assigned to the siderochromes are based mainly on analysis of the hydrolysis products of the desferri-siderochromes. Vigorous acid or alkaline hydrolysis yields rather simple molecules, which are involved in various numbers in the structure of the siderochrome. Table 2 shows a list of the simple hydrolysis products that have been found. The siderochromes are evidently built up from compounds which play a role in intermediary metabolism or from those which can easily be derived through simple reactions from metabolites of widespread occurrence.

Under milder conditions of hydrolysis, more complex fragments are obtained, which are important for determining the constitution. Under acid conditions, the hydroxamic acid groups are much more easily saponified than the amide groups, and the resulting larger fragments yield information about the sequence of the simpler units in the molecule.

Table 2. *Simple hydrolysis products of ferrioxamines and sideramines*

Hydrolysis products of	
ferrioxamines	sideramines from fungi
CH_3COOH	CH_3COOH
$HOOC(CH_2)_2COOH$	$HOCH_2CH_2C(CH_3) = CHCOOH$, cis- and trans-
$H_2N(CH_2)_5NHOH$	$HOOCCH_2C(CH_3) = CHCOOH$, trans-
$H_2N(CH_2)_4NHOH$	H_2NCH_2COOH
	$HOCH_2CH(NH_2)COOH$, L-
	$HONH(CH_2)_3CH(NH_2)COOH$, L-

The constitutions which have been determined so far for siderochromes are represented in the following figures. The formulae of ferrioxamine B (*12*), D_1 (*13*), and G (*13*) (shown in Fig. 1) indicate that, in these compounds, the corresponding hydroxamates are long, thread-like particles which wrap themselves round the iron

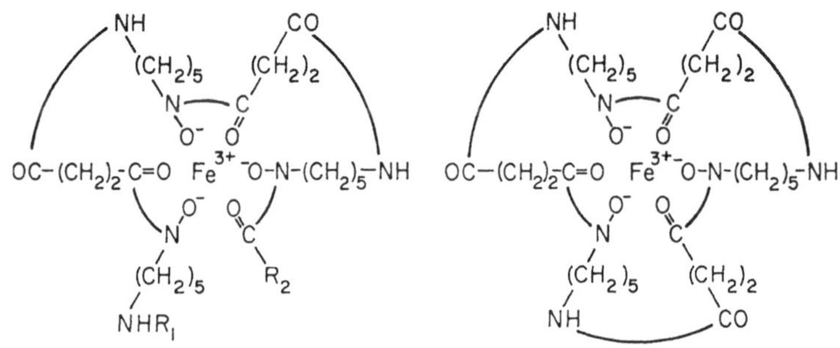

FERRIOXAMINE B
$R_1=H$ $R_2=CH_3$

FERRIOXAMINE D_1
$R_1=CH_3CO$ $R_2=CH_3$

FERRIOXAMINE G
$R_1=H$ $R_2=CH_2CH_2COOH$

FERRIOXAMINE E

Fig. 1. Structures of ferrioxamines B, D_1, G, and E

(III) ion. Ferrioxamine B contains a basic amino group, by means of which stable, water-soluble salts can be prepared. Ferrioxamine D_1, on the other hand, is neutral, since the amino group is acetylated. Ferrioxamine G_1 is amphoteric and forms water-soluble salts with acids as well as bases. In the trihydroxamate part of ferrioxamine E (*13*), the long thread has been closed into a circle, and the iron (III) ion is embedded in a large 33-membered ring. This kind of constitution and the neutral character of ferrioxamine E are the reason for its low solubility.

Ferrioxamine A (*25*) (shown in Fig. 2) is very closely related to ferrioxamine B, the only difference being that a 1-amino-5-hydroxylaminopentane residue is replaced by a 1-amino-5-hydroxylaminobutane residue, so that the length of the thread is somewhat

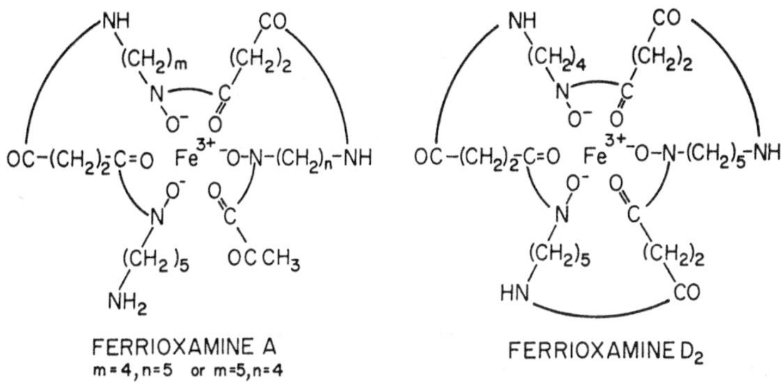

Fig. 2. Structures of ferrioxamines A and D_2

reduced. Ferrioxamine D_2 (*25*) (Fig. 2) is the corresponding lower homologue of ferrioxamine E; the loss of a methylene group means that the ring is only 32-membered.

The siderochromes which have been isolated from fungi have a different constitution from the ferrioxamines. The corresponding trihydroxamic acids are cyclohexapeptides, built up from 3 mono-amino acids (glycine and L-serine) and from 3 molecules of L-δ-N-hydroxyornithine. The exact sequence of the 6 amino acids in the cyclohexapeptide is still unknown; we assume, however, contrary to Emery and Neilands (*15*), that the L-δ-N-hydroxyornithine residues alternate with the mono-amino acids. The constitutions that have been established for some of these compounds are shown in Figs 3 and 4. The large 18-membered ring of the cyclohexapeptide has three tentacles, each holding a hydroxamic acid residue, which surround the iron (III) ion.

Up till now it has not been possible to establish the constitution of a sideromycin complete with all details. In the case of ferrimycin A_1, our investigations have enabled us to establish the partial constitution shown in Fig. 5 (*17*). This indicates that ferrimycin is a derivative of ferrioxamine B. It is therefore not surprising that the antibiotic is transformed – even under mild conditions (e.g.

when left to stand with sodium acetate) or by the action of micro-organisms – into compounds of the sideramine type. According to

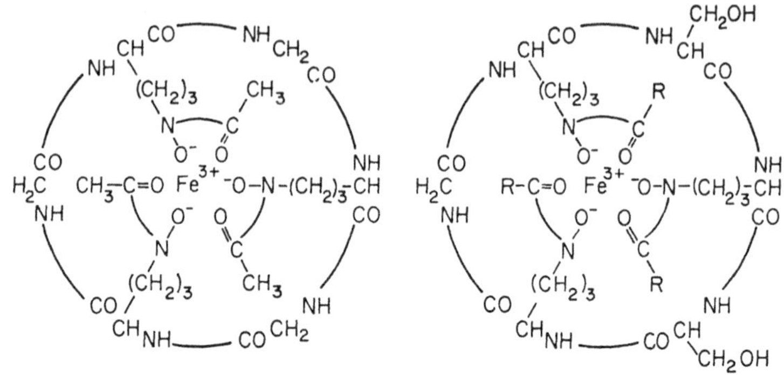

FERRICHROME

FERRICHROME A
R = $CH{=}C(CH_3)CH_2COOH$

Fig. 3. Structures of ferrichromes

recent investigations, δ-albomycin seems to be more closely related to the sideramines from fungi than to the ferrioxamines (*18*, *19*).

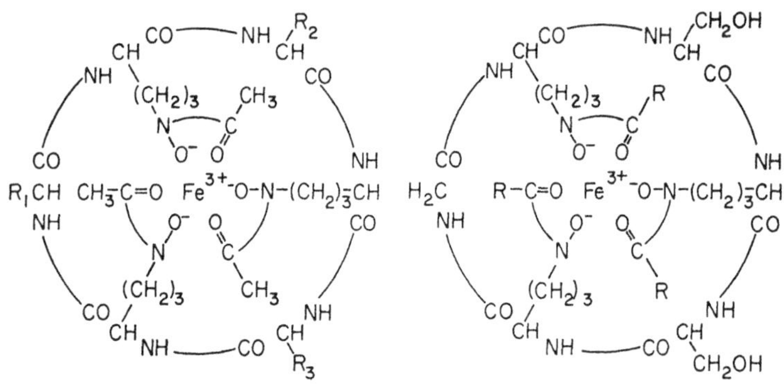

FERRICHRYSIN
$R_1{=}H \quad R_2{=}R_3{=}CH_2OH$

FERRICROCIN
$R_1{=}R_2{=}H \quad R_3{=}CH_2OH$

FERRIRHODIN
R=cis-$CH{=}C(CH_3)CH_2CH_2OH$

FERRIRUBIN
R=trans-$CH{=}C(CH_3)CH_2CH_2OH$

Fig. 4. Structures of sideramines from fungi

Biological activity and function of sideramines (*24*). The activity of sideramines as growth-factors may be demonstrated directly with sideramine-heterotrophic strains of certain micro-organisms such as *Pilobolus kleinii*, *Arthrobacter terregens*, and *Microbacterium lacticum*. Fig. 6 shows the result of such a test, in which the growth of *Microbacterium lacticum* ATCC 8181 in response to added ferrioxamine B was determined by measuring the optical extinction.

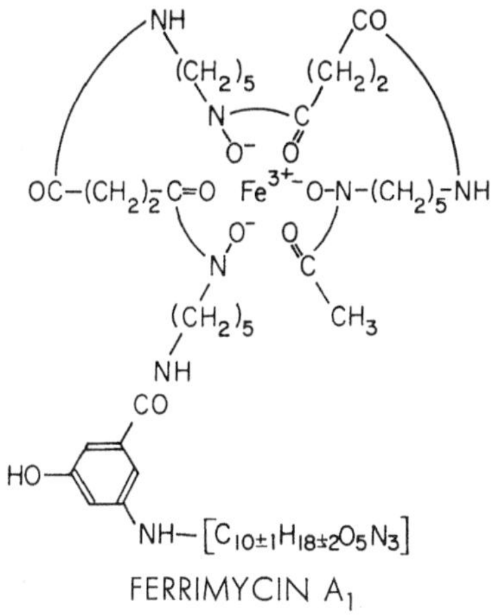

Fig. 5. Partial structure of ferrimycin A_1

Technically simpler than experiments designed to demonstrate growth promotion directly is the antagonism test against sideromycins as represented schematically in Fig. 7. A strip of filter paper (Y), impregnated with a sideromycin solution, is laid perpendicular to a second strip (X), impregnated with the sideramine solution, on an agar plate which is then inoculated with a suitable micro-organism. After incubation, there appears in the sterile zone (y), due to the diffusion of the antibiotic into the agar, a wedge (x), whose size – under standard experimental conditions – provides a means by which the two antagonists can not only be detected but also determined quantitatively. The antagonism is strongly specific for sideramines and sideromycins and is competitive over a wide range of concentrations. It is not due to a chemical reaction between the two antagonists, since the latter – still displaying their full biological activity – can be separated by electrophoresis from an inactive mixture in which the antibiotic activity of the sideromycin is completely neutralised by the sideramine.

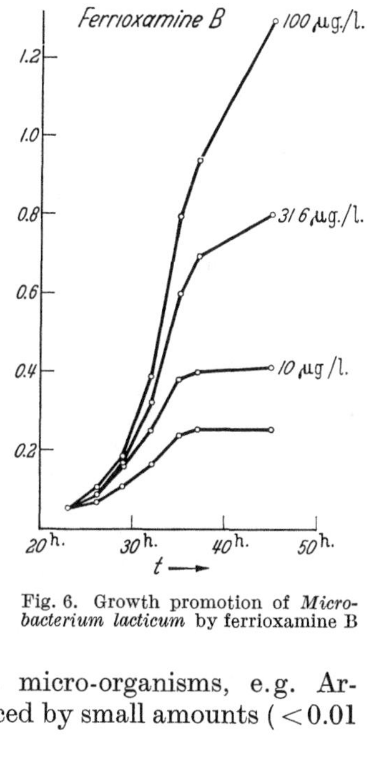

Fig. 6. Growth promotion of *Microbacterium lacticum* by ferrioxamine B

In certain haemin-heterotrophic micro-organisms, e.g. Arthrobacter JG-9, haemin can be replaced by small amounts (<0.01

mol) of sideramine; this activity can, in turn, be stopped by sideromycins. On the other hand, the growth-factor activity of haemin is not checked by sideromycins. Haemin cannot be replaced by sideramines in the case of all haemin-heterotrophic micro-organisms; for example, *Haemophilus influenzae* will not grow in the absence of protoporphyrin or haemin, even if sideramines are present.

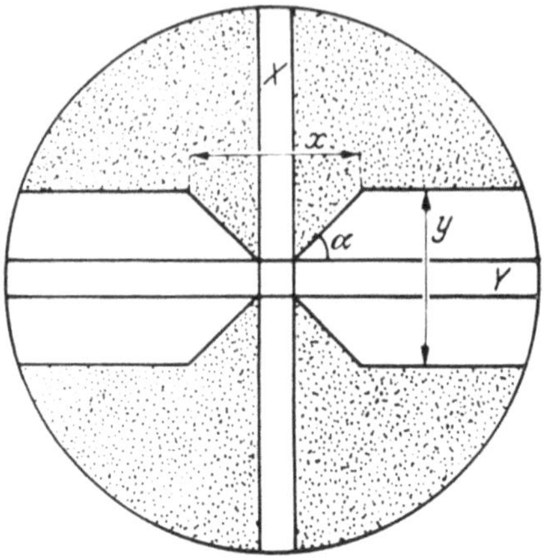

Fig. 7. Antagonism test. X: filter-paper strip with sideramine; Y: strip with sideromycin; y: sterile zone; x: wedge due to antagonistic action of sideramine; α: angle indicating activity of x

The haemin-heterotrophic Arthrobacter JG-9 reacts to the addition of haemin by increasing its catalase activity; such an increase is also induced by sideramines. The reaction to haemin in this case is again not inhibited by sideromycins, whereas the reaction to sideramines is completely blocked. An increase in catalase activity following the addition of

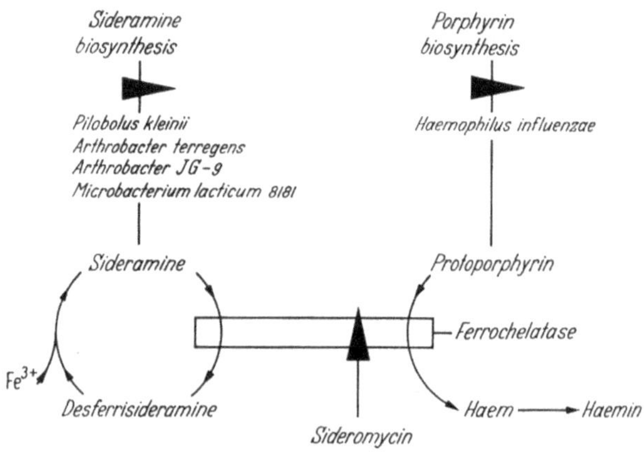

Fig. 8. Biological function of sideramines (*8*)

sideramines is also shown by cell-free extracts of *Rhodopseudomonas spheroides* (*26*); this makes it seem very unlikely that sideramines are iron-transporting factors whose role it is to transport iron (III) ions through the cell membranes, as had been suggested earlier.

All the facts mentioned can, however, be explained on the assumption that, at least in micro-organisms, the sideramines play an important part in the enzymatic incorporation of iron into porphyrins, as shown, according to ZÄHNER (*24*), in Fig. 8. The formation of haem (or haemin) and of the corresponding iron-containing enzymes, such as catalase, can, according to this hypothesis, be inhibited by blocking the biogenesis of sideramines, by blocking the biogenesis of porphyrin, or by blocking the enzymatic incorporation of iron (III) ions into porphyrin through sideromycins.

Desferri-sideramines as specific chelating agents for iron (III) ions (*27*, *28*). Desferri-sideramines form very stable complexes with iron (III) ions in the pH range 3–9. In Table 3, the logarithms of the stability constants of desferri-ferrioxamine B [or simply desferrioxamine B (*29*)] for iron (III) ions and for certain other biologically important ions are compared with the corresponding values for the well-known complexing agent, ethylene-diamine tetra-acetic acid (E.D.T.A.). It will be seen that not only the stability constant of ferrioxamine B is several powers of ten greater than that of the E.D.T.A.-iron (III) complex, but also the desferrioxamine complexes of the other biologically important ions, especially Ca^{+2}, are much less stable than those of E.D.T.A. This high specificity for the iron (III) ion, coupled with the extremely low acute and chronic toxicity and rapid elimination of soluble ferrioxamine B salts by the kidneys, forms the basis for the clinical use of desferrioxamine B, which will be discussed in other contributions to this Symposium.

Table 3. *Comparison of the stability constants (log. K) of desferri-ferrioxamine and E.D.T.A. with respect to various metallic ions*

	Desferri-ferrioxamine	E. D. T. A.
Fe^{3+}	30.6	25.1
Ca^{2+}	2.5	10.6
Co^{2+}	10.3	16.1
Zn^{2+}	11.1	16.1
Cu^{2+}	14.1	18.3

Summary

Siderochromes are naturally occurring iron (III) trihydroxamates. Many of them are either microbial growth-factors (sideramines) or antibiotics (sideromycins). The occurrence, isolation, identification, constitution, and properties, as well as the biological activities and functions of siderochromes are reviewed.

Zusammenfassung

Siderochrome sind natürlich vorkommende Eisen(III)-trihydroxamate. Viele von ihnen sind entweder mikrobielle Wuchsfaktoren (Sideramine) oder Antibiotica (Sideromycine). Es wird eine Übersicht über Vorkommen, Isolierung, Identifizierung, Konstitution, Eigenschaften sowie über biologische Wirkungen und Aufgaben der Siderochrome gegeben.

Résumé

Les sidérochromes sont des trihydroxamates de fer trivalent naturels. Beaucoup d'entre eux sont soit des facteurs de croissance de micro-organismes (sidéramines), soit des antibiotiques (sidéromycines). La présence, l'isolement, l'identification, la constitution, les propriétés, ainsi que l'activité biologique et la fonction des sidérochromes sont passés en revue.

Acknowledgements

I should like to express my gratitude to my colleagues, Dr. W. KELLER-SCHIERLEIN and Dr. H. ZÄHNER in Zurich, and to Dr. H. BICKEL and Dr. E. VISCHER in Basle, as well as to the many co-workers mentioned in the references.

References

1. BICKEL, H., E. GÄUMANN, W. KELLER-SCHIERLEIN, V. PRELOG, E. VISCHER, A. WETTSTEIN, and H. ZÄHNER: Experientia (Switz.) **16**, 129 (1960). — 2. Cf. review article by PRELOG, V.: Pure Appl. Chem. (G.B.) **6**, 327 (1963). — 3. REYNOLDS, D. M., A. SCHATZ, and S. A. WAKSMAN: Proc. Soc. Exper. Biol. Med. (U.S.A.) **64**, 50 (1947). — 4. GAUSE, G. F., and M. G. BRAZHNIKOVA: Nov. med. Akad. med. nauk S.S.S.R. **23**, 3 (1951). — 5. NEILANDS, J. B.: J. Amer. Chem. Soc. **74**, 4846 (1952). — 6. HESSELTINE, C. W., C. PIDACKS, A. R. WHITEHILL, N. BOHONOS, B. L. HUTCHINGS, and J. H. WILLIAMS: J. Amer. Chem. Soc. **74**, 1362 (1952). — 7. LOCHHEAD, A. G., M. O. BURTON, and R. H. THEXTON: Nature (G.B.) **170**, 282 (1952). — 8. BICKEL, H., E. GÄUMANN, G. NUSSBERGER, P. REUSSER, E. VISCHER, W. VOSER, A. WETTSTEIN, and H. ZÄHNER: Helvet. chim. acta **43**, 2105 (1960). — 9. BICKEL, H., R. BOSSHARDT, E. GÄUMANN, P. REUSSER, E. VISCHER, W. VOSER, A. WETTSTEIN, and H. ZÄHNER: Helvet. chim. acta **43**, 2118 (1960). — 10. ZÄHNER, H., R. HÜTTER, and E. BACHMANN: Arch. Mikrobiol. (G.) **36**, 325 (1960). — 11. BICKEL, H., B. FECHTIG, G. E. HALL, W. KELLER-SCHIERLEIN, V. PRELOG, and E. VISCHER: Helvet. chim. acta **43**, 901 (1960). — 12. BICKEL, H., G. E. HALL, W. KELLER-SCHIERLEIN, V. PRELOG, E. VISCHER, and A. WETTSTEIN: Helvet. chim. acta **43**, 2129 (1960). — 13. KELLER-SCHIERLEIN, W., and V. PRELOG: Helvet. chim. acta **44**, 709, 1982 (1961); **45**, 590 (1962). — 14. PRELOG, V., and A. WALSER: Helvet. chim. acta **45**, 631, 1732 (1962). — 15. EMERY, T., and J. B. NEILANDS: J. Amer. Chem. Soc. **83**, 1626 (1961). — 16. KELLER-SCHIERLEIN, W., and A. DEER: Helvet. chim. acta **46**, (in press, 1963). — 17. BALENOVIĆ, K., J. BECK, and A. WALSER: Unpublished results. — 18. MIKEŠ, O., and F. ŠORM: Symposium Antibiotics, Prague, 1959, p. 30. — 19. TURKOVÁ, J., O. MIKEŠ, and F. ŠORM: Collection Czech. Chem. Commun. **27**, 591 (1962). —

20. STOLL, A., J. RENZ, and A. BRACK: Helvet. chim. acta **34**, 862 (1951). — 21. TWORT, F. W., and G. L. Y. INGRAM: Johne's Disease. Baillière, Tindall and Cox, London, 1913. — 22. FRANCIS, J., H. M. MACTURK, J. MADINAVERTIA, and G. A. SNOW: Biochem. J. (G.B.) **55**, 596 (1953). — 23. SNOW, G. A.: J. Chem. Soc. London **1954**, 2588. — 24. Cf. review by ZÄHNER, H., E. BACHMANN, R. HÜTTER, and J. NÜESCH: Path. et microbiol. (Switz.) **25**, 708 (1962) and references therein. — 25. KELLER-SCHIERLEIN, W., and A. WALSER: Unpublished results. — 26. BURNHAM, B. F.: Arch. Biochem. Biophysics (U.S.A.) **97**, 329 (1962). — 27. SCHWARZENBACH, G., and K. SCHWARZENBACH: Helvet. chim. acta **46**, 1390 (1963). — 28. ANDEREGG, G., F. L. EPPLATENIER, and G. SCHWARZENBACH: Helvet. chim. acta **46**, 1400, 1409 (1963). — 29. BICKEL, H., H. KEBERLE, and E. VISCHER: Helvet. chim. acta **46**, 1385 (1963).

Introduction to the General Discussion

By

I. M. London

In opening this discussion I should like to make one general remark to which I am sure we all subscribe: that is that we are all most grateful to our hosts and our chairmen for having invited us to participate in this extremely pleasant and interesting Symposium.

In this general discussion I cannot hope to cover all the various questions that have been raised or that we would like to consider. Dr. Eichhorn has provided us with a very lucid exposition of the role of the electronic configurations of iron and has properly emphasized the fact that the specificity of the biological functions of the heme proteins depends on the protein to which the heme is linked. In the case of most of the hemoproteins, the precise nature of the heme-protein linkage remains to be determined, and I believe this is a subject which certainly deserves further study. I hope that Dr. Schubert will be willing to discuss hemocyanin and its relation to cytochrome oxidase and the evolution of the heme proteins.

In Dr. Yoshikawa's very interesting discussion of the enzyme concerned with the incorporation of iron into protoporphyrin, there were a number of points which may be re-emphasized. You will recall that he did not observe any stimulatory effect of globin on the incorporation of iron into protoporphyrin such as has previously been reported. This represents a divergence of results which should be studied further. Secondly, he did not find that the vinyl groups are essential for the incorporation of iron into protoporphyrin. This, too, constitutes a departure from previously accepted knowledge. Also still to be settled is the question whether, in the synthesis of hemoglobin, heme is formed which is then bound to globin, whether one forms a protoporphyrin globin which then accepts the iron, or whether iron is first bound to globin and then the protoporphyrin is added to form hemoglobin. I should be interested to know if anyone here has any information on this specific point. I think we would all view with considerable interest any additional information on the phospholipid which is said to enhance the activity of this enzyme and on its precise chemical character.

Of general interest with regard to the synthesis of heme is the work of BURNHAM and LASCELLES at Oxford, who have shown recently that heme or protoporphyrin has a marked inhibitory effect on δ-aminolevulinic acid synthetase. This enzyme, which acts at the first step in porphyrin biosynthesis, may well be the site at which porphyrin biosynthesis is normally controlled. This would be another example in which the control of a biosynthetic pathway may reside in the first enzyme in the pathway and in which the final product of the biosynthetic pathway may exercise a regulatory function by its inhibitory effect on the first enzyme in the series.

Dr. HARRISON's important observations on the structure of ferritin answer many questions but pose others. We should like to have information on the precise mechanism of the movement of iron into the ferritin molecule and on the role of the reduction of iron in its entry into the ferritin molecule. There is also the question as to how iron accelerates the synthesis of apoferritin. Given the present state of our knowledge of the mechanism of protein synthesis, we should be able to answer this question quite precisely. There is the further question of whether iron enhances the metabolic stability of apoferritin, as has been suggested by Dr. HARRISON. One would like to know to what extent metabolic stability is enhanced and what the mechanism for such stabilization may be. We shall also look forward to studies designed to determine to which amino acid, or acids, in the apoferritin the iron is preferentially bound.

Dr. BEARN's stimulating discussion on the genetics of the transferrins indicates the value of having another system for the study of human genetics. It would be of interest to obtain information on the kinetics of iron binding in transferrins that are free of carbohydrate, as for example in the transferrins of cord serum, and in the genetic variants in which the amounts of carbohydrates bound to the transferrins are different. Dr. BEARN has raised the difficult question of the search for amino-acid differences in these genetic variants of the transferrins. The fact that electrophoretic differences exist, and the fact that up to now there has been no demonstrable difference in amino-acid composition, are reminiscent of earlier findings with respect to the human hemoglobin variants. You will recall that, when electrophoretic differences were demonstrated in human hemoglobins, the earliest work did not succeed in revealing differences in amino-acid compositions, and one can readily understand how a difference in one amino-acid residue may not be picked up by these techniques. It would be interesting to know whether these electrophoretic differences are modified by raising or lowering the pH, so that one may change the charge on the molecule and perhaps under these circumstances get a clue as to which amino acids might possibly be substituted in these variants.

Dr. PRELOG's very intriguing paper leaves me frankly speechless with admiration. I was hoping that Dr. ZÄHNER would respond to the invitation to discuss this work further. I wonder whether Dr. EICHHORN would care to comment on Dr. PRELOG's discussion of the sideramines and sideromycins in terms of how the electronic configuration of the iron may differ in these two kinds of compound.

Reference

BURNHAM, B. F., and J. LASCELLES: Biochem. J. (G.B.) 87, 462 (1963).

General Discussion

Eichhorn: I find it interesting that these micro-organisms use the same functional groups as have been employed in analytical schemes to achieve specificity with iron. Otherwise I do not know that very many conclusions can be reached concerning the electronic configuration of iron in these complexes.

I do want to make a remark on the question as to the possible reason why iron leaves and enters the ferritin molecule in the bivalent state; this is something that everyone probably understands, but I think that perhaps it nevertheless calls for comment. Presumably the ferric iron inside the ferritin molecule is in the form of this tremendous iron (III) hydroxide macromolecule or micelle, or whatever one prefers to call it, which is produced at a pH as low as 2. When reduced to the + 2 state, the iron can probably leave such a micelle at higher pH's. I forget exactly at what pH, but the ferrous ion certainly does not precipitate until a pH much higher than 2 is reached. For this reason ferrous iron can presumably enter the micelle at reasonable pH levels, at which iron (III) would be in the form of this huge ferric hydroxide macromolecule which would not manage to get inside the ferritin structure. Thus it is understandable why iron should be in the + 2 state so as to be able to get in and out of ferritin.

Harrison: As you say, the micelles, once formed inside the protein shell, may be too large to pass through the channels between subunits. But there may be some form of binding between the outer surface of the micelles and the inner surface of the protein. Anderegg has studied, by low-angle scattering of X-rays in solution, a ferritin fraction which contains a very small amount of iron per molecule. On the basis of these unpublished studies, he has arrived at the tentative conclusion that the iron has a radius of about 40 Å. This suggests that the iron is bound to the protein, which has an average inner radius of about 37 Å. Mazur[1] suggested that a few iron atoms at the surface of the micelles are bound to the protein through a mercaptide linkage. We have confirmed his finding that the number of reactive sulphydryl groups is rather greater in ferritin fractions containing little iron than in those with a high iron content. (The actual values were between about 1 and $1^1/_2$ active sulphydryl groups per subunit, the number increasing to 2 per subunit on denaturation.) Of course, this correlation does not in itself prove that there is a direct linkage, but it does suggest this possibility.

Schubert: I should like to make two brief comments. One is about the channels in ferritin. These are very small, about 10 Å, as Dr. Harrison indicated. So when the hydrated iron enters, water must be "squeezed out". Now for iron to precipitate compounds like ferric hydroxide or ferric phosphate, you have to have a concentration in excess of roughly 10^{-4}M, i.e. the mononuclear barrier. Hence, one of the functions one might associate with ferritin is that of removing water from iron salts and thus raising the concentration of iron within the channels to the point at which precipitation occurs.

---

[1] Mazur, A., and S. Green: In: Sulfur in Proteins. Academic Press, New York and London, 1959, p. 189.

Secondly, a comment on a relation between haemocyanin and haemoglobin. As you go up the evolutionary scale, the oxygen-carrying agent of the blood changes from haemocyanin, which is a copper protein, to haemoglobin, which is an iron protein. However, copper does not lose its function in the evolutionary sense of combining directly with oxygen, because it is the principal metal for combining with molecular oxygen and other 4-electron transfer oxidases. The copper may be linked with iron, but the function of copper enzymes is quite unique and cannot be fulfilled by any other enzyme, including iron enzymes; this function consists in the reduction of molecular oxygen to water, a process which requires four electron steps. Iron enzymes only go as far as hydrogen peroxide, requiring two electrons. In point of fact, there is no general rule as to which primitive organisms have haemocyanin and which have haemoglobin; the latter is not pre-eminent, it is merely much more widely distributed[1].

EICHHORN: I should like to amend the remarks I made a while ago to this extent: it seems, really, upon reflection, that one might predict that complexes having the stabilities that Dr. PRELOG has indicated should be strong field complexes.

PRELOG: A determination of magnetic susceptibility carried out in the laboratory of Prof. R. S. NYHOLM[2] at University College, London, showed that ferrioxamine B (and therefore also the other siderochromes) is a so-called ionic complex with five unpaired electrons (magnetic moment: calc. 5.92, found 5.86 Bohr magnetons).

KRUH: I should like to ask Dr. YOSHIKAWA if the following observations fit in with his results. When we incubate intact rabbit reticulocytes with radioactive glycine, we increase the incorporation of the radioactive precursor into the globin as well as into the haem of haemoglobin by a factor of 2 or 3, if we add a mixture of amino acids to the medium[3]. It is easy to understand how this mixture could stimulate the biosynthesis of globin. It would seem reasonable to assume that the increase in the biosynthesis of haem is directly related to the increase in globin biosynthesis.

YOSHIKAWA: I am afraid I have had little experience with experiments using mammalian reticulocytes, but I should just like to add a brief comment to what I have already said. I think that the globin prepared from haemoglobin is not identical with the globin which is supposed to be present in haemolysate and to accept the haem produced by the iron-incorporating enzyme.

SCHAPIRA: May I ask Dr. BEARN two questions? Firstly, among the different variants of transferrin, are there any which offer any special advantages with regard to the metabolism of iron, iron deficiency, or iron overload? Dr. BOTHWELL could perhaps answer this question as far as iron overload in Negroes is concerned. Secondly, I think the finger-printing method should certainly enable one to make a clear distinction between the transferrin of human beings and the transferrin of monkeys, because there are eight differences between them with respect to their content of arginine and lysine.

BEARN: There are still insufficient studies to answer Dr. SCHAPIRA's question.

---

[1] ANSON, M. L., and A. E. MIRSKY: Physiol. Rev. (U.S.A.) **10**, 506 (1930).
[2] NYHOLM, R. S.: Personal communication.
[3] KRUH, J., and H. BORSOOK: J. Biol. Chem. (U.S.A.) **220**, 965 (1956).

Physiology of iron

Digestive absorption of iron

By

Sheila T. Callender

One of the first difficulties encountered by anyone who attempts to measure absorption of dietary iron is in trying to decide the best technique to use. Various methods have their advocates, but arguments may be raised against all of them. With the introduction of radioactive tracers, there was a hasty dismissal of data derived from the tedious and time-consuming iron balance studies of the thirties. But, as Josephs (1958) has pointed out, much of the criticism of these early studies was unjustified. Indeed, since it is well-nigh impossible to label all the iron in the diet uniformly, we are driven back to the conclusion that, ideally, chemical iron balance studies are the only means of truly assessing the iron retention from any mixed diet. However, the intricacies of carrying out such chemical balances accurately have inevitably made workers turn to the use of radioactive iron.

Earlier investigators using labelled inorganic iron were perhaps too ready to assume that the retention of the oral dose reflects the ability to absorb food iron. The St. Louis group of workers, realising that this might not be so, introduced the *in vivo* labelling of individual foods such as eggs and greens (Moore and Dubach, 1951). The Seattle group had a different approach; they have added a tracer quantity of labelled iron to a standard meal, and have assumed that this will act as a true label (Pirzio-Biroli, Bothwell, and Finch, 1958). The first method has the disadvantage that one can only study the absorption from one type of food or from a combination of a very limited number of foods. With the second method the question arises: can we really be sure that the radioactive iron can be regarded as a true label for the standard meal? Is one not rather studying the effect of a meal on the absorption of a tracer quantity of iron which is chelated to an unknown substance in the food? Can we assume that the iron is always chelated to the same substance, and, if not, can this affect absorption?

With regard to the actual methods used to determine iron absorption, here again we meet with controversy. In the absence of a whole-body counter, we in Oxford still determine absorption of iron by measuring the unabsorbed radioactivity in the faeces. With any negative method such as this, which relies so much on the cooperation of the patient, one must constantly be on the look-out for possible errors.

Simple use of the amount of radioactivity appearing in the red cells as a measure of absorption provides at best only a crude guide and may lead to gross errors. BOTHWELL, PIRZIO-BIROLI, and FINCH (1958) have attempted to solve the difficulty by using the double isotope technique, which assumes that the proportion of absorbed iron which will ultimately appear in red cells is the same as the proportion utilised from an intravenous tracer dose of labelled iron. This has certainly been shown to be a valid assumption for inorganic iron, but does it always hold good also for food iron?

Using the method of measuring unabsorbed radioactivity in the faeces and the 14-day utilisation of the absorbed iron in the blood, we have found evidence that iron is less well utilised when given as labelled haemoglobin than when given as inorganic iron.

Thus, in non-anaemic control subjects given 5 mg. iron in the form of ferrous sulphate, a mean of 77% of the retained iron was utilised for red-cell formation; with haemoglobin iron the mean was 69%. Comparable figures for iron-deficiency anaemia were 100% for inorganic iron and 76% for haemoglobin iron. There is no reason to suppose that those receiving iron in the form of haemoglobin were less reliable in their collection of faeces.

Examination of the data published by CHODOS et al. (CHODOS, ROSS, APT, POLLYCOVE, and HALKETT, 1958) for iron absorption from Fe^{59}-labelled eggs reveals an even more striking difference.

Their control subjects utilised 84% of the retained iron from an oral dose of ferrous chloride, but only 12% of the retained iron given in eggs. Iron-deficient subjects utilised 63% of the retained iron from eggs, in contrast to 100% for ferric chloride.

Unfortunately, most of the other published data for absorption of food iron give figures for blood uptake only, on the assumption that this would produce little error in normal and iron-deficient subjects. It would seem desirable to make further studies on the retention from individual labelled foods, preferably with a reliable whole-body counter, so that this problem may be further elucidated.

In our own studies on absorption of food iron, we have made extensive use of labelled haemoglobin. It has the great advantage of being easy to prepare and is easily standardised (CALLENDER, MALLETT, and SMITH, 1957).

We now have a considerable number of observations on the absorption of haemoglobin iron in non-anaemic control subjects and in iron-deficiency states. Since for some time we had used a dose of 5 mg. as our standard test of absorption of inorganic iron, we used the equivalent of 5 mg. iron when the iron was given in the form of labelled haemoglobin.

In 45 non-anaemic control subjects, absorption of inorganic iron varied from 8% to 70%, with a mean of 30%. Nineteen subjects with iron deficiency absorbed 14% to 94%, with a mean of 56%, all but two showing an absorption higher than the mean for the non-anaemic group.

Comparable figures for the absorption of iron from haemoglobin are 1% to 32% in 17 non-anaemic controls, with a mean of 13%, and 1% to 68% in 27 iron-deficient subjects, with a mean of 25%.

It is clear that the majority of subjects show an increased absorption of iron in response to iron deficiency, as has been found repeatedly by other workers, but there are a few in whom this compensatory mechanism seems inefficient, and this is particularly so when one considers the figures for absorption from haemoglobin iron. Although undoubtedly deficient in iron, 10 of the 27 iron-deficient subjects absorbed less than the mean for the non-anaemic group. None had any evidence of general malabsorption.

If one compares the absorption of inorganic iron and haemoglobin iron in the same individuals it appears that, although in general haemoglobin iron is about half as well absorbed as inorganic iron, occasional subjects show a far greater difference. Such subjects might well repay more detailed study.

We have throughout been careful to standardise our dose, as it is well known that, with inorganic iron, the greater the amount of iron given the more will be absorbed, although the percentage will drop (SMITH and PANNACCIULLI, 1958). The relationship is expressed as a straight line when plotted on a log. log. scale. Dr. BANNERMAN has found the same relationship to hold in rats given varying doses of labelled haemoglobin, using total-body counting to assess absorption (personal communication).

It is remarkable to note that, when the reported figures for retention of food iron as determined by chemical balance studies are plotted in the same way, the same overall conclusion may be reached, although the scatter is considerably greater (data from JOSEPHS, 1958) (Fig. 1).

This observation is interesting in view of the finding of TURNBULL and others (TURNBULL, CLETON, and FINCH, 1962) that, when inorganic iron is added to labelled haemoglobin to increase the total amount of iron given, there is no apparent effect on the proportion of labelled iron which is absorbed. BANNERMAN has made similar observations in rats (personal communication). It

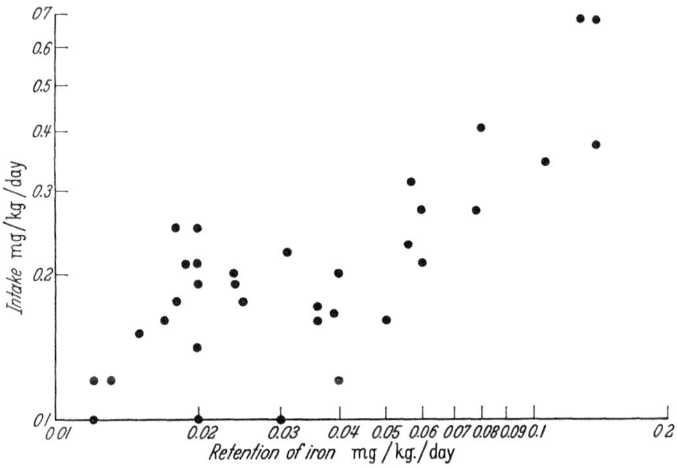

Fig. 1. Relationship between iron intake and iron retained in adult subjects. Data derived from chemical balance studies quoted by JOSEPHS (1958)

seems reasonable to attribute this to the different rates of absorption of iron from the two different sources, the peak of absorption from haemoglobin iron being considerably later than that from inorganic iron.

Substances such as phytates, which interfere with absorption of inorganic iron, do not appear to influence the absorption of haemoglobin iron (TURNBULL, CLETON, and FINCH, 1962). Their effect on various other forms of dietary iron still warrants investigation. Similarly, the effect of amino acids in enhancing absorption of inorganic iron (KROC, KINNEY, KAUFMAN, and KLAVINS, 1963) has yet to be investigated with food iron.

The question of the significance of gastric acidity in relation to absorption of iron from food still remains a problem. We were unable to show any reduction in the absorption of haemoglobin iron in the presence of achlorhydria, nor were we able to increase absorption by the addition of 100 ml. of normal gastric juice of pH 2 to the test dose. More recently, however, GOLDBERG and his colleagues (GOLDBERG, LOCKHEAD, and DAGG, 1963), using the labelled meal technique, have suggested that absorption may be depressed in the presence of achlorhydria, and clearly the debate is not yet closed.

One of the most interesting facets of the digestive absorption of iron is the part played by pancreatic secretion. Although experimental work in animals (TAYLOR, STIVEN, and REID, 1935; KINNEY, KAUFMAN, and KLAVINS, 1955) showed that the pancreas was

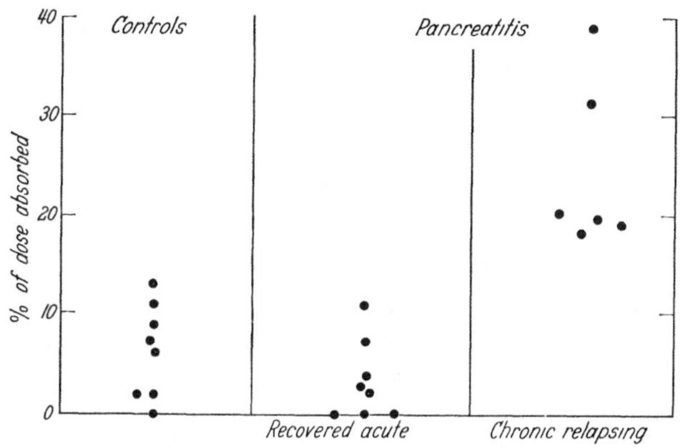

Fig. 2. Iron absorption from a standard meal containing 4.7 mg. iron in non-anaemic controls and patients with pancreatic disease (data from DAVIS and BADENOCH, 1962)

concerned in iron absorption, little attention had been given to these observations in relation to human disease.

Recently, however, DAVIS and BADENOCH (1962) studied a series of patients with pancreatic disease, testing the iron absorption with a standard labelled meal. Those who had an isolated attack of acute pancreatitis from which they had recovered, or who had had repeated attacks of acute pancreatitis relieved by biliary surgery, showed normal absorption of iron. In contrast, those who had evidence of severe and chronic pancreatic damage showed increased absorption (Fig. 2). In one of this latter group, the test was repeated with the addition of pancreatin. This resulted in a reduction in the amount absorbed.

It would appear that the pancreatic secretion must contain some substance which normally inhibits iron absorption. In the absence of this substance, uncontrolled absorption is likely to occur with resulting siderosis.

More recently, Dr. MALPAS and I have turned our attention to chronic liver disease, a condition in which siderosis has long been noted. We now have observations on 7 patients suffering from cirrhosis of the liver. Two were alcoholics; in the remainder, the aetiology was unknown. All had evidence of considerable liver damage, but were in a relatively stable clinical condition. None had had a recent haemorrhage (Fig. 3).

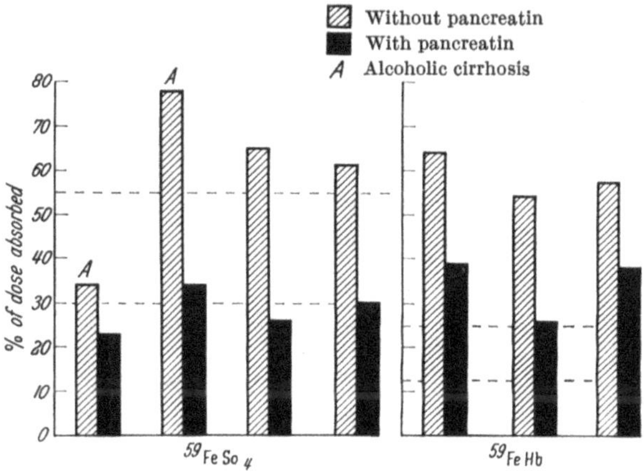

Fig. 3. Iron absorption from ferrous sulphate or from haemoglobin in patients with cirrhosis of the liver and the effect of the addition of pancreatic extract to the test dose. The dotted lines indicate the mean absorption for control subjects and for patients with iron deficiency

In 4, the iron absorption was tested with labelled ferrous sulphate; the other 3 were given labelled haemoglobin. All but one of those given ferrous sulphate showed a high absorption, higher in fact than the mean for iron-deficient subjects. With the labelled haemoglobin, the increased absorption was even more striking, all three giving values at the upper limit of that found in iron deficiency.

We thought it might be interesting to see whether pancreatin would have any effect on this high iron absorption. In every case when pancreatin was given with the test dose, absorption was reduced. It is of particular interest that the inhibitory effect was just as evident in those individuals given labelled haemoglobin as in those receiving inorganic iron, as this seems to indicate that the effect cannot simply be one of precipitating an insoluble iron salt.

I would emphasise that this is of the nature of a preliminary report. We have as yet no idea what the inhibitory factor is, although, in one experiment, heating the pancreatin abolished its effect, and it is therefore probably heat-labile. Clearly much more work is needed, but it does appear as if the pancreatic secretion may eventually be found to play a key role in the regulation of the digestive absorption of iron.

In closing, I should like to mention that much of what I have said is based on the collaborative work of several past and present members of our department, and I am especially indebted to Dr. MALPAS for allowing me to quote our recent unpublished results.

Summary

The methods used to assess the digestive absorption of iron are discussed and criticised. Evidence is given that methods depending on blood values only may give false low results for absorption of food iron, even in patients with iron deficiency.

Factors which influence the absorption of inorganic iron, e.g. phytates, may not play an important part in the absorption of food iron.

The part played by gastric secretion is still debatable. Those who have used *in vivo* labelled foods have been unable to show reduced absorption in achlorhydria, but others using a standard labelled meal have managed to do so.

The pancreatic secretion appears to contain an inhibitor of iron absorption. In severe chronic pancreatitis and cirrhosis of the liver, iron absorption is greatly increased. The addition of pancreatin to the test dose reduces iron absorption in both these conditions.

Zusammenfassung

Die heute üblichen Methoden für die Bestimmung der gastrointestinalen Resorption von Eisen werden besprochen und kritisiert. Es hat sich gezeigt, daß die Methoden, welche lediglich die Blutkonzentration berücksichtigen, falsche, zu niedrige Werte für die Resorption von Nahrungseisen geben können, und zwar auch bei Patienten mit Eisenmangel.

Faktoren, die die Absorption von anorganischem Eisen beeinflussen, z. B. Phytate, haben keine wesentliche Bedeutung für die Resorption von Nahrungseisen.

Die Rolle der Magensaftsekretion ist noch nicht klargestellt. Bei Gabe von *in vivo* markierten Nahrungsmitteln war keine verminderte Absorption bei Achlorhydrie festzustellen, dagegen war dies der Fall bei Nahrungsmitteln, die in üblicher Weise radioaktiv markiert waren.

Der Pankreassaft scheint ein Prinzip zu enthalten, das die Absorption von Eisen hemmt. Bei Patienten mit schwerer chronischer Pankreatitis oder mit Leberzirrhose ist die Eisenresorption deutlich gesteigert. Die Zugabe von Pankreatin zu einer Testdosis von Eisen setzt dessen gesteigerte Resorption bei den beiden genannten Erkrankungen herab.

Résumé

L'auteur fait la critique des méthodes utilisées pour la détermination de l'absorption digestive du fer. Elle rapporte des faits montrant que les méthodes basées uniquement sur des valeurs sanguines peuvent conduire, en ce qui concerne l'absorption du fer alimentaire, à des résultats erronés, trop bas, même chez des malades en hyposidérose.

Les facteurs influençant l'absorption du fer inorganique, par exemple les phytates, ne jouent probablement pas un rôle important dans l'absorption du fer alimentaire.

L'influence de la sécrétion gastrique est encore discutée. Ceux qui ont utilisé des aliments marqués *in vivo* n'ont pas pu démontrer une diminution de l'absorption de fer au cours des achlorhydries, diminution qu'ont par contre pu mettre en évidence ceux qui ont utilisé des aliments marqués de la manière habituelle.

Il semble que la sécrétion pancréatique contienne un inhibiteur de l'absorption du fer. Dans les pancréatites chroniques sévères et dans les cirrhoses hépatiques l'absorption du fer est nettement augmentée. Dans ces deux états pathologiques, l'adjonction d'extrait pancréatique à la dose-test de fer administrée en diminue l'absorption.

References

Bothwell, T. H., G. Pirzio-Biroli, and C. A. Finch: J. Laborat. Clin. Med. (U.S.A.) **51**, 24 (1958). — Callender, S. T., B. J. Mallett, and M. D. Smith: Brit. J. Haemat. **3**, 186 (1957). — Chodos, R. B., J. F. Ross, L. Apt, M. Pollycove, and J. A. E. Halkett: J. Clin. Invest. (U.S.A.) **26**, 314 (1957). — Davis, A. E., and J. Badenoch: Lancet (G.B.) **1962/II**, 6. — Goldberg. A., A. Lockhead, and J. H. Dagg: Lancet (G. B.) **1963/I**, 848. — Josephs, H. W.: Blood (U.S.A.) **13**, 1 (1958). — Kinney, T. D., N. Kaufman, and J. Klavins: J. Exper. Med. (U.S.A.) **102**, 151 (1955). — Kroc, D., T. D. Kinney, N. Kaufman, and J. Klavins: Blood (U.S.A.) **21**, 546 (1963). Moore, C. V., and R. Dubach: Transact. Ass. Amer. Physicians **64**, 245 (1951). — Pirzio-Biroli, G., T. H. Bothwell, and C. A. Finch: J. Laborat. Clin. Med. (U.S.A.) **51**, 37 (1958). — Smith, M. D., and I. M. Pannacciulli: Brit. J. Haemat. **4**, 428 (1958). — Taylor, J., D. Stiven, and E. W. Reid: J. Path. Bact. (G.B.) **41**, 397 (1935). — Turnbull, A., F. Cleton, and C. A. Finch: J. Clin. Invest. (U.S.A.) **41**, 1897 (1962).

Discussion

J.-C. Dreyfus: Do you know in what form haemoglobin iron is absorbed? Is it still a haem compound or not?

Callender: I don't think we know that as yet.

Moore: Did those of your patients who absorbed haem iron so poorly have any abnormality of gastric hydrochloric acid?

Callender: No, they were not achlorhydric.

Gajdos: Iron absorption is indeed a very complicated problem. It seems that the metal can be absorbed from any segment of the intestinal tract, as was suggested by Dr. Moore. Following rectal administration of ferrous salts labelled with radioactive iron, we observed within only 4 to 6 hours a highly significant degree of radioactivity in haemin isolated from red blood cells.

Wöhler: Dr. Finch has shown that haemoglobin iron is absorbed as haem, and he has no proof that haemoglobin is absorbed. There seems to be a difference between your experience, Dr. Callender, and that of Dr. Finch. Your investigation appears to show that the haemoglobin molecule is broken down in the gastro-intestinal tract to iron itself, and that no haem and no haemoglobin is absorbed.

Callender: I think this is a very difficult problem. *In vitro* we were unable to split off sufficient iron to account for the absorption by incubation with coliform organisms or by tryptic digestion, and it may well be that the iron is absorbed as a haem compound. We have, however, no definite evidence for this.

Wöhler: This is a very important question as regards therapy. If the iron is completely split from the haemoglobin, then it is presumably possible to block its absorption in the gastro-intestinal tract by administering desferrioxamine. If haem is absorbed as such, then there is no chance of the desferrioxamine binding iron.

Beutler: Your studies, Dr. Callender, show that hydrochloric acid seems to make very little difference to the absorption of haemoglobin iron. In the case of other forms of food iron, Dr. Moore and his associates[1] demonstrated some time ago that hydrochloric acid makes no difference to absorption. On the other hand, it is well known that many patients who have undergone partial gastrectomy develop iron-deficiency anaemia, and there is suggestive evidence in the literature that such patients may respond to inorganic iron therapy. Yet they develop an iron-deficiency anaemia when they are given a diet which seems to have a relatively normal iron content. I wonder whether you had an opportunity to study patients with partial gastrectomy to see if there is, indeed, a greater difference in their ability to absorb iron which is incorporated in haemoglobin, as opposed to inorganic iron, than appears to be the case with non-gastrectomised individuals.

[1] Moore, C. V., and R. Dubach: Science (U.S.A.) **116**, 527 (1952).

Callender: We haven't made any observations with haemoglobin iron in patients who had undergone partial gastrectomy, but we are currently studying some patients with total gastrectomy, and so far we have not been able to show much difference as compared with normal controls. It may be that, if you give iron in another form, e.g. with a bulky meal, the decreased transit time may reduce absorption and hence contribute to the development of anaemia.

Undritz: What haemoglobin preparation did you use? Pure, fresh rat blood with an iron content equivalent to the required therapeutic dose of an organic iron preparation — e.g. iron gluconate — is completely ineffective in experimental iron-deficiency anaemia in the rat. The iron in the haemoglobin of fresh blood is apparently so firmly bound that it cannot be split and absorbed in the rat intestine. On the other hand, it is possible with haemoglobin preparations to split off a certain percentage of the iron by means of haemolysis, partial predigestion and decomposition, and thus to render it absorbable. The failure of iron to be absorbed from fresh blood is all the more remarkable since the rat intestine displays great digestive powers: iron-E.D.T.A. complex is partly split and used for the synthesis of haemoglobin if it is administered orally, whereas similarly large amounts administered intravenously or subcutaneously are simply excreted again by the kidneys without improving the haemoglobin levels. It would be interesting to know if Dr. Callender also carried out tests with myoglobin and vegetable iron preparations, which perhaps play a more important role than haemoglobin as organic dietary iron in human nutrition.

Salera: I should like to make a remark on a point that has been raised by Dr. Dreyfus and Dr. Wöhler. I remember a patient who suffered from repeated blood losses from the intestinal tract and who showed very high excretion levels of faecal stercobilinogen. I don't think the latter was derived from haemoglobin present in the intestinal lumen. Perhaps it was porphyrin that had been absorbed and metabolised. Maybe the iron is absorbed from haemoglobin in the form of haem and not as free iron.

Hallberg: I don't know if it is necesary to assume that haem iron is absorbed as haem. The fact that there are great differences in the rate of absorption of haem iron and ionised iron may explain some of the confusions. In one case of iron deficiency, which Dr. Sölvell and I studied, we gave simultaneously Fe^{55}-labelled haemoglobin and Fe^{59}-labelled ferrous sulphate orally, each corresponding to 5 mg. of elemental iron.

The plasma activity of Fe^{59} increased rapidly and reached a maximum after about $2^1/_2$ to 3 hours, whereupon it rapidly declined. The Fe^{55} activity, however, increased more slowly and stayed on a plateau level for the remainder of the 4 hours during which we recorded the plasma activities. These data not only indicate differences in rates of absorption, but also show that iron from haemoglobin is absorbed over a much longer period of time.

Moeschlin: Dr. Callender, I think we have all been very impressed by the results you obtained using pancreatin. Have you done any studies in primary haemochromatosis (homozygote form) and, if so, could you also inhibit the increased iron absorption in this disease by the oral addition of pancreatin?

Bothwell: I should like to make three remarks about the effects of luminal factors on iron absorption. We have tested the effects of hydrochloric acid on absorption in achlorhydric subjects, using a double isotope technique in which each individual served as his own control. In this way we found, as Dr. CALLENDER has done, that acid has no effect on haemoglobin absorption. In contrast, ferric iron absorption was increased about fourfold by the presence of acid, and the absorption of ferrous iron was increased about twofold. Haemoglobin thus seems to behave differently in this particular system. Secondly, with regard to pancreatic secretions, we stimulated the pancreas in rats with pancreozymin and secretin and tested the effects on iron absorption. With pancreatic stimulation, there was a 50% drop in the rate of absorption in rats. The third observation is related to the effects of alcohol on iron absorption in healthy young volunteers. We tested the absorption of a ferric salt given with and without 3 ozs whisky. The rate of absorption was increased severalfold by the giving of alcohol.

VENTURA: On the basis of our investigations with different radioactive iron compounds and also haemoglobin labelled with Fe^{59}, we agree with Dr. CALLENDER that the administration of radioactive haemoglobin yields interesting information on what proportion of the iron present in the food may be absorbed. However, negative results may sometimes be obtained in human beings, despite a normal iron balance. For this reason, I think we should not neglect the more conventional techniques of investigation.

In our clinical department we use a method specially designed to analyse the gastro-intestinal digestion and absorption of dietary iron. It is based on oral administration of 5 mg. iron as Fe^{59} reduced by H_2 (10 μc. of radioactivity), plus intramuscular injection of 1 mg. histamine, followed some days later by another dose of the same quantity of $Fe^{59}Cl_2$ + vitamin C[1].

The former iron compound is not spontaneously soluble and ionisable. It liberates Fe ions only if gastro-intestinal secretion and motility are normal. Thus we find (Fig. 1, above) that absorption is better in cases with gastric hyperchlorhydria and hypomotility. On the other hand, some patients with hypochlorhydria, gastric hypermotility, or sprue-like syndromes show no absorption.

Unlike the first iron compound, $Fe^{59}Cl_2$ is spontaneously ionised, and can thus be normally absorbed even in the presence of alterations affecting gastro-intestinal secretory function and motility (Fig. 1, below). Impairment of the absorption of this iron salt is observed only in cases where there are modifications of the intestinal contents or changes in the duodenal-jejunal mucosa.

By simultaneously determining the rate of absorption of Fe^{59} reduced by H_2 and of $Fe^{59}Cl_2$, one can therefore obtain some insight into the factors which play a part in reducing iron absorption, into the factors that are involved in the ionisation of dietary iron compounds, and into factors interfering with the mucosal absorption of Fe ions.

Fig. 2 shows that by this method it is possible to demonstrate — in some iron-deficiency anaemias — an impairment of iron absorption due to alteration either of the ionising phase or of the absorption phase.

SHERLOCK: I was particularly interested in Dr. CALLENDER's observations in cirrhotic patients. The quantity of pancreatin she is giving can in no way be regarded as replacement therapy. I should like to know what she thinks is the active substance in the pancreatic juice, because it clearly must be present in almost trace amounts. This links up, too, with her observation that cirrhotics, other than alcoholics, show the same effect. The non-alcoholics, in contrast to the alcoholics, would not be expected to show pancreatic

[1] VENTURA, S.: Arch. stud. fisiopat. ricambio (It.) **25**, 1 (1961).

dysfunction. How can she correlate the effect on iron absorption with the dosage of pancreatin she gives and with the actual changes in the pancreas that are known to occur in the different types of cirrhosis?

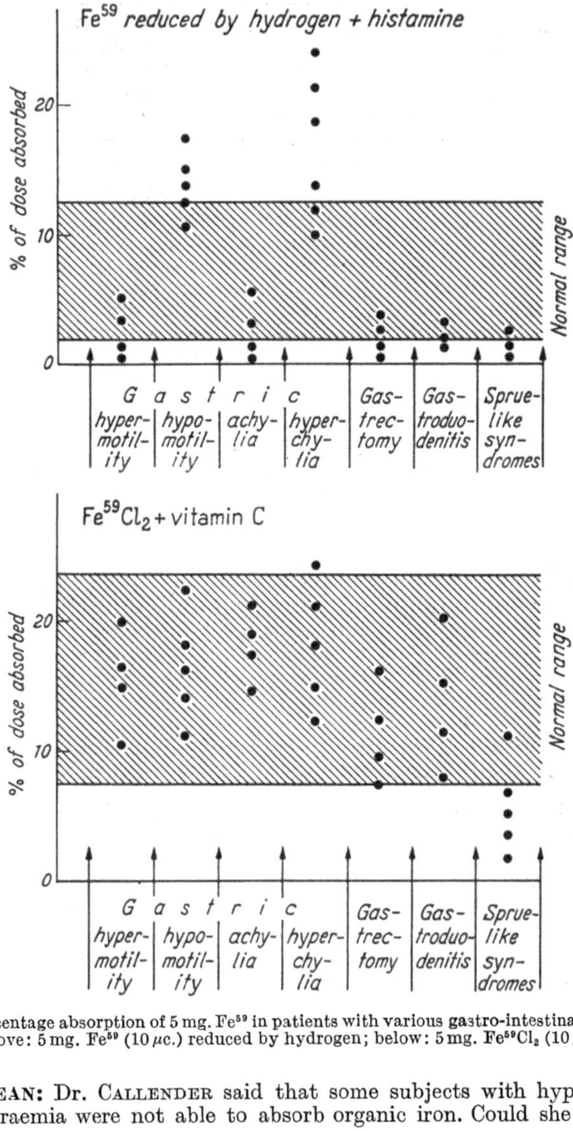

Fig. 1. Percentage absorption of 5 mg. Fe^{59} in patients with various gastro-intestinal disorders, Above: 5 mg. Fe^{59} (10 μc.) reduced by hydrogen; below: 5 mg. $Fe^{59}Cl_2$ (10 μc.)

Najean: Dr. Callender said that some subjects with hypochromic hyposideraemia were not able to absorb organic iron. Could she tell us if these subjects had the same clinical pictures or the same aetiology of the syndrome as the other subjects? I presume these patients were cured by giving them inorganic iron; if so, did Dr. CALLENDER explore them after they had been cured? Is the absorption of dietary iron restored to normal or not?

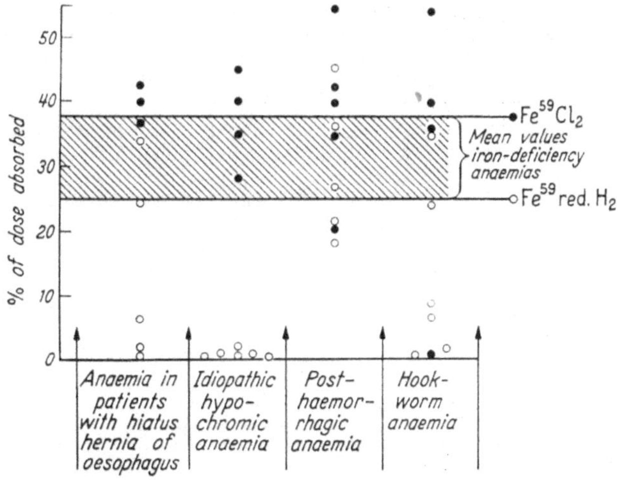

Fig. 2. Percentage absorption of Fe^{59} reduced by hydrogen (open circles) and of $Fe^{59}Cl_2$ (full circles) in patients with various iron-deficiency anaemias

BRICK: This observation of Dr. CALLENDER's as to the increased absorption of iron in chronic pancreatitis with lithiasis interests me. We have had an opportunity to study punch and surgical liver-biopsy specimens in a fair number of these patients. We haven't been impressed by the amount of iron in the liver. I wonder if you had any experience along these lines?

FINCH: I think this attention to secretion is most appropriate. A little over a year ago, Dr. TURNBULL in our laboratory started studies on gastrectomy and various other surgical alterations in the upper gastro-intestinal tract, and these studies seemed to be pointing more to the conclusion that trace amounts of iron added to food are greatly affected by gastric secretion. I should like to ask Dr. CALLENDER about the interesting difference in percent utilisation that she showed in haemoglobin iron. The studies by TURNBULL dealing with haemoglobin iron indicate that, once it has appeared in the serum, it is dialysable to the same degree that transferrin iron would be; his results seem to exclude the possibility that absorbed iron in the plasma is present in a different form, such as haem. It would be most interesting if there were a mechanism which operated to alter utilisation by these two different compounds, i.e. haemoglobin and free iron.

KRUH: Do you think that pancreatin could inhibit the absorption of iron simply by combining with it and making it insoluble?

J.-C. DREYFUS: It has quite often been observed that, after a porta-caval surgical shunt, haemochromatosis develops. Have any absorption studies been done in such cases?

Callender: In reply to Dr. Undritz's question concerning the preparation of haemoglobin, we prepared the labelled haemoglobin by injecting rabbits with radioactive iron and subsequently bleeding them when the label had been incorporated into the haemoglobin.

Regarding Dr. Moeschlin's question about primary haemochromatosis, we have not as yet studied the effect of pancreatin in this condition, but of course are anxious to do so. It is conceivable that primary haemochromatosis might simply be due to a genetic abnormality in the pancreas which leads to lack of a normal inhibitor to iron absorption. Recently, I heard that X-ray surveys in Africa have revealed a very high proportion of subjects with pancreatic calcification, so I think once again that pancreatic disease may be an important contributory factor in the development of the haemosiderosis seen there.

Dr. Bothwell's remarks about the effect of pancreozymin stimulation in rats are most interesting. We have planned similar studies in humans, but have not yet had the opportunity to do them.

I agree with Dr. Sherlock that the dose of pancreatin we are giving is quite minute in relation to what the patient would normally produce. We haven't any idea of what the substance is which causes this strong inhibition. As I mentioned, there is a suggestion that it is heat labile, but we have done only one experiment following heat treatment of the pancreatin. We have tested absorption in a few patients with simple iron deficiency with or without pancreatin. We chose such subjects, because they would be expected to have a high iron absorption, and in 2 out of 3 the addition of pancreatin led to a striking reduction in absorption. In these cases, inorganic iron was used in the test.

In reply to Dr. Najean, from the clinical point of view the patients with hypochromic anaemia who showed poor absorption from haemoglobin were not recognisably different from other subjects with hypochromic anaemia. Most of them responded adequately to treatment with inorganic iron. We have, however, at the moment two patients, both of whom show a very low absorption without any other evidence of malabsorption syndrome. In our experience this is extremely rare; in fact, the only other patients we have come across who showed a similar poor absorption of inorganic iron, with a lack of response to treatment, were suffering from amyloid disease or thalassaemia minor. In these two recent patients, there is no evidence of such conditions, but we hope to be able to investigate them further.

With regard to Dr. Finch's comments on the percent of utilisation of haemoglobin iron, it seems possible that the slower rate of absorption of haemoglobin iron determines a different pattern of distribution of the iron, with perhaps a greater proportion being taken up by the liver, but this is pure speculation.

Dr. Dreyfus, we haven't yet made any studies on patients with portacaval shunt, but again we are naturally anxious to do so, especially if we can study patients before and after operation.

Finally, in reply to Dr. Kruh, we don't think that the effect of the pancreatin has anything to do with the simple precipitation of an insoluble iron salt, because pancreatin has a marked influence on the haemoglobin iron absorption as well as on the absorption of inorganic iron.

The role of transferrin in the transport of iron into the developing red cell

By

J. H. Katz and J. H. Jandl

I should like today to review some of the work that Dr. Jandl and I have been doing over the last few years in an attempt to define the role of transferrin in the transport of iron in the plasma and its delivery to erythroid cells.

Under physiologic conditions, the iron of plasma is tightly bound to transferrin, each molecule of which is capable of complexing two atoms of the metal in its ferric oxidation state. The tenacity of this binding at pH 7.4 exceeds that of even the more powerful synthetic chelating substances (*3*, *4*). Indeed, it has been suggested that the particular structural configuration of the binding sites enables them to function as efficient chelators (*25*).

Despite this very tight union, plasma iron turnover is, even in normal circumstances, quite rapid, and almost all the iron that leaves the plasma is taken up by the marrow (*22*). Erythroid stimulation leads to a further increase in this turnover, and erythroid suppression has the opposite effect. Since there is no evidence of any alteration in the nature of the binding sites of transferrin in these conditions, it must be presumed that the rate of removal of iron from the plasma is regulated primarily by the demands of red-cell production.

In order to study how transferrin-bound iron is utilized by hemoglobin-synthesizing cells, we have, for the most part, utilized crystalline transferrin, prepared from Cohn-Fraction IV-4 by the method of Inman and co-workers (*9*). Moving boundary electrophoretic, ultracentrifugal, and immunologic analysis indicated that this protein was at least 97% pure. Each mg. of protein was able to bind 1.30 μg. of iron to form a reddish-colored complex.

The crystalline transferrin, completely saturated with stable iron, was "lightly" labeled with I^{131}, the final product containing less than one equivalent of iodide per mol of protein. The stable iron was then removed and replaced by Fe^{59} with sufficient carrier to bring the transferrin to any desired level of saturation. The labeling procedure did not appear to produce any gross alterations in the physical and immunologic properties of the protein. Less than 0.1% of the I^{131} was inorganic as determined by trichloracetic acid precipitation.

In vivo studies

The doubly-labeled transferrin was injected intravenously into eight normal subjects (*13*). The Fe^{59} disappeared from the plasma at an exponential rate, the half-time of which was found to range from 58 to 149 minutes. These figures, as well as the plasma iron turnover and red-cell utilization, as calculated by the equations of HUFF et al. (*8*), were within the same range as is obtained when radio-iron is bound to "whole" plasma. The I^{131} radioactivity, representing the protein moiety of the transferrin-iron complex, left the plasma at only one-sixth to one-twentieth the rate at which the Fe^{59} was cleared over the first few hours (Fig. 1). This initial component of transferrin disappearance was thought to be due to diffusion through capillary walls. After three or four days, during which the intra- and extravascular pools of transferrin became equilibrated, the I^{131} disappeared at a second exponential rate corresponding to the excretion of I^{131} from the body as measured with a total-body counter (*7*). The half-time of protein degradation was 6.7 to 8.4 days. When these data were analyzed according to the methods of STERLING (*24*), it appeared that the total exchangeable pool of transferrin

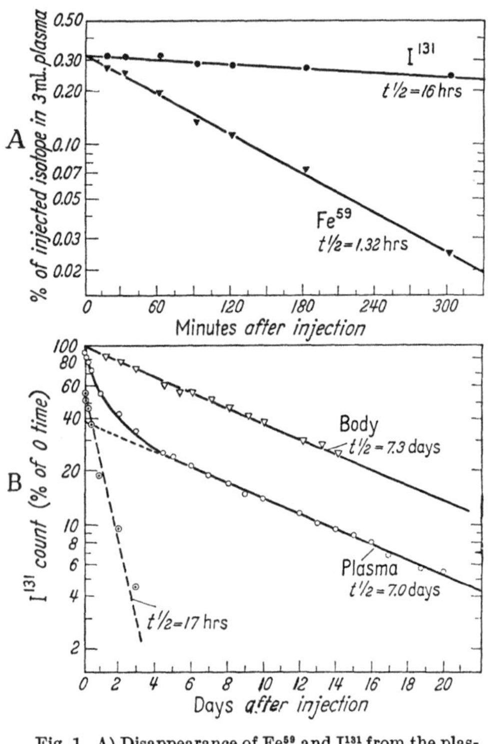

Fig. 1. A) Disappearance of Fe^{59} and I^{131} from the plasma over the first 5 hours after injection of doubly-labeled transferrin. Abscissa units are in minutes. B) Disappearance of I^{131} from plasma and "body". Abscissa units are in days (*13*)

was about 0.3 g./kg. body-weight and that 56 to 62% of this was located extravascularly.

Other investigators have found that radio-iron bound to commercially available Cohn-Fraction IV-7 has a significantly slower clearance rate than iron bound to native plasma (*2*, *17*). We have recently repeated these studies using crystalline transferrin (*14*). Either Fe^{59} or Fe^{55} was bound to the subject's own plasma and the other isotope to the purified protein. They were injected simultaneously, and the activity of each isotope in the plasma was followed for several hours[1].

In three of the four subjects studied, the clearance of the iron isotopes was quite similar. The data from two of these subjects are shown in Fig. 2. In the fourth subject, the slopes were somewhat more divergent, the half-times of transferrin and plasma-bound iron being 86 and 72 minutes, respectively.

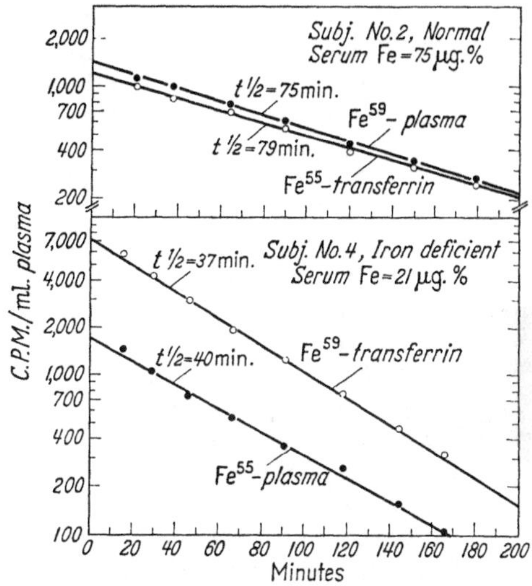

Fig. 2. Simultaneous clearances of radio-iron bound to plasma and purified transferrin in two subjects

Thus, the *in vivo* studies suggested that the isolation and labeling of crystalline transferrin did not affect its functional integrity in a physiologic setting. This left unanswered the question of how iron, so firmly attached as judged by *in vitro* criteria, was able to be cleared from the plasma at a much more rapid rate than the binding protein itself. LAURELL (*16*) suggested some years ago that this dissociation might occur as a result of a simple equilibrium between intra- and extravascular ionic iron. However, at the time, the stability of the iron-transferrin complex was thought to be considerably lower than recent estimates (*4*), and certain dialysis experiments (*13*) have made it seem unlikely that ionic diffusion can account for the rapidity with which iron is cleared.

[1] We are indebted to Dr. RAYMOND J. DERN for the assay of the radioactivity, which was carried out by his previously published method (*5*).

In vitro studies

When red cells are incubated in solutions of $Fe^{59}Cl_3$, iron is taken up indiscriminately by both mature red cells and reticulocytes (*10*). However, when the radio-iron is bound to transferrin, either in plasma (*18*, *20*) or in solutions of the purified protein, only the reticulocytes are capable of incorporating the metal. Thus, transferrin, in some manner, directs the entry of iron into those cells which are still actively synthesizing hemoglobin and prevents its presumably needless accumulation by mature cells. Transferrin itself is not consumed during the process of iron transfer. Inhibition of intracellular metabolism and enzymatic alteration of the reticulocyte membrane markedly depress iron uptake (*10*). The latter findings suggested that not only was iron accumulation by reticulocytes an energy-dependent process, but that some particular property of their membrane surface was responsible for its specificity. A further clue was provided by the observation that Coombs serum was able to agglutinate the reticulocytes of patients whose mature red cells were Coombs-negative, and that this agglutination could be inhibited by prior adsorption of the serum with purified transferrin (*11*).

With these data in mind it was decided to use the I^{131}-Fe^{59} labeled transferrin to gain further insight into the mechanism of the interaction between the protein and the reticulocyte (*12*).

Red cells were generally obtained from patients with pernicious anemia who were undergoing a reticulocytosis in response to therapy. The cells were washed 2 or 3 times with cold saline before being suspended in a modified Krebs-bicarbonate buffer containing glucose. The labeled transferrin, diluted to a concentration of 0.5 g./100 ml. in the same buffer, was mixed with an aliquot of the red-cell suspension at 37° C. The mixture was gassed with 95% O_2—5% CO_2, and the incubation continued with constant shaking until it was terminated by flushing the flask with a large volume of cold saline.

The cells were washed 4 or 5 times, the last washing containing little, if any, radioactivity. The activity of the cells and appropriate standards were then measured in a well-type scintillation counter equipped with a dual scaler, each of the two being set at different levels of discrimination. It was thus possible to determine the activity of each isotope simultaneously (*6*).

When the red cells of seven normal subjects and eight patients with varying degrees of reticulocytosis were incubated with doubly-labeled transferrin, a definite relationship was obtained between the reticulocyte concentration and the amount of I^{131}

adhering to the cells. Since the I^{131} activity represented a known amount of protein, the results could be expressed in terms of the amount of transferrin bound per ml. of cells, as shown in Fig. 3. By extrapolating this regression line, we calculate that on the average about 75 μg. of transferrin was bound to each ml. of reticulocytes and that about 0.6 μg. adhered per ml. of mature red cells. Thus, it would appear that reticulocytes have an affinity for transferrin at least 100 times greater than that of mature red cells. By contrast, when I^{131}-labeled human serum albumin was incubated with the cells, no such correlation existed, less than 1 μg. being bound per ml. of cells, regardless of the reticulocyte concentration.

When albumin was added to a mixture of labeled transferrin and reticulocytes, there was no effect on either the uptake of Fe^{59} or the binding of I^{131}. However, when autologous serum was added, there was a decrease in the binding of the labeled protein, which was about the same as would be expected if the specific activity of the labeled protein were reduced in proportion to the amount of serum transferrin added. This serves to illustrate the fact that the purified protein was equivalent to the native material in terms of its affinity for reticulocytes.

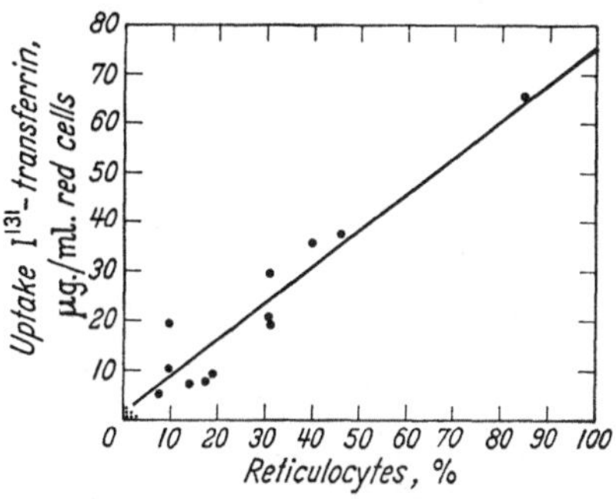

Fig. 3. The relation between uptake of I^{131}-transferrin by red-cell suspensions and their concentration of reticulocytes (*12*)

To determine the site of attachment of the transferrin, we hemolyzed the cells of a reticulocyte-rich suspension which had been incubated with the doubly-labeled protein for one hour. The hemolysate was then subjected to differential centrifugation. About 90% of the I^{131} activity in the original cells was recovered in the large particle fraction (stroma), whereas more than half of the Fe^{59} was located in the small particle (mitochondria and microsomes) and soluble supernatant fractions.

Thus, it appears that during the process of iron transfer the transferrin remains on the surface of the reticulocyte, while the greater part of the iron enters the interior of the cell, where it is incorporated into hemoglobin or precursors thereof.

Inhibition of the metabolic processes of the cell was achieved either by incubation at 2° C. or by addition of cyanide or dinitrophenylphenol. Under these circumstances, both Fe^{59} incorporation and transferrin binding were diminished, though the former was more markedly affected than the latter. When the reticulocyte suspensions were pre-treated with various concentrations of trypsin, which was then removed by washing the cells, a marked and approximately equal decrease in Fe^{59} and I^{131} uptake was observed. It is significant that this enzymatic alteration of the reticulocyte membrane had previously been shown not to interfere with lactate production or O_2 consumption by these cells (*10*). We therefore consider that specific "receptors" for transferrin exist on the reticulocyte surface, which can be split off by trypsinization. Such receptors may also depend on active cellular metabolism for their maintenance.

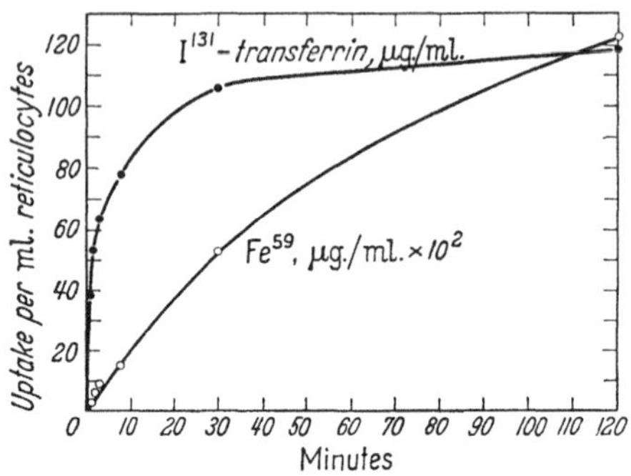

Fig. 4. Comparison of uptake by reticulocytes of transferrin-bound iron (Fe^{59}) and of transferrin itself (*12*)

We now turned to a study of the kinetics of transferrin binding to the reticulocyte. Attachment of the labeled protein was very rapid, about half of the maximum uptake occurring within a minute or two of the addition of the transferrin. Thereafter, the rate of attachment decreased exponentially, as illustrated in Fig. 4. On the other hand, Fe^{59} accumulation was more or less linear with respect to time. When reticulocytes, which had previously been incubated with labeled transferrin, were washed and placed in solutions of the *un*labeled protein, there was a rapid elution of I^{131}. The rate of detachment of the protein appeared to be identical to the rate of the initial attachment. This is shown in Fig. 5, which

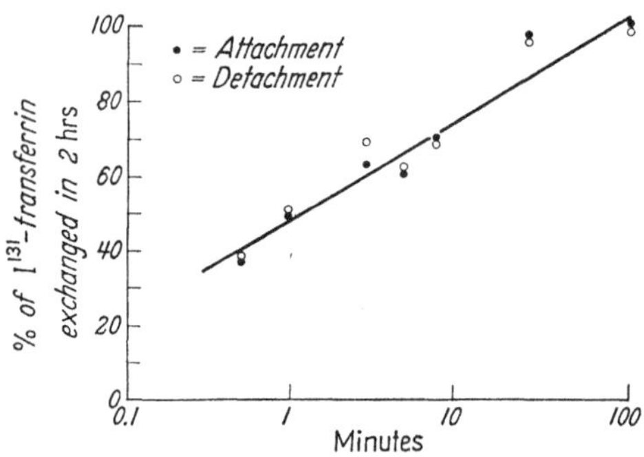

Fig. 5. Rate of uptake ("attachment") of I^{131}-transferrin by reticulocytes compared with its rate of release ("detachment") in solutions of unlabeled transferrin (*12*)

again emphasizes the exponential relationship of both processes to time. These findings indicate that the transferrin molecules bound to the surface of the reticulocyte are in dynamic equilibrium with those in its environment and that, on the average, a given molecule remains bound for about one minute. During this interval, the iron which is complexed to the transferrin is removed by a mechanism which remains to be elucidated, although it apparently requires a source of metabolic energy.

It might be added at this point that, in our experience, the uptake of iron from pure transferrin solutions does not differ significantly from that of plasma under comparable conditions. We therefore can find no evidence for a plasma factor which accelerates iron incorporation such as has been reported by others (*18*).

We next turned our attention toward the effect of the relative degree of iron saturation on transferrin binding to reticulocytes. It was found that the greater the saturation of the transferrin, the greater was the amount bound at any given time after addition of the I^{131}-labeled protein. A series of studies was then carried out to determine if we could quantitate these differences in the avidity of binding. Unlabeled transferrin, either iron-free or iron-saturated, was added in equal amounts to solutions of the labeled protein, which in turn was either iron-free or iron-saturated. The data, when analyzed in terms of the known uptake of I^{131} and the estimated uptake of the unlabeled protein, appeared to indicate that the iron-saturated transferrin had an avidity about five times greater than that of the iron-free form. However, in a similar experiment, in which unlabeled protein, variously saturated with iron, was added to labeled transferrin of a fixed (34%) saturation, it appeared that unsaturated transferrin had little or no inhibitory effect. With increasing saturation of the unlabeled protein, there was more and more inhibition of I^{131} binding, and the extent of inhibition was very close to that which would be predicted if only the iron-laden protein were competing for binding (Fig. 6).

Thus, while there was some ambiguity in the quantitation of the difference, it appeared that molecules of transferrin which were complexed to iron had a much greater affinity for the receptor sites on the reticulocytes than did those which were not complexed to the metal. This might indicate that iron is involved in the bond between transferrin and the receptor. On the other hand, the binding of iron is known to produce alterations in the physical properties of the transferrin molecule which indicate that a change in charge and configuration is produced (*1*, *15*). Conceivably, such changes may favor binding to the reticulocyte.

There has been a good deal of interest in the effect which the relative degree of saturation of transferrin with iron exerts on the uptake of this metal by immature red cells and other tissues (*10, 19*). Previous investigations had appeared to demonstrate that there is a gradual rise in the rate of iron uptake by reticulocytes as the saturation of pure transferrin is increased, the change becoming most pronounced at saturations greater than 60%. We have recently attempted to re-study this phenomenon.

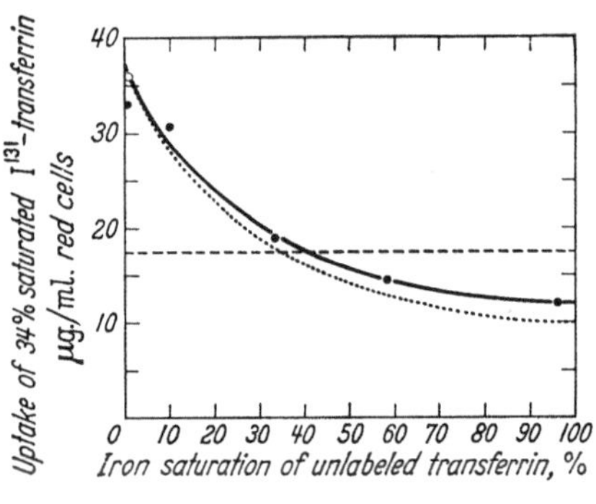

Fig. 6. Influence of iron saturation on the uptake of transferrin by reticulocytes. The uptake of 34% saturated I^{131}-transferrin (solid line) was inhibited more effectively by the more highly saturated unlabeled transferrin. The dotted line shows the uptake of I^{131}-transferrin predicted if only the iron-complexed transferrin were competing for the reticulocyte receptor sites. The dashed line shows the uptake predicted if both the iron-free and iron-complexed forms of transferrin competed equally (*12*)

Although we find no evidence for any peculiarities in the behavior of our crystalline transferrin either *in vivo* or *in vitro*, it has been suggested by others that at least certain preparations do not act like the native protein (*23*). Therefore, in some of these studies, we have used whole plasma as a source of transferrin. The plasma was obtained from patients with pernicious anemia, several days after they had received large doses of vitamin B_{12}. Plasma iron is generally quite low at this stage of the therapeutic response. Ten ml. aliquots of the plasma were placed in sterile flasks, and 0.5 ml. of 0.5 M $NaHCO_3$ was added, followed by 1 ml. of a mixture of Fe^{59} with an appropriate amount of carrier iron. Aliquots of the plasma were then removed for use as counting standards and for determination of the iron concentration and binding capacity. The plasma was allowed to remain at room temperature for several hours and was then left in the refrigerator overnight. The following morning, cells were obtained from the same donor, washed and added to the radioactive plasma. The initial pH of the plasma was about 7.6 and did not fall below 7.2 during the course of the incubation. Aliquots of cells were removed at intervals and, after washing, were counted together with the standards. The specific activity was calculated on the basis of the chemically determined iron concentration in the standards and thus took into consideration both indigenous and added iron.

As shown in Fig. 7, iron accumulation increased as the saturation of the plasma was raised, though, if anything, the rate of change tended to decrease at the higher saturations. In two other experiments of this type, the same effects were observed.

These results can be explained by two alternate hypotheses. 1) Molecules of transferrin which are not complexed with iron compete for the reticulocyte receptor site with those molecules which are so complexed. As saturation is increased, there are fewer of the first class of molecules available for such competition, and hence the binding of the second class is favored. 2) The effect of saturation may be due solely to the effect of increasing the concentration of the Fe-transferrin complex, there being essentially no competitive effect from the metal-free protein.

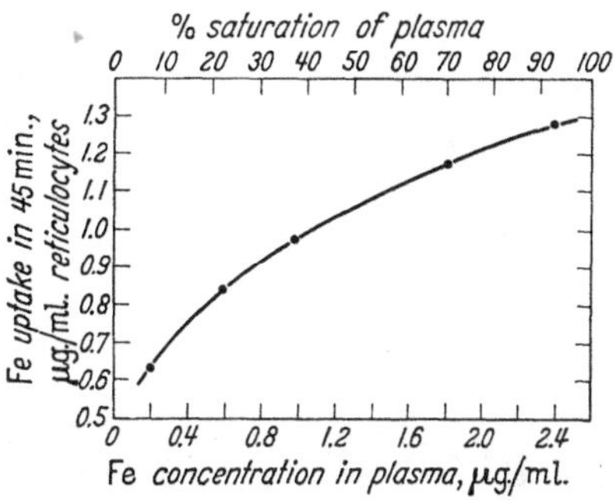

Fig. 7. Effect of relative plasma saturation on uptake of iron by reticulocytes. The uptake is shown plotted against the concentration of iron in the incubating plasma or its equivalent in terms of percentage saturation of the total iron-binding capacity (2.61 µg./ml.)

In order to resolve these possibilities, the following experiments were carried out. The plasma was divided into two aliquots, and Fe^{59} with carrier was added to each, so as to produce different levels of saturation. The two plasmas were then added in varying amounts to a set of flasks, following which they were brought to a constant volume with a modified Krebs-bicarbonate buffer. Thus, there were two sets of flasks, each set containing dilutions of plasma of a given saturation. Aliquots of the same red-cell suspension were then added to all flasks.

The results of two such experiments are shown in Fig. 8, in which the uptake of iron by the reticulocytes is plotted as a function of the extracellular iron concentration. Is should be noted that, even at the lowest concentrations, the *amount* of iron available for utilization was not limiting, since, at the conclusion of the relatively short incubations, at least five times as much Fe remained in the bathing medium as had been taken up by the cells. There was little or no difference in the uptake at any given level of extracellular iron concentration, regardless of the initial plasma saturation. We would conclude that iron-free transferrin molecules do not compete to any significant extent for the reticulocyte receptors; the influence of increasing transferrin saturation appears to be entirely due to the effect of increasing the concentration of the metallo-protein complex. This same dependence on concentration can also be demonstrated for solutions of crystalline transferrin incubated with reticulocytes (Fig. 9).

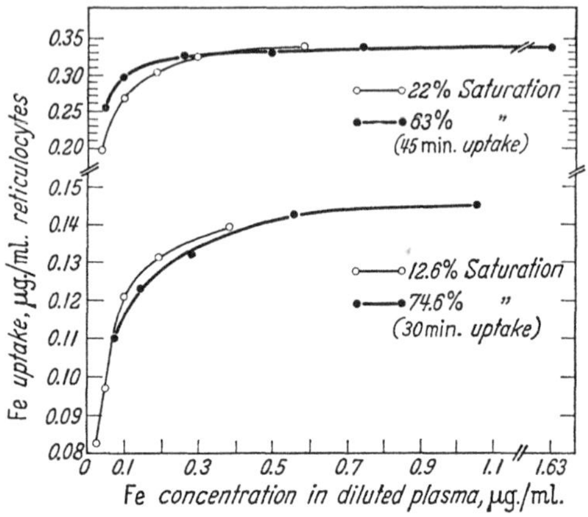

Fig. 8. Effect of dilution of plasma on iron uptake by reticulocytes. Results in two separate experiments are shown. There was little difference in uptake at any given level of iron concentration in the incubating plasma, regardless of its relative saturation initially

It is of some interest that all of these curves are quite similar to those obtained when increasing amounts of substrate are added to a system with a constant amount of enzyme. Indeed, from a conceptual point of view, there are many features in the receptor-transferrin interaction which are analogous to an enzyme-mediated process. We calculate that there are about 50,000 receptor sites per reticulocyte. The number of such sites which are occupied at any given time can be considered to be a function of the concentration of Fe-transferrin ("substrate") in the surrounding medium. Since the momentary attachment of this complex to the receptor ("enzyme") appears to be necessary for iron to be incorporated within the cell, it would be expected that the rate of iron accumulation by the reticulocyte would in turn depend on the concentration of Fe-transferrin in the medium. When, at relatively high concentrations, all receptor sites are occupied, further increases would no longer influence iron incorporation. However, if the number of reticulocytes

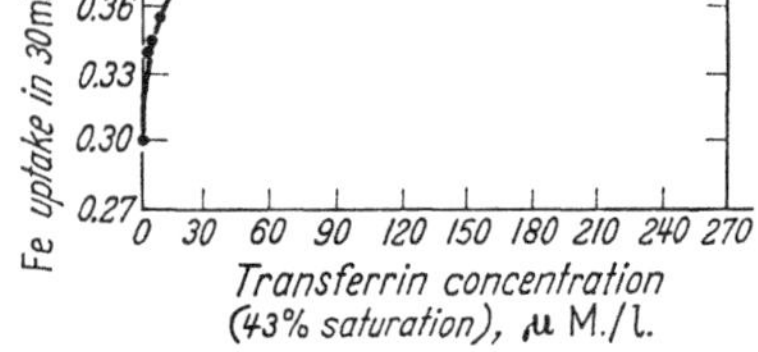

Fig. 9. Effect of the transferrin concentration on iron uptake by reticulocytes. The cells were incubated in solutions of purified transferrin which was 43% saturated with iron. Concentration of transferrin is plotted as micromols per liter

and therefore the number of receptor sites were changed, the concentration of the Fe-transferrin complex necessary to produce this maximum uptake of iron would change proportionately. This analogy is, of course, largely speculative, but seems to offer a reasonable explanation for our findings.

We were puzzled by the fact that, as noted above, previous investigations (*10*) had indicated that there was a sharp rise in iron uptake by reticulocytes (and also by liver slices) when transferrin saturation was greater than 60%. On examining the data, the principal difference in technique was found to be related to the length of time the iron and transferrin were allowed to interact in solution before being added to the reticulocytes. In our recent experiments, the iron was added to the plasma or transferrin solution about 18 hours before its addition to the cells, whereas in the previous studies they had been mixed only an hour or two before the beginning of the incubation. Experiments were then carried out to determine whether this was the decisive factor.

An aliquot of the same plasma was placed in each of a pair of flasks. One ml. of a solution of Fe^{59}, pre-mixed with carrier iron, was added to the first of these, bringing the saturation to 19%. An identical amount of stable iron without Fe^{59} was added to the second flask. The same procedure was carried out with another set of flasks, except that the saturation of this pair was brought to 63%. Seventeen hours later, the essentially carrier-free Fe^{59} was mixed with the second flask of both pairs. Thus, the plasma in both flasks of each set was now virtually the same, except for the order of addition of isotope and carrier. All flasks were then incubated at 37° C. for an additional hour before the red-cell suspension was added.

The results are shown in Table 1. The uptake of iron by the cells in the first pair of flasks (19% saturation) was similar. However, in the other pair (63% saturation), there was a much greater uptake of Fe^{59} by cells in the flask to which the carrier and radioactive iron had been added sequentially. Therefore the apparent iron accumulation was about three times greater when calculated on the basis of the specific activity of the initial plasma mixtures. Similar results were obtained in two other studies of this type.

It could be shown that this disparity at the higher saturations was not due to the order of addition *per se*, but rather to the length of time the tracer was allowed to stand with the plasma before incubation with the cells. Thus, the uptake in paired flasks was identical if 12 hours were allowed to elapse following the separate additions of carrier and Fe^{59}, even when saturation was as high as 85%.

Table 1. *Effect of adding Fe^{59} to plasma 1 hour before incubation with reticulocytes*

Flask	Saturation %	Spec. act.[1] c.p.m. /µg. Fe	Activity c.p.m./ml. cells	Apparent uptake µg. Fe/ml. retics
1A[2]	19	160,000	5,201	0.21
1B[3]	19	158,000	4,950	0.20
2A[2]	63	52,400	2,536	0.30
2B[3]	63	46,500	6,325	0.87

[1] Specific activity of incubating plasma.

[2] Carrier added pre-mixed with Fe^{59} 18 hours before incubation with cells.

[3] Carrier added 18 hours before and Fe^{59} 1 hour before incubation with cells.

Iron unbound to transferrin is rapidly taken up by both mature and immature red cells (*10*). Therefore the results of these studies suggest to us that, when iron is added to plasma or to solutions of purified transferrin in amounts which approach (but do not exceed) its binding capacity, the time it takes for complete complex formation to be accomplished is increased. If the solution is added to the reticulocytes before complex formation is completed, some of the iron will enter the cells in a non-specific fashion. Of course, we have exaggerated the apparent degree of this incomplete binding in our experiments, since the specific activity of the uncomplexed Fe^{59} is much higher than that of the bound isotope, but the general conclusion still would appear to be valid. Although we have as yet no experimental evidence in this regard, on theoretical grounds it seems reasonable to expect that the rate of complex formation in mixtures of transferrin and iron would follow second-order kinetics. If this is the case, then the more iron one were to add so as to approach complete saturation of a fixed amount of protein, the greater would be the quantity which was uncomplexed at a given time following admixture. In any event, it would appear that incomplete binding may account for some of the anomalous findings in previous studies of iron uptake by reticulocytes. One may also conjecture about its significance in hemochromatosis and other diseases associated with high serum iron levels. For example, when iron absorption from the small bowel is rapid, binding to transferrin in the portal blood may also be incomplete as a consequence of the already high saturation. Under such circumstances, the iron bound loosely to proteins other than transferrin may be deposited in the liver, as has recently been reported (*27*).

Conclusions

It is always difficult to correlate *in vitro* findings with the far more subtle processes of physiologic regulation. We believe, however, that the attachment of transferrin to the developing red cells of the marrow explains certain of our *in vivo* observations. There is abundant evidence from electron-microscopic studies that the reticulo-endothelial cells which line the sinusoids of the marrow are normally discontinuous (*21, 26*). The erythroid tissue which surrounds these sinusoids is thus being constantly bathed by plasma (*28*). Transferrin may therefore be adsorbed from the functional confines of the "vascular space" and, after giving up its iron to the immature cells, return directly to the plasma pool. Such a phenomenon would account for the discrepant disappearance of Fe^{59} and the labeled protein from the plasma. It is also consistent with the fact that, in the final analysis, the rate of removal of iron from the plasma by the marrow is related to the number of active red-cell precursors present. The data of POLLYCOVE and MORTIMER (*22*) indicate that plasma perfusion of the marrow is sufficiently great to account for even the most rapid iron clearance, were it accomplished solely by the mechanism of transferrin adsorption to these cells.

In summary, our findings suggest that iron is delivered to developing red cells by means of the specific adherence of the iron-transferrin complex to the surface of these cells. This attachment permits the active removal of the metal from the transferrin and its incorporation into the cells. The transferrin, freed of its iron, is displaced by other iron-bearing molecules which are taken up directly from the plasma. The displaced transferrin re-enters the plasma, where, in the course of its circulation, it acquires more iron from storage sites, enabling it to repeat the cycle once more.

Summary

Under physiologic conditions, the iron of plasma is tightly bound to transferrin. However, when the metallo-protein complex was injected intravenously, it was found that the iron was cleared at a rate which was at least six times greater than that at which the transferrin itself leaves the vascular compartment.

When doubly-labeled transferrin was incubated with reticulocytes and mature erythrocytes, the protein specifically adhered to the surface of the younger cells. A study of the kinetics of this transferrin binding indicated that, on the average, a given molecule remained on the reticulocyte surface for one minute, during which time the iron it bore was removed and incorporated into the cell. This process required a source of metabolic energy. Enzymatic alteration of the reticulocyte membrane with trypsin markedly interfered with both transferrin attachment and iron uptake. Certain other studies indicated that transferrin molecules to which iron is complexed have a much higher affinity for the hypothesized "transferrin receptor site" than do molecules which lack the metal.

Evidence was obtained that, when iron is added to plasma in amounts which approach its binding capacity, the time it takes for the completion of complex formation is greatly increased. Anomalous results may be obtained if this factor is not taken into consideration in studies of iron incorporation into developing red cells.

The implications of these investigations and their bearing on the mechanisms of bone-marrow utilization of transferrin-bound iron are discussed.

Zusammenfassung

Unter physiologischen Bedingungen ist Eisen im Plasma fest an Transferrin gebunden. Wenn jedoch dieser Metall-Eiweißkomplex intravenös injiziert wurde, fand sich, daß Eisen mindestens sechsmal schneller aus dem intravaskulären Raum verschwand als Transferrin.

Wenn doppelt radioaktiv markiertes Transferrin mit Retikulozyten und reifen Erythrozyten inkubiert wurde, fixierte sich das Protein spezifisch an der Oberfläche der jungen Zellen. Eine Untersuchung der Kinetik dieser Transferrinbindung ergab, daß ein einzelnes Molekül im allgemeinen für eine Minute auf der Retikulozytenoberfläche verblieb. Während dieser Zeitspanne wird das an ihm haftende Eisen abgelöst und in die Zelle eingebaut. Dieser Vorgang benötigt eine Energiequelle. Enzymatische Veränderung der Retikulozytenmembran durch Trypsin störte sowohl die Anlagerung von Transferrin als auch die Eisenaufnahme beträchtlich. Aus anderen Untersuchungen ging hervor, daß Transferrinmoleküle, an welche Eisen komplex gebunden ist, eine viel höhere Affinität für den hypothetischen „Transferrinrezeptor" besitzen als metallfreie Moleküle.

Wenn man Eisen zu Plasma in Mengen hinzufügt, die dessen Bindungskapazität erreichen, so wird dadurch die Zeit bis zur Beendigung der Komplexbildung stark verlängert. Berücksichtigt man diesen Faktor bei Untersuchungen über den Einbau von Eisen in sich entwickelnde Erythrozyten nicht, können sich abweichende Resultate ergeben.

Die Schlußfolgerungen aus diesen Untersuchungen und ihre Bedeutung für die Mechanismen, die der Nutzung von an Transferrin gebundenem Eisen im Knochenmark zugrunde liegen, werden besprochen.

Résumé

Dans les conditions physiologiques, le fer plasmatique est étroitement lié à la transferrine. Pourtant, si on injecte par voie intra-veineuse le complexe métallo-protéique, on trouve que le fer disparaît de l'espace vasculaire dans une proportion au moins six fois plus grande que la transferrine elle-même.

Si de la transferrine doublement marquée est incubée en présence de réticulocytes et d'érythrocytes adultes, la protéine adhère spécifiquement à la surface des cellules les plus jeunes. Une étude de la cinétique du phénomène montre qu'une molécule reste en moyenne une minute à la surface du réticulocyte, temps pendant lequel le fer qu'elle contient est détaché et incorporé à la cellule. Ce phénomène nécessite une source d'énergie métabolique. Une altération enzymatique, par de la trypsine, de la membrane cellulaire, perturbe profondément aussi bien la fixation de la transferrine sur la cellule que l'incorporation du fer dans celle-ci. D'autres études montrent que les molécules de transferrine porteuses de fer ont une plus grande affinité que les molécules dépourvues de ce métal pour l'hypothétique «zone réceptrice de transferrine».

Si on ajoute du fer au plasma en quantités voisines de la capacité de fixation, le temps nécessaire à la formation du complexe métallo-protéique est considérablement augmenté. On peut ainsi trouver des résultats insolites si l'on ne tient pas compte de ce facteur dans les études d'incorporation du fer dans les globules rouges en développement.

Les conséquences de ces investigations, leurs répercussions sur les mécanismes de l'utilisation par la moelle osseuse du fer lié à la transferrine sont discutées.

Acknowledgement

These investigations were supported in part by Grant RG-3507 from the National Institutes of Health, Bethesda, Md., and by training grant 2A-5155 from the National Institute of Arthritis and Metabolic Diseases, Bethesda, Md. (U.S.A.)

References

1. Azari, P. R., and R. E. Feeney: J. Biol. Chem. (U.S.A.) **232**, 293 (1958). — 2. Bothwell, T. H., A. V. Hurtado, D. M. Donohue, and C. A. Finch: Blood (U.S.A.) **12**, 409 (1957). — 3. Cleton, F., A. Turnbull, and C. A. Finch: J. Clin. Invest. (U.S.A.) **42**, 327 (1963). — 4. Davis, B., P. Saltman, and S. Benson: Biochem. Biophys. Res. Commun. (U.S.A.) **8**, 56 (1962). — 5. Dern, R. J., and W. L. Hart: J. Laborat. Clin. Med. (U.S.A.) **57**, 322 (1961). — 6. Hine, G. J., B. A. Burrows, L. Apt, M. Pollycove, J. F. Ross, and L. A. Sarkes: Nucleonics (U.S.A.) **13**, 23 (1955). — 7. Hine, G. J., P. L. Jagger, and B. A. Burrows: J. Laborat. Clin. Med. (U.S.A.) **55**, 476 (1960). — 8. Huff, R. L., T. G. Hennessy, R. E. Austin, J. F. Garcia, B. M. Roberts, and J. H. Lawrence: J. Clin. Invest. (U.S.A.) **29**, 1041 (1950). — 9. Inman, J. K., F. C. Coryell, K. B. McCall, J. T. Sgouris, and H. D. Anderson: Vox sang. (Switz.) **6**, 34 (1961). — 10. Jandl, J. H., J. K. Inman, R. L. Simmons, and D. W. Allen: J. Clin. Invest. (U.S.A.) **38**, 161 (1959). — 11. Jandl, J. H.: J. Laborat. Clin. Med. (U.S.A.) **55**, 663 (1960). — 12. Jandl, J. H., and J. H. Katz: J. Clin. Invest. (U.S.A.) **42**, 314 (1963). — 13. Katz, J. H.: J. Clin. Invest. (U.S.A.) **40**, 2143 (1961). — 14. Katz, J. H.: Unpublished observations. — 15. Koechlin, B. A.: J. Amer. Chem. Soc. **74**, 2649 (1952). — 16. Laurell, C. B.: Blood (U.S.A.) **6**, 183 (1951). — 17. Monti, A., M. F. Glynn, and R. J. Dern: J. Laborat. Clin. Med. (U.S.A.) **61**, 272 (1963). — 18. Najean, Y., R. Ardaillou, and J. Bernard: Rev. franç. étud. clin. biol. **5**, 783 (1960). — 19. Najean, Y.: Rev. franç. étud. clin. biol. **7**, 605 (1962). — 20. Paoletti, C.: Compt. rend. Acad. sc. (Fr.) **245**, 377 (1957). — 21. Pease, D. C.: Blood (U.S.A.) **11**, 501 (1956). — 22. Pollycove, M., and R. Mortimer: J. Clin. Invest. (U.S.A.) **40**, 753 (1961). — 23. Schade, A. L.: Personal communication. — 24. Sterling, K.: J. Clin. Invest. (U.S.A.) **30**, 1228 (1951). — 25. Warner, R. C.: Transact. N. Y. Acad. Sc. **16** Ser. 2, 182 (1954). — 26. Weiss, L.: Bull. Johns Hopkins Hosp. (U.S.A.) **108**, 171 (1961). — 27. Wheby, M. S., and L. G. Jones: Clin. Res. (U.S.A.) **10**, 211 (1962). — 28. Zamboni, L., and D. C. Pease: Ultrastructure Res. (U.S.A.) **5**, 65 (1961).

Discussion

SCHAPIRA: Are there any variants of transferrin that are capable of acting on certain types of reticulocyte?

KATZ: I don't know. I might add that the transferrin we have used is of the transferrin C phenotype. I don't know whether this is a result of the particular process that we used for purification, but our preparations show only one transferrin band when run on starch-gel electrophoresis.

J.-C. DREYFUS: Did you work with transferrins from different species, and did you, for example, study the action of human transferrin on animal reticulocytes?

TUBIANA: A few years ago, together with C. PAOLETTI[1], we studied *in vitro* the incorporation into reticulocyte haemoglobin of iron bound to transferrin obtained from different animal species. We found that iron incorporation differed, depending on whether the iron was bound to transferrin of the same species or to transferrin of another species.

KATZ: Yes, I believe Dr. JANDL and co-workers[2] some years ago observed that human tissues could take up iron from conalbumin and rabbit transferrin. I think one of the points which emerges from this is something that may be generally applied to transport proteins, i.e. that they may have a dual function. They may not only serve to carry the transported substance in the plasma, but they may also ensure its delivery to those cells which have a specific need for it. This might be brought about by the sort of interaction I have described with special cell surfaces. Lest transferrin be considered simply as a vehicle for the transport of iron, I would point out that it plays a much more direct role in bringing the iron to those cells which specifically require it for haemoglobin synthesis and in preventing its release to cells which have no need for it.

LONDON: Is there any information available on the extent to which the transferrin which has been treated by neuraminidase will combine with the reticulocytes?

KATZ: No, I only have the qualitative type of data Dr. BEARN mentioned. Despite treatment of transferrin with neuraminidase, the bound iron is still undialysable over a period of 48 or 72 hours. Treatment of the reticulocytes with neuraminidase does depress iron uptake from transferrin, however.[2]

LONDON: Do you have any information on the relative numbers of receptors in erythroid cells younger than reticulocytes as compared with the reticulocytes themselves?

KATZ: It is very difficult, as you know, to handle marrow cells and to get them into suspension satisfactorily. But on the basis of our calculation we would suspect that the number of membrane receptor sites is larger. Dr. JANDL[2] has calculated that, if iron came into all cells at the rate at which it comes into reticulocytes, it would take 14 days to produce the full comple-

---

[1] PAOLETTI, C., M. BOIRON, M. TUBIANA, R. TRUHAUT, and J. BERNARD: Sang (Fr.) **29**, 492 (1958).

[2] JANDL, J. H., J. K. INMAN, R. L. SIMMONS, and D. W. ALLEN: J. Clin. Invest. (U.S.A.) **38**, 161 (1959).

ment of haemoglobin. Since we think that younger cells are much more active in this process, we would guess that they have more receptor sites than do reticulocytes, or that the bound transferrin is turned over more rapidly.

NAJEAN: What proof is there that the uptake of iron from transferrin to reticulocytes requires energy? Many enzymatic inhibitors — for instance, iodo-acetate — are able to block cell respiration, glucose utilisation, and the synthesis of haem without blocking the uptake of iron to any significant degree. A second question I should like to ask is: are the kinetics governing the uptake of transferrin and its release the same with reticulo-endothelial cells as with reticulocytes? Is it conceivable that the receptors of the stroma may be the same in the two kinds of cells, with only a quantitative difference from one cell to another?

TUBIANA: Does the dissociation constant of the bond between iron and transferrin vary in the different physico-chemical conditions?

FINCH: I should just like to emphasise that an understanding of the relationship between the saturation of transferrin and the uptake of iron by the reticulocytes is of considerable clinical significance. Dr. BAINTON[1] carried out a clinical study in which the number of sideroblasts as one parameter was related to the saturation of transferrin, and an excellent correlation was found, suggesting that the amount of excess iron in the developing red cell is correlated to the percent saturation of transferrin.

SALERA: Do you have any information about the kinetic behaviour of different variants of transferrin?

If I understood correctly, you take the slope of the last part of the curve as a measure of the turnover rate of the iodine-labelled transferrin. In this way you find that the half-life varies from 7 to 8 days. This is very similar to the situation in turnover studies with iodine-labelled albumin. The model is represented at least by two pools, A and B, which change with one another. We introduce the tracer into pool A, in which there is a continuous turnover of the substance. At the beginning, all the tracer is found in A and none in B. Subsequently, owing to the change and especially to the transfer of the tracer to B, the radioactivity decreases in A and increases in B until a point of equilibrium is reached, i.e. when the specific activites in A and in B are equal and the same amount of tracer is transferred from A to B as from B to A. After this point of equilibrium is attained, the amount of tracer transferred from A to B is less than that transferred from B to A. So I think that, as a measure of the turnover rate of the substance, it is necessary to take into account the rate at the point of equilibrium, when the amount of the tracer transferred from A to B is equal to that transferred from B to A. The turnover rate is in fact measured from the slope of the tangent at the point of equilibrium.

The problem is in reality still more complex, because part of the protein transferred to the interstitial space (pool B) returns to the plasma (pool A) via the lymphatic pathway.

PETERS: The experiments of Dr. KATZ and Dr. JANDL clearly demonstrate that iron transferrin is readily bound to receptors on the surface of reticulocytes, whereas iron-free transferrin is bound to a much lesser extent. So something must change in the properties of transferrin when it takes up one (or two) atoms of iron. The change could be related to the presence of iron in the molecule. This leads to the question already raised by Dr. FINCH:

[1] BAINTON, D. L.: Amer. J. Med., in press (1964).

how do chelating agents with a particular affinity for iron influence the binding of iron transferrin to reticulocytes? The presence of iron may, however, also induce changes in the molecular configuration of transferrin. This hypothesis would raise another question: transferrin may presumably also form (less stable) complexes with other cations. Are such complexes bound to the surface of reticulocytes?

KATZ: Let me answer Dr. SALERA's question first. The analysis of the transferrin degradation curves that I showed is very unsophisticated. There have been many more complicated analyses of these curves in the last few years. On the other hand, we measured the actual I^{131} excretion from the body with a total-body counter, and the measurements agreed very well with this plasma disappearance curve. TURNBULL and GIBLETT[1] published a paper some years ago on this. They found no difference in the rate of disappearance of iron from transferrin variants as compared with a given individual's own transferrin type.

In answer to Dr. NAJEAN, when a variety of anaerobic or aerobic inhibitors are added to the system of reticulocytes and transferrin, there is a decrease in iron accumulation by reticulocytes. This is accompanied by a somewhat less marked depression in the binding of the protein itself to the surface of the reticulocytes. Also, MAZUR and co-workers[2] postulated some time ago that A.T.P. plays an important role in the transfer of iron from transferrin into liver cells. I have no information as to whether reticulo-endothelial cells are capable of taking up iron from transferrin.

Regarding Dr. TUBIANA's question, we have not determined the stability constants ourselves. Recently, one group of workers[3] calculated it at about 10^{30}. Now if I understood the question correctly, you asked whether there was a change in the stability constants under different physiological conditions. Of course there is a very marked dependence on the pH. However, it is not very noticeable until the pH becomes less than 7.

TUBIANA: My idea was to ask whether the dissociation constant varies with the amount of iron bound to transferrin; because, if iron is first bound by the sites with the tighter bonds, when the transferrin is nearly saturated the iron could become bound to the sites with the looser bonds.

KATZ: No, I do not think this is the case. The workers who calculated the stability constants for the two iron-transferrin binding sites made certain assumptions which led them to conclude that the stability of the first binding site was higher than that of the second. More than 10 years ago, WARNER and WEBER[4] arrived at just the opposite conclusion. They felt that the stability constant of the second iron which was attached to conalbumin was much higher than that of the first. As you know, conalbumin is very similar in its properties to transferrin. This is an important point, because it means that, when we say that a solution is 50% saturated, this would imply that, for all practical purposes, half of the molecules of transferrin contain two iron atoms and half have none. If, however, the first stability constant exceeds the second by a significant amount, then in a 50% saturated solution all of the transferrin molecules would carry only one iron atom.

[1] TURNBULL, A., and E. R. GIBLETT: J. Laborat. Clin. Med. (U.S.A.) **57**, 450 (1961).

[2] MAZUR, A., S. GREEN, and A. CARLETON: J. Biol. Chem. (U.S.A.) **235**, 595 (1960).

[3] DAVIS, B., P. SALTMAN, and S. BENSON: Biochem. Biophys. Res. Commun. (U.S.A.) 8, 56 (1962).

[4] WARNER, R. C., and I. WEBER: J. Amer. Chem. Soc. **75**, 5094 (1953).

Mechanisms of iron storage

By

P. Sturgeon and A. Shoden

> "In this the reader will have several biological and pathological questions which can be answered only with the help of knowledge in which form and combination the iron in organs is deposited. But the answering of this, even with the isolation of ferritin, will be premature, because the absolute topography of iron in organs is needed."
>
> [Laufberger, 1934]

Introduction

With his report on the isolation from horse spleen of a brown-colored iron-heavy compound which he called "ferritin", Laufberger in 1934 established the existence of a new form of storage iron. In the same report it was clearly set forth that the water-solubility of this new material distinguished it from the small, dark, water-insoluble granules known as hemosiderin. The latter could be separated from horse spleen with the help of centrifugation after moderate alkalinization. This water-insoluble iron is generally thought to be identical with the microscopic, Prussian-blue positive granules seen in tissue sections. Originally, these granules were assumed to result from the excessive and rapid destruction of red cells; thus, they were given the name "hemosiderin" by histologists (Cook, 1929).

During the intervening thirty years, study of these compounds has tended to fall into separate scientific disciplines. Ferritin, because of its water-solubility and the fact that it has to attain a high concentration before it can be demonstrated with the Prussian-blue stain *in situ* (Shoden and Richter, 1960), has required biochemical methods for its study. Hemosiderin, in contrast, because of the facility with which it can be seen microscopically and its lack of susceptibility to conventional biochemical methods, has been studied instead by histological methods. Thus, the studies of ferritin have gravitated towards its physico-chemical, biochemical, and immunological properties, while those of hemosiderin have tended to remain in the realm of the anatomist. Combined investigations of both substances have been scarce.

In the last decade, the electron microscope has made possible the study of ferritin in its anatomical sites, as well as of the chemically isolated material. However, lack of attention to the biochemical criteria which LAUFBERGER established in the original definition of ferritin, and failure to distinguish ferritin clearly from hemosiderin in electron-microscopic terms, have introduced a measure of ambiguity into these reports.

During the course of the last ten years, we have conducted, on iron-loaded rabbits, a series of studies dealing with the physical, chemical, and anatomical interrelationships of hemosiderin and ferritin. The fundamental basis for our distinction between these two compounds has been the difference in their water-solubility. This report will review our studies in an attempt to show how the criterion of water-solubility clearly distinguishes between two classes of iron storage compounds which are not only distinct chemically, but are also distinct in the physiological, pharmacological, and anatomical senses. In addition, a theory on the relationship of ferritin to hemosiderin will be advanced, which is in consonance with our own observations as well as with those obtained by means of electron microscopy.

Methods

For the most part, New Zealand white rabbits over six months of age are used in these studies. At the appropriate time, the animals are killed and the livers or other organs are excised and perfused with 0.9% saline. In studies on organs which cannot be readily perfused, the hemoglobin content is measured and subtracted from the total iron determination (SHODEN and STURGEON, 1958). The total wet weight of the organ is determined, and analyses are made on aliquots of the homogenized organ, thus permitting calculation of the total content of the substance under examination.

Fractionation into ferritin and hemosiderin is done by homogenizing the sample in a Waring blendor for approximately five minutes and then extracting with twice its weight of distilled water for one minute in the blendor. The resultant suspension is centrifuged for thirty minutes at 1,400 × G. and the supernatant fluid decanted. Iron determinations are done on the latter for the ferritin content (water-soluble iron). The hemosiderin content (water-insoluble iron) is calculated by subtracting the latter from the total iron.

Separation of the sedimented hemosiderin granules is accomplished by re-suspending the homogenized tissue in twice the weight of distilled water, centrifuging, and discarding the supernatant. This procedure is repeated a total of four times to remove any remaining traces of ferritin. After the last extraction, the residue is again homogenized in twenty volumes of distilled water and then filtered through one layer of gauze. The debris from the tissue cling to the gauze, but the main portion of the hemosiderin granules filters through. The filtering process is repeated four times with progressively increasing layers of gauze up to twenty. The isolated hemosiderin granules are purified further by differential centrifugation. They are suspended in water and centrifuged for five minutes; this permits the heavier particles to settle. The turbid supernatant fluid, which contains the lighter particles, is decanted and discarded. This procedure is repeated until the supernatant fluid is clear.

Iron determinations (LORBER, 1927) are done by digesting the samples in sulfuric and nitric acid 1:1 for fifteen minutes, followed by oxidation with hydrogen peroxide and boiling with distilled water to dissolve completely all iron sulfate. Sulfosalicylic acid is added to develop the color, which is read in a spectrophotometer at 424 mμ.

The above procedures and determinations are common to all studies; the special methods used in specific experiments are described in detail in the individual publications dealing with them.

Results

A. General observations

Normal content of hemosiderin and ferritin in rabbit liver (SHODEN and STURGEON, 1959).

The livers from eleven animals were perfused; they weighed an average of 89.7 g. The means and ranges for total iron, ferritin iron, and hemosiderin iron are given in Table 1. In general, it can be stated that the average rabbit liver contains 9.0 mg. iron with 7 mg. in the form of ferritin and 2 mg. as hemosiderin.

Table 1. *Normal values for rabbit[1] livers*

	Weight (g.)	Iron (mg.)		
		Total	Ferritin	Hemosiderin
Mean	89.7	8.6	6.8	1.8
Range	56—137	5.5—13.2	3.5—9.9	0.9—3.3

[1] Based on 11 animals of 2.5 kg. body-weight or greater.

The iron content of the liver is dependent on the quantity of iron injected rather than on liver size (SHODEN and STURGEON, 1958).

Ten animals were paired at random into five sets, and each set was given a different quantity of iron intravenously, but animals within the sets each received the same quantity. When duplicate animals or organs are compared in terms of iron concentration (mg./100 g. tissue), the agreement is poor (Table 2). However, when total organ contents are compared, irrespective of differences in weights, the agreement is good. This type of relationship is to be expected in view of the fact that the dose of iron in these experiments is not adjusted in proportion to size and that essentially all iron injected is permanently held within the animal. Therefore, after our first series of experiments, all results were analyzed according to total iron rather than iron concentration.

Table 2. *Comparison of liver iron concentration with total liver iron*[1]

Weight. of liver (g.)	Mg. Fe per 100 g. tissue	Total iron in organ (mg.)
68	467	319
106	275	293
121.5	714	868
85.5	982	840
165.5	660	1,090
116	912	1,060
166	747	1,240
133	950	1,260
144	1,080	1,572
116	1,295	1,501

[1] Paired experiments; both animals received the same quantity of iron parenterally.

Physical properties of isolated hemosiderin granules and of ferritin crystals (SHODEN and STURGEON, 1960).

Observations were made under the light microscope of the filtrate obtained after repeated gauze filtrations. The hemosiderin sediment was prepared for histological examination. No identifiable cytological structures are seen in conjunction with individual hemosiderin granules. A few strands of fine, amorphous, fibrillar material are scattered throughout. The individual granules vary in size from less than 1 micron to approximately 5 microns in diameter. The bulk of the preparation consists of dense aggregates of granules which fill an entire oil immersion field. "Purified" material from the final differential centrifugation reveals little alteration in the microscopic character of the hemosiderin granules; however, all of the amorphous material is eliminated. Fig. 1 is a photomicrograph of a "purified" hemosiderin preparation as seen under the microscope after fixation and staining. Grossly, this material, when unstained, makes a uniform brown suspension homogeneous in appearance. In a few hours, however, the heavier granules gradually settle out. Thus, hemosiderin, as defined and presented in these studies, is grossly a relatively homogeneous material, composed microscopically of granules of varying size and degrees of aggregation.

The water-soluble ferritin extract from iron-heavy tissues makes a clear, dark-brown solution. With cadmium sulfate, LAUFBERGER (1937) crystallized a portion of the ferritin; the remainder is referred to as "non-crystallizable ferritin". Under the microscope, the crystals are the shape of a regular octahedron and have a deep reddish-brown color; these are also shown in Fig. 1.

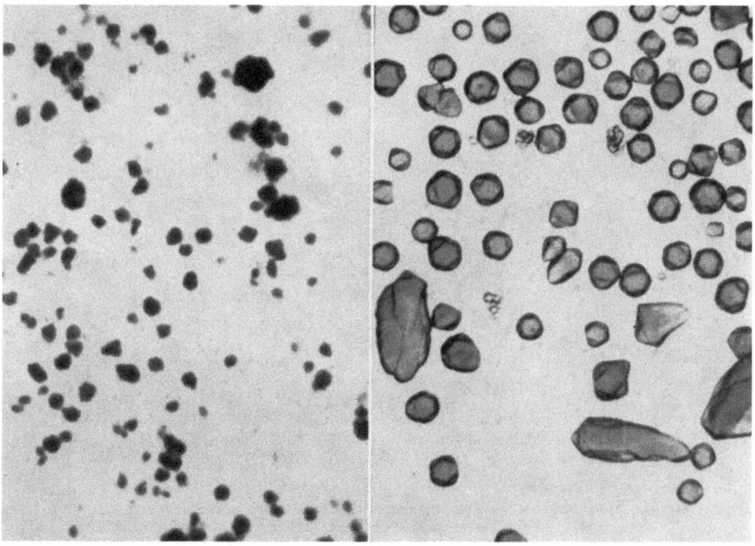

Fig. 1. Left: Hemosiderin granules isolated from rabbit liver, embedded and stained with eosin-hematoxylin and Prussian blue, 100 ×. Right: Ferritin crystals, 100 ×

B. The chemistry of hemosiderin and ferritin

From the preceding it is seen that ferritin and hemosiderin, as defined in these studies, are distinctly different in their gross and microscopic characteristics and in their water-solubility. This could result from alterations in molecular configuration, without any change in basic chemical composition; alternatively, there could be any degree of chemical differences to the extent that, other than iron, the two would have little in common.

Iron-heavy rabbit livers were prepared by injecting 2,000 mg. iron as iron dextran over a period of ten weeks. Human livers were obtained *post mortem* from cases of transfusion hemosiderosis secondary to congenital hypoplastic anemia. In one case, more than 100 liters of blood had been given over an 18-year period.

Hemosiderin granules were subjected to the process of differential centrifugation until the iron/nitrogen ratio reached a maximum. The granules obtained by this procedure were analyzed quantitatively for iron, nitrogen, phosphorus, and sulfur. Their magnetic susceptibility was also measured. In addition, it was found

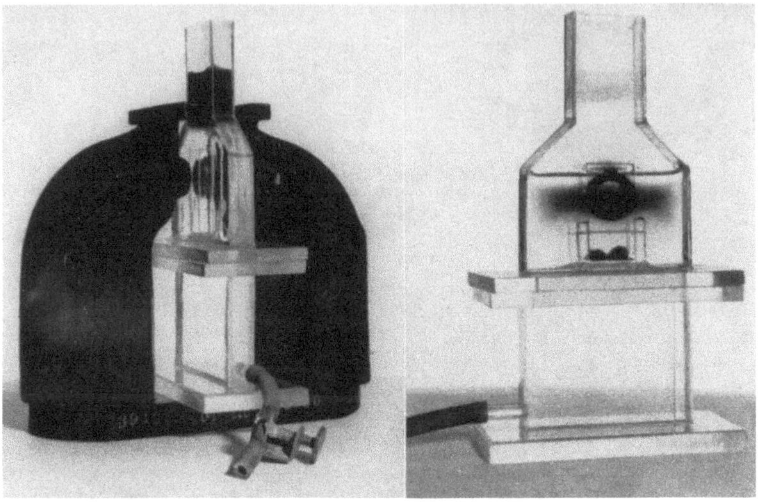

A B

Fig. 2. Magnetic separation cell for isolation of hemosiderin granules directly from tissue homogenates. (A) cell in position; (B) cell showing hemosiderin collection

that these granules as well as ferritin crystals could be dissolved in mercapto-acetic acid, thus making comparative absorption spectra and dialysis experiments possible[1].

Further purification of hemosiderin granules from the last differential centrifugation was attempted with a specially designed apparatus, based on a separation cell positioned between the poles of a 5,000 gauss magnet (Figs 2 A and B). In this procedure, the hemosiderin was separated on the basis of the magnetic susceptibility of its iron. In general, this method did not achieve any further purification over the differential centrifugation method.

Results of chemical analysis of ferritin and hemosiderin are compared in Table 3. The iron content of hemosiderin is sub-

[1] It is realized that mercapto-acetic acid probably acts by splitting S = S bonds, thus effecting a chemical change. However, if the two compounds had an identical matrix, they should behave in the same manner in this medium; therefore comparisons of the dissolved materials are valid.

stantially greater than that of ferritin. The nitrogen content for both human and rabbit hemosiderin is approximately half of that for ferritin, phosphorus is greater, and sulfur is approximately the same. In hemosiderin, the iron/nitrogen ratio is approximately

Table 3. *Chemical analysis of crystallized ferritin and "purified" hemosiderin samples*

Preparation	Percent composition				Ratios		
	Fe	N	P	S	Fe/N	P/N	S/N
Human hemosiderin.	29.0	5.1	2.2	1.14	5.70	0.43	0.223
Human hemosiderin.	24.9	5.8	2.9	1.0	4.30	0.50	0.173
Human hemosiderin.	23.9	5.0	1.9	0.82	4.77	0.38	0.164
Rabbit hemosiderin.	26.7	5.7	3.6	—	4.68	0.63	—
Rabbit hemosiderin.	25.8	7.8	3.4	0.84	3.30	0.44	0.108
Human ferritin . . .	15.3	11.2	1.0	1.06	1.37	0.090	0.094
Human ferritin . . .	16.7	11.7	1.3	0.90	1.42	0.120	0.077
Human ferritin . . .	15.8	11.7	1.0	0.97	1.32	0.086	0.083
Rabbit ferritin . . .	14.9	11.3	1.3	0.90	1.32	0.115	0.080

four times that of ferritin; the phosphorus/nitrogen ratio is four to six times greater, and the sulfur/nitrogen ratio is twice as great. If hemosiderin were simply an iron-heavy ferritin or simply crystallized ferritin, the last two ratios should be the same for both compounds, since it is assumed that they would form part of the organic supporting matrix.

Comparative studies on the magnetic properties of hemosiderin and ferritin show for ferritin ranges of value that are closely grouped between 3.9 and 4.2 Bohr magnetons, while the variations for hemosiderin are significantly greater (3.5 to 4.7).

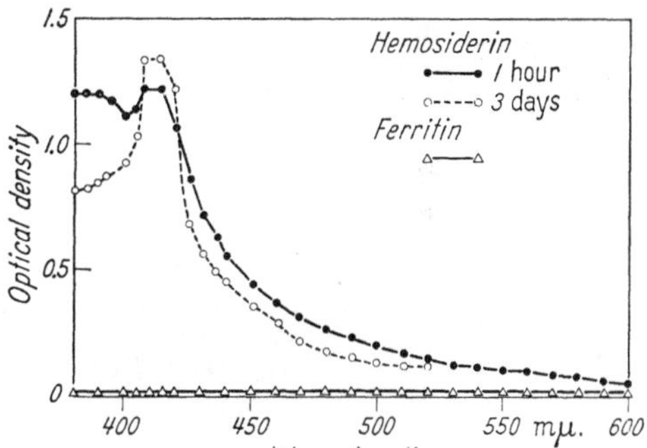

Fig. 3. Comparative light-absorption spectra of storage compounds dissolved in mercapto-acetic acid.

The absorption spectrum of hemosiderin in mercapto-acetic acid is shown in Fig. 3. For comparison, a ferritin curve is also shown; the difference is evident. The peak at 412 mμ appears to be similar to that from hemoglobin; further studies show that this is due to a two carboxyl porphyrin. The porphyrin peak is much less conspicuous in hemosiderin formed as the result of iron injection than in that formed from red-cell destruction.

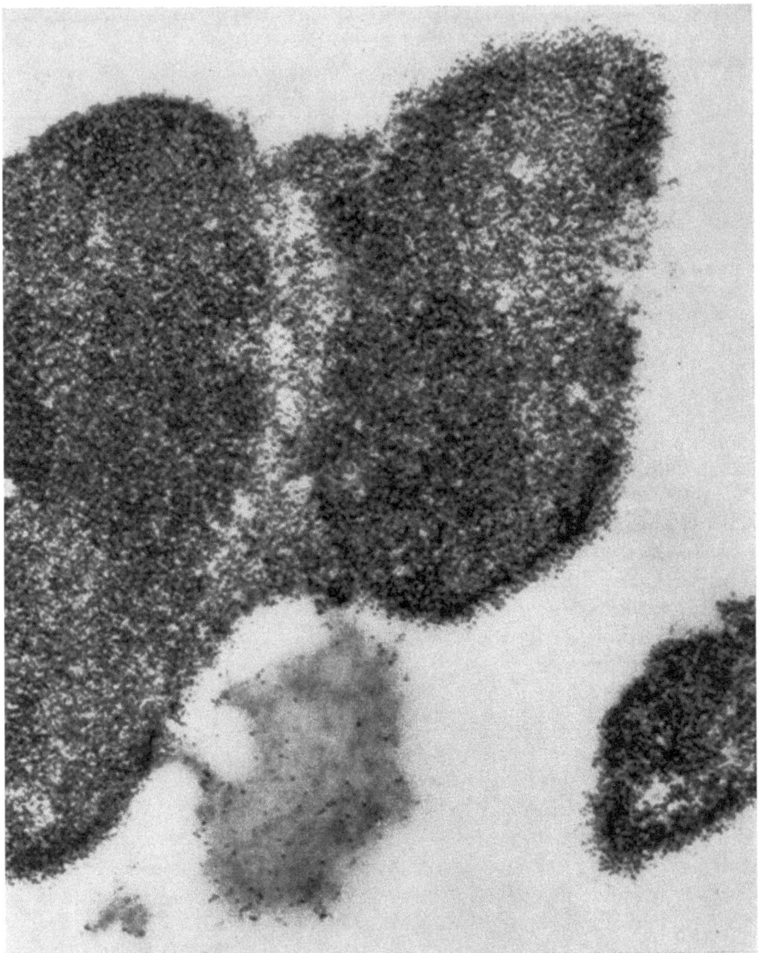

Fig. 4. Electron micrograph of hemosiderin granule from a water-extracted liver homogenate showing closely aggregated electron-dense particles, but no ferritin

Dialysis experiments also show distinct differences between the two compounds when they are dissolved in mercapto-acetic acid (Table 4). It is apparent that the protein component of ferritin has an affinity for iron approximately ten times greater than that of the organic components of hemosiderin.

Table 4. *Affinity, in mercapto-acetic acid, of iron for apoferritin and "hemosiderin protein"*

% iron recovered in dialysate, 2° C.		
Dialysis periods	Ferritin 3 mg. Fe/ml.	Hemosiderin 3 mg. Fe/ml.
First 24 hours	0.84	74.0
Second 24 hours	1.78	17.8
Third 24 hours	1.00	7.2
Total, combined dialysates	3.62	99.0

From these comparative physical and chemical observations on purified hemosiderin and crystallized ferritin, distinct differences are evident in inorganic composition, affinity for iron, absorption spectrum, magnetic susceptibility, and association with porphyrin. It would seem beyond any reasonable doubt, therefore, that hemosiderin represents more than a molecular re-arrangement of ferritin associated with the absorption of additional iron (GRANICK, 1949) or that it is crystallized ferritin, as may be deduced (SHODEN and STURGEON, 1961) from electron-microscopic studies by others. In this latter connection, we submitted purified hemosiderin granules to Dr. RICHTER, who kindly subjected them to electron-microscopic examination (Fig. 4). The electron micrographs showed closely aggregated electron-dense particles, but neither ferritin crystals nor even isolated "tetrads" were evident (SHODEN and STURGEON, 1961).

C. Factors influencing the biochemical distribution of iron in storage compounds

The influence of the quantity of iron injected on the proportion of hemosiderin and ferritin (SHODEN, GABRIO, and FINCH, 1953).

Rabbits were given progressively increasing doses of saccharated iron oxide intravenously until concentrations of 1,500 mg. iron/100 g. tissue were reached. The iron content of the ferritin and hemosiderin fractions was determined; Fig. 5 depicts the results. As the total liver iron load approaches 500 mg./100 g. tissue, the fraction of iron in ferritin exceeds that in hemosiderin. As 250 to 300 mg. ferritin iron is reached, further increases in iron are associated with a leveling off of the ferritin curve; the hemosiderin iron, however, increases indefinitely. These experiments establish that the capacity of the organism to store excess iron as ferritin has definite limits, while its capacity to store hemosiderin is relatively unlimited. Our studies on human tissues, both of adults with hemochromatosis and of children with transfusion hemosiderosis, show the same pattern.

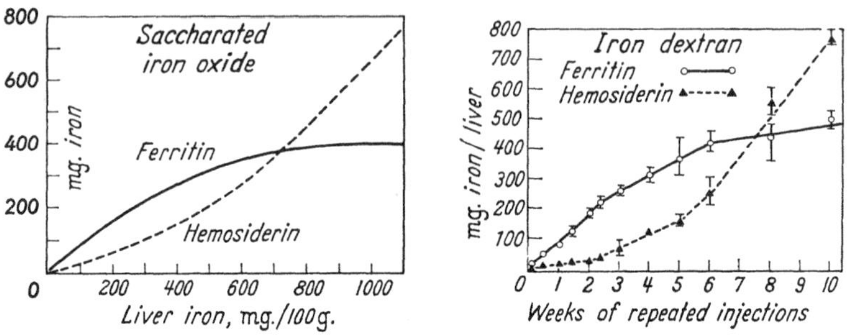

Fig. 5. Pattern of distribution of iron between hemosiderin and ferritin in relation to increasing iron loads established with different preparations

In later experiments it was found that the iron from iron dextran given intravenously followed a different pattern of distribution between ferritin and hemosiderin, particularly at low levels of total liver iron (less than 150–200 mg.), i. e. there is relatively scant hemosiderin formation. Nevertheless, as high loads are reached, the ferritin curve levels off, and hemosiderin rises indefinitely.

The influence of time on the re-distribution of excess storage iron (SHODEN and STURGEON, 1958).

Rabbits were given 2,000 mg. saccharated iron oxide intravenously over a period of six weeks. After the last injection, pairs of animals were killed at one week and at 3, 6, 10, and 14 months. The livers at one week contain 1,250 mg. iron; over the succeeding months, this increases to 1,500 mg., while the iron content of bone marrow, spleen, and kidney decreases; 85% of the injected iron is recovered from these four organs. Within the liver, the total iron and hemosiderin iron increase with time, and ferritin iron decreases; this characteristic sequence of events is summarized in Fig. 6.

These experiments show that re-distribution occurs for the most part during the first three to six months following the loading period. Within the liver, the increase in hemosiderin iron results not only from the intraconversion of ferritin to hemosiderin, but also from the accumulation of iron from other sites. Thus, the time interval between administration of an iron preparation and study of the pattern of iron distribution is a significant variable.

The influence of the type of iron preparation administered on the distribution of iron between ferritin and hemosiderin (SHODEN and STURGEON, 1959).

Five groups of rabbits were started on a series of injections of iron given in 50 mg. doses once a week; a different iron preparation was given to each group. One animal from each group was killed at

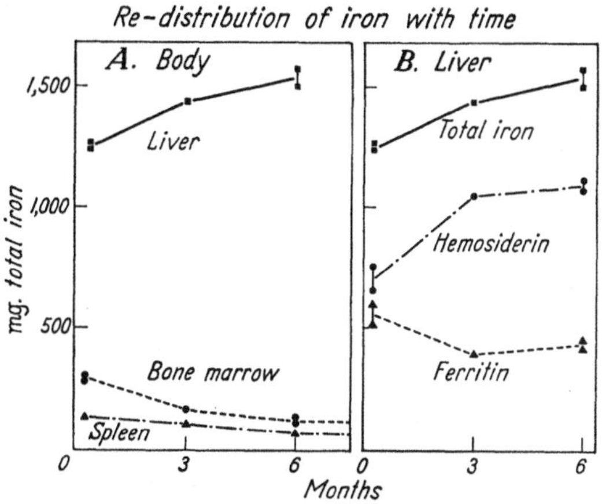

Fig. 6. Influence of time after cessation of iron loading on the pattern of iron distribution in storage compounds at high iron loads

weekly intervals (3–4 days after the last injection) and the livers analyzed for ferritin and hemosiderin as well as total iron. Fig. 7 compares the results from the group that received saccharated iron oxide with those from the group that received iron dextran; these two groups showed the maximum differences. With iron dextran, there is no significant increase in hemosiderin until the quantity of iron injected exceeds 300 mg., whereas with saccharated iron oxide, hemosiderin and ferritin formation go on simultaneously. As the quantity of iron injected brings the total liver iron toward 800 mg. (SHODEN and STURGEON, 1962a), the content of hemosiderin and ferritin becomes equal; once this point is reached, all further increases in liver iron are associated with rising hemosiderin and a steady liver ferritin, irrespective of the type of compound injected.

The question arises whether the water-soluble iron from livers of animals given iron dextran, as in the above experiment, might not be simply native iron dextran temporarily stored intracellularly. That this is not the case is seen in data from subsequent radioisotopic studies (SHODEN and STURGEON, 1963). There it was found that the specific activity of water-soluble iron in animals studied within four days of receiving a large dose of iron dextran, preceded several weeks by a tracer dose of $Fe^{55}Cl_3$, was the same as that of the crystallized ferritin.

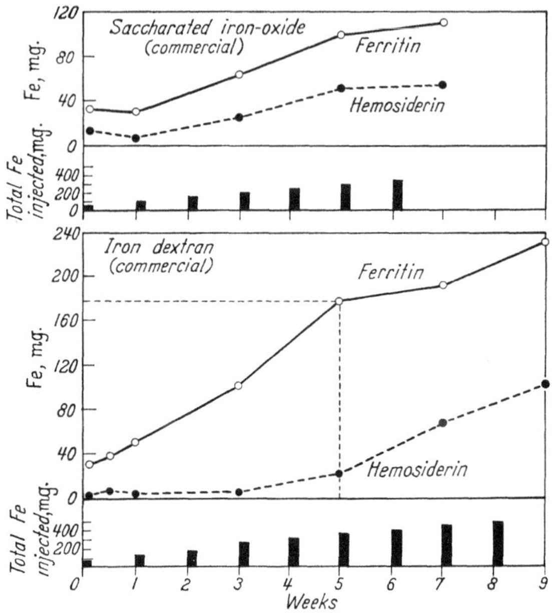

Fig. 7. Influence of the type of preparation administered on the pattern of distribution of iron in storage compounds at low iron loads

From these last experiments, where levels of iron load and intervals after injection are kept constant, it is evident that the types of preparation injected also influence the distribution of iron between hemosiderin and ferritin. Among numerous considerations on the properties of such preparations that could influence the distribution of iron, there was the possibility that the rate of release of iron might be a factor.

In this connection the observation was made that tracer doses of $Fe^{59}Cl_3$, given along with the injection of each preparation, followed clearance and utilization patterns of the accompanying iron compound. These findings are summarized in Table 5. The counts given along with the iron dextran cleared at approximately $^1/_3$ the rate of those given with an equal quantity of saccharated iron; nevertheless, red-cell utilization of the dextran counts was substantially faster. This latter phenomenon, however, probably bears little relation to deposition of iron in storage forms; but the slow rate of clearance of iron from the dextran preparation could account for the preference of its iron for ferritin rather than for hemosiderin.

Table 5. *Distribution of radioactivity*[1] *in plasma during the first week following intravenous injection of 50 mg. iron as saccharated iron oxide and iron dextran*

	1 hr	3 hrs	6 hrs	1 day	3 days	1 week
Sacc. iron oxide . .	114,000	82,500	36,700	2,000	0	0
Iron dextran . . .	—	144,000	103,000	37,700	1,500	0

[1] c.p.m. per 100 ml.

The influence of rates of administration of iron on its distribution between ferritin and hemosiderin (SHODEN and STURGEON, 1962a).

This series of experiments was designed to test the hypothesis that hemosiderin formation occurs not only when the total iron load is great, but also when the influx of iron exceeds the capacity of the ferritin mechanism to clear the circulation. An acute experiment was designed around two groups of thirty-two animals each; the groups were given iron dextran and saccharated iron oxide, respectively. Within the groups, four sub-groups received the intravenous preparations in quantities to provide in a single dose 25, 50, 100, and 200 mg. iron. Four animals from each subgroup were killed at 24 hours and one week following the injections. The results from the study of all 64 animals are given in Fig. 8. On the left are those from the 32 animals used in the 24-hour experiment and on the right those from the 32 animals of the one-week experiment.

From the 24-hour experiment it is apparent that ferritin formation approximates its maximum with a 50 mg. dose of either preparation. A fourfold increase in this dose increases the 24-hour ferritin production little, if any. Thus, for the full-grown rabbit, the maximum rate of liver ferritin iron production is in the order of 1 mg./hour. It also bears emphasis, with iron dextran, that despite the presence in the circulation of iron in excessive amounts, there is no stimulus to hemosiderin formation. Thus, this experiment does not support the hypothesis that hemosiderin formation is activated under all conditions of rapid loading. With saccharated iron oxide, hemosiderin formation begins substantially before the rate of ferritin synthesis reaches its maximum. Nevertheless, when the latter's maximum is reached, hemosiderin formation continues to increase with increasing dose. It is apparent that the two compounds, when injected intravenously, are handled differently by the liver.

At the one-week interval, after the preparations clear the serum, the iron dextran curve shows further deposition of iron, but essentially all as ferritin; the net rate of the latter is 10 to 11 mg./day. With the saccharated iron oxide, the total liver iron remains

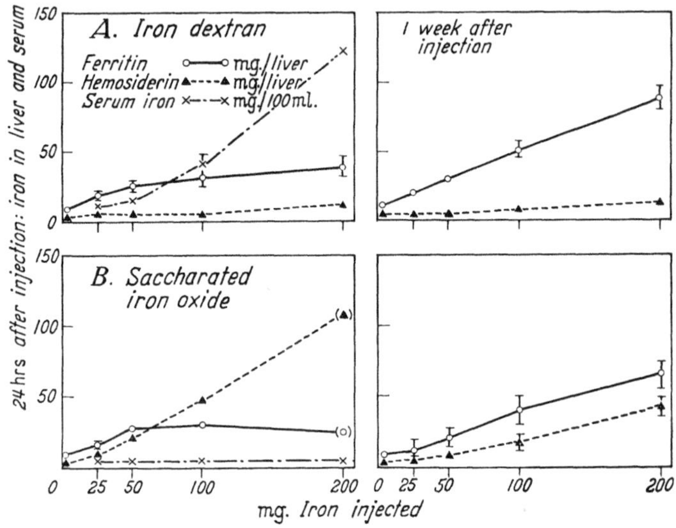

Fig. 8. Influence of dose and type of preparation on the pattern of iron distribution at different times after single injections

essentially constant, but there is an internal re-distribution, i.e. hemosiderin iron shifts to ferritin. This, incidentally, is just the opposite in direction of the "shift with time" seen at higher levels of iron loading. This latter sequence of events, when viewed independently of the iron dextran observation, would tend to indicate that hemosiderin formation represents a mechanism for clearance of iron from the serum. However, when the two series are compared, it appears that the early deposition of hemosiderin is a unique pharmacological property of saccharated iron oxide rather than being dependent on the rate at which the liver cells are presented with iron. This is confirmed by the fact that the same rate of ferritin production was achieved with iron dextran at one day, yet no hemosiderin deposition occurred in spite of a great excess of this preparation in the serum.

To further substantiate this point, a group of rabbits was given saccharated iron oxide in a dose which would supply to the liver 10 mg. iron per day; that is, at approximately one-half of the liver's ferritin iron production capacity of approximately 24 mg./day. This dose was given for five consecutive days per week for a four-week period. Therefore, were hemosiderin formation rate-dependent, none should occur under these circumstances. An experiment was conducted in parallel with the week's dose given as a single injection. The rates of hemosiderin formation under both conditions were identical, as shown in Fig. 9. This again confirms that the formation of hemosiderin with saccharated iron oxide, in the early phase of loading, is more an inherent pharmacological property of the preparation than it is dependent upon the rate of release of iron from its carrier.

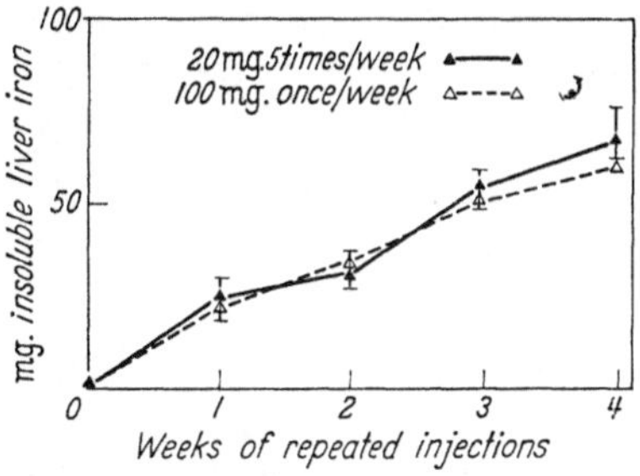

Fig. 9. Influence of the rate of injection of saccharated iron oxide on the rate of hemosiderin formation at low iron loads

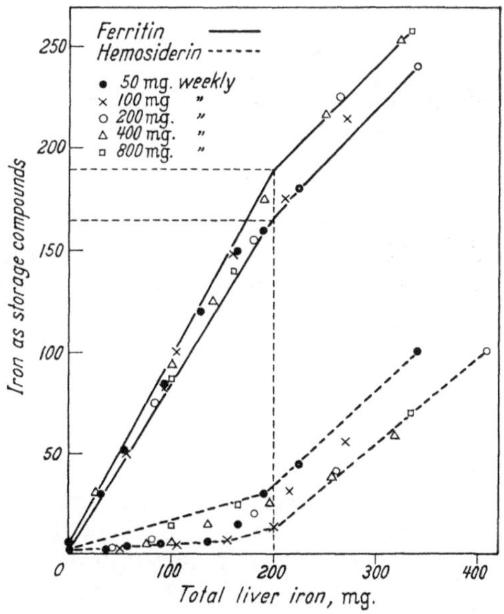

Fig. 10. Composite curve from five experiments on the influence of increasing doses of iron dextran on the formation of ferritin and hemosiderin in relation to total liver iron

Finally, as the rate of injection was gradually increased from 50 to 800 mg. iron per week, the observation was made, particularly from examination of the iron dextran curves, that hemosiderin deposition begins at time intervals inversely proportional to the rate of the injection. Thus, when all the curves are re-plotted as a composite with ferritin and hemosiderin iron as functions of total liver iron, Fig. 10 is obtained. It shows, after the ferritin iron approximates 150–200 mg., that there is a sharp increase in the rate of hemosiderin formation. Again this confirms that hemosiderin formation, with the injection of iron dextran, is essentially independent of the rate of administration, but that it is triggered when the total ferritin iron reaches the "critical ferritin level" of 150–200 mg.

D. The anatomy of hemosiderin formation

The preceding quantitative biochemical studies bring to light two important phases in the course of iron loading experiments. Each phase is related to the total iron load and is associated with characteristic phenomena.

At low levels of iron storage (in the range of 0–150 mg. total liver iron), with the injection of iron dextran, approximately 90% of the iron goes to ferritin. When the "critical" 150–200 mg. ferritin iron level is reached, only then does the proportion going to hemosiderin increase. This sequence is not influenced by size or frequency of dose. With saccharated iron oxide, the rate of ferritin formation has an upper limit, which is comparable to that seen with iron dextran. However, at these low levels, hemosiderin deposition goes on simultaneously with ferritin synthesis, but it tends to shift rapidly to ferritin; thus, upon cessation of injection, ferritin iron continues to increase at the expense of hemosiderin. The second characteristic phase is approached as further loading brings both the ferritin and hemosiderin iron to 400 mg. each, i.e. from the point of ferritin-hemosiderin equivalence and beyond. Further administration of either iron dextran or saccharated iron oxide results only in additional hemosiderin formation.

In view of the above "preparation" and "load" related phenomena, as seen with quantitative biochemical studies, it becomes evident that knowledge of their anatomic counterparts could lead to a better understanding of them. Therefore several of the previous experiments were repeated in parallel with conventional histochemical studies.

The sequence of events, with the injection of increasing doses of iron dextran, is summarized in Table 6 and Fig. 11. The outstanding feature of these experiments is the absence of stainable iron in both the Kupffer and parenchymal cells up to a total liver iron load in excess of 100 mg. The appearance of substantial numbers of positive Prussian-blue granules occurs at the "critical point" where, with biochemical methods, the water-insoluble fraction makes its first sharp increase. Thus, with iron dextran, it is evident that hemosiderin formation is a phenomenon of the parenchymal cell and that a substantial excess of iron may be present in the liver as ferritin, negative histochemical evidence notwithstanding.

Table 6. *Iron dextran. Comparison of biochemical data and anatomic pattern of iron deposition with increasing iron load*

	Iron injected (mg.)						
	(Control) 0	50	100	200	400	800	1,600
Total liver iron, mg.	7	30	54	98	210	408	1,048
Total water-soluble iron, mg.	6	28	51	88	191	290	494
Total water-insoluble iron, mg.	1	2	3	10	19	118	554
Parenchymal-cell granules .	0	0	0	±	+	+++	++++
Kupffer-cell granules. . . .	0	0	0	±	±	±	±

With the injection of saccharated iron oxide, the anatomic pattern is distinctly different; this is summarized in Table 7 and in Fig. 12. Prussian-blue positive granules become immediately evident in the Kupffer cells with the 50 mg. injection. At the 400 mg. dose level, a large proportion of Kupffer cells contains stainable granules. The ferritin iron meanwhile reaches 152 mg. and, for the first time, granules begin to appear in the parenchymal cells.

Table 7. *Saccharated iron oxide. Comparison of biochemical data and anatomic pattern of iron deposition with increasing iron load*

	Iron injected (mg.)						
	(Control) 0	50	100	200	400	800	1,600
Total liver iron, mg.	7	38	49	94	213	495	1,055
Total water-soluble iron, mg. .	6	20	28	65	152	354	534
Total water-insoluble iron, mg.	1	18	21	28	61	141	521
Parenchymal-cell granules . .	0	0	0	0	±	++	+++
Kupffer-cell granules.	0	+	+	+	++	++	+++

These observations account for the difference in the pattern of biochemical distribution noted previously with iron dextran and saccharated iron oxide. At the early stages of iron loading with saccharated iron oxide, hemosiderin formation is confined to the

Kupffer cells, which it would appear — along with other reticulo-endothelial cells — have the capacity to clear it, whereas iron dextran tends to remain in the circulation with its rate of clearance

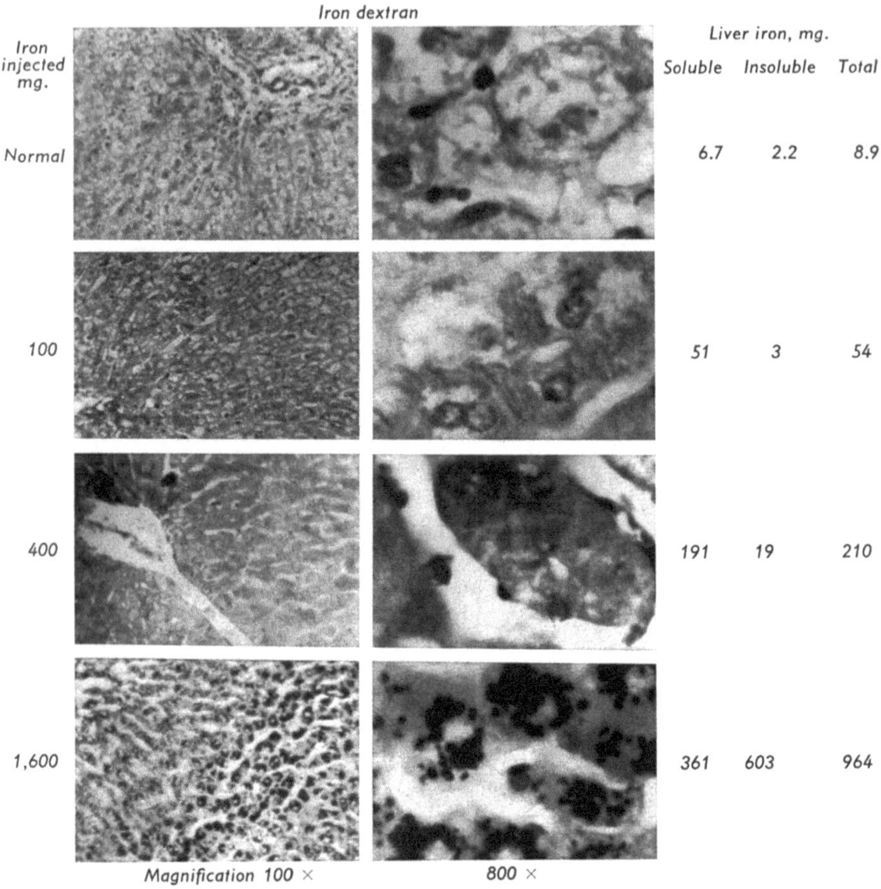

Fig. 11. Influence of increasing doses of iron dextran on the anatomic distribution of hemosiderin; comparison with the biochemical distribution of storage compounds

limited by the capacity of the liver to form ferritin. The explanation for the difference in behavior between these two compounds has been advanced that saccharated iron oxide is, or upon injection forms, a colloid which is susceptible to the phagocytic activity of Kupffer cells. Conversely, iron dextran is in a class of colloid which, when given intravenously, is not cleared by the reticulo-endothelial system (Shoden and Sturgeon, 1962a). In this connection, note

Saccharated iron oxide

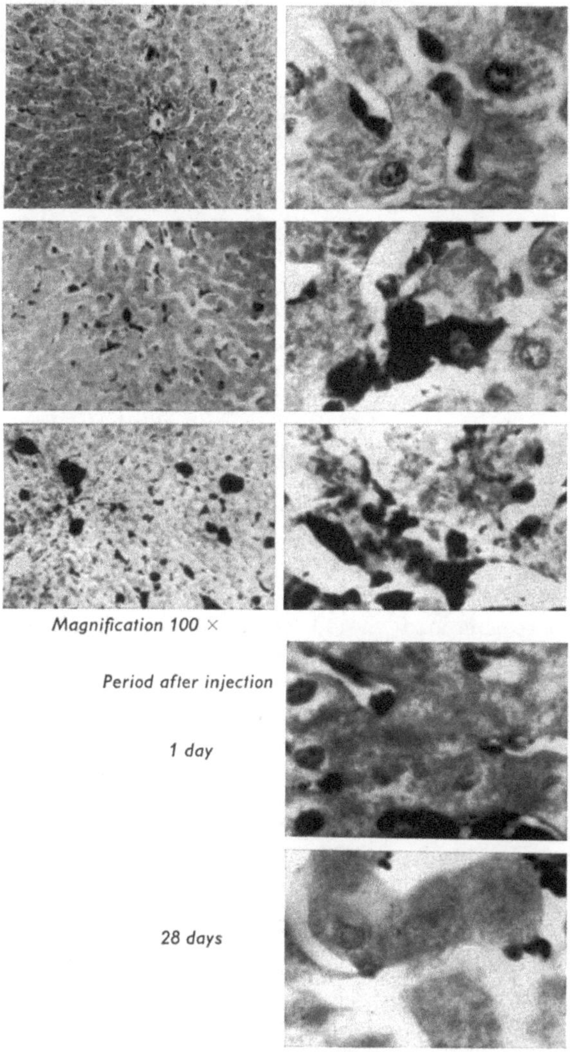

Iron injected mg.	Period after injection	Liver iron, mg. Soluble	Insoluble	Total
100		28	21	49
400		152	61	213
1,600		468	543	1,011
300	1 day	91	60	151
300	28 days	125	36	161

Magnification 100 ×

Magnification 800 ×

Fig. 12. Influence of increasing doses of saccharated iron oxide on the anatomic distribution of hemosiderin; comparison with the biochemical distribution of storage compounds should also be taken of the electron-microscopic studies by RICHTER (1959) on iron preparations given intraperitoneally to rats. These indicate that the histochemically demonstrable iron ("hemosiderin") in liver macrophages at the early stage may be for the most part the native preparation, or iron released from it, rather than aggregates of iron micelles which characterize indigenous hemosiderin. In our studies, saccharated iron oxide may have followed such a pattern of utilization; however, with iron dextran given intravenously to rabbits, essentially no Kupffer-cell iron deposits are formed.

The transient nature, as seen in our quantitative biochemical studies, of the early hemosiderin deposits associated with the injection of saccharated iron oxide, is also evident in these anatomic studies as shown at the bottom of Fig. 12. At the liver iron load associated with the injection of 300 mg. iron, Kupffer-cell hemosiderin is plainly evident; however, it diminishes distinctly over a 28-day interval. Simultaneously, the amount of liver ferritin iron, as demonstrated biochemically, increases from 91 to 125 mg. It is particularly noteworthy that, histochemically, as this latter ferritin level is attained, there is an associated early appearance of faint blue parenchymal-cell vacuoles.

Finally, it should also be noted that, with both preparations, the appearance of the faint blue vacuoles occurs characteristically when the liver ferritin iron reaches its critical 150–200 mg. level. These vacuoles are particularly prominent in the periphery of liver lobules. With increasing load, these become the sites of formation of typical dense blue staining hemosiderin granules. Water extraction, prior to fixation of tissues heavily laden with such granules, reveals that all of the water-soluble iron can be recovered. Subsequent histochemical studies show no diminution in the intensity of staining or in the size or number of these parenchymal-cell hemosiderin granules. Thus, these granules could not simply be crystallized ferritin but, if derived from ferritin, they must represent a more fundamentally altered form and, having lost their water-solubility, they can no longer be ferritin according to the original chemical definition by LAUFBERGER.

In view of the above observations, along with the evidence from electron microscopy, we have advanced the hypothesis that the above intracellular faint blue vacuoles represent regions of ferritin saturation or even "crystallization", which then undergo denaturation and finally become relatively protein-free aggregates of ferritin iron micelles. We propose that these aggregates are the biochemical equivalent of hemosiderin granules (SHODEN and

STURGEON, 1961) and might be designated "true" or "mature" hemosiderin. Thus, these combined studies suggest a theory which provides an adequate explanation for all of the biochemical quantitative phenomena observed previously and for the qualitative difference in the biochemical pattern of distribution when iron dextran and saccharated iron oxide are injected. It also reconciles any differences between our studies and those done with the electron microscope.

Table 8 diagrams this theory on the stages in the transformation of parenchymal-cell ferritin into hemosiderin and relates these to the histochemical, biochemical, and electron-microscopic properties at the various stages. From the diagram it is suggested that at the second and third stages of iron loading, a faintly positive Prussian-blue reaction may be obtained. Histochemically, therefore, the term "hemosiderin" is applicable and, as a consequence, in histochemical terms, hemosiderin does encompass iron compounds that are water-soluble and may show in the electron microscope typical ferritin iron-micelle structures. Nevertheless, it bears considerable emphasis that these are, according to the theory, transition forms between ferritin (stage 1) and the fully developed or "mature" hemosiderin granule (stage 4). It must also be emphasized that in heavily iron-laden states (where the water-insoluble iron content is substantially greater than the soluble or where histochemically typical dark blue staining parenchymal-cell hemosiderin granules are in abundance) a significant part of the iron may be in the stage of dispersed ferritin, but the bulk of it will be in the form of mature hemosiderin granules. Under these circumstances, transition forms should be relatively infrequent; in the early phases of iron loading, they should also be essentially absent. The preceding theory and related concepts on the evolution of iron storage compounds, as induced artificially in the rabbit, are in essential agreement with those arrived at independently by RICHTER (1960) from electron-microscopic, histochemical, chemical, and serological studies of storage iron from cases of hemochromatosis and hemosiderosis in humans.

E. The kinetics of iron storage

As a corollary to the theoretical model advanced above, it follows that ferritin formation in parenchymal cells should always precede that of hemosiderin; thus, iron movement within parenchymal cells would be first to ferritin, thence to hemosiderin. To test this corollary, a series of radio-isotopic experiments was done,

Table 8. *Comparative classification and nomenclature of stages in the evolution of iron storage compounds as observed with various techniques*

Technique	Stages of iron loading			
	1st (0—100)[1]	2nd (100—150)	3rd (150—200)	4th (200 and greater)
Histochemistry (Prussian blue)	Negative	Negative to faint vacuoles	Faint vacuoles	Dark blue granules
Biochemistry (water-solubility)	Soluble; apoferritin matrix	Soluble; apoferritin matrix	Insoluble; denatured matrix	Insoluble; degenerated matrix
Electron microscopy (ferritin hexads)	Dispersed	Clusters or crystals	Clusters or crystals	Powder aspect (1) Aggregated micelles (2)
Nomenclature				
Histochemistry		Hemosiderin ("pre")	Hemosiderin ("pre")	Hemosiderin ("mature")
Biochemistry	Ferritin	Ferritin	Hemosiderin	Hemosiderin
Electron microscopy	Ferritin	Hemosiderin ? / Ferritin ?	Hemosiderin ? / Ferritin ?	Ferruginous micelles (1) / Indigenous hemosiderin (2)

[1] Numbers in brackets are hypothetical liver iron load in mg. (1) Bessis (1959) (2) Richter (1959, 1960).

taking advantage of the properties of intravenously administered iron dextran as the loading preparation. This avoids the complication of early deposition of hemosiderin in Kupffer cells.

As an example of one such experiment, eight rabbits were injected with 2,000 mg. iron; three were studied five days after the last injection to establish the control level of iron compounds in the liver. The remaining five were given, on four consecutive days, 10 mg. iron as iron dextran; this was mixed with a few μc. of $Fe^{59}Cl_3$ (activity: 625,000 c.p.m.). Two of the radio-isotope tagged rabbits were studied 16 days and two others 67 days after the last injection. Table 9 briefly summarizes the results. It shows the characteristic biochemical changes in the pattern of iron distribution with time. At these high levels, slightly more than one-half of the total iron injected is found in the liver (1,257 mg.). In spite of the fact that during the 16-day interval following injection of the

Table 9. *Comparison, in iron-loaded rabbits, of the shifts from ferritin to hemosiderin of iron and radioactivity during 67 days*

	Iron, mg.			Fe^{59} c.p.m. × 10^3	
	Control	+ 16 days	+ 67 days	+ 16 days	+ 67 days
Ferritin	497	415	373	1,090	515
Hemosiderin. .	760	900	968	690	1,200
Total	1,257	1,315	1,341	1,780	1,715

Fe^{59} there is absolutely no increase in the ferritin compartment, 61% of the activity is found in ferritin. This indicates that, even at these high levels, new iron is used for ferritin formation; concomitantly, because there is an actual decrease in ferritin iron, there must be a transfer of older ferritin iron to hemosiderin. Over the subsequent 67 days, without injection of additional iron, the hemosiderin compartment increases further in size at the expense of the ferritin compartment; there is an associated shift of radioactivity. It should be noted, during this 16 to 67-day interval, that half of the remaining radioactivity moves from ferritin to hemosiderin, while somewhat less than one-tenth of the iron follows the same path. This latter sequence was also noted in double isotope experiments, where recently administered Fe^{59} shifts more rapidly from ferritin to hemosiderin than does earlier administered Fe^{55}.

Analysis of these data and those from several similar experiments leads to the conclusion that there is a direct transformation of ferritin iron into parenchymal-cell hemosiderin and that the more recently administered iron has a higher priority for transfer. In view of our histochemical studies, which show that the cells in the periphery of the liver lobule participate more actively in hemosiderin production than the centrally located cells, an explanation for this phenomenon of rapid transfer of more recently administered iron is suggested. While all cells may be approaching saturation with ferritin, the peripheral cells, being more active in the uptake of iron, will have reached their saturation point (critical level) first. These cells would thus be converting their ferritin to hemosiderin and, in turn, more actively synthesizing new ferritin. It follows, then, that recently administered iron would tend to be taken up as ferritin in these cells and to go through the transformation to hemosiderin, while ferritin iron in the balance of the cells remains relatively static.

The interpretations of the data on kinetic studies of iron storage are therefore also consistent with the theory we have proposed for the evolution of iron storage compounds, at least as found in the rabbit liver parenchymal cell.

Summary

Ferritin and mature hemosiderin are physically, biochemically, and physiologically distinctly different. For the study of these two classes of compound, and of iron storage mechanisms in general, the difference in their water-solubility provides a most useful tool. Water-solubility was the original basis on which iron storage compounds were distinguished, and it remains the least ambiguous as well as a very practical basis for their classification.

Biochemically, several variables influence the pattern of iron distribution in storage compounds of the liver when iron preparations are injected intravenously into rabbits; these include: the rate of injection, the amount and type of preparation injected, and the time interval from injection to observation.

Histochemically, ferritin iron may be demonstrable by the Prussian-blue technique when the ferritin becomes sufficiently concentrated to be near or at its saturation point. However, quantities of iron greatly in excess of normal may be present as ferritin, despite negative histochemical evidence. Kupffer-cell hemosiderin formation is observed only when certain types of preparation are administered. At low levels of loading, Kupffer-cell hemosiderin shows a tendency to diminish with time in a reciprocal relationship with ferritin. Parenchymal-cell hemosiderin formation is observed only when higher iron loads are reached; it is independent of the preparation administered and occurs only after the liver ferritin reaches a critical level.

From these observations the theory has been advanced that the formation of parenchymal-cell storage compounds begins with intracellularly dispersed ferritin which, as the iron level increases, becomes concentrated in vacuoles and may form "clusters" or "crystals". At this point, denaturation of the apoferritin matrix is associated with loss of water-solubility, which in biochemical terms marks the change from ferritin to hemosiderin. This is followed by degradation of the apoferritin matrix, then aggregation of the iron micelles into what we propose should be called true or mature hemosiderin. The fact that iron-kinetic studies show that radioactivity invariably goes first to ferritin, thence to hemosiderin, is in good agreement with this theory.

Zusammenfassung

Ferritin und „reifes“ Haemosiderin sind physikalisch, biochemisch und physiologisch voneinander verschieden. Für die Untersuchung dieser beiden Klassen von Verbindungen und der der Eisenspeicherung im allgemeinen zugrunde liegenden Mechanismen stellt ihre verschiedene Wasserlöslichkeit ein geeignetes Hilfsmittel dar. Die ursprünglich für die Unterscheidung der Speichereisenverbindungen als Grundlage herangezogene Wasserlöslichkeit ist auch heute noch die am wenigsten zweideutige und gleichzeitig zweckmäßige Basis für ihre Einteilung.

In biochemischer Hinsicht beeinflussen mehrere Veränderliche die Art der Eisenverteilung in Speicherverbindungen, die in der Leber des Kaninchens nach intravenöser Injektion von Eisenpräparaten auftreten. Die pro Zeiteinheit injizierte Menge, die Art und die Dosis des Präparates sind dafür ebenso von Bedeutung wie die Zeitspanne, die von der Injektion bis zur Beobachtung verstreicht.

Histochemisch kann Ferritineisen mit der Berlinerblau-Reaktion nachgewiesen werden, vorausgesetzt, daß es genügend konzentriert wird, um nahe beim oder am Sättigungspunkt zu sein. Ferritineisen kann jedoch auch in übernormalen Mengen vorhanden sein und sich trotzdem dem histochemischen Nachweis entziehen. Eine Haemosiderinbildung in den Kupfferschen Sternzellen ist nur nach Gabe bestimmter Eisenpräparate zu beobachten. Bei geringer Beladung der Kupfferschen Zellen zeigt Haemosiderin mit der Zeit eine Tendenz zur Abnahme, und zwar in einem reziproken Verhältnis zu Ferritin. Haemosiderinbildung in Parenchymzellen ist nur unter stärkerer Eisenbelastung zu beobachten; sie ist unabhängig von der Art des verabreichten Eisenpräparates und tritt erst auf, nachdem Ferritin in der Leber einen kritischen Wert erreicht hat.

Diese Beobachtungen haben zu der Theorie geführt, daß die Bildung von Speicherverbindungen in Parenchymzellen mit intrazellulär dispers verteiltem Ferritin beginnt, welches sich bei Zunahme des Eisengehaltes in Vakuolen konzentriert und zu „Haufen“ oder „Kristallen“ zusammenballt. In diesem Stadium geht die Denaturierung der Apoferritinmatrix mit einem Verlust der Wasserlöslichkeit einher, was in biochemischer Hinsicht den Wechsel von Ferritin zu Haemosiderin bedeutet. Anschließend kommt es zu einem Abbau der Apoferritinmatrix und dann zu einer Aggregation von Eisenmicellen, für die wir die Bezeichnung „echtes“ oder „reifes“ Haemosiderin vorschlagen. Der bei Untersuchungen über die Eisenkinetik erhobene Befund, daß die Radioaktivität stets zuerst an Ferritin und erst dann an Haemosiderin geht, stimmt mit dieser Theorie gut überein.

Résumé

La ferritine et l’hémosidérine «à maturité» sont nettement différentes des points de vue physique, biochimique et physiologique. Leur différence de solubilité dans l’eau est un critère très utile pour l’étude de ces deux classes de composés ainsi que pour l’étude des mécanismes du stockage du fer en général. La solubilité dans l’eau a été la première base de distinction entre les différentes formes de dépôts du fer, et elle reste encore le principe de classification le moins aléatoire en même temps que très pratique.

Sur le plan biochimique, plusieurs facteurs influencent la distribution du fer dans les divers composés qui sont déposés dans le foie après injection intra-veineuse de fer au lapin, à savoir: la vitesse d'injection, la quantité et la nature de la préparation injectée, le temps écoulé entre l'injection et l'observation.

On peut mettre en évidence histochimiquement le fer de la ferritine par le bleu de Prusse quand la concentration de la ferritine approche ou atteint la saturation. Mais des quantités de fer de beaucoup supérieures à la normale peuvent exister sous forme de ferritine malgré une réaction histochimique négative. La formation d'hémosidérine dans les cellules de Kupffer ne s'observe après administration que de certaines préparations. A de basses concentrations, l'hémosidérine des cellules de Kupffer montre une tendance à diminuer avec le temps, inversement proportionnellement à la ferritine. La formation d'hémosidérine dans le parenchyme ne s'observe que pour des hautes concentrations; elle est indépendante de la nature de la préparation administrée et ne survient qu'une fois que la ferritine a atteint dans le foie un seuil critique.

De ces observations on a déduit une théorie selon laquelle le point de départ de la formation des composés déposés dans les cellules parenchymateuses est la ferritine disséminée dans les cellules, ferritine qui, lorsque le taux de fer augmente, se concentre dans des vacuoles en pouvant former des «amas» ou des «cristaux». A ce stade, la dénaturation de la matrice d'apoferritine s'accompagne d'une perte de solubilité dans l'eau, c'est-à-dire, en termes biochimiques, d'une transformation de la ferritine en hémosidérine. Puis vient la dégradation de la matrice d'apoferritine suivie de l'assemblage des micelles ferriques pour former ce que nous proposons d'appeler l'hémosidérine «vraie» ou «à maturité». Le fait que, comme le montrent les études sur la cinétique du fer, la radioactivité aille invariablement d'abord sur la ferritine, puis sur l'hémosidérine, est en parfait accord avec cette théorie.

References

BESSIS, M. C., and J. BRETON-GORIUS: Blood (U.S.A.) **14**, 423 (1959). — COOK, S. F.: J. Biol. Chem. (U.S.A.) **82**, 595 (1929). — GRANICK, S.: Bull. N. Y. Acad. Med. **25**, 403 (1949). — LAUFBERGER, V.: Biol. listy (Czech.) **19**, 73 (1934). — LAUFBERGER, V.: Bull. Soc. chim. biol. (Fr.) **19**, 1575 (1937). — LORBER, L.: Biochem. Zschr. (G.) **181**, 391 (1927). — RICHTER, G. W.: J. Exper. Med. (U.S.A.) **109**, 197 (1959). — RICHTER, G. W.: J. Exper. Med. (U.S.A.) **112**, 551 (1960). — SHODEN, A., B. W. GABRIO, and C. A. FINCH: J. Biol. Chem. (U.S.A.) **204**, 823 (1953). — SHODEN, A., and G. W. RICHTER: Fol. hemat. (G.) **4**, 180 (1960). — SHODEN, A., and P. STURGEON: Amer. J. Path. **34**, 1139 (1958). — SHODEN, A., and P. STURGEON: Acta haemat. (Switz.) **22**, 140 (1959). — SHODEN, A., and P. STURGEON: Acta haemat. (Switz.) **23**, 376 (1960). — SHODEN, A., and P. STURGEON: Nature (G.B.) **189**, 846 (1961). — SHODEN, A., and P. STURGEON: Acta haemat. (Switz.) **27**, 33 (1962a). — SHODEN, A., and P. STURGEON: Amer. J. Path. **40**, 671 (1962b). — SHODEN, A., and P. STURGEON: Brit. J. Haemat. (in press, 1963).

Discussion

CHATTERJEA: I should like to know from Dr. STURGEON the pattern of distribution of haemosiderin in the Kupffer cells and in the liver parenchyma in chronic haemolytic anaemias. Do you have any observation to make on the trend and sequence of distribution of haemosiderin in haemolytic syndromes?

STURGEON: We have not studied pathological conditions. I think one could set up an experimental model in rabbits which might duplicate clinical conditions. Blood and blood products could be given intravenously to rabbits and the pattern of iron distribution followed both histochemically and biochemically. In such experiments it should be kept in mind that Kupffer-cell iron does get to the liver from the destruction or the elaboration of free iron both outside the liver as well as *in situ*. The pattern of distribution may be related to the site of destruction, to the use of haemoglobin versus whole-blood cells, to the destruction of cells by antibodies or by chemicals, etc.

Iron kinetics

By

M. Pollycove

More than twelve years ago, Huff and his colleagues demonstrated that tracer iron-kinetic studies of plasma, red-cell, and organ radioactivity in human subjects could be used to localize sites of red-cell production and destruction; rates of erythropoiesis were calculated from plasma iron turnover determinations (*1*–*3*). It is now apparent that plasma iron turnover must be analyzed into its component parts before it can be used for quantitative determination of hemoglobin synthesis. For this purpose, a mathematical model was developed — for the quantitation of plasma-erythropoietic and plasma-storage iron exchange, labile erythropoietic and storage iron pools, erythron and storage fixation of iron, hemoglobin synthesis, mean erythron life-span, and mean effective erythron hemoglobinization time — which permits distinct differentiation between *in situ* marrow hemolysis and hemolysis after entry into the circulation (Fig. 1) (*4*). Mathematical analysis of tracer plasma radio-iron data in humans disclosed three distinct exponential components, from which it was theoretically predicted that there exist two distinct pools, whence there is a relatively rapid feedback of iron to plasma. Body-surface measurements suggested that the larger, predominant labile pool is normally associated with erythropoiesis, whereas the smaller labile pool is normally associated with storage (*4*). The concepts of erythropoietic and storage labile iron pools are of central importance to the proposed model. Before presenting quantitative results obtained with this model let us consider experimental data indicating the existence of physiologic entities corresponding to the labile iron pools predicted theoretically from the above-mentioned model (*4*).

Erythropoietic labile iron pool. A series of studies was performed in dogs, injected intravenously with tracer amounts of radio-iron bound to plasma transferrin, to determine whether a considerable non-heme iron pool was present in the marrow, whether the directly measured rate of fixation in heme of iron from this non-heme pool corresponds to the rate constant calculated from iron-kinetic studies employing a mathematical model, and whether there was cellular localization of non-heme iron (*5*). Complete iron-kinetic studies were made in two dogs for a period of ten days in order to calculate the intercompartmental transfer rate of iron from the erythropoietic labile iron pool to iron irreversibly fixed for heme synthesis. Eight other dogs were serially killed 4 to 10 hours after injection to obtain marrow for measurement of specific activity of

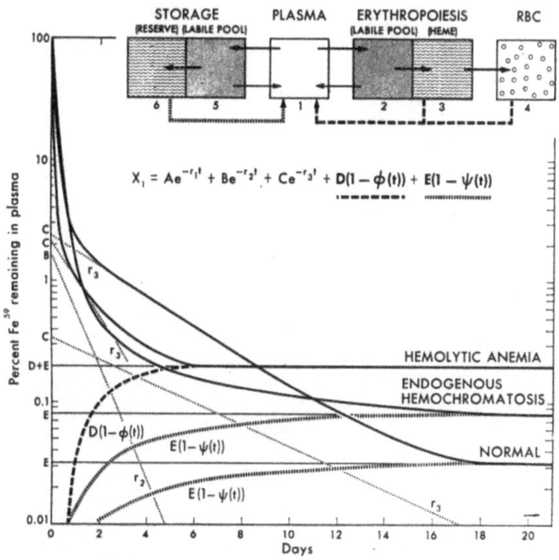

Fig. 1. General iron-kinetics model. In normal subjects plasma radio-iron equilibrates at a constant level after approximately two weeks as a result of the slow feedback of radio-iron to the plasma from the reserve miscible storage iron pool (E [1—ψ(t)]); patients with endogenous hemochromatosis similarly feed back radio-iron from storage reserve, but to a greater degree, with a resultant higher level of radio-iron equilibration. In patients with hemolytic anemia, however, plasma radio-iron equilibrates relatively rapidly at a still higher level, this being a result of the hemolysis of maturing erythrons or circulating erythrocytes (D [1—ϕ(t)]). When plasma-storage iron exchange is greatly increased, as in patients with endogenous hemochromatosis or hypoplastic anemia, the intermediate exponential component (r_2 with intercept B) is markedly prolonged and must be used when applying the model

doubly crystallized heme. This measurement was used to determine the fraction of marrow radio-iron remaining in the non-heme compartment. The calculated rate constants obtained from analysis of plasma iron removal were in close agreement with the direct measurements of marrow as shown in Fig. 2. After freeze-thawing and centrifugation of the marrow, supernatant radio-iron from the cell interior was found to be almost entirely in heme, while radio-iron in the sedimented cell stroma was found to be predominantly non-heme iron (Table 1). The lability of this non-heme iron was demonstrated by another series of experiments in which human reticulocytes were labeled *in vivo* and *in vitro* with Fe^{59} derived

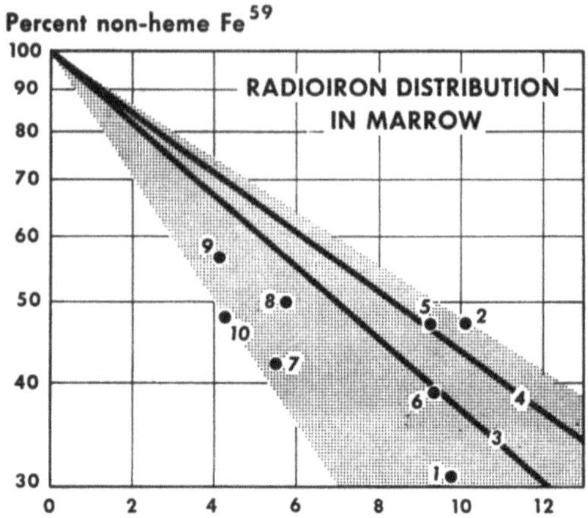

Fig. 2. Radio-iron distribution in marrow. Points for dogs 1, 2, and 5—10 were obtained from direct analysis of red marrow, including measurement of Fe^{59} specific activity of doubly crystallized heme. The slopes for dogs 3 and 4 are the calculated intercompartmental transfer rates from the erythropoietic labile iron pool to irreversible fixed erythron iron, α_{23}. These rate constants were calculated by analysis in accordance with the mathematical model (Fig. 1) of plasma radio-iron data

from plasma transferrin (*6*). The washed labeled reticulocytes were incubated at 37° C. for 1 hour with plasma containing transferrin of determined iron saturation as well as with control solutions such as deproteinized plasma, acid-citrate-dextrose solution, and isotonic saline. Approximately one-quarter of the non-heme radio-iron became transferred from the reticulocytes to the plasma, regardless of the degree of saturation of the transferrin; there was a negligible transfer of radio-iron to the control solutions (Table 2). These studies suggest that an erythropoietic labile iron pool is present in the stroma of immature red cells, being labile in the sense that it may feed back to plasma transferrin and may also become incorporated into heme, as shown

Table 1. *Distribution of radio-iron between non-heme and heme in cell stroma and cell interior. Data correspond to times after injection and distribution of radio-iron in intact cells shown in Fig. 2*

Radio-iron distribution in marrow cells		
Dog	% non-heme Fe^{59}	
	Cell stroma	Cell interior
6	61	21
7	80	—
9	59	9
10	68	22

diagrammatically in Fig. 3. This erythropoietic labile iron pool provides an excess of iron substrate for heme synthesis during development of the immature red cell, while also permitting rapid removal of excess iron from the red cell during further maturation with cessation of hemoglobin synthesis.

Table 2. *Transfer of reticulocyte radio-iron to plasma after incubation for 1 hour at 37° C. Reticulocytes of the same subject (hereditary telangiectasia with severe iron-deficiency anemia responding to iron administered intravenously) were initially labeled by in vitro or in vivo transfer of* Fe^{59} *from plasma transferrin.* (T.I.B.C. = total iron-binding capacity; L.I.B.C. = latent iron-binding capacity; A.C.D. = acid-citrate-dextrose; T.C.A. = trichloro-acetic acid; P = plasma; P_D = deproteinized plasma; P_N = normal plasma)

In vitro

Conditions: 30 min. *in vitro* labeling
73.5% Fe^{59} non-heme

Reticulocytes incubated in:	Fe	T.I.B.C.	L.I.B.C.	Reticulocyte Fe^{59} feedback	
				% of total Fe^{59}	% of non-heme Fe^{59}
A.C.D.	0	—	—	1.4	1.9
P + T.C.A.	0	0	0	1.6	2.2
P_D	19	419	400	20.9	28.5
P_D (saturated)	408	411	3	19.1	26.0
P_N	92	399	307	17.0	23.1
P_N (saturated)	400	400	0	21.7	29.5
			Mean:	19.7	26.8

In vivo

Conditions: 45 min. *in vivo* labeling
55.6% Fe^{59} non-heme

Reticulocytes incubated in:	Fe	T.I.B.C.	L.I.B.C.	Reticulocyte Fe^{59} feedback	
				% of total Fe^{59}	% of non-heme Fe^{59}
A.C.D.	0	—	—	3.5	6.3
Saline	0	—	—	3.2	5.8
P_D	20	458	438	12.6	22.6
P_D (saturated)	456	468	12	15.6	28.1
P_N	118	355	237	14.5	26.1
P_N (saturated	357	355	0	14.7	26.5
			Mean:	14.4	25.9

Storage labile iron pool and the hepatic plasma protein "shunt". The presence of a storage labile iron pool was investigated in our laboratory by Dr. H. S. WINCHELL utilizing measurements of thoracic-duct and hepatic lymph in dogs (*6a*). Following the simultaneous intravenous injection of I^{131}-albumin and Fe^{59}-transferrin, both isotopes appear rapidly in thoracic-duct lymph (Fig. 4). The thoracic-duct lymphatic I^{131}-albumin rapidly reaches an asymptotic plateau at a single exponential rate corresponding to the function: $I^{131} = A(1-e^{-kt})$. By subtracting the observed values of lymph I^{131} from the asymptote we obtain a $t^1/_2$ of 26 minutes for washout of this compartment in dog No. 70. The thoracic-duct Fe^{59}-transferrin increases similarly, except that its asymptote decreases exponentially with a single slope similar to that

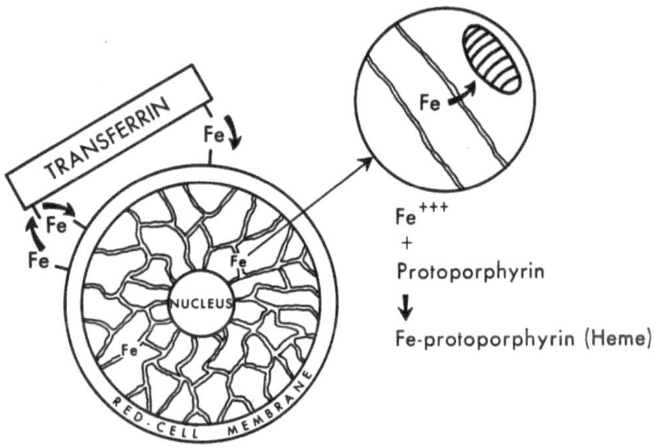

Fig. 3. Diagram of the erythropoietic labile iron pool in the stroma of immature erythrons. Transfer of iron is shown from and to transferrin, as well as irreversible incorporation of iron into heme after movement from the stroma into the cell interior

of the plasma Fe^{59} curve. In all dogs studied, the lymph radio-iron also follows a similar single exponential function with a half-time slightly less than that obtained with I^{131}-albumin, thus indicating similar pool sizes for I^{131}-albumin and Fe^{59}-transferrin (Fig. 4). A maximum volume of "washout" pool may be obtained by measurement of the flow rate of thoracic-duct lymph from the relationship: volume = flow rate $\times$ $T^1/_2/0.693$. In this way we determined that the total quantity of albumin and transferrin contained in this rapidly equilibrating "thoracic-duct lymph" pool is approximately 2% of that contained in the plasma. Serial comparison of the ratio R_{Tr}/R_A of lymph Fe^{59}: plasma Fe^{59} to lymph I^{131}: plasma I^{131} demonstrates that for a few hours there is proportionately less Fe^{59} than I^{131} in the lymph, and that subsequently the ratio is reversed, with a relative excess of Fe^{59}, which after 12 hours was twice the concentration of Fe^{59} in the plasma

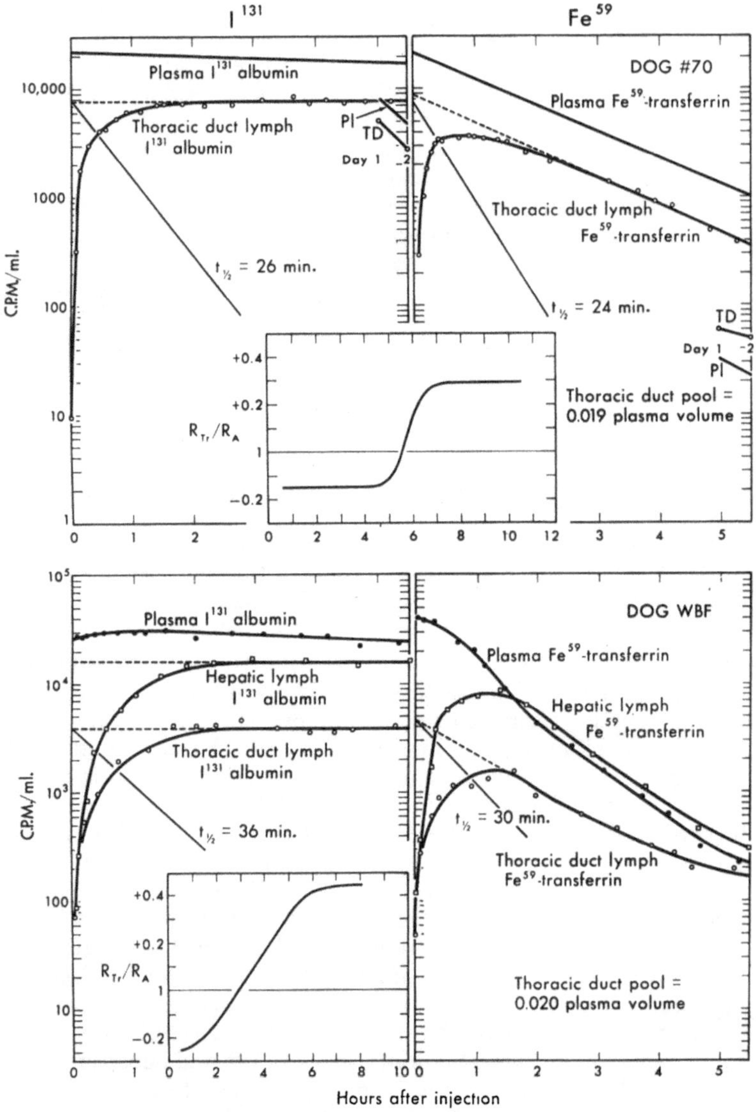

Fig. 4. Measurements of I^{131}-albumin and Fe^{59}-transferrin in plasma, thoracic-duct lymph, and hepatic lymph after simultaneous intravenous injection of I^{131}-albumin and Fe^{59}-transferrin. The concentration of Fe^{59} in thoracic-duct lymph is more than twice that in the plasma between days 1 and 2, while the concentration of I^{131} in thoracic-duct lymph remains less than the plasma I^{131} concentration, being approximately half that of the plasma concentration (Dog 70)

(Fig. 4). This indicates an initial net uptake of Fe^{59} from the plasma transferrin with a subsequent net feedback of Fe^{59} to transferrin. Since the half-time of plasma-albumin exchange with extravascular fluid in this experiment was 14 hours, in agreement with other studies (*7*, *8*), and since others have shown that the half-time of plasma-transferrin exchange is approximately 20 hours (*9*–*11*), these data suggest the presence of a small shunt through which albumin and transferrin leak rapidly into a specific small lymphatic pool that empties rapidly into the thoracic duct. Because of its small size and relatively rapid return of I^{131}-albumin and Fe^{59}-transferrin to the plasma via the thoracic duct, this pool does not significantly alter the size of the plasma volume as calculated from measurements of plasma I^{131}-albumin or Fe^{59}-transferrin, nor does it significantly modify the proposed mathematical models in which plasma-lymph Fe^{59} exchange is neglected.

The location of the "shunt" and its small lymphatic pool was demonstrated by simultaneous sampling of hepatic lymph, thoracic-duct lymph, and plasma after intravenous injection of I^{131}-albumin and Fe^{59}-transferrin. The hepatic-lymph I^{131}-albumin and Fe^{59}-transferrin concentrations are parallel to, and approximately triple those of, the thoracic-duct lymph. Since others have demonstrated that approximately 25–50% of the thoracic-duct lymph is derived from the liver in the dog (*12*–*14*), these results suggest that the liver is the major, if not sole, source of I^{131}-albumin and Fe^{59}-transferrin during the first few hours after intravenous injection. Further evidence indicating that the liver is the major site of rapid shunting of plasma proteins into thoracic-duct lymph was obtained when the porta hepatis containing the hepatic artery, portal vein, and hepatic lymphatic ducts was clamped prior to intravenous injection of the labeled proteins: none of the injected radioactivity appeared in the thoracic-duct lymph during a 30-minute period following injection of I^{131}-albumin and Fe^{59}-transferrin. In three totally hepatectomized dogs the amount of radioiron appearing in the thoracic-duct lymph within 1 hour after Fe^{59} injection was approximately one-fourth of the corresponding prehepatectomy levels.

Comparison of hepatic-lymph I^{131} and Fe^{59} with plasma I^{131} and Fe^{59} again demonstrated an initial net uptake and subsequent net release of Fe^{59} from the liver (Fig. 4). As presented so clearly by Dr. KATZ, it has been shown that the transfer of plasma iron to cells involves the attachment of iron-saturated transferrin to the cell surface, the transfer of iron to a material other than transferrin, and the release of unsaturated transferrin (*15*). The finding of more iron in the hepatic lymph than can be accounted for by the shunting of plasma transferrin through the liver is evidence that iron in the liver is in equilibrium with extracellular fluid and that there is an active feedback of iron to plasma — some of which occurs via hepatic and thoracic-duct lymph — from a storage labile iron pool in the liver as outlined in Fig. 5. Additional evidence obtained

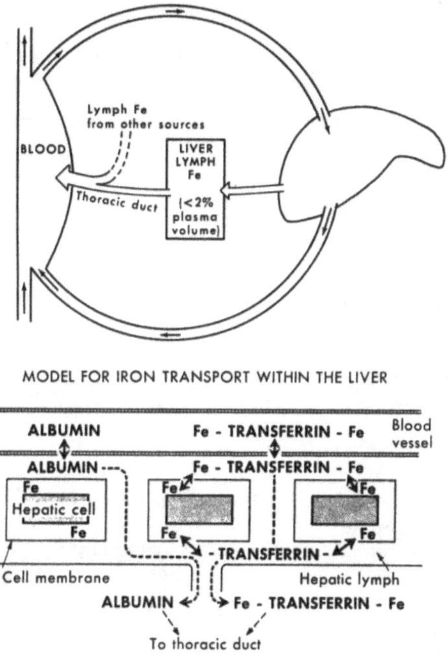

Fig. 5. Diagram showing the rapid hepatic plasma protein shunt from circulating blood back to circulating blood, via hepatic lymph and thoracic-duct lymph pools, and the uptake and feedback of iron by the storage labile iron pool in the liver

in humans, indicating the presence of a storage labile iron pool in the liver, will be presented in the section concerning hemochromatosis.

Normal iron kinetics. Let us now examine results obtained by using this mathematical model with erythropoietic and storage labile iron pools (Fig. 1) to quantitate iron kinetics. Solution of the corresponding differential equations permits calculation of the rate constants, pool sizes, and amounts of iron transferred, utilizing as primary data the plasma iron concentration, the fraction of radio-iron fixed in marrow erythrons, and the exponential com-

Table 3. *Data obtained from normal subjects, patients with endogenous*

Subjects (number studied)		Age and body-weight Yrs	Kg.	Hb. g./100 ml.	Hct %	M.C.H.C.[1] %	R.C.V.[2] ml.
Normal (*13*)	Mean	35	71.5	15.2	45.4	33	2,150
Endogenous hemochromatosis (*5*) . .	Mean	56	63.7	14.0	42.1	34	2,020
Iron-deficiency anemia (*20*)	Mean	44.5	62	7.9	28.4	28	1,099

Subjects (number studied)		Intercompartmental rate constants[4] f[3]	$\alpha_{1/2}$	$\alpha_{2/3}$	$\alpha_{2/1}$	$\alpha_{1/5}$	$\alpha_{5/6}$
Normal (*13*)	Mean	~1	9.21	0.258	0.131		
Endogenous hemochromatosis (*5*) . .	Mean	0.58	4.60	0.223	0.056	2.98	1.348
Iron-deficiency anemia (*20*)	Mean	~1	49.817	3.884	0.494		

[1] Mean corpuscular hemoglobin concentration
[2] Red-cell volume
[3] Fraction of radio-iron fixed in maturing erythrons
[4] $\alpha_{i/j}$ = fraction of iron in compartment i transferring to compartment j per day (see Fig. 1)
[5] Mean erythron life-span
[6] Mean effective erythron hemoglobinization time

ponents of the plasma radio-iron disappearance curve (Table 3) (*4*). Hemoglobin synthesis is readily calculated from the irreversible fixation of iron in maturing erythrons, since non-hemoglobin iron in normal erythrocytes is negligible and 1 g. hemoglobin contains 3.4 mg. iron. The mean erythron life-span is calculated by relating daily hemoglobin synthesis to total body hemoglobin, as measured with P^{32}-labeled red cells at the beginning and end of the 2-week period of study (*4*). All studies were performed with serial measurements of radio-iron in the plasma, circulating red cells, sacral bone marrow, liver, and spleen after intravenous injection of transferrin-bound tracer Fe^{59} as described previously (*4*). Investigation of normal subjects yielded the following observations (Fig. 6). Plasma *hemochromatosis, and patients with iron-deficiency anemia*

Total body Hb. g.	$t^1/_2$ hrs	Serum iron µg./100 ml.	Blood volume ml.	Plasma volume ml.	Total plasma iron X_1	First plasma slope r_1	Second plasma slope r_2	Third plasma slope r_3	First intercept A	Second intercept B	Third intercept C
738	1.88	132	5,010	2,810	3.6	9.3		0.254	0.984		0.0165
679	2.20	217	5,320	3,300	7.0	7.70	1.483	0.241	0.981	0.0142	0.0053
313	0.35	20	4,569	3,470	0.648	50.54		3.794	0.981		0.0190

α_{51}	Fe leaving plasma/day $(\alpha_{12} + \alpha_{15})X_1$ mg.	Erythropoietic labile iron pool X_2 mg.	Storage labile iron pool X_5 mg.	Miscible storage iron X_{ms} g.	Daily Fe for storage deposition $\alpha_{56} X_5$ mg.	Daily Fe for Hb. synthesis $\alpha_{23}X_2$ mg.	Daily Hb. synthesis g.	Daily Hb. synthesis g./L.	M.E.L.S.[5] days	M.E.E.H.T.[6] days
	32.5	84.9				21.4	6.3	1.3 ±0.2	117 ±7.5	1.4 ±0.2
0.225	51.9	109.1	15.6	4.98	18.0	24.7	7.2	1.4 ±0.2	108 ±5	1.6 ±0.5
	31.037	10.099				26.76	7.87	1.7 ±0.8	44.8 ±15.5	2.5 ±0.4

radio-iron initially maintains a constant rapid exponential rate of decrease for approximately 4–8 hours, after which the rate of decrease diminishes progressively. After approximately 2 days, a second, much slower, constant exponential rate of radio-iron decrease is established, which persists for the next 8–12 days. This exponential component is associated with the fractional rate of transfer of iron from the erythropoietic labile iron pool to iron fixed for heme synthesis ($\alpha_{2/3}$ in Fig. 1 and Table 3). Another exponential component of intermediate rate, associated with a small amount of normal plasma-storage iron exchange, is detectable between 8 and 36 hours, but may be neglected in normal subjects. Hemoglobin synthesis is 6.3 g./day, and the derived mean erythron life-span is 118 days in this subject. Virtually all tracer radio-iron moves rapidly from plasma to bone marrow, remaining there for approximately $1^1/_2$ days (Fig. 6). During the next 4–6 days, radio-iron leaves the marrow while simultaneously appearing in circulating erythrocytes; 85–100% of the removed plasma iron is incorporated into circulating erythrocytes within 7–10 days. The rate of irreversible fixation of radio-iron in marrow erythrons, as calculated from analysis of plasma radio-iron disappearance, is shown by the dotted line in Fig. 6. The mean time interval between fixation

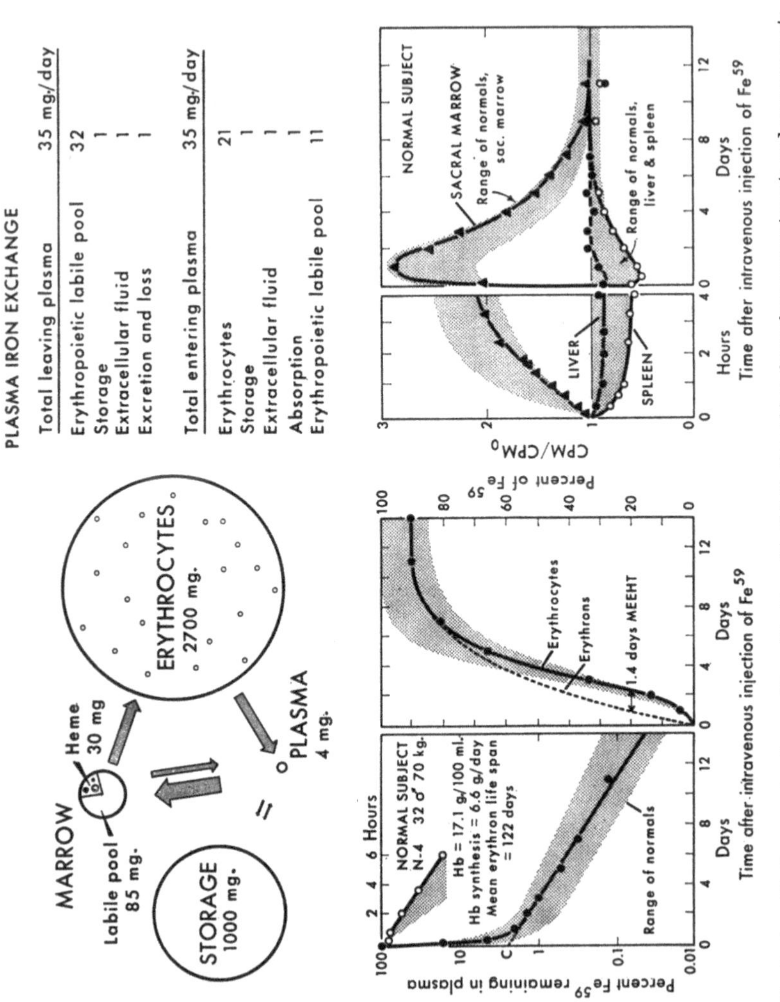

Fig. 6. Quantitative aspects of normal iron kinetics with distribution of iron in various compartments and measurements of radio-iron in the plasma and erythrocytes and surface radioactivity in a normal subject. The interrupted curve, showing cumulative fixation of radio-iron in the erythrons, and the mean effective erythron hemoglobinization time (M.E.E.H.T.) are calculated

of radio-iron in marrow erythrons at all stages of development and its appearance in circulating erythrocytes is designated as the "mean effective erythron hemoglobinization time" (M.E.E.H.T.), the normal range being 1.0–1.8 days (Table 3). Prolongation of the M.E.E.H.T. is a result of intramedullary hemolysis of maturing erythrons, since the time interval between the initial fixation of some radio-iron in maturing erythrons and the appearance of this label in a cell that reaches the circulation may span two or more passages through the marrow maturational pathway (*4*). The M.E.E.H.T. is greatly increased, to 4–6 days, in severely anemic patients with marked intramedullary hemolysis, such as may occur in pernicious anemia, thalassemia major, and refractory anemia with erythroid hyperplasia (*16–18*).

Body surface measurements trace the movement of iron after it leaves the plasma by detecting the gamma-ray emission of radio-iron over the sacrum (marrow), liver (representing iron stores), and spleen. Fig. 6 shows the data so obtained, the surface radioactivity at any time being expressed as a ratio to extrapolated zero-time radioactivity, when all radio-iron is in the plasma. The spleen and liver counting rates decrease exponentially as the marrow accumulates iron, with active uptake of iron persisting at the end of 4 hours. Subsequently, as radio-iron leaves the marrow, the increase in splenic and hepatic radioactivity towards their initial level indicates the reappearance of radio-iron in the circulating erythrocytes. An increase in splenic radioactivity at this time to above the initial level, i.e. exceeding the previous decrease, would indicate splenic sequestration and destruction of erythrocytes, which is frequently observed in hemolytic anemias. Extramedullary erythropoiesis is present whenever the accumulation and release of iron, characteristic of marrow, occurs ectopically in the spleen or liver.

After 8–12 days, erythrocyte radio-iron remains constant for approximately 100 days (Fig. 7). Subsequently, as erythrocyte death occurs, erythrocyte radio-iron slowly decreases. Because of re-incorporation, this decrease is transient, after which erythrocyte radio-iron increases to near its original value. The amount of radio-iron in the circulating erythrocytes can be calculated from a normal distribution curve of erythrocyte longevity, assuming that after a period of delay radio-iron re-enters the plasma and re-incorporation proceeds as measured initially. In this subject, the *calculated* amount of radio-iron in the erythrocytes, shown by the heavy line, is derived from the normal distribution curve shown in Fig. 7 with a delay of reappearance in the plasma of 0 days. This calculated curve fits the experimental data well. The erythrocyte life-span *distribution of this subject* is thus determined as being 115.5 ± 7.0 (1 SD) days. In two other normal subjects studied in this way, the delay in the reappearance of radio-iron in the plasma for re-incorporation into another generation of red cells was less than half a day and 2 days, respectively (*19*).

The main pathways of normal iron kinetics and the compartments and rates of iron transfer are shown in Fig. 6 and Table 3. The main flow of iron is from the plasma to the marrow erythrocytes and then, following death of the erythrocyte, back to the plasma. Approximately 32 mg./day leaves the plasma for the marrow; of this, 21 mg. goes on to the erythrocytes and 11 mg. returns to the plasma (*4*). Plasma iron exchange also occurs with: 1) absorption from the intestine and excretion in the bile, urine, and stools (approximately 1 mg./day) (*20*–*25*); 2) storage exchange (approximately 1 mg./day) (*4*); and 3) exchange with extracellular fluid, myoglobin, and heme enzymes (approximately 1 mg./day) (*4*). The daily amount of iron involved in all these exchanges, however, is less than 10% of the daily amount of iron going to the marrow. In Fig. 6 the area of each compartment corresponds to the amount of iron in it. Plasma iron exchange is not proportional to the amount of iron in the compartment involved. A storage iron reserve of 1,000 mg. is equivalent to approximately 25% of total iron, yet storage iron exchange accounts for less than 5% of total iron exchange (Fig. 6). The erythropoietic labile pool, though containing only 85 mg. iron, receives 90% of the iron leaving the plasma; two-thirds of this iron is used in hemoglobin formation, the remainder re-entering the plasma.

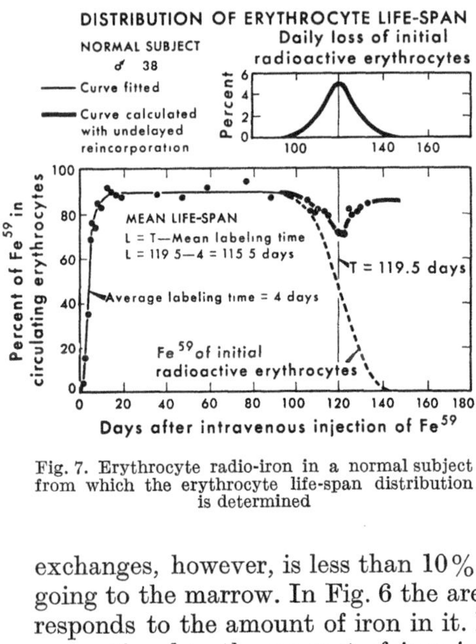

Fig. 7. Erythrocyte radio-iron in a normal subject from which the erythrocyte life-span distribution is determined

Hemochromatosis. Though plasma-storage iron exchange is normally very small, it may become a major component of plasma iron turnover in patients with increased iron stores and/or decreased erythropoiesis. Patients with endogenous hemochromatosis have a 30 to 60-fold increase in storage iron and are thus a useful source of information about alterations in iron kinetics associated

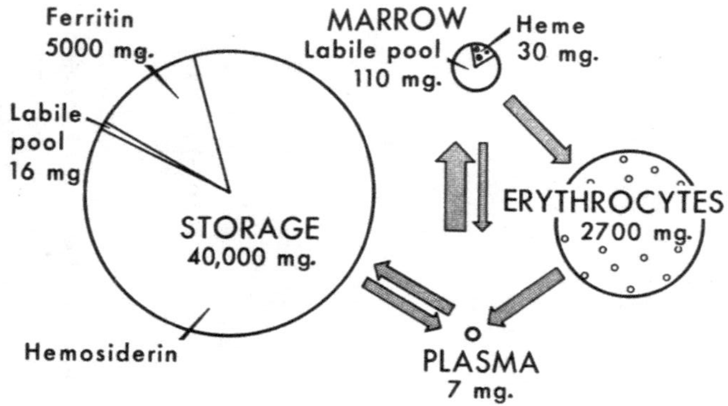

PLASMA IRON EXCHANGE

Total leaving plasma	56 mg./day
Erythropoietic labile pool	32
Storage	20.5
Extracellular fluid	2
Excretion and loss	1.5
Total entering plasma	**56 mg./day**
Erythrocytes	21
Storage	18
Extracellular fluid	2
Absorption	4
Erythropoietic labile pool	11

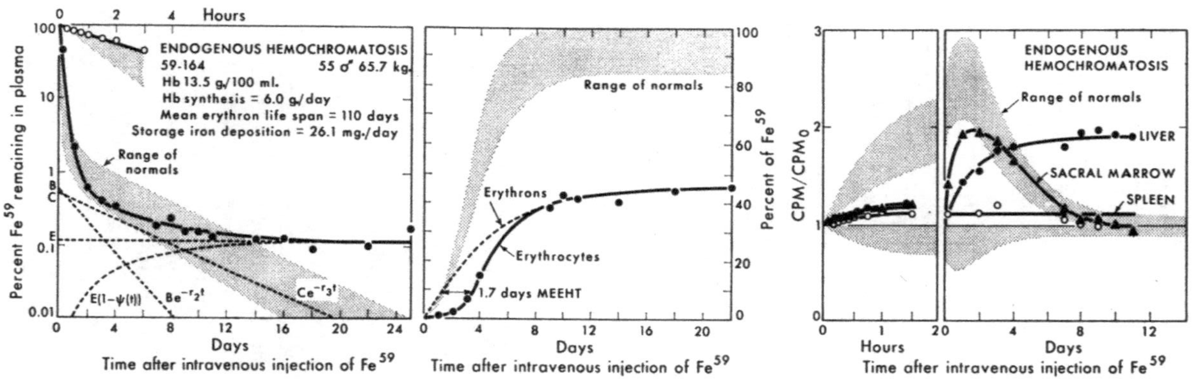

Fig. 8. Quantitative aspects of iron kinetics in patients with endogenous hemochromatosis with distribution of iron in various compartments and measurements of radio-iron in the plasma and erythrocytes and surface radioactivity in a patient with endogenous hemochromatosis. The interrupted curve, showing cumulative fixation of radio-iron in the erythrons, and the mean effective erythron hemoglobinization time (M.E.E.H.T.) are calculated

with increased iron stores. Fig. 8 shows the iron kinetics of a non-anemic patient with endogenous hemochromatosis. The slow feedback of radio-iron from storage reserve — E $[1-\psi(t)]$ from compartment 6, Fig. 1 — is shown as a dashed curve increasing exponentially towards its asymptote. The plasma radio-iron curve reveals three distinct constant exponential rates indicating considerable plasma-storage iron exchange. Measurement of the three

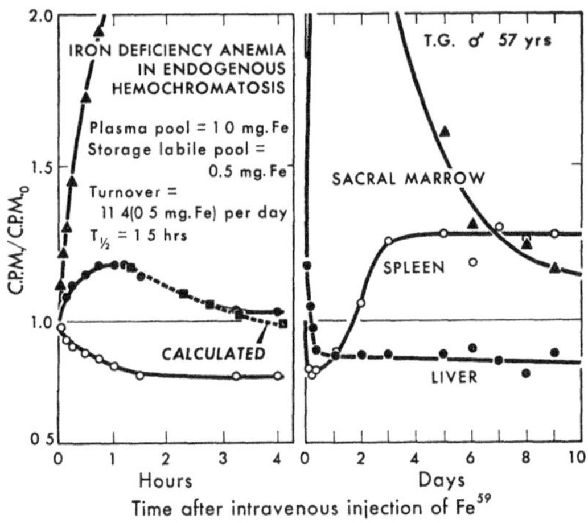

Fig. 9. Body surface radioactivity in a patient with endogenous hemochromatosis and iron-deficiency anemia (therapeutically induced). The interrupted hepatic curve shown between one and four hours (almost completely superimposed upon the measured hepatic curve) is a plot of the storage labile iron pool ($X_5 = 0.5$ mg.) washout rate ($\alpha_{51} = 11.4$ per day) calculated from analysis of plasma radio-iron data ($\alpha_{56} = X_6 = 0$)

slopes and the zero-time intercepts permits quantitation of the iron kinetics. Hemoglobin synthesis (6.4 g./day) and mean erythron life-span (103 days) are normal in this patient.

Measurements *in vivo* show an initial accumulation of radio-iron in the liver as well as the marrow (Fig. 8). Subsequently, liver accumulation continues, ultimately remaining constant at a high level. These findings indicate increased plasma-storage iron exchange. The incorporation of radio-iron into circulating erythrocytes is correspondingly low.

The main pathways of iron kinetics and the compartments and rates of iron transfer in patients with endogenous hemochromatosis are shown in Fig. 8 and Table 3 (*4*). The principal abnormal finding is a 20-fold increase in the movement of iron from plasma to storage, i.e. 20 mg./day. This metabolic abnormality is associated with a

40-fold increase in storage iron, i.e. 40,000 mg. That the increase in plasma-storage iron exchange is not merely a passive consequence of the size of the storage pool, but is largely the result of an active affinity of storage cells for iron, is demonstrated by the following patient. In this male patient with endogenous hemochromatosis and iron-deficiency anemia resulting from systematic venesection therapy (*6*), a sixfold increase in the movement of iron from plasma to storage (6 mg./day) was measured (Fig. 9). Body surface measurements in this patient disclosed a rapid net hepatic uptake and release of plasma radio-iron (not observed previously in other subjects) at a rate corresponding closely to the rate constant ($\alpha_{5/1} = 11.4$/day, $T^1/_2 = 1.46$ hours) of feedback from the storage labile iron pool ($X_5 = 0.52$ mg.) to the plasma ($X_1 = 1.06$ mg.) calculated from mathematical analysis of plasma radio-iron measurements (Fig. 9). It is remarkable that the hepatic cells in this patient are able to remove iron from the plasma at six times the normal rate despite a slightly increased marrow uptake of plasma iron (36 mg./day) and despite the complete absence of storage iron deposits with a low plasma iron concentration of 38 μg./100 ml. and a transferrin saturation of only 10%. This abnormal tissue avidity for iron is probably an inherited disorder, which may result in the increased absorption of iron present in persons with endogenous hemochromatosis.

Storage iron, which equilibrates with plasma iron fairly rapidly within a month, is probably in the form of ferritin and comprises approximately one-eighth of total storage iron (Fig. 8). The storage labile iron pool is a small fraction of the stores (16 mg.) yet it contains more than twice the iron in the plasma (7 mg.). Increases in the plasma and erythrocyte labile iron (110 mg.) pools produce only slight alterations in the iron kinetics involved in erythropoiesis. Patients with superimposed hemolysis show splenic sequestration together with destruction of red cells and increased erythropoiesis.

Iron-deficiency anemia. The kinetics of iron-deficiency anemia is in many respects the reverse of that of hemochromatosis, but with additional changes resulting from defective erythropoiesis (*26*). Fig. 10 shows the iron kinetics of a patient with iron-deficiency anemia. Because plasma iron is markedly decreased, removal of radio-iron is extremely rapid. Within a few hours, equilibrium is established between the plasma iron and the erythropoietic labile iron pool, as contrasted with 2 days in a normal subject. At the end of $1^1/_2$ days, the plasma radio-iron reaches a constant equilibrium level, signifying additional rapid re-entry of radio-iron from hemolyzed erythrons, shown as a dashed curve increasing exponentially towards its asymptote: $D[1-\phi(t)]$ from compartment 3 or 4. Graphical analysis of plasma radio-iron into two distinct compo-

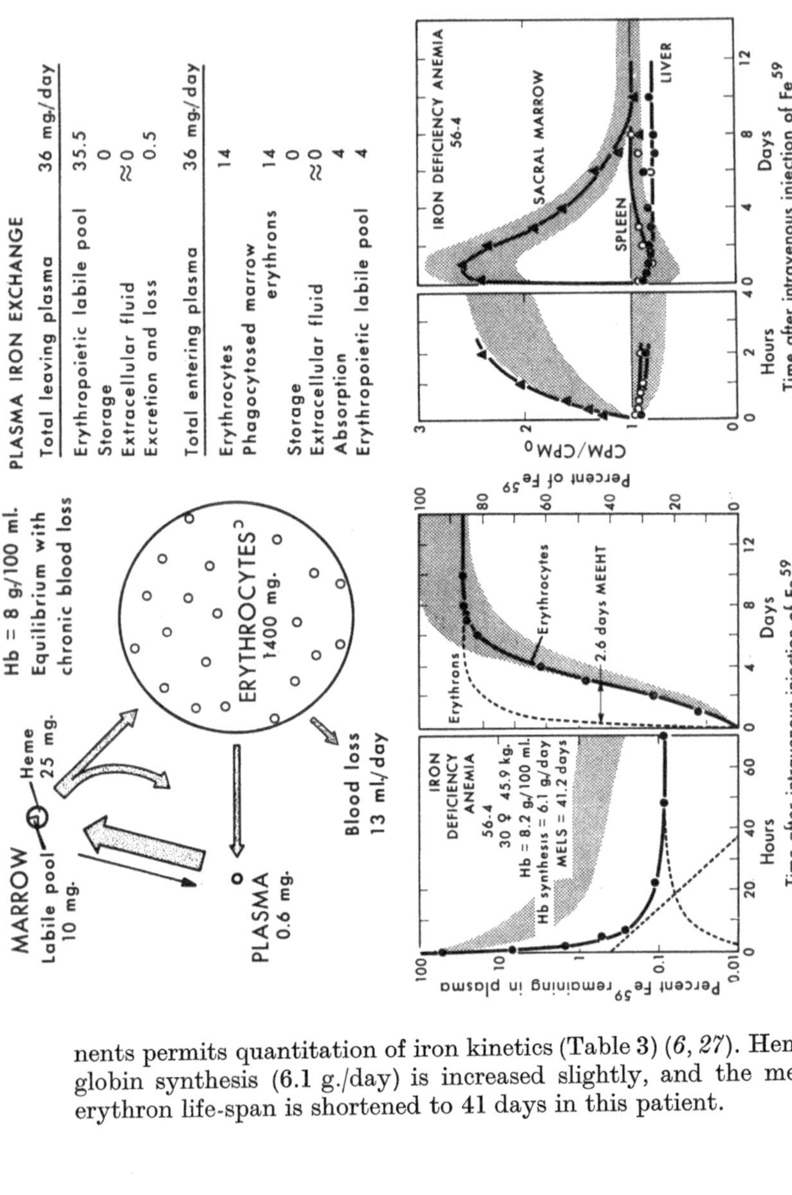

Fig. 10. Quantitative aspects of iron kinetics in patients with iron-deficiency anemia with distribution of iron in various compartments and measurements of radio-iron in the plasma and erythrocytes and surface radioactivity in a patient with iron-deficiency anemia. The interrupted curve, showing cumulative fixation of radio-iron in the erythrons, and the mean effective erythron hemoglobinization time (M.E.E.H.T.) are calculated

nents permits quantitation of iron kinetics (Table 3) (*6, 27*). Hemoglobin synthesis (6.1 g./day) is increased slightly, and the mean erythron life-span is shortened to 41 days in this patient.

Measurements *in vivo* show a rapid accumulation of radio-iron in the marrow which is complete in 2 hours (Fig. 10). No significant accumulation of radio-iron takes place elsewhere. Subsequently, marrow release occurs promptly, and is complete in 7 days. In patients with severe iron-deficiency anemia, slight to moderate splenic sequestration and destruction of red cells frequently occur. Incorporation of radio-iron into the circulating erythrocytes is also rapid and complete (Fig. 10). There is a prolonged time-lag between the incorporation of radio-iron into the marrow erythrons — which occurs very rapidly because the labile pool is small — and the appearance of radio-iron in the circulating erythrocytes. The mean erythron "hemoglobinization" time is thus increased (2.6 days) despite the prompt appearance of radio-iron in the erythrocytes. The considerably shortened mean erythrocyte life-span and the increased M.E.E.H.T. indicate that destruction of maturing erythrons occurs within the marrow. The morphology of marrow erythrons — small, distorted normoblasts with ragged, ill-defined borders and cytoplasmic hemoglobinization lagging behind nuclear condensation — is also suggestive of the breakdown of marrow erythrons. Phagocytosis of immature erythrons by marrow reticuloendothelial cells was repeatedly observed in patients with iron-deficiency anemia, but is not seen in the marrow of normal subjects (*28*). This intramedullary hemolysis is compatible with the results of Ashby and Cr^{51} studies, showing relatively slight shortening of the life-span of *circulating* erythrocytes (75–90 days), as well as with measurements of breath carbon-monoxide indicating over-all hemoglobin catabolism corresponding to a red-cell life-span of 40–60 days (*29–31*).

The main pathways of iron kinetics and the compartments and rates of iron transfer in patients with iron-deficiency anemia are shown in Fig. 10 and Table 3 (*6*, *27*). Though storage iron is absent and plasma iron is reduced to one-sixth of normal (0.6 mg. plasma iron), transfer to the marrow is increased (35 mg./day), and since feedback to the plasma from the small erythropoietic labile pool (10 mg.) is small (4 mg./day), iron fixed in heme is also increased (31 mg./day). This seeming paradox becomes understandable, however, when it is realized that the increased amount of iron utilized for heme synthesis is derived from the increased destruction of red cells. Assuming a survival of 2 days for erythrons hemolyzed in the marrow, and relating the survival of *circulating* erythrocytes (approximately 80 days) to the mean erythron life-span of 41 days, it may be estimated that approximately half of the erythrons formed are destroyed by intramedullary hemolysis or very shortly after their entry into the circulation.

Conclusions

The major changes in iron kinetics which occur in several common disorders are summarized diagrammatically in Fig. 11. Plasma iron normally proceeds from plasma to marrow, to erythrocytes, and back to plasma. The movement, however, is not linear, because approximately one-third of the iron initially leaving for the marrow returns from the marrow without being involved in erythropoiesis during that cycle. The amount of iron in storage is 250 times greater than the plasma iron; nevertheless, plasma exchange with stores is normally quite small.

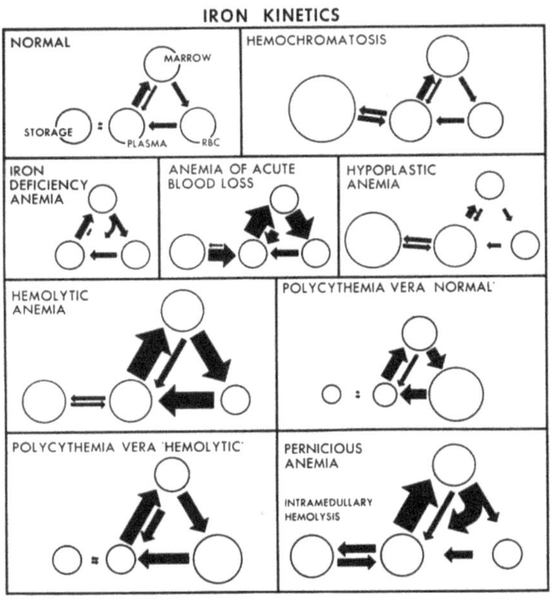

Fig. 11. Iron kinetics in various disorders. The change in the area of each compartment, as compared with normal, is suggestive of the change in the amount of iron contained

In patients with hemochromatosis, storage iron is 30 to 60 times greater than normal, and plasma iron is doubled (Fig. 11). Erythrocyte iron usually remains normal. The greatly increased tissue avidity for iron in these patients results in an increase in plasma-storage iron exchange, so that it constitutes a large fraction of total plasma iron exchange. This increased exchange, added to the normal exchange related to hemoglobin synthesis, results in an increased total plasma iron exchange.

In iron-deficiency anemia, iron stores are no longer present and plasma and erythropoietic labile iron pools are decreased (Fig. 11). Though erythrocyte iron is also decreased, the amount of iron involved in hemoglobin synthesis is normal or even slightly increased. Near-normal survival of circulating erythrocytes, associated with a considerable reduction in the mean erythron life-span and an increase in the mean effective erythron hemoglobinization time, indicates that shortened erythron survival is chiefly the result of intramedullary hemolysis, premature destruction of circulating erythrocytes contributing to a lesser extent. This destruction of red cells may result from structural defects secondary to an inadequate iron transfer *per cell* (the number of marrow erythrons is considerably increased), this being a consequence of the abnormally low saturation of transferrin. Though hemoglobin synthesis is quantitatively normal or even increased, it is inadequate to compensate for the moderate cell destruction occurring chiefly in the marrow. Defective and subnormal compensatory erythropoiesis is the basic defect, as shown by the cessation of intramedullary hemolysis and the marked increase in hemoglobin synthesis following iron therapy.

The anemia of acute blood loss occurs when a considerable fraction of the erythrocytes is removed from the body (Fig. 11). This decrease in erythrocyte iron normally produces a marked increase in hemoglobin synthesis, which, in turn, diminishes the labile marrow pool and plasma iron. In this way, a large amount of iron is removed from stores. Continuation of this process, as in chronic blood loss, will eventually exhaust the iron stores and result in iron-deficiency anemia.

Hypoplastic anemia results from insufficient erythropoiesis associated with decreased marrow erythrons (Fig. 11). The reduction in erythrocyte iron is usually greater than the reduction in hemoglobin synthesis, since generally there is also some decrease in the mean erythron life-span. The decrement of erythrocyte iron is added to the stores through the plasma; hence plasma and storage iron are increased, even without transfusion. As a result, plasma-storage exchange is increased as plasma-erythropoiesis exchange is decreased. Total plasma exchange, though somewhat lessened, is consequently not reduced proportionately to the decrease in hemoglobin synthesis (*32*).

Hemolytic anemia develops when destruction of erythrocytes is greater than compensatory erythropoiesis (Fig. 11). The anemia progressively worsens until hemoglobin synthesis and destruction become equal. The decrement of erythrocyte iron is added to the stores, thus increasing plasma and storage iron. The increased plasma-storage exchange, however, still remains very small as compared with plasma-erythropoiesis exchange, which may be increased by 6—14 times. Marked splenic sequestration and destruction of erythrocytes is frequently present and may be used as an indication for splenectomy (*32*).

Anemia in patients with myeloid metaplasia, chronic myelogenous leukemia, or chronic lymphatic leukemia is usually the result of an increase in the destruction of circulating erythrocytes. Erythropoiesis, though usually increased, frequently constitutes a subnormal response to the degree of anemia and is inadequate to compensate for the shortened erythrocyte survival (*33*). The "secondary" anemias of infection, inflammation, and malignancy manifest a similar inadequacy in the erythropoietic response to hemolysis (*34*). Here, the diagram for hemolytic anemia in Fig. 11 is applicable. Extramedullary erythropoiesis occurs in the spleen and liver of patients with myeloid metaplasia or chronic myelogenous leukemia, but not in patients with chronic lymphatic leukemia (*32*).

Typical of patients with polycythemia vera is the increased red-cell volume. Early in the course of this disorder, erythropoiesis is usually increased in proportion to the red-cell volume, the red-cell life-span being normal (Fig. 11). Subsequently, the red-cell life-span becomes shortened and erythropoiesis further increased, thus maintaining an increased red-cell volume. Finally, many patients develop myelosclerosis and extramedullary erythropoiesis, and the further shortening of the red-cell life-span is not balanced by the further increase in erythropoiesis. Though frequently appearing anemic, the red-cell volume still remains increased, although considerably less so than in the earlier stages of polycythemia vera (*32*, *35*). Splenic destruction of red cells may at times exceed splenic erythropoiesis, indicating the therapeutic value of splenectomy in these patients.

In pernicious anemia, the etiology of the defective erythropoiesis is known. Although marrow release of erythrocytes is reduced, plasma-erythropoiesis iron exchange is greatly increased (Fig. 11). Here again, the deficit of iron in the erythrocyte compartment, as compared with normal, is added to the stores. Plasma and storage iron, and their exchange, are increased. Plasma-storage exchange nevertheless remains small as compared with the great amount of iron passing from the plasma to the large erythropoietic labile pool and becoming fixed in heme. At this point, erythron destruction largely prevents effective delivery of hemoglobin to the circulation, and, after erythrophagocytosis by reticular cells, the iron returns to the plasma (*4*, *32*, *36*). Intramedullary hemolysis is also present in patients with thalassemia major, erythremic myelosis, and refractory anemias with erythroid hyperplasia (*6*, *17*, *18*).

Summary

The availability of radio-iron of highly specific activity, sensitive instruments, and appropriate mathematical models permits the quantitative determination of plasma-storage iron exchange, labile iron pools, miscible storage iron, erythron fixation of iron, hemoglobin synthesis, mean effective erythron hemoglobinization time, mean erythron life-span, and erythrocyte life-span distribution. Since iron kinetics is largely controlled by erythron metabolism, this method of analyzing iron metabolism is also very useful in studying the alterations in erythropoiesis and red-cell survival which occur in a wide variety of disorders. Iron-kinetic studies serve to establish clinical diagnoses and pathophysiology, as well as to provide objective indications for therapy in patients with anemia, polycythemia, and endogenous hemochromatosis.

Zusammenfassung

Die Anwendung von markiertem Eisen hoher spezifischer Radioaktivität, von empfindlichen Instrumenten und von geeigneten mathematischen Modellen erlaubt eine quantitative Bestimmung des Austausches zwischen Plasma- und Depoteisen, der labilen Eisenvorräte, des mischbaren Speichereisens, der Fixierung von Eisen im Erythron, der Haemoglobinsynthese, der mittleren effektiven Zeitspanne für die Haemoglobinisierung des Erythrons, der mittleren Lebensdauer des Erythrons und der Erythrozyten. Da die Eisenkinetik weitgehend durch den Stoffwechsel des Erythrons kontrolliert wird, eignet sich diese Methode der Analyse des Eisenstoffwechsels auch für Untersuchungen über Änderungen der Erythropoiese und der Überlebenszeit der Erythrozyten bei ganz verschiedenen Störungen. Studien der Eisenkinetik können für die Erkennung pathophysiologischer Vorgänge und die Sicherung der klinischen Diagnose herangezogen werden. Sie geben außerdem objektive Hinweise für die Behandlung von Patienten mit verschiedenen Formen von Anaemie, von Polycythaemie und von endogener Haemochromatose.

Résumé

L'existence de fer hautement radioactif, d'instruments d'une grande sensibilité, de formules mathématiques adéquates permet aujourd'hui de déterminer quantitativement: les échanges de fer entre le plasma et les dépôts, les *pools* du fer échangeable, le fer miscible des dépôts, la fixation du fer dans la lignée rouge, la synthèse de l'hémoglobine, le temps moyen d'hémoglobinisation efficace des éléments rouges, la vie moyenne de ces éléments, la distribution des durées de vie des érythrocytes. Puisque la cinétique du fer est en grande partie conditionnée par le métabolisme des éléments rouges, cette méthode d'analyse du métabolisme du fer est également très utile pour l'étude des troubles de l'érythropoièse et de la survie des hématies, que l'on rencontre dans divers états pathologiques. Les études de la cinétique du fer peuvent aussi bien servir à poser des diagnostics cliniques et physiopathologiques que donner des indications objectives pour le traitement d'anémies, de polyglobulies et d'hémochromatoses endogènes.

References

1. HUFF, R. L., T. G. HENNESSY, R. E. AUSTIN, J. F. GARCIA, B. M. ROBERTS, and J. H. LAWRENCE: J. Clin. Invest. (U.S.A.) **29**, 1041 (1950). — 2. HUFF, R. L., P. J. ELMLINGER, J. F. GARCIA, J. M. ODA, M. C. COCKRELL, and J. H. LAWRENCE: J. Clin. Invest. (U.S.A.) **30**, 1512 (1951). — 3. ELMLINGER, P. J., R. L. HUFF, C. A. TOBIAS, and J. H. LAWRENCE: Acta haemat. (Switz.) **9**, 73 (1953). — 4. POLLYCOVE, M., and R. MORTIMER: J. Clin. Invest. (U.S.A.) **40**, 753 (1961). — 5. POLLYCOVE, M., and M. MAQSOOD: Nature (G.B.) **194**, 152 (1962). — 6. POLLYCOVE, M.: Unpublished observations. — 6a. WINCHELL, H. S., M. POLLYCOVE, N. KUSUBOV, and J. H. LAWRENCE: Iron and Albumin Kinetics of Thoracic Duct Lymph. To be published. — 7. BERSON, S. A., R. S. YALOW, S. S. SCHREIBER, and J. POST: J. Clin. Invest. (U.S.A.) **32**, 746 (1953). — 8. TAKEDA, Y., and E. B. REEVE: J. Laborat. Clin. Med. (U.S.A.) **61**, 183 (1963). — 9. GITLIN, D., C. A. JANEWAY, and L. E. FARR: J. Clin. Invest. (U.S.A.) **35**, 44 (1956). — 10. GITLIN, D.: Ann. N. Y. Acad. Sc. **70**, 122 (1957). — 11. KATZ, J. H.: J. Clin. Invest. (U.S.A.) **40**, 2143 (1961). — 12. CAIN, J. C., J. H. GRINDLAY, J. L. BOLLMAN, E. V. FLOCK, and F. C. MANN: Surg. Gyn. Obstetr. (U.S.A.) **85**, 559 (1947).— 13. NIX, J. T., E. V. FLOCK, and J. L. BOLLMAN: Amer. J. Physiol. **164**, 117 (1951). — 14. NIX, J. T., F. C. MANN, J. L. BOLLMAN, J. H. GRINDLAY, and E. V. FLOCK: Amer. J. Physiol. **164**, 119 (1951). — 15. JANDL, J. H., and J. H. KATZ: J. Clin. Invest. (U.S.A.) **42**, 314 (1963). — 16. WALLERSTEIN, R. O., and M. POLLYCOVE: A. M. A. Arch. Int. Med. **101**, 418 (1958). — 17. POLLYCOVE, M.: In: Proceedings of the 7th Congress of the International Society of Hematology, Vol. I. Grune & Stratton, New York, 1960, p. 465. — 18. POLLYCOVE, M., and J. H. LAWRENCE: In: Proceedings of the 8th International Congress of Hematology, Tokyo, 1960. Pan-Pacific Press, Tokyo, 1962, p. 42. — 19. POLLYCOVE, M., P. J. ELMLINGER, L. A. SARKES, L. APT, and J. F. ROSS: Clin. Res. Proc. **4**, 79 (1956). — 20. CHODOS, R. B., J. R. ROSS, L. APT, J. HALKETT, and M. POLLYCOVE: Clin. Res. Proc. (U.S.A.) **2**, 53 (1955); J. Clin. Invest. (U.S.A.) **36**, 314 (1957). — 21. DUBACH, R., C. V. MOORE, and S. CALLENDER: J. Laborat. Clin. Med. (U.S.A.) **45**, 599 (1955). — 22. JOSEPHS, H. W.: Medicine (U.S.A.) **32**, 125 (1953). — 23. MOORE, C. V.: Amer. J. Clin. Nutrit. **3**, 3 (1955). — 24. JOSEPHS, H. W.: Blood (U.S.A.) **13**, 1 (1958). — 25. CALLENDER, S. T.: Brit. Med. Bull. **15**. 5 (1959). — 26. POLLYCOVE, M.: Iron Kinetics in Iron in Clinical Medicine. Ed. by R. O. WALLERSTEIN. Univ. of Calif. Press, Berkeley, 1958, p. 43. — 27. POLLYCOVE, M., and J. H. LAWRENCE: In: Proceedings of the 9th Congress of the International Society of Hematology, Mexico City, 1962 (in press). — 28. FEICHTMEIER, T., and M. POLLYCOVE: Unpublished observations. — 29. ASHBY, W.: Blood (U.S.A.) **3**, 486 (1948). — 30. HARRIS, J. W.: Personal communication. — 31. LAURELL, C. B.: Personal communication. — 32. POLLYCOVE, M.: In: Eisenstoffwechsel. Ed. by W. KEIDERLING. Thieme, Stuttgart, 1959, p. 20. — 23. VAN DYKE, D., M. LAYRISSE, J. LAWRENCE, J. GARCIA, and M. POLLYCOVE: Blood (U.S.A.) **18**, 201 (1961). — 34. TURA, S., M. POLLYCOVE, and A. GELPI: Clin. Res. (U.S.A.) **8**, 113 (1960); J. Nuclear Med. **3**, 110 (1962). — 35. POLLYCOVE, M., and J. H. LAWRENCE: Clin. Res. (U.S.A.) **6**, 191 (1958). — **36**. PEABODY, F. W., and G. O. BROUN: Amer. J. Path. **1**, 169 (1925).

Discussion

SAADI: The second patient that you showed with haemochromatosis had been venesected, and his liver biopsy had revealed no iron deposits. His transferrin was 10% saturated, and still the liver was taking eight times the normal amount of iron. Is that correct?

POLLYCOVE: Yes, except that it was six times more than normal. This iron, however, did not pass from the storage labile pool into the storage reserve pool (Fig. 1, p. 149), as demonstrated by the absence of a significant amount of radio-iron in the liver at 10 hours (Fig. 9, p. 162). The rate of transfer from the storage labile pool to the storage reserve pool was zero ($\alpha_{5/6} = 0$). There was no transfer of iron to storage reserve; examination of marrow and hepatic tissues demonstrated the absence of storage reserve iron. Under these circumstances it is very surprising that hepatic cells were able to remove iron from transferrin rapidly, i.e. at six times the normal rate, with only a 10% saturation of transferrin, thereby competing successfully with a hyperplastic erythroid series for plasma iron. I have never seen this plasma-storage exchange occur in any other disorder associated with iron-deficiency anaemia.

SAADI: How did you make sure that the iron didn't actually stay in the liver?

POLLYCOVE: The liver biopsy showed no stainable iron. Also in Fig. 9 (p. 162) it is apparent that, though the liver initially accumulated radio-iron, subsequently there occurred a rapid hepatic wash-out and a decrease of radio-iron to as low a level as in other iron deficiencies at 10 hours. Radio-iron was removed from the liver with a half-time of approximately $1^1/_2$ hours, which is in close agreement with the intercompartmental rate constant of transfer from the storage labile iron pool to the plasma iron pool ($\alpha_{1/5}$) calculated from mathematical analysis of the plasma radio-iron curve.

KRUH: In your model you don't take into account the fact that iron from the dead red cells is utilised preferentially for the biosynthesis of the new molecules of haemoglobin.

POLLYCOVE: The model is centred on the plasma. When the red cells die, they are phagocytosed by reticulo-endothelial cells, which rapidly return almost all the iron to the plasma (Fig. 7, p. 160). As iron re-enters the plasma it is attached to transferrin and is normally again used chiefly to make new red cells.

KRUH: But iron from dead red blood cells is not diluted by the pool of iron.

POLLYCOVE: Radio-iron entering the plasma from erythrophagocytic reticulo-endothelial cells is diluted in the plasma iron pool.

KRUH: When you inject radioactive iron into an animal, the radioactivity remains constant for weeks and weeks.

POLLYCOVE: Do you mean in the plasma or in the blood?

KRUH: In the red blood cells.

POLLYCOVE: Yes, that's right; whole-blood radio-iron remains essentially constant, since circulating erythrocyte radio-iron remains constant (Fig. 7, p. 160).

KRUH: So the iron which is released after the first life-span is ready to be re-utilised in the next life-span without any dilution. There is no decrease in the radio-activity?

POLLYCOVE: Well, there is a slight decrease in red-cell radio-iron after recycling, because normally when you inject tracer radio-iron into the plasma, an average of 92% of the radio-iron will become incorporated into circulating red cells. The next time it goes around the cycle, only 92% of that 92%, or 84.6% of the injected radio-iron, will be present in the circulating erythrocytes (Fig. 7, p. 160). In six studies of erythrocyte radio-iron undertaken during periods of six months or longer, i.e. similar to the one shown in Fig. 7, virtually all the erythrocyte radio-iron was returned to the plasma, as judged by the final level of erythrocyte radio-iron. You are quite right in supposing that, for several generations after each cycle, erythrocyte radio-iron will be slightly less.

FINCH: One key aspect of this interesting model of Dr. POLLYCOVE's is the assumption that the bone marrow takes up the bulk of the iron going through the plasma, and this seems correct. The point that has concerned us has been the assumption of the existence of a labile pool, before haemoglobin synthesis, of sufficient size to affect the plasma iron kinetics. The data that NOYES and HOSAIN[1] have obtained differ from those presented by Dr. POLLYCOVE. In studies done in man, dog, rabbit, and rat, there was an almost immediate synthesis of haemoglobin to a level of 90% or so within an hour. While these direct measurements of haem synthesis in biopsied marrow have a certain margin of error — perhaps ±10 or 15% — the data obtained nevertheless indicate that there cannot be a large pool of iron before haemoglobin.

KATZ: I just want to comment that perhaps the difference in these results is due to the type of cells NOYES and HOSAIN were investigating as compared with the reticulocytes studied by Dr. POLLYCOVE, which after all are not synthesising haemoglobin at the same rate as normoblasts are. Therefore, even though the Fe^{59} uptake is slower in reticulocytes than in normoblasts, a larger portion of it might be present as non-haem iron.

POLLYCOVE: Actually, in our analyses we found a more rapid fixation of iron into the haem of reticulocytes than into the haem of immature red cells in the marrow. The uptake of iron from transferrin, and the amount of non-haem iron, is much less in reticulocytes than in more immature red cells, so it is understandable that the fixation of non-haem iron into haem proceeds more rapidly.

With regard to Dr. FINCH's comment that the measurements made by NOYES and HOSAIN indicated that essentially all of the marrow radio-iron was found in haem, I might add that our own initial measurements also gave these results. Subsequently, however, when the bones were rapidly excised, immediately iced, and the marrow suspended in a 10^{-3} molar concentration of lead ions to block haem synthesis, we obtained the results presented today. MAZUR and CARLETON[2] have recently studied the relationship between ferritin iron and haem synthesis in marrow and reticulocytes of the intact rat and in systems *in vitro* by the use of serum-bound Fe^{59} and 2-C^{14}-glycine.

[1] NOYES, W. D., and F. HOSAIN: Fed. Proc. (U.S.A.) **20**, 67 (1961) and unpublished data.

[2] MAZUR, A., and A. CARLETON: J. Biol. Chem. (U.S.A.) **238**, 1817 (1963).

Their findings support the conclusion that there is a precursor labile iron pool in the marrow and in the reticulocytes and that "the iron released by the ferritin either is incorporated into heme by combination with protoporphyrin or is returned to the serum".

CHATTERJEA: I was impressed by the evidence presented by Dr. POLLYCOVE on the presence of intramedullary haemolysis in iron deficiency. Dr. POLLYCOVE said that in some cases there is slight shortening of the erythrocyte life-span and also a certain degree of splenic sequestration. These facts are not widely known and deserve our attention. In a few cases we do have clinical evidence pointing to a haemolytic component. Does Dr. POLLYCOVE have any information as to the mechanism of this haemolysis? Has the degree or the duration of anaemia any contributory role in this haemolysis?

POLLYCOVE: I believe not. I think that intramedullary haemolysis usually, if not always, arises from some metabolic or structural defects that develop in the cell as it matures. The defects associated with vitamin B_{12} deficiency are widely recognised. Though this is still not well understood, we know that there is impairment of nucleoprotein synthesis, that D.N.A. synthesis, although increased, is defective, and that consequently most of the immature red cells do not survive to enter the circulation. The cellular defects associated with iron-deficiency anaemia may be a result of inadequate haemoglobin per cell. I think that haemoglobin is not just inert baggage carried by the red cell for the transportation of oxygen and carbon dioxide, but that it probably contributes to the structural stability of the cell. If the haemoglobin content of a maturing red cell is markedly reduced, the cell may not be able to survive long enough to enter the circulation. If a critical minimal amount of haemoglobin is not synthesised by some of the cells, they may lose their viability, begin to decompose, and be phagocytosed by the reticulo-endothelial cells. The intramedullary haemolysis demonstrated in iron-kinetic studies of anaemic iron-deficient patients may be detected morphologically by the presence in the marrow of erythrophagocytosis of nucleated cells. Erythrophagocytosis of immature cells is not observable in normal marrow but can be seen, with both the light and the electron microscope, in marrow from patients with iron-deficiency anaemia. This erythrophagocytosis is probably a scavenging operation and not an active attack by sensitised cells or anything of that nature.

VANNOTTI: In connection with the problem of trying to explain how it is that in haemochromatosis iron from the blood becomes accumulated in excessive quantities in the tissues, I should like to ask Dr. POLLYCOVE whether he thinks this mechanism could be partly attributable to a severe decrease in the transferrin content of the serum due to the haemochromatosis. Using a quantitative immunochemical method, myself and Dr. BLANC[1], of the Biochemical Institute (Dr .H. C. ISLIKER) in Lausanne, measured the transferrin levels in the blood of normal subjects and of patients suffering from haemochromatosis, infectious hepatitis, and liver cirrhosis. We found a very marked reduction in the transferrin levels in the patients with haemochromatosis as well as in those with infectious hepatitis and in some cases of cirrhosis.

POLLYCOVE: Yes, I would agree with Dr. VANNOTTI that an increased plasma-storage iron exchange is associated with an increased or virtually complete saturation of transferrin. However, I would regard this saturation

[1] VANNOTTI, A., and B. BLANC: Schweiz. med. Wschr. **34**, 1189 (1963).

as secondary to the accumulation of very large abnormal amounts of body iron as a result of increased iron absorption persisting for several decades. Using a whole-body counter, we have recently demonstrated increased iron absorption and increased iron stores in young asymptomatic, non-cirrhotic relatives of patients with florid endogenous haemochromatosis. These relatives also showed a normal saturation of transferrin with a normal plasma iron concentration and latent iron-binding capacity. We have not measured transferrin immunologically. Our measured values for the transferrin concentration, as determined by the ion-exchange resin method of PETERS and his associates[1], correspond to total iron-binding capacity values of 200—280 μg./100 ml. With superimposed infection, inflammation, or malignancy, one would expect a further reduction in the transferrin concentration.

FIGUEROA: I should like to ask Dr. POLLYCOVE how he managed to determine that the liver was able to take up six times more iron than normal livers. We have studied 3 or 4 patients with haemochromatosis following venesection. My recollection is that, once the excessive iron stores had been removed and slight to moderate anaemia had been produced, we were unable to demonstrate any excessive affinity of the liver for Fe^{59}. The liver looked fairly normal and showed no excessive localisation of Fe^{59}.

POLLYCOVE: Hepatic body-surface measurements in the patient with endogenous haemochromatosis and iron-deficiency anaemia secondary to venesection therapy clearly demonstrate a large increase in plasma-storage iron exchange. Normally, hepatic counting rates decrease initially as radio-iron leaves the plasma and accumulates predominantly in the marrow. Subsequently, as almost all the radio-iron returns to the blood within the reticulocytes, *in vivo* counting rates usually return to their initial value, c.p.m.$_0$. Hepatic and splenic radioactivity, expressed for convenience as the ratio c.p.m./c.p.m.$_0$, normally do not exceed unity. An initial increase in surface hepatic radioactivity that persists indicates abnormal plasma-storage iron exchange and iron deposition in the storage reserve. Rapid initial hepatic accumulation and subsequent release of radio-iron, simulating the characteristic erythropoietic pattern of the marrow, indicates extra-medullary erythropoiesis in the liver. In this patient, though complete secondary release of radio-iron occurs, it is far too rapid to be attributable to erythropoiesis. This initial accumulation of radio-iron has not been seen in similar studies of over 50 other patients with iron-deficiency anaemia but without endogenous haemochromatosis. This very unusual hepatic accumulation and complete release of radio-iron is compatible with increased plasma-storage iron exchange without deposition of iron in the storage reserve. Graphic analysis of the plasma radio-iron curve does, indeed, reveal a prominent exponential component clearly and accurately demonstrable for 9 hours. The slope of this component, r_2, is characteristic of that associated with plasma-storage iron exchange, being intermediate between the rapid initial component, r_1, and the considerably slower component, r_3, associated with plasma-erythropoietic iron exchange. Using these three slopes, their intercepts at time zero — assuming that approximately all the injected radio-iron becomes incorporated into maturing erythrons, i.e. that $F = 1$ (since there was no significant hepatic net retention of radio-iron, the rate of transfer of iron from the storage labile iron pool to the storage

[1] PETERS, T., T. J. GIOVANNIELLO, L. APT, and J. F. ROSS: J. Laborat. Clin. Med. (U.S.A.) 48, 274 (1956).

reserve iron pool approximates zero, i.e. $\alpha_{5/6} = 0$, and the measured plasma iron pool = 1.06 mg.) — the intercompartmental rate constants, storage and erythropoietic labile iron pools, and the daily intercompartmental transfer of iron were calculated on the basis of the general iron-kinetics model shown in Fig. 1 (p. 149). In this way the storage labile pool was calculated to comprise 0.52 mg. iron, as compared with 10 mg. iron before venesection, with an intercompartmental transfer rate of iron from the storage labile pool to the plasma pool ($\alpha_{5/1}$) of 11.4/day; hence, since $\alpha_{5/6} = 0$, plasma-storage iron exchange $= \alpha_{1/5}X_1 = \alpha_{5/1}X_5 = 11.4 \times 0.52 = 5.7$ mg./day. This is approximately six times the mean normal plasma-storage iron exchange of 1 mg./day. The calculated wash-out of the storage labile iron pool, determined by mathematical analysis of the plasma radio-iron measurements (corresponding to the turnover rate of 11.4/day, $t^1/_2 = 1.46$ hours), is in close agreement with the wash-out of hepatic iron determined by hepatic surface measurements, as shown in Fig. 9 (p. 162).

Beutler: May I ask you something else about your model? How can you distinguish, by measuring only plasma radioactivity, the difference between, on the one hand, exchange between plasma and what you are calling the labile storage pool and, on the other hand, plasma and the labile erythropoietic pool?

Pollycove: Serial analyses of plasma radio-iron content demonstrate three exponential components: a rapid initial component, a second component of intermediate rate, and a third relatively slow component. Normal individuals show a relatively brief second exponential component as compared with that observed in patients with endogenous haemochromatosis, while patients with erythroid aplasia show a very prominent, prolonged second exponential component with absence of the third exponential component. From these and numerous similar correlations it has become clear that the second exponential component, Be^{-r_2t}, is associated with plasma-storage iron exchange, while the third exponential component, Ce^{-r_3t}, is associated with plasma-erythropoietic iron exchange. By measuring the slopes r_1, r_2, and r_3, the intercepts A, B, and C, the fraction of tracer radio-iron fixed in maturing red cells, F, and the total plasma iron, and by using the solutions of the differential equations corresponding to the general mathematical model, it is possible to calculate the six rate constants and the amounts of iron in the storage and erythropoietic labile iron pools. For example, the previously discussed patient with endogenous haemochromatosis and iron-deficiency anaemia had calculated iron content values of 148 mg. and 10 mg. in the erythropoietic and storage labile iron pools, respectively, before venesection therapy when the total plasma iron was 6.8 mg., whereas the corresponding values after the production of iron-deficiency anaemia were 93 mg. and 0.5 mg., respectively, with a total plasma iron of 1.1 mg.

Tubiana: In what form was the iron injected? Was it bound to the patient's own plasma?

Pollycove: Yes, in our usual way.

Tubiana: How high was the level of iron in the plasma? Was all the iron bound to the transferrin?

Pollycove: We incubated the radio-iron with the patient's plasma in our usual manner for half an hour. The amount of iron that we use to label the plasma transferrin is always less than half of the latent iron-binding capacity. In this case the latent iron-binding capacity of 312 μg./100 ml.

(or 15.6 μg. in 5 ml. injected) was high, so that the added amount of iron, 2.7 μg. (corresponding to 40 μc.), utilised only a sixth of the available plasma iron-binding capacity. We did not ascertain directly that in this patient all of the radio-iron was bound to transferrin; but this technique has been consistently satisfactory in the past, except for rare occasions when some colloidal radio-iron was present in the material received from our supplier. Under these circumstances, however, the movement of radio-iron from the plasma is very different. It does not decrease in a continuous smooth fashion, but disappears very rapidly with a simultaneous abrupt and marked deposition in the liver. In this patient, the usual exponential components of the plasma radio-iron were clearly demonstrable, with excellent agreement between the *in vivo* hepatic surface measurements and the rate constants calculated by analysis of the plasma radio-iron measurements.

NAJEAN: If the erythropoietic labile pool is as high as you said and if these movements are so slow, how do you explain the fact that the feed-back of iron from the reticulocytes to the plasma in your observation was so fast and that so much iron was incorporated into the haem in half an hour? These processes can be observed *in vitro*, where they proceed at the same rate with normal reticulocytes as with reticulocytes from patients suffering from hyposideraemic anaemia; however, the intermediate pool in normal reticulocytes is presumably greater than in hypochromic reticulocytes.

POLLYCOVE: As I mentioned before when discussing the remark of Dr. KATZ, the non-haem iron content of the circulating reticulocytes is relatively very small in comparison with that of the less mature red cells developing in the marrow. Consequently, the rate constants for the fixation of labile iron in haem, $\alpha_{2/3}$, and the feed-back of labile iron to plasma, $\alpha_{2/1}$, i.e. the *fractions* of the reticulocyte labile iron pool transferred per hour, are probably much greater, although the amounts transferred are less. This would explain the much more rapid fixation of radio-iron in haem (26.5% in 30 minutes, 44.4% in 45 minutes) and the more rapid feed-back of radio-iron to the plasma (26.4% in 60 minutes) occurring in reticulocytes as compared with the correspondingly slower rates occurring in marrow erythroid cells. It is interesting to note that the rate of feed-back of radio-iron from the reticulocytes to the plasma transferrin was entirely unaffected by the degree of saturation of the transferrin; the feed-back to completely saturated transferrin was equal to the feed-back to transferrin with only 4.5% saturation. This suggests that iron from immature red cells is transferred to the attached transferrin at binding sites that have become vacant owing to the prior transfer of iron from transferrin to the immature red cell. Probably almost all plasma transferrin molecules are either saturated with 2 atoms of iron or bind no iron. Since, as JANDL and KATZ[1] have shown, the saturated transferrin is attached preferentially to the reticulocyte, it is understandable that the rate of feed-back would not be affected by the degree of transferrin saturation.

NAJEAN: I should just like to point out that, where the iron supplies are normal, the speed of the movements is exactly the same in other reticulocytes, e.g. in reticulocytes from patients with haemolytic anaemia. This presumably means that the reticulocyte labile pool is small in all cases.

POLLYCOVE: Yes, we have had similar results with reticulocytes from patients with haemolytic anaemia and from patients with pernicious anaemia

[1] JANDL, J. H., and J. H. KATZ: J. Clin. Invest. (U.S.A.) **42**, 314 (1963).

during a therapeutic reticulocyte response to vitamin B_{12}. The erythropoietic labile iron pool of the reticulocyte is quite small as compared with that of the more immature red cell. The data shown may be regarded as having been obtained with relatively "normal" reticulocytes, although they constitute 30% of the circulating red cells. This degree of reticulocytosis is present continuously in a patient with hereditary telangiectasia bleeding approximately 900 ml. blood daily, with a haemoglobin concentration of 7 g./100 ml., while receiving 1,500 mg. iron per week intravenously.

BEUTLER: I wonder whether you have any comment to make, Dr. POLLYCOVE, on the suggestion put forward by BESSIS[1] that iron may possibly be transported directly in the form of ferritin to the developing erythroblasts. This would result in a short-circuit around the plasma iron pool.

POLLYCOVE: BESSIS postulated a direct transport of iron from phagocytosed red cells via ferritin micropinocytosis by immature red cells derived from reticular cells; this implies bypassing the plasma. One can, of course, always raise the question as to how we know, by means of electron microscopy, which way the ferritin is moving. Assuming that the direction of movement of iron from reticulo-endothelial cells into red cells is correct, the amount of iron so transferred may not be significant. Quantitation of haemoglobin synthesis from plasma iron in normal subjects yields amounts which, when related to the circulating haemoglobin, indicate erythrocyte life-spans of 102—132 days. Any additional iron for haemoglobin synthesis would be associated with a shorter life-span. It would seem, then, that the amount of iron transferred directly from the reticulo-endothelial cells to the red cells cannot constitute a considerable fraction of the total iron entering the red cells, because this would entail a red-cell life-span that is much shorter than the established normal range. I think the evidence BESSIS himself has presented also leads to the conclusion that iron entering directly from the reticulo-endothelial cells constitutes an insignificant fraction of the total iron entering the red cell. He has observed that this direct transfer of ferritin from reticulo-endothelial cells to immature red cells is very greatly increased in the secondary anaemia of infection, i.e. to approximately 10—20 times the normal figure. Using the electron microscope, BESSIS has confirmed observations made with the light microscope to the effect that during infection the developing erythroid cells are iron deficient. If, then, despite a ten to twentyfold increase in the amount of direct iron transfer by micropinocytosis, the red cells are still iron deficient, it would seem that this possible iron bypass of the plasma is quantitatively insignificant as compared with plasma iron transfer into the red cells.

BEUTLER: Maybe it is difficult to measure rates by electron microscopy.

POLLYCOVE: Yes, it seems quite difficult.

KATZ: I should also like to add that we believe marrow perfusion to be sufficiently great to account for even the most rapid plasma clearance rates observed in the various hyperkinetic anaemias. We feel, therefore, that transferrin adsorption to erythroid cells is the primary route by which iron enters such cells.

POLLYCOVE: This is especially clear in man, where normally only a very small fraction of the iron removed from the plasma (approximately 10%) is not involved in haemoglobin synthesis.

---

[1] BESSIS, M. C., and J. BRETON-GORIUS: Nouv. rev. franç. hémat. 1, 569 (1961).

Introduction to the General Discussion

By

U. Salera

In introducing the general discussion on the physiology of iron I should like to begin by turning to the problem of the digestive absorption of iron. I think it would be profitable to make certain criticisms regarding the methods by which the absorption of iron has been studied. Perhaps Dr. Najean, who has given us a new technique for the study of iron absorption, would like to discuss this question. We are, of course, faced not only with the quantitative aspects of the problem but also with the task of assessing those factors which influence the absorption of iron in the form both of iron salts as well as of iron from food; these factors include the gut itself, the mucosal wall, the plasma iron-binding protein, the iron-storage mechanisms, and erythropoietic function.

There are certainly many factors operative in determining how much iron has to be absorbed to satisfy the needs of the organism. But, as Dr. Callender has said, the actual mechanisms of absorption and regulation still remain obscure.

Moreover, it is very difficult to assess the relative importance of certain factors in the absorption of iron, because many of the data derived from different experiments are in complete disagreement with one another. For instance, the plasma iron-binding globulin was until recently accepted as being a regulating factor, or at least a limiting factor, in the digestive absorption of iron. Crosby and co-workers (*1*), however, have meanwhile furnished experimental data demonstrating that the absorption of iron from an isolated intestinal loop continues despite saturation or near-saturation of the iron-binding capacity of transferrin. This finding seems incompatible with Hallberg's concept (*2*) that the degree of saturation of transferrin plays a direct or immediate role in the regulation of iron absorption. This is but one example among many. I think Dr. Heilmeyer and Dr. Moore will probably have other views on this subject, especially as regards the so-called "mucosal block".

Transferrin is the main factor active in the second stage of iron metabolism, i.e. the transport of iron and its transfer to the iron stores and active fractions, including first of all the erythroblasts (for haemoglobin formation). Here, once again, different methods have led to different interpretations. Dr. BESSIS (*3*) thinks that the reticular cell fulfils the function of a nurse, with ferritin serving as the milk. Many others think that the main source of iron for the erythroblasts is transferrin. We all know that, by means of autoradiography, one can demonstrate that the erythroblasts are able to take up radioactive iron when incubated in a plasma containing labelled iron. On the other hand, we are confronted with the brilliant experimental demonstration which Dr. BESSIS has given. I suspect that, as is so often the case, the real truth probably lies somewhere half-way between the two opposing concepts.

With regard to iron storage, we must take into consideration the relationship between ferritin and haemosiderin and the factors governing the biochemical and anatomical distribution of iron, including particularly the iron introduced into the body via physiological pathways rather than iron administered in the form of a drug. Here, too, conflicting evidence has been presented by different research workers, depending on whether they have approached the problem as chemists, isotope specialists, anatomists, etc.

The whole problem of research on iron metabolism is fundamentally one of ferrokinetics, which at present is still a highly specialised subject. During recent years, Dr. POLLYCOVE has treated us to such a wealth of intriguing mathematics in this connection that I fear it would be presumptuous of me even to touch on this complicated topic.

The finer mechanism of iron transfer to the erythroblasts was studied by JANDL (*4*) and by KATZ (*5*). Dr. KATZ has just given us a complete report on this subject. But I think it would be worthwhile to add something about the iron proteins as distinct from the stroma proteins and particulate matter which, according to JANDL, may act as an intermediate in haemoglobin formation. Dr. YOSHIKAWA thinks that the non-protein bound form of iron may be the direct precursor of haem and haemoglobin iron – a supposition which is in agreement with the data of SONDHAUS and THORELL (*6*).

Two years ago, we isolated in our laboratory a bone-marrow iron protein from rabbit bone-marrow homogenate by means of electrophoresis (*7*). We suggested that the iron protein in question might be a precursor of haemoglobin. One year later, GREENOUGH et al. (*8*) published a report also describing an intracellular iron

Fig. 1

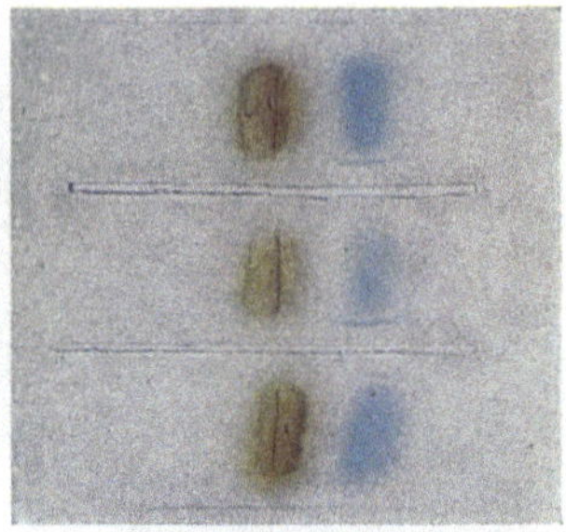

Fig. 2

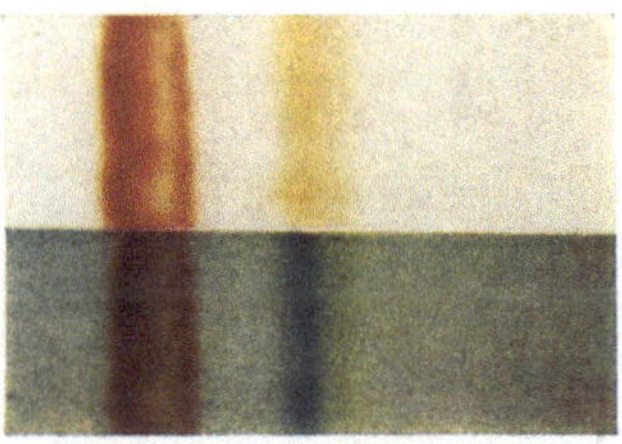

Fig. 3

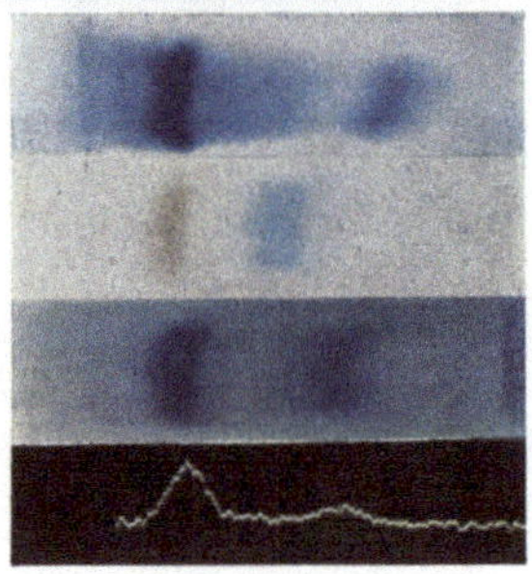

Fig. 4

Fig. 1. Paper-electrophoretic pattern of the supernatant of rabbit bone-marrow homogenate: strips stained with amidoschwarz (above) and Prussian blue reaction (below)

Fig. 2. Immuno-electropherogram of a bone-marrow homogenate tested with antiferritin antiserum

Fig. 3. Starch-block electrophoresis of the supernatant of rabbit bone-marrow homogenate before (above) and after (below) Prussian blue reaction

Fig. 4. Electropherogram of bone-marrow homogenate of a rabbit sacrificed 3 hours after intravenous injection of Fe^{59}. Radioactivity is located in the migration zone of the haemoglobin and of another iron protein fraction with intermediate mobility between the ferritin and the albumin. a) strip stained with amidoschwarz; b) strip stained with Prussian blue reaction; c) radio-autogram of b; d) radioscan of b

protein isolated by chromatography which they concluded to be an intermediate in haemoglobin formation. The characteristics of this iron protein are almost the same as those of the protein which we had isolated in our laboratory and to which I would like to refer now.

Fig. 1 shows the paper-electrophoretic pattern of the supernatant of a rabbit bone-marrow homogenate. Besides a band of haemoglobin, there is a protein fraction stained with Prussian blue. The same phenomenon can be observed when separation is effected by means of agar or starch-block electrophoresis.

In Fig. 2 the agar-electrophoretic pattern of the supernatant of a horse bone-marrow homogenate is given. The pherogram was tested with antiferritin antiserum and stained with Prussian blue. Since there is a precipitation band corresponding to the Prussian blue zone, we can conclude that the protein fraction which takes up Prussian blue is ferritin.

In Fig. 3 we have the starch-block electrophoretic pattern of the supernatant of a rabbit bone-marrow homogenate before (above) and after (below) applying Prussian blue.

If a rabbit is given an intravenous dose of radioactive iron, the distribution of the radioactivity on the pherogram varies depending on the time intervals between the injection of the iron and the sacrifice of the animal. The distribution of the radioactivity can be studied on the paper-electropherogram by means of autoradiography or radio-scanning and on the starch-block electropherogram by cutting out the supporting medium into slices and measuring the radioactivity of the corresponding eluates.

A few minutes after the injection, only a fraction corresponding to the transferrin-migration zone is radioactive, as demonstrated by experiments using electrophoresis of radioactive rabbit plasma on the same starch block. Half an hour after injection of the tracer, the radioactivity begins to appear in the haemoglobin, as well as in an electrophoretic fraction which has an intermediate mobility between the ferritin and the albumin. The ferritin, however, is not yet labelled. The phenomenon is even more clearly evident three hours after the injection, by which time the radioactivity is no longer measurable in the transferrin and can be detected by autoradiography only in the haemoglobin and in a fraction showing faster mobility than the ferritin (Fig. 4).

This new bone-marrow iron protein displays the following properties:

a) In an aqueous solution it appears colourless and does not stain either with Prussian blue or with benzidine.

b) It does not react to EHRLICH's reagent.

c) By means of dialysis against buffers at different pH's, as well as by cold and warm acid hydrolysis, it has been possible to demonstrate a strong link between the metal and the protein – a link which is far stronger than in the case of transferrin and ferritin.

d) The absorption spectrum shows a peak at 280 mμ and another at 320–330 mμ, whereas no absorption is observed at 415 mμ.

e) Immuno-electrophoresis of a bone-marrow homogenate does not show a cross-reaction with antiferritin antiserum at the site corresponding to the migration zone of this fraction.

f) A comparison between electrophoresis of a bone-marrow homogenate and of Fe^{59}-labelled serum shows that the fraction identified by us has a migration rate different from that of transferrin.

The new iron protein is a fraction peculiar to bone marrow. It is in fact impossible to find any radioactivity in the corresponding zone of the pherogram of a liver homogenate, even at the time when in the bone marrow the radioactivity of the fraction attains its maximum. Nor were we able to trace this fraction in the pherograms of homogenates prepared from various segments of the intestine.

Ferrokinetic studies on the bone-marrow iron proteins were undertaken in experiments on rabbits both *in vivo* and *in vitro*. In these experiments we studied the incorporation of radioactive iron in the iron proteins separated by starch-block electrophoresis from bone-marrow homogenate incubated in Fe^{59}-labelled plasma. The study was carried out at different periods of incubation both in normal plasma and in plasma to which lead acetate had been added. During the first 10 minutes more radioactivity was incorporated into our protein fraction than into the haemoglobin. Afterwards, however, the radioactivity in our fraction increased at a much slower rate than in the haemoglobin, with the result that after 3 hours the radioactivity in the haemoglobin was much higher (almost double) than in the other fraction. On the other hand, when lead acetate was added to the substrate, the radioactivity in the haemoglobin was very small after 3 hours, whereas in our fraction it reached higher values than in the control.

These findings suggest that our bone-marrow iron protein may be a precursor of haemoglobin similar to, or identical with, the intracellular iron protein described by GREENOUGH et al. (*8*).

References

1. POLLACK, S., S. P. BALCERZAK, and W. H. CROSBY: Blood (U.S.A.) **21**, 33 (1963). — 2. HALLBERG, L., and L. SÖLVELL: Acta med. Scand. Suppl. 358 (1960). — 3. BESSIS, M. C., and J. BRETON-GORIUS: Blood (U.S.A.) **14**, 423 (1959). — 4. ALLEN, D. W., and I. H. JANDL: Blood (U.S.A.) **15**, 71 (1960). — 5. KATZ, J. H.: J. Clin. Invest. (U.S.A.) **40**, 2143 (1961). — 6. SONDHAUS, C. A., and B. THORELL: Blood (U.S.A.) **16**, 1285 (1960). — 7. SALERA, U., P. MAGNANELLI, R. D'AVINO, I. ZECCA, and A. L. MATCOVICH: Proceedings of the 8th Congress of the European Society of Haematology, Vienna, 1961, 240a. — 8. GREENOUGH, W. B., T. PETERS, Jr., and E. D. THOMAS: J. Clin. Invest. (U.S.A.) **41**, 1116 (1962).

General Discussion

SALERA: I should like to put a question to Dr. POLLYCOVE. When you speak of the average life-span, are you referring to the erythrocytes or to the erythron? I mention this because we did not succeed in finding any reduction in the life-span of the erythrocytes in iron-deficiency anaemia[1].

POLLYCOVE: Mean erythron life-span is used to designate the mean survival of all erythroid cells from the time they are capable of rapidly removing iron from transferrin, i.e. the nucleated and reticulocyte stages of development. The mean erythron life-span may be considerably shorter than the mean erythrocyte life-span, the latter being the mean survival of the circulating red-cell population. Normally the mean erythron life-span is 2—3 days longer than the mean erythrocyte life-span. However, there may be a considerable difference between these two red-cell life-spans in various pathological conditions with intramedullary haemolysis. Iron-deficiency anaemia is a common disorder in which intramedullary haemolysis occurs with a resultant large discrepancy between mean erythron and mean erythrocyte life-spans. The average mean erythron life-span in 20 patients with iron-deficiency anaemia was found by iron-kinetic studies to be 45 days as compared with mean circulating erythrocyte survivals of 75—95 days as determined by Ashby survival, Cr^{51} and D.F.P.^{32} studies. The red cells of patients with pernicious anaemia in severe relapse are markedly defective, with pronounced intramedullary haemolysis, the Fe^{59}-determined mean erythron life-span being 4—8 days as compared with a D.F.P.^{32}-determined mean circulating erythrocyte survival of 15—35 days.

FIGUEROA: Dr. DREYFUS was asking a question about studies following portacaval shunt. It was TUTTLE[2] who reported the first case of haemochromatosis developing about three years after portacaval shunt. We have studied an additional 5 patients who had had a portacaval shunt, but here there was no evidence of excessive tissue iron. We were also unable to demonstrate any excessive iron absorption in these cases. Similarly, we have studied 5 or 6 dogs with portacaval shunt, and here again we failed to find any evidence of excessive iron absorption following the shunt.

I should also like to make a remark concerning the pancreas. Some 8 or 9 years ago, we studied 3 patients who had undergone total pancreatectomy for chronic relapsing pancreatitis. In these patients, too, we were unable to show any excessive iron absorption. I should like to ask Dr. CALLENDER if she knows where the iron goes to. Does she have any evidence that it enters the liver, or does it perhaps go into the red blood cells? We had one particular patient with primary haemochromatosis to whom we gave several grammes of Viocase a day; studies with Fe^{59} showed that the patient was absorbing 30 to 35% of iron by mouth; in this case we did not observe any reduction in the absorption of iron with the Viocase. I was struck by the fact that you

[1] ZECCA, I., H. KOYUNCUOGLU, G. ANDREUCCI, N. A. SERAFINI, and U. SALERA: Progr. Méd. (Fr.) **17**, 852 (1961).

[2] TUTTLE, S. G., W. G. FIGUEROA, and M. I. GROSSMAN: Amer. J. Med. **26**, 655 (1959).

were able to demonstrate excessive iron absorption in chronic relapsing pancreatitis. Does this occur in all patients with chronic pancreatitis? I notice that DAVIS[1] found excessive iron absorption in only 6 out of 14 patients suffering from pancreatitis associated with calcification; 6 out of 7 patients with cirrhosis also showed excessive iron absorption. Is this the case with all cirrhotics, or were these patients something of an exception? We have seen excessive iron absorption only in one out of 10 cases of cirrhosis.

CALLENDER: These are the first cirrhotics we have studied. They were unselected cases referred to us with chronic liver disease. As to the question where the iron goes to, we have no definite data on this point. One would expect a high liver uptake, as very little iron appears in the blood.

VENTURA: I should like to refer again to the function of transferrin in the absorption of iron. While some people believe that transferrin plays no part in iron absorption, others — including myself — think that it does.

We know that there are some pathological conditions in which a low transferrin value is accompanied by a normal absorption of iron, but in all cases where a high transferrin value is found, e.g. iron-deficiency anaemia, an increase in iron absorption is evident. That transferrin has something to do with the absorption of iron can easily be proved by the following method. The plasma transferrin of a patient with iron-deficiency anaemia is saturated with Fe ions by intravenous infusion of a readily ionisable iron compound. The infusion is continued for 24 hours, the infusion rate being varied in order to maintain a constant degree of saturation. Two hours after the saturation reaches a constant value, 5 mg. iron in the form of $Fe^{59}Cl_2$ is administered orally. The resultant iron absorption is invariably found to be lower than that observed in the same patient without transferrin saturation.

POLLYCOVE: Is this measured by analysis of stool collections or blood samples?

VENTURA: It is measured from the stools, which are collected over a period of 5—10 days, i.e. until such time as the faecal iron excretion falls to below 0.1% of the dose of radioactivity administered. The presence of non-absorbed fractions of Fe^{59} in the intestinal lumen is excluded by surface counting rates.

ROSA: Dr. SALERA, did you check the specific activity of your protein and the specific activity of the haemoglobin in relation to time?

SALERA: Yes, but we only checked that of the haemoglobin and only at 10-minute, 30-minute, and 3-hour intervals in *in vitro* experiments. In the experiments *in vivo* one is dealing with a different animal at each interval; this makes it very difficult to compare one experiment with another because of the biological variability.

[1] DAVIS, A. E., and J. BADENOCH: Lancet (G.B.) **1962**/II, 6.

Iron deficiency

Experimental hyposiderosis

By

E. H. Morgan

Hyposiderosis may be defined as a reduction in the storage or reserve iron present in the body. This iron is found in most of the different tissues in the form of the two non-haem iron protein compounds, ferritin (water-soluble) and haemosiderin (water-insoluble). It is available for use elsewhere in the body when required for haemoglobin, cellular enzyme, or myoglobin synthesis and therefore acts as a reserve against the possibility of an inadequate dietary iron supply or of increased iron loss due to bleeding. The iron is also available when requirements are increased by a period of rapid growth or by the need to transfer iron to the foetus or suckling young.

The present paper will be concerned very briefly with the means by which hyposiderosis can be produced in experimental animals, and then with the changes which occur in the iron stores and the accompanying alterations in certain other aspects of iron metabolism.

Experimental production of hyposiderosis

Hyposiderosis may be produced by restriction of dietary iron intake or absorption or by causing excess iron loss from the body. For the rapid development of dietary hyposiderosis it is necessary to feed a low-iron diet to young, rapidly growing animals, whose iron requirements are high, or to combine an iron-deficient diet with increased iron loss, usually produced by bleeding. Many low-iron diets have been described. Most consist of milk in one form or another with or without supplements of vitamins and salts (Waddel, Steenbock, Elvehjem, and Hart, 1928; Chappelle, Gabrio, Stephens, and Finch, 1955; Beutler and Blaisdell, 1958; McCall, Newman, O'Brien, Valberg, and Witts, 1962). Hallgren (1953) described a low-iron diet using dried egg-white as the protein source. The most critical examination of an iron-deficient diet so far published was that by MCCALL and his colleagues, who showed that, supplemented with iron, their diet would support normal growth, blood formation, and reproduction in rats for at least three generations. Using this diet, the minimum iron content of the diet for normal growth was found to be approximately 50 mg./kg., but it was considered necessary to increase this to 240 mg./kg. to provide for the increased requirements of pregnancy and lactation.

To produce hyposiderosis at all rapidly in adult animals it is necessary to increase the iron loss from the body. This is usually achieved by bleeding, which may be combined with a low-iron diet. Partial hepatectomy has also been used (VENKATACHALAM and KALDOR, 1957). The disadvantage of producing hyposiderosis by increasing iron losses is that other body materials are removed in addition to iron, and this may produce changes not due solely to iron depletion.

Hyposiderosis may also be studied under physiological conditions in pregnant, lactating, and rapidly growing young animals fed normal diets. In these conditions, iron is mobilised from the stores to meet the additional requirements of growth, increased blood formation, and iron transfer to the young.

Changes in the iron stores in hyposiderosis

The highest concentrations of storage iron are found in the spleen, liver, and bone marrow, which are therefore generally considered to represent the main iron-storage organs. However, considerable storage iron is to be found elsewhere in the body, especially in the muscles and skin, which in some animals may contain as much or more storage iron than the liver and spleen combined (KOOYMAN, 1949; ROTH, JASINSKI, and v. BIDDER, 1951; HALLGREN, 1953; HEVESY and LOCKNER, 1962). These facts may explain why, in normal human males, the liver, spleen, and bone marrow together have been found to contain only about 700 mg. storage iron (TOMPSETT, 1935; BRÜCKMAN and ZONDEK, 1939; SCHAIRER and RECHENBERGER, 1948; MEIER, BENEKE, and AHLERT 1959; BOTHWELL and FINCH, 1962), and yet the iron stores, as measured by phlebotomy, have been assessed at between 1,000 to 1,500 mg. (HASKINS, STEVENS, FINCH, and FINCH, 1952).

Because of the difficulty in measuring the entire storage iron content of the bone marrow, muscles, or skin of an animal, most experimental studies on storage iron have been concerned with the liver and spleen only. It is therefore important to know how well the changes in storage iron in hyposiderosis in one organ reflect those in other organs. Fig. 1 shows the relation found between liver

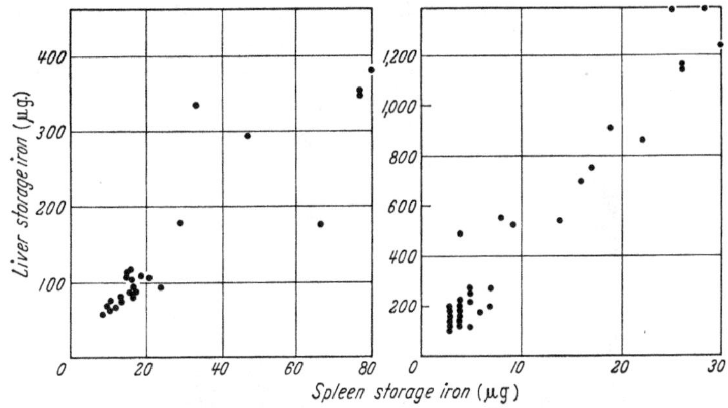

Fig. 1. The relation between liver and spleen storage iron in dietary (left) and haemorrhagic (right) hyposiderosis in rats (adapted from HALLGREN, 1953, and MORGAN, 1961a)

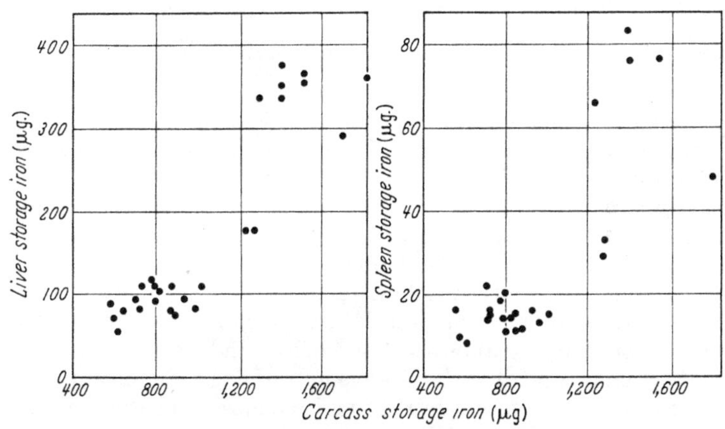

Fig. 2. The relation between carcass storage iron and liver and spleen storage iron in dietary hyposiderosis in rats (HALLGREN, 1953)

and spleen storage iron in rats with dietary (HALLGREN, 1953) or haemorrhagic (MORGAN, 1961a) iron depletion. Fig. 2, also taken from HALLGREN's work, shows the relation found between the storage iron of the carcass and that of the liver and spleen. With only a few exceptions, there appears to be a close linear relationship between liver and spleen iron stores, while that between the carcass and liver or spleen is not quite so close. In addition, Hallgren states, without giving actual results, that the changes in bone-marrow storage iron found in his iron-deficient rats followed closely those of the liver and spleen. It may therefore be safe to conclude that, with the development of hyposiderosis, storage iron is reduced more or less proportionately in all organs.

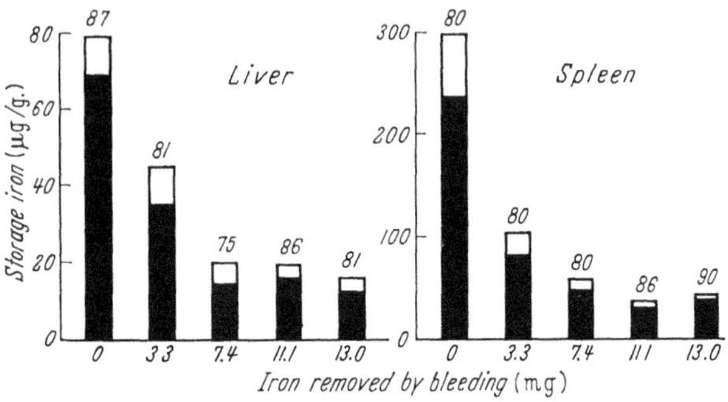

Fig. 3. Mean liver and spleen storage iron concentrations and their relative distribution between ferritin (■) and haemosiderin (□) in rats with hyposiderosis produced by repeated bleeding from the tail over a period of 8 weeks. The severity of hyposiderosis was varied by removing different amounts of iron from different groups of rats as indicated under each column. The figure above each column gives the percentage of the total storage iron which was present as ferritin iron (Morgan, 1961a)

Storage iron is present in the tissues as both ferritin and haemosiderin. Shoden, Gabrio, and Finch (1953), using chemical, isotopic, and immunochemical methods, showed that ferritin and haemosiderin iron may each be estimated quantitatively by a simple chemical technique based on their different solubilities in water. Furthermore, Kaldor (1958) has shown that the sum of the water-soluble and water-insoluble non-haem iron fractions equals the total tissue non-haem iron. If non-haem iron is equated with storage iron, then it appears that ferritin and haemosiderin iron together constitute all of the storage iron. Using a chemical method for total storage iron and ferritin and haemosiderin iron based on these principles (Kaldor, 1958), the relative distribution of liver and spleen storage iron between its two forms has been studied in several different types of experimental hyposiderosis. Fig. 3 shows the results obtained in rats with haemorrhagic hyposiderosis (Morgan, 1961a). It can be seen that, as the degree of hyposiderosis was increased by greater severity of bleeding, the total storage iron values became progressively less. However, no significant alteration was found in either liver or spleen in the relative distribution of the iron between ferritin and haemosiderin. These results suggest that, in response to haemorrhage, iron is released equally readily from the two compounds. Similarly, in rats where the iron stores were depleted by the natural stresses of pregnancy or lactation alone, or combined with haemorrhage, the relative distribution of liver and spleen storage iron between its two forms remained constant (MORGAN, 1961b). Also, after partial hepatectomy in the rat, the storage iron concentration of the regenerating liver is at first low, rising slowly during 3 to 4 weeks to the pre-operative level. The proportion of the storage iron present as ferritin and haemosiderin was found to remain constant during this process (Fig. 4).

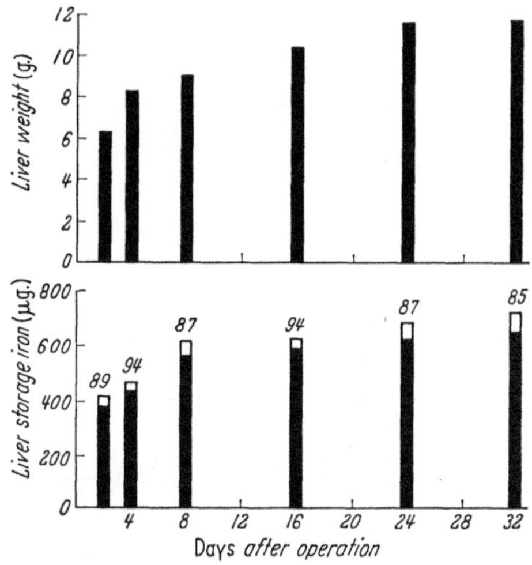

Fig. 4. Mean liver weights, storage iron concentrations, and relative distribution of the iron between ferritin (■) and haemosiderin (□) in rats at different time intervals after removal of approximately 65% of the liver. Each column indicates the mean values from 4 rats, and the figures above the columns give the percentage of the storage iron present as ferritin

The degree of storage iron depletion found in experimental animals depends on the stress applied to their iron status, i.e. on the iron content of the diet and the duration of dietary iron restriction, or on the frequency and severity of bleeding. However, several workers have found that the iron stores cannot be lowered below a certain minimum level (BOGNIARD and WHIPPLE, 1932; HAHN and WHIPPLE, 1936; WAKEHAM and HALENZ, 1936; MCCALL, NEWMAN, O'BRIEN, and WITTS, 1962). Fig. 5, from HALLGREN (1953), illustrates this. It shows the liver, spleen, and carcass storage iron of rats reared for about 40 days from the time of weaning on diets containing varying amounts of iron. With diets providing 70, 35 or 0 µg. iron/day, liver and spleen storage iron remained at a constant minimum level, as did carcass storage iron with the 35 or 0 µg. diets. The term "parenchyma iron" has been used to describe tissue non-haem iron which is not mobilised despite severe iron depletion (BOGNIARD and WHIPPLE, 1932). Its exact relationship to true storage iron is not clear. HALLGREN considers that this residual iron should not be regarded as storage iron, but that it should be subtracted from the non-haem iron value found in any tissue, in order to obtain the true storage iron. However, since the "parenchyma iron" of the liver and spleen is only a small fraction of the

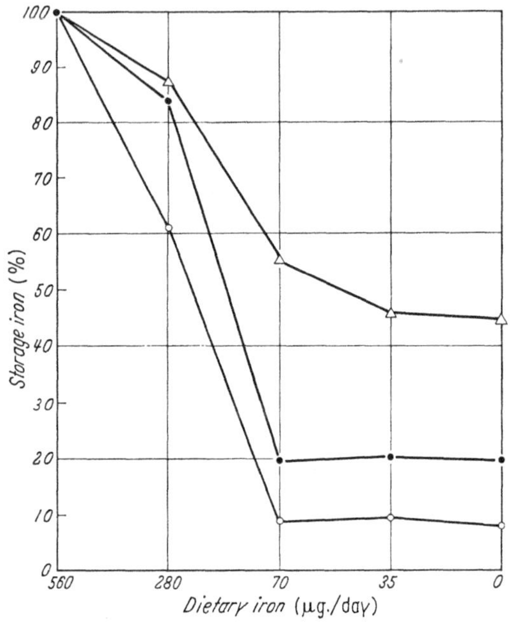

Fig. 5. Liver (●), spleen (○), and carcass (△) storage iron in rats fed differing amounts of iron for about 6 weeks from the time of weaning. The results for each organ are given as % of the mean amount of storage iron found in the rats which received 560 µg. iron in their diet each day (adapted from HALLGREN, 1953)

total non-haem iron, it is probably justifiable to call the non-haem iron of these organs "storage iron" as long as it is remembered that a small proportion may not be mobilisable in time of need.

Alterations in other aspects of iron metabolism accompanying hyposiderosis

Plasma iron concentration. This is usually found to be reduced in animals with depleted iron stores. It is rather difficult to assess the exact relationship between storage and plasma iron and to know what degree of storage iron reduction must occur before the plasma value changes. There is evidence, however, that the plasma iron concentration commences to fall before the iron stores are completely mobilised (HALLGREN, 1953; McCALL, NEWMAN, O'BRIEN, and WITTS, 1962). Indeed, McCALL and his co-workers found a direct linear relationship between plasma iron and carcass non-haemoglobin iron concentrations.

Plasma transferrin concentration. Iron deficiency in animals, as in man, is usually accompanied by an increase in plasma transferrin concentration (measured by the plasma total iron-binding capacity, T.I.B.C.); but, in rats and rabbits, at least, there does not appear to be a very close relationship between transferrin concentration and iron stores (MORGAN 1961c, 1962). Fig. 6 shows the relation found between T.I.B.C. and storage iron, and T.I.B.C. and blood haemoglobin concentration in rats with haemorrhagic iron deficiency. Although there is a good inverse linear relationship between T.I.B.C. and haemoglobin, there is no evidence of such between T.I.B.C. and iron stores. Similarly, when a large number of rats treated in a variety of ways (haemorrhagic and dietary iron depletion, copper depletion, acute and chronic haemolysis, iron feeding, and blood transfusion) were examined, a good correlation was found between T.I.B.C. and haemoglobin values, but not between T.I.B.C. and storage iron (Fig. 7). The relationship between T.I.B.C. and haemoglobin is probably due to the fact that, in the rat, the main factor regulating plasma transferrin concentration is the balance between tissue supply and requirements for oxygen – relative oxygen

Table 1. *Factors regulating T.I.B.C. (plasma total iron-binding capacity) in the rat. Summary of the changes in several measured and inferred values found in rats treated as indicated*
(For details see MORGAN, 1962, 1963)

Treatment	Changes measured				Changes inferred		
	T.I.B.C.	Iron stores	Blood haemoglobin concentration	Reticulocyte count	Rate of erythropoiesis	Supply of erythropoietin	Relative tissue oxygen supply
Haemorrhage . . .	+	—	—	+	+	+	—
Haemolysis	+	+	—	+	+	+	—
Thyroxine	+	0	+	+	+	+	—
X-irradiation	0	0	0	—	—	0	0
Blood transfusion . .	—	+	+	—	—	—	+
Plasma from anaemic rabbits	—		+	+	+	+	+
Propylthiouracil . .	—	0	—	—	—	—	+

+ indicates an increase, — indicates a decrease, and 0 indicates no change with respect to values from untreated rats.

supply (Morgan, 1962, 1963). Some of the evidence for this hypothesis is summarised in Table 1. It can be seen that an increase in

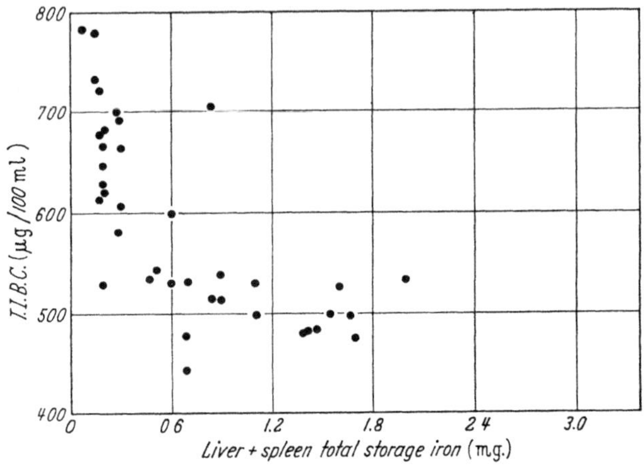

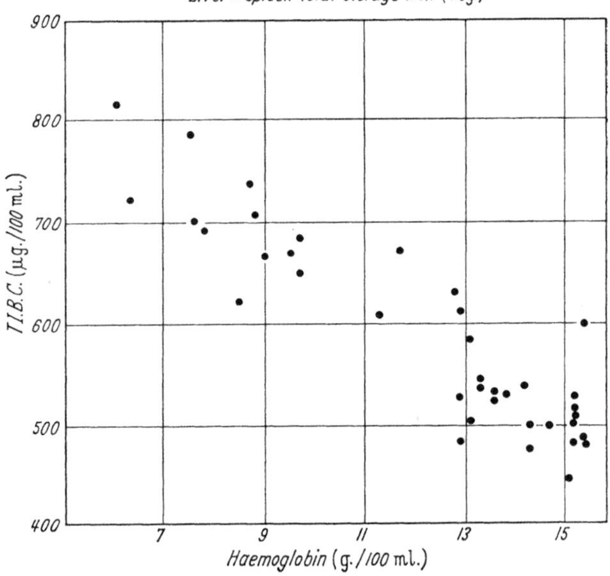

Fig. 6. Relation between T.I.B.C (plasma total iron-binding capacity) and liver plus spleen storage iron, and between T.I.B.C. and blood haemoglobin concentration in control male rats and male rats with differing degrees of haemorrhagic iron depletion

Fig. 7. Relation between T.I.B.C. (plasma total iron-binding capacity) and liver plus spleen storage iron, and between T.I.B.C. and blood haemoglobin concentration in male rats. The rats were treated in a variety of ways, including the production of iron and copper depletion, haemolysis, blood transfusion, and the feeding of extra-dietary iron

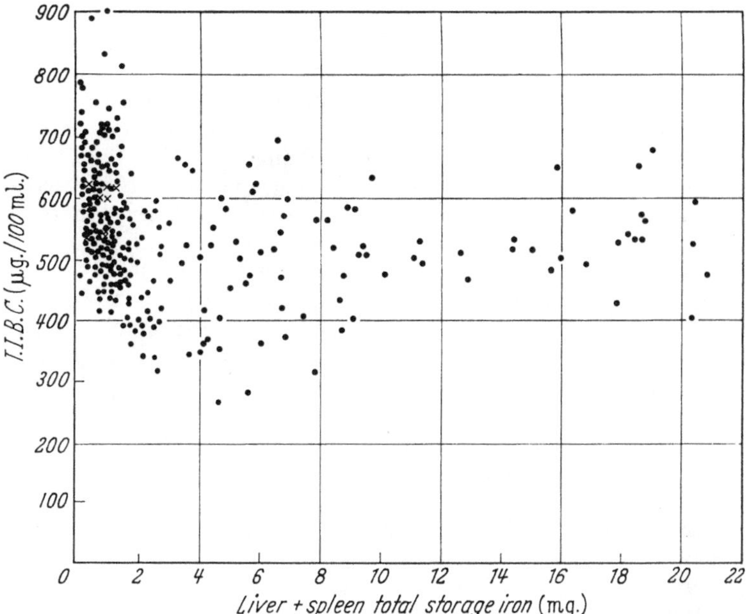

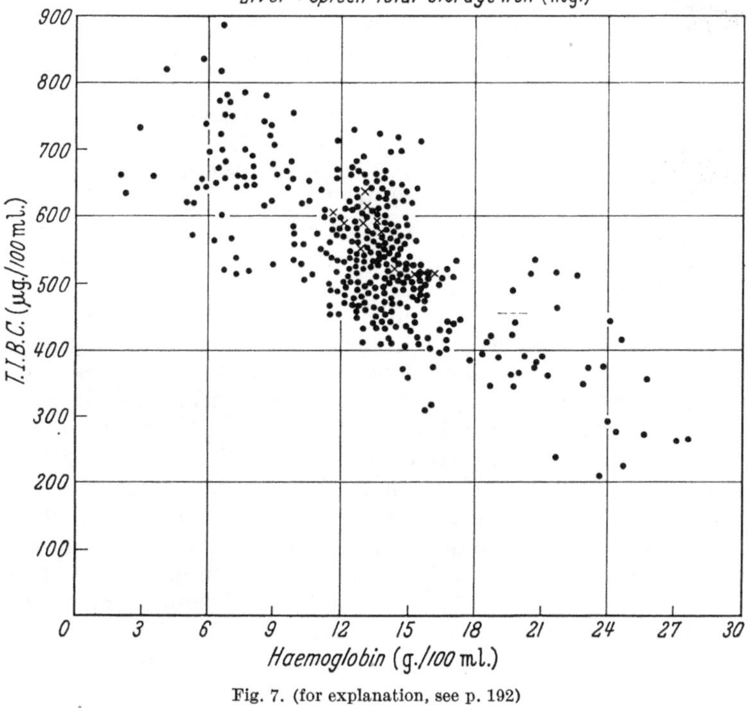

Fig. 7. (for explanation, see p. 192)

T.I.B.C. may be accompanied by increased, decreased, or unchanged iron stores and by increased as well as decreased blood haemoglobin concentrations. Of the changes shown in the table, only those of relative tissue oxygen supply fit the changes of T.I.B.C. in a constant manner. Further experiments have shown that the effects of oxygen supply on the serum proteins are exerted only on transferrin and not on the other protein fractions (Morgan and Brackenridge, 1962; Morgan and Lynch, 1963). Additional work is required before it will be known whether regulation of the plasma transferrin concentration in other animal species is similar to that in the rat and rabbit. It may be noted, however, that, in iron-deficient humans with little or no anaemia, the T.I.B.C. may be normal and that, with the development of anaemia, the T.I.B.C. appears to be related inversely to the haemoglobin concentration (Beutler, Robson, and Buttenwieser, 1958; Pirzio-Biroli and Finch, 1960).

Blood haemoglobin concentration. It is generally believed that the iron stores must be depleted before a reduction in haemoglobin occurs (Bothwell and Finch, 1962; Beutler, Fairbanks, and Fahey, 1963). However, there is some evidence that the haemoglobin concentration may commence to fall before the iron stores have been completely mobilised (Hallgren, 1953). Similarly, stainable iron is found in the bone marrow of a small proportion of patients with untreated iron-deficiency anaemia (Davidson and Jennison, 1952; Bothwell and Finch, 1962). It therefore seems likely that, with the development of hyposiderosis, the haemoglobin level remains constant until the iron stores are largely depleted, but may commence to fall while some storage iron still remains. The exact relationship between haemoglobin and storage iron has yet to be elucidated.

Iron absorption and excretion. Iron deficiency is accompanied by increased efficiency of iron absorption both in humans (Balfour, Hahn, Bale, Pommerenke, and Whipple, 1942; Dubach, Callender, and Moore, 1948; Pirzio-Biroli and Finch, 1960) as well as in experimental animals (Austoni, Rabinovitch, and Greenberg, 1940; Wintrobe, Greenberg, Humphreys, Ashenbrucker, Worth, and Kramer, 1947; Bothwell, Pirzio-Biroli, and Finch, 1958; Bannerman, O'Brien, and Witts, 1962). Indeed, the two most important intrinsic factors influencing iron absorption are thought to be the state of the iron stores and the rate of erythropoiesis (Bothwell, Pirzio-Biroli, and Finch, 1958). The increased absorption found in hyposiderosis appears to be relatively independent of the blood haemoglobin or plasma iron concentrations, or of the plasma latent iron-binding capacity (BOTHWELL, PIRZIO-BIROLI, and FINCH, 1958; PIRZIO-BIROLI and FINCH, 1960; WHEBY and JONES, 1962). It appears likely that the storage iron level has a direct effect on iron absorption. The mechanism by which this is achieved is not yet properly understood. Recent experiments by BANNERMAN and co-workers (1962) suggest that it is not the iron content of the main storage organs, but of the intestine itself, which affects iron absorption. They found in rats that switching from a low to a high iron diet, or vice versa, produced changes in iron absorption within 1 or 2 days. Because of the rapidity of onset of these changes it appeared that local factors, such as the amount of iron in the intestinal tissues, were of greater importance in their production than general changes in the iron stores.

Iron excretion in the urine and faeces is reduced in iron deficiency (HAHN, BALE, HETTIG, KAMEN, and WHIPPLE, 1939; DUBACH, MOORE, and CALLENDER, 1949). CHAPPELLE and co-workers (1955) found that, in the mouse, iron excretion was directly proportional to the total body iron content. The mechanism of this is probably that iron excretion depends mainly on desquamation of cells from the surfaces of the body, and the iron content of these cells is closely related to the total amount of iron and to the amount of storage iron in the body.

Iron metabolism in pregnancy and iron transfer to the foetus. During pregnancy, the iron requirements of the foetuses and the placentae and the increase in maternal haemoglobin mass are met partly by enhanced absorption of dietary iron and increased food intake and partly by mobilisation of the iron stores (SMYTHE and MILLER, 1929; WIDDOWSON and MCCANCE, 1948; HAHN, CAROTHERS, DARBY, MARTIN, SHEPPARD, CANNON, BEAM, DENSEN, PETERSON, and MCCLELLAN, 1951; MANIS and SCHACHTER, 1962). A physiological type of hyposiderosis results. This is illustrated in Fig. 8, which shows changes in liver and spleen storage iron during pregnancy in normal rats and rats whose iron stores were depleted by haemorrhage prior to mating (MORGAN, 1961b). Both groups of rats were fed a normal laboratory rat diet, and the iron-depleted animals were not bled after the commencement of pregnancy. The iron stores of the normal rats decreased greatly during pregnancy. The stores of the depleted rats, low at the commencement of pregnancy, remained considerably lower than those of the controls throughout. This experimentally produced hyposiderosis, however, had no effect on maternal blood haemoglobin or plasma iron concentrations or T.I.B.C., or on placental or foetal iron.

Apparently the depleted rats were able to absorb increased amounts of iron from their diet so as to maintain the normal maternal values and normal iron transfer to the foetuses.

The effect of a more severe degree of iron depletion during pregnancy on iron transfer to the foetuses has been studied by Nylander (1953). He bled rats from the tail, removing approximately 2 ml. blood daily from the time of mating until the 15th to 21st days of pregnancy. All the rats were fed a normal diet. The

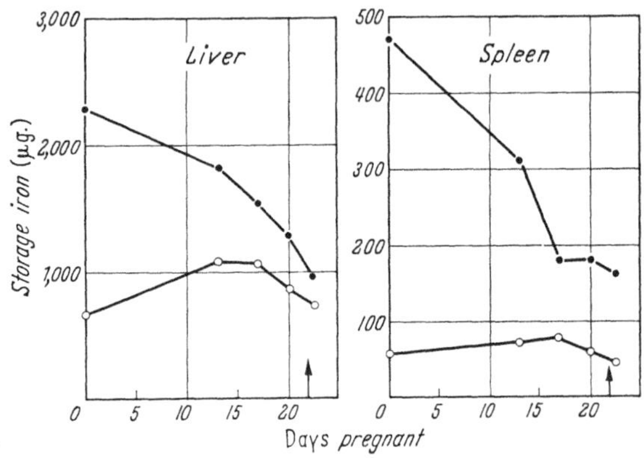

Fig. 8. Changes in liver and spleen storage iron during pregnancy in controls rats (●) and in rats whose iron stores were depleted by bleeding during the two weeks immediately preceding mating (○). The arrows indicate the time of parturition (Morgan, 1961b)

bled rats had considerably lower liver storage iron values throughout pregnancy than did control animals. Some of his results are summarised in Fig. 9. It can be seen that the bleeding produced a reduction in maternal haemoglobin and plasma iron and placental and foetal iron values. The reduction in iron transfer to the foetuses was probably a consequence of the low plasma iron concentration of the bled rats. This in turn was probably due, in part at least, to the accentuation of erythropoiesis caused by the anaemia. The possibility cannot be excluded, however, that some of the decrease in plasma iron and placental iron transfer may not have been a direct consequence of the hyposiderosis.

The results of these two experiments show that, in the rat, hyposiderosis need not lead to reduced iron transfer to the foetuses, provided the diet contains adequate iron. Furthermore, the fall in haemoglobin and plasma iron during pregnancy is probably not a consequence of the reduced iron stores. Other experiments, where additional iron was given to pregnant rats, support the latter conclusion (MITCHELL and MILLER, 1931; VAN DONK, FELDMAN, and STEENBOCK, 1934; MORGAN, 1961b). However, if the iron status of the pregnant rat is subjected to additional stress due to bleeding or to restriction of dietary iron intake (ALT, 1938), then the passage of iron to the foetuses may be reduced.

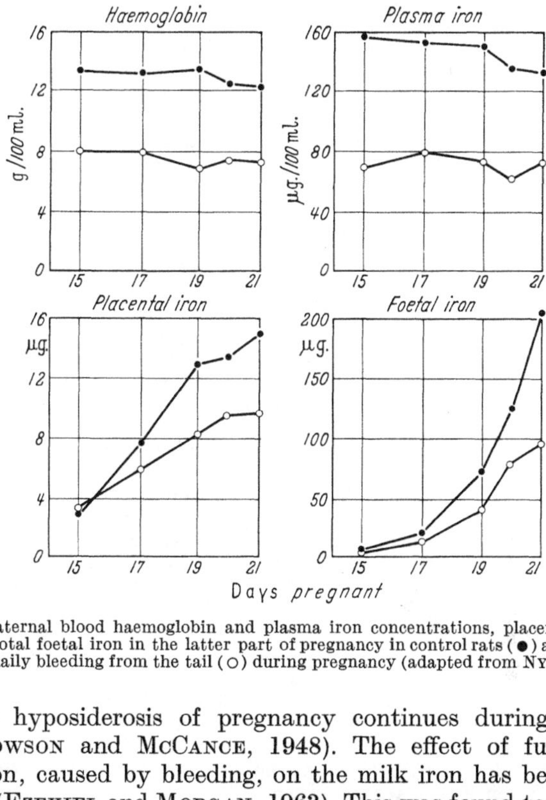

Fig. 9. Maternal blood haemoglobin and plasma iron concentrations, placental non-haem iron and total foetal iron in the latter part of pregnancy in control rats (●) and in rats subjected to daily bleeding from the tail (○) during pregnancy (adapted from NYLANDER, 1953)

The hyposiderosis of pregnancy continues during lactation (WIDDOWSON and McCANCE, 1948). The effect of further iron depletion, caused by bleeding, on the milk iron has been studied in rats (EZEKIEL and MORGAN, 1963). This was found to produce a significant reduction in milk iron concentration, while the feeding of additional dietary iron produced the opposite change. It is not known whether the change in milk iron was in any way related to alterations in the iron stores.

Summary

Hyposiderosis, which may be defined as a reduction in the body's iron reserves, can be produced experimentally by restriction of dietary iron in young animals or by increasing iron loss from the body as by haemorrhage.

During the development of hyposiderosis, iron is mobilised from the main storage organs, at approximately equal rates and with equal readiness from its water-soluble (ferritin) and water-insoluble (haemosiderin) fractions.

Hyposiderosis is commonly associated with reduced blood haemoglobin and plasma iron concentrations and with elevated plasma total iron-binding capacity and accentuated iron absorption. Although a reduction in haemoglobin and plasma iron values does not occur until the iron stores have been considerably reduced, it is probable that the two values commence to fall before the iron stores are completely depleted. The increase in iron-binding capacity appears to be due, not to the reduction in iron stores, but to a fall in the blood haemoglobin concentration. Accentuation of iron absorption may be directly due to a decrease in the storage iron in the intestinal mucosa.

Iron stores normally decrease during pregnancy and lactation. The effect of accentuation of this hyposiderosis on iron transfer to the foetuses and to the milk depends on the severity of iron depletion and on the amount of iron available from the diet.

Zusammenfassung

Hyposiderose, definiert als eine Verminderung der Eisenreserven des Organismus, kann experimentell bei jungen Tieren entweder durch Einschränkung des Nahrungseisens oder durch vermehrten Eisenverlust infolge wiederholter Blutungen hervorgerufen werden. Während der Entwicklung einer Hyposiderose wird Eisen aus den hauptsächlichen Speicherorganen mobilisiert, und zwar zu ungefähr gleichen Teilen und mit gleicher Geschwindigkeit aus seiner wasserlöslichen (Ferritin) und seiner wasserunlöslichen (Haemosiderin) Speicherform.

Hyposiderose geht gewöhnlich mit verminderten Konzentrationen von Haemoglobin im Blut und von Plasmaeisen einher sowie mit einer erhöhten Gesamtbindungsfähigkeit für Eisen im Plasma und gesteigerter Eisenresorption. Obgleich keine Verminderung von Haemoglobin und von Plasmaeisen auftritt, bevor die Eisenspeicher erheblich abgenommen haben, ist wahrscheinlich, daß beide Werte bereits vermindert sind, ehe die Eisenspeicher vollständig entleert sind. Die Zunahme der Eisenbindungsfähigkeit scheint nicht auf einer Verminderung der Eisenspeicher zu beruhen, sondern auf einer Abnahme der Haemoglobinkonzentration im Blut. Die gesteigerte Eisenresorption kann direkt auf eine Abnahme des in der Darmmucosa gespeicherten Eisens zurückzuführen sein.

Die Eisenspeicher sind normalerweise während der Schwangerschaft und während der Laktation vermindert. Der Einfluß einer Verstärkung dieser Hyposiderose auf den Übergang von Eisen in den Fetus und in die Milch ist vom Grad der Eisenverarmung und von der Menge des in der Nahrung verfügbaren Eisens abhängig.

Résumé

L'hyposidérose, que l'on peut définir comme une diminution des réserves de fer de l'organisme, peut être reproduite expérimentalement en réduisant l'apport alimentaire de fer chez de jeunes animaux ou en augmentant les déperditions de fer par saignées par exemple. Au cours du développement de l'hyposidérose, le fer est mobilisé de ses principaux organes de mise en réserve, dans des proportions à peu près équivalentes et avec une égale facilité qu'il s'agisse de sa fraction soluble dans l'eau (ferritine) ou de sa fraction insoluble (hémosidérine).

L'hyposidérose s'accompagne habituellement d'une baisse de l'hémoglobine et du fer sérique, avec augmentation de la capacité totale de fixation du sérum et augmentation de l'absorption du fer. Bien que les taux d'hémoglobine et de fer sérique ne s'abaissent que lorsque les réserves de fer sont considérablement réduites, il est probable qu'ils commencent à baisser avant que ces réserves soient complètement épuisées. L'augmentation de la capacité de fixation du sérum semble liée non pas à la baisse des réserves de fer, mais à la diminution de la concentration d'hémoglobine dans le sang. L'accroissement de l'absorption du fer est peut-être lié directement à la baisse de la réserve de fer dans la muqueuse intestinale.

Normalement, les réserves de fer diminuent pendant la grossesse et la lactation. Les conséquences, sur le transport de fer au foetus et au lait, de l'accentuation de cette hyposidérose dépendent de sa gravité et de la quantité de fer présente dans le régime alimentaire.

References

ALT, M. L.: Amer. J. Dis. Child. **56**, 975 (1938). — AUSTONI, M. E., A. RABINOVITCH, and D. M. GREENBERG: J. Biol. Chem. (U.S.A.) **134**, 17 (1940). — BALFOUR, W. M., P. F. HAHN, W. F. BALE, M. D. POMMERENKE, and G. H. WHIPPLE: J. Exper. Med. (U.S.A.) **76**, 15 (1942). — BANNERMAN, R. M., J. R. P. O'BRIEN, and L. J. WITTS: Blood (U.S.A.) **20**, 532 (1962). — BEUTLER, E., and R. K. BLAISDELL: J. Laborat. Clin. Med. (U.S.A.) **52**, 694 (1958). — BEUTLER, E., V. F. FAIRBANKS, and F. L. FAHEY: Clinical Disorders of Iron Metabolism. Grune & Stratton, New York/London, 1963. — BEUTLER, E., M. J. ROBSON, and E. BUTTENWIESER. Ann. Int. Med. (U.S.A.) **48**, 60 (1958). — BOGNIARD, R. P., and G. H. WHIPPLE: J. Exper. Med. (U.S.A.) **55**, 653 (1932). — BOTHWELL, T. H., and C. A. FINCH: Iron Metabolism. Little, Brown & Co., Boston, 1962. — BOTHWELL, T. H., G. PIRZIO-BIROLI, and C. A. FINCH: J. Laborat. Clin. Med. (U.S.A.) **51**, 24 (1958). — BRÜCKMANN, G., and S. G. ZONDEK: Biochem. J. (G.B.) **33**, 1845 (1939). — CHAPPELLE, E., B. W. GABRIO, A. R. STEPHENS, and C. A. FINCH: Amer. J. Physiol. **182**, 390 (1955). — DAVIDSON, W. M., and R. F. JENNISON: J. Clin. Path. (G.B.) **5**, 281 (1952). — DUBACH, R., S. T. CALLENDER, and C. V. MOORE: Blood (U.S.A.) **3**, 526 (1948). — DUBACH, R., C. V. MOORE, and S. T. CALLENDER: Fed. Proc. (U.S.A.) **8**, 353 (1949). — EZEKIEL, E., and E. H. MORGAN: J. Physiol. (G. B.) **165**, 336 (1963). — HAHN, P. F., and G. H. WHIPPLE: Amer. J. Med. Sc. **191**, 24 (1936). — HAHN, P. F., W. F. BALE, R. H. HETTIG, M. D. KAMEN, and G. H. WHIPPLE: J. Exper. Med. (U.S.A.) **70**, 443 (1939). — HAHN, P. F., E. L. CAROTHERS, W. J. DARBY, M. MARTIN, C. W. SHEPPARD, R. O. CANNON, A. S. BEAM, P. M. DENSEN, J. C. PETERSON, and G. S. MCCLELLAN: Amer. J. Obstetr. Gynec. **61**, 477 (1951). — HALLGREN, B.: Acta Soc. med. Uppsal. **59**, 79 (1953). — HASKINS, D., A. STEVENS, S. FINCH, and C. A. FINCH: J. Clin. Invest. (U.S.A.) **31**, 543 (1952). — HEVESY, G., and D. LOCKNER: Ark. Kemi (Sweden) **19**, 303 (1962). — KALDOR, I.: Austral. J. Exper. Biol. **36**, 173 (1958). — KOOYMAN, J. C.: Acta med. Scand. **134**, 205 (1949). — MANIS, J. G., and D. SCHACHTER: Amer. J. Physiol. **203**, 81 (1962). — MEIER, W., G. BENEKE, and G. AHLERT: Zschr. inn. Med. (G.) **14**, 1065 (1959). — MITCHELL, M. S., and L. MILLER: Amer. J. Physiol. **98**, 311 (1931). — MORGAN, E. H.: Austral. J. Exper. Biol. **39**, 371 (1961a). — MORGAN, E. H.: J. Physiol. (G.B.) **158**, 573 (1961b). — MORGAN, E. H.: Quart. J. Exper. Physiol. (G.B.) **46**, 220 (1961c). — MORGAN, E. H.: Quart. J. Exper. Physiol.

(G.B.) **47**, 57 (1962). — MORGAN, E. H.: Quart. J. Exper. Physiol. (G.B.) **48**, 176 (1963). — MORGAN, E. H., and C. J. BRACKENRIDGE: Quart. J. Exper. Physiol. (G.B.) **47**, 66 (1962). — MORGAN, E. H., and W. LYNCH: Quart. J. Exper. Physiol. (G.B.) **47**, 181 (1963). — MCCALL, M. G., G. E. NEWMAN, J. R. P. O'BRIEN, L. S. VALBERG, and L. J. WITTS: Brit. J. Nutrit. **16**, 297 (1962). — MCCALL, M. G., G. E. NEWMAN, J. R. P. O'BRIEN, and L. J. WITTS: Brit. J. Nutrit. **16**, 305 (1962). — NYLANDER, G.: Acta physiol. Scand., Suppl. 107 (1953). — PIRZIO-BIROLI, G., and C. A. FINCH: J. Laborat. Clin. Med. (U.S.A.) **55**, 216 (1960). — ROTH, V. O., B. JASINSKI, and M. v. BIDDER: Helvet. med. acta **18**, 159 (1951). — SCHAIRER, E., and J. RECHENBERGER: Virchows Arch. path Anat. (G.) **315**, 309 (1948). — SCOTT, E. M., and R. H. MCCOY: Arch. Biochem. (U.S.A.) **5**, 349 (1944). — SHODEN, A., B. W. GABRIO, and C. A. FINCH: J. Biol. Chem. (U.S.A.) **204**, 823 (1953). — SMYTHE, C. V., and R. C. MILLER: J. Nutrit. (U.S.A.) **1**, 209 (1929). — TOMPSETT, S. L.: Biochem. J. (G.B.) **29**, 480 (1935). — VAN DONK, E. C., M. FELDMAN, and H. STEENBOCK: Amer. J. Physiol. **107**, 616 (1934). — VENKATACHALAM, P. S., and I. KALDOR: Austral. J. Exper. Biol. **35**, 25 (1957). — WADDEL, J., H. STEENBOCK, C. A. ELVEHJEM, and E. B. HART: J. Biol. Chem. (U.S.A.) **77**, 769 (1928). — WAKEHAM, G., and H. F. HALENZ: J. Biol. Chem. (U.S.A.) **115**, 429 (1936). — WHEBY, M. S., and L. G. JONES: Clin. Res. (U.S.A.) **10**, 240 (1962). — WIDDOWSON, E. M., and R. A. MCCANCE: Biochem. J. (G.B.) **42**, 577 (1948). — WINTROBE, M. M., G. R. GREENBERG, S. R. HUMPHREYS, H. ASHENBRUCKER, W. WORTH, and R. KRAMER: J. Clin. Invest. (U.S.A.) **26**, 103 (1947).

Human hyposideraemia

By

L. Heilmeyer

Fundamentally, there are three ways in which plasma iron may be reduced below the normal level:

1. By an increased outflow of iron from the plasma, with the result that outflow exceeds inflow.

2. By a delayed release of iron into the plasma.

3. By a general iron deficiency in the organism as a whole.

It is with these three possibilities that the present paper will be concerned.

1. An increased outflow of iron is most frequently seen during a sudden acceleration of haemoglobin synthesis. This occurs as a result of acute blood loss. Here, hyposideraemia usually appears on the third or fourth day after a transitory increase. The iron outflow from the plasma is likewise increased during the regenerative phase of many other anaemias. The first effect of vitamin B_{12} in the treatment of pernicious anaemia, for example, is to decrease the serum iron. Hyposideraemia occurs earlier than the reticulocyte crisis. In anaemias responsive to treatment with vitamin B_6, hyposideraemia is also seen as an early effect of treatment after administration of pyridoxine.

Conditions are different in chronic haemolytic anaemia. Here, the increased outflow of iron is usually balanced by an increased inflow, so that the iron values are frequently normal or even increased owing to erythrocyte destruction. However, hyposideraemia may also be found in cases of haemolytic anaemia. Hypersideraemia, normosideraemia, and hyposideraemia are, in fact, all possible in this type of anaemia (Fig. 1).

An increased outflow of iron is also encountered in anaemias associated with infectious diseases. This is due to acceleration of a partially inefficient erythropoiesis and also to an increase in the incorporation of iron into the reticulo-endothelial system and into inflammatory foci. However, the increased outflow is only one factor in the development of this type of hyposideraemia. An additional mechanism involved is the fixation of iron in the reticulo-endothelial system, which will be discussed in the next section.

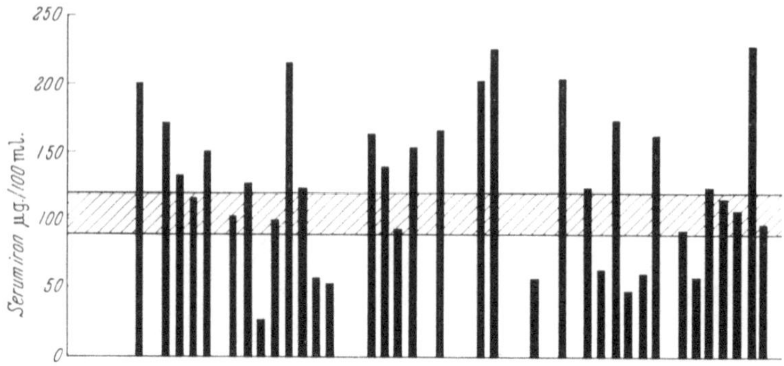

Fig. 1. Serum iron levels in 35 unselected cases of haemolytic anaemia; the hatched area indicates the normal range

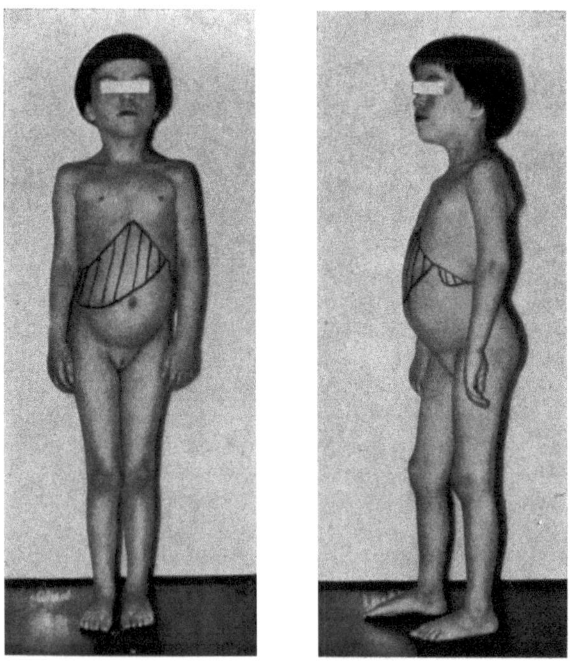

Fig. 2. Hepatic and splenic enlargement in a 7-year-old girl with congenital atransferrinaemia

An increase in the outflow of iron from the plasma also takes place if the levels of the transporting protein, transferrin, are extremely reduced. A classic example is the clinical picture of *congenital atransferrinaemia*, one case of which I should like to describe briefly here.

The case is that of a 7-year-old girl who was markedly retarded in her physical development (Fig. 2). She was 106 cm. tall (normal height for her age: 126 cm.) and weighed 15.6 kg. (normal: 22.6 kg.). Anaemia had already been diagnosed at the age of 3 months and had proved completely refractory to any therapy. The child could only be kept alive by blood transfusions. The blood count upon admission showed 9.1 g.% Hb. and 4.1 mill. erythrocytes; mean cell haemoglobin was 22.2 pg. The blood smear revealed severe

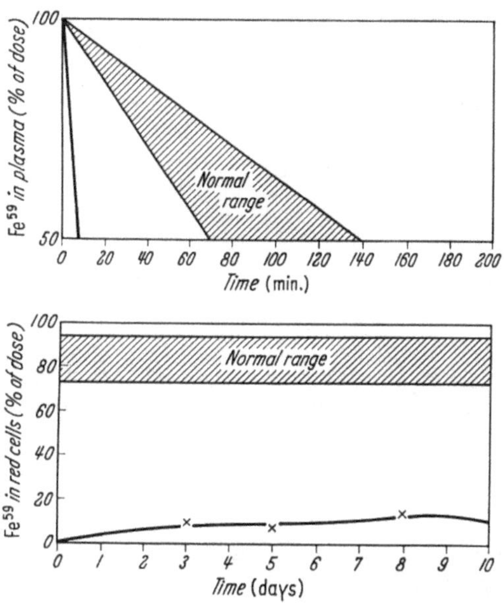

Fig. 3. Plasma iron clearance and iron utilisation, determined with Fe^{59}, in congenital atransferrinaemia

hypochromia with ring-shaped erythrocytes and target cells. Thalassaemia could definitely be excluded. In the bone marrow there was a pronounced increase in the number of immature erythroblasts. Sideroblasts, as well as iron-storing reticular cells, were completely absent. In contrast to the iron deficiency of the bone marrow, liver biopsy showed extreme siderosis with cirrhosis.

Serum iron was between 14 and 20 μg. %. The total iron-binding capacity varied between 20 and 33 μg./100 ml. plasma. Radioactive iron injected after incubation of Fe^{59} with the child's own plasma displayed a half-life of 5 minutes. Iron utilisation worked out at about 12% in 8 days (Fig. 3). Plasma iron turnover and non-haemoglobin iron turnover were increased about three to fourfold. Measurement of Fe^{59} activity from the outside yielded the highest concentration over the liver, less over the spleen, and only very

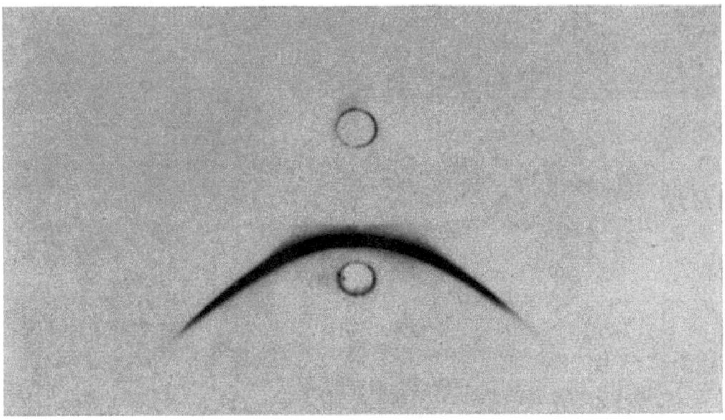

Fig. 4. Immuno-electrophoresis with anti-transferrin serum, showing no precipitation with the serum of the child (above) as compared with the precipitation observed using normal serum (below)

little over the sacrum, thus showing a complete reversal of normal conditions. Immuno-electrophoresis of the child's serum gave no transferrin band. Nor was there any reaction between an anti-transferrin serum and the child's serum (Fig. 4). Serum electrophoresis with simultaneous addition of Fe^{59} demonstrated an increased activity in the area of one gamma-globulin peak (Fig. 5). Here, a transferrin antibody is probably involved, resulting from frequent transferrin transmission due to numerous blood transfusions with simultaneous total endogenous deficiency of transferrin. This antigen-antibody complex could be split with mercaptopyridoxine and cysteine, forming a precipitation band with the anti-transferrin serum. The child was treated with plasma infusions, which effected an increase in the reticulocyte count, probably as the result of an improvement in the iron supply to the bone marrow by the transferrin transferred with the plasma. The child suddenly died of acute circulatory failure. Autopsy revealed severe siderosis in all organs, particularly in the liver, pancreas, kidneys, myocardium, and thyroid gland; strange to say, the spleen was less affected, and iron was completely absent from the bone marrow.

The explanation for these findings is that iron could not be bound in the bloodstream owing to absence of the specific iron-transporting protein. The iron therefore diffused into all the organs of the body. As a consequence, the bone marrow received too little. In other words, we are confronted here with the paradoxical picture of an iron-deficiency anaemia occurring in an organism overloaded with iron.

This case of complete atransferrinaemia also enables us to answer some theoretical questions concerning iron metabolism. Transferrin is not required for the mechanism of iron absorption. Furthermore, the half-life of transferred transferrin in this case was found to be 3 to 5 days. Both the child's parents were healthy persons; they showed, however, a plasma transferrin concentration of about half the normal value. Thus, the child was a homozygote, whereas the parents were heterozygotes, which accounts for the extraordinary rarity of this interesting disease.

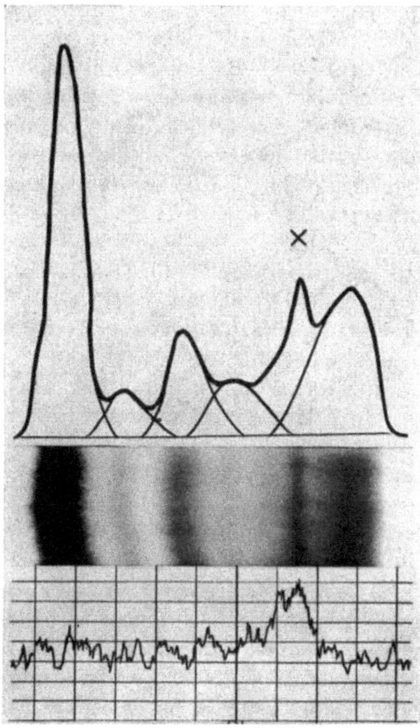

Fig. 5. Paper electrophoresis with the serum of the child and (below) Fe^{59}-activity curve

2. Now I should like to discuss decreases in plasma iron due to a delay in the release of iron into the plasma. It has already been mentioned above that in infectious or malignant diseases and also in severe allergic inflammations or rheumatic diseases – in short, in all conditions associated with extensive inflammation – plasma iron will decrease. In these diseases, a complete reversal of total iron metabolism occurs, which I have previously described as a "stimulated state of iron metabolism". This change in iron meta-

bolism forms part of the general inflammatory reaction. It is accompanied in the plasma by an alteration of the plasma colloids, by an increased erythrocyte sedimentation rate, and by an increase in plasma copper. In this form of hyposideraemia, we also always find a decrease in total iron-binding capacity, as distinct from a decrease in plasma iron resulting from an increased outflow of iron or from iron deficiency. Thus, not only the serum iron, but also the transferrin concentration decreases. This fact, in addition to the simultaneous increase in plasma copper, is very important for differential diagnosis. The decrease in plasma iron which is associated with the general inflammatory reaction is partly due to the strong fixation of iron in the reticulo-endothelial system and in the inflammatory area. If Fe^{59} is given by injection to an animal with a turpentine abscess, one hour later an accumulation of the iron in the marginal zone of the abscess can be detected, i.e. at first in the collagenous fibrils and later in the phagocytosing cells. The increased fixation of iron can be particularly well demonstrated in animal experiments with diphtheria toxin.

Besides a decrease in the supply from the reticulo-endothelial system and the inflammatory areas, we also find an increased turnover of plasma and haemoglobin iron in infections (Fig. 6), as well as increased erythrocyte destruction with simultaneously increased erythropoiesis. The processes occurring in infections are thus extraordinarily complicated. When the inflammation is terminated, all processes of iron metabolism revert to normal.

3. The most frequent and severest forms of hyposideraemia are those associated with general iron deficiency in the organism as a whole. In cases of this kind, the available iron deposits are completely depleted not only in the spleen and liver but also in other organs, such as the storage cells of the bone marrow. These findings are also of diagnostic importance. In bone-marrow smears stained with Prussian blue, no stored iron is found in the reticular cells. Sideroblasts are likewise markedly depleted or are even absent altogether. Whereas iron granules of normal size are detected in 30 to 40% of all nucleated red cells in the bone marrow, these are extremely decreased in states of iron deficiency.

One problem of iron deficiency which has recently been studied by us (HEILMEYER and CLOTTEN) concerns the effects which the decreased iron supply has upon porphyrin metabolism. It has been known since 1934 that the protoporphyrin content of the erythrocytes is increased in iron-deficiency anaemias (SEGGEL), and this finding has been frequently confirmed (WATSON and others). The increase in protoporphyrin cannot be due to the presence of a larger number of immature erythrocytes, as hardly any rise in the reticulocyte count occurs in iron deficiency. An increase in protoporphyrin is also seen in bone-marrow blood. Fig. 7 outlines our findings in 16 cases of iron deficiency; a regular pattern of changes can be clearly seen. The free protoporphyrin shows a fairly considerable increase, attaining values of between 135 and 680 μg./

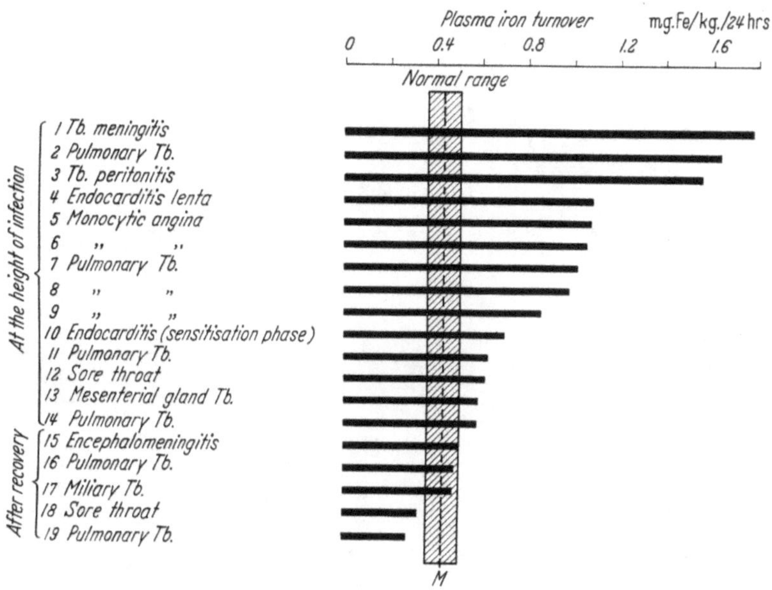

Fig. 6. Plasma iron turnover in 19 cases of various infectious or other inflammatory diseases; 1—14 at the height of the infection; 15—19 after recovery

100 ml. red-cell mass. Erythrocyte coproporphyrin also shows a rise in the majority of cases (1.5 to 37μg./100 ml. red-cell mass), as has already been demonstrated by WATSON. In 3 cases examined in this connection, uroporphyrin was also slightly augmented (up to 10 μg.). Furthermore, we detected in all cases an increase in the excretion of δ-aminolaevulinic acid (δ-A.L.A.), of which up to 12 mg. may be excreted daily. On the other hand, porphobilinogen (P.B.G.) is not increased, but, on the contrary, may even be decreased in many cases. The ratio of δ-A.L.A. to P.B.G. shows a shift in favour of δ-A.L.A. excretion in all cases. Moreover, enhanced urinary excretion of coproporphyrin is also encountered in all cases, whereas the values for uroporphyrin

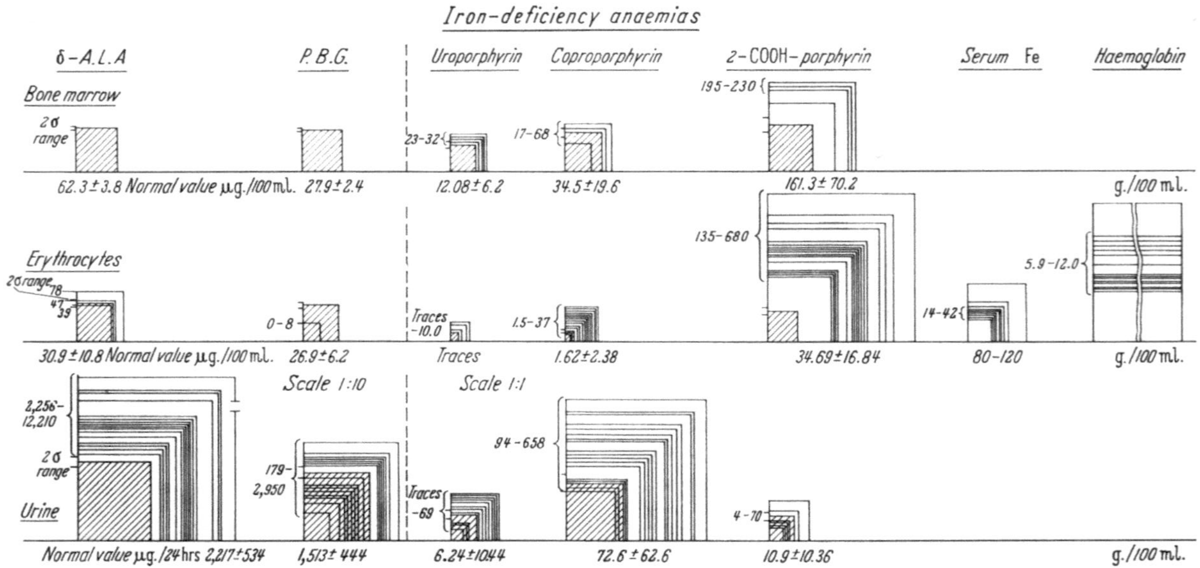

Fig. 7. Pattern of haem precursors in 16 cases of iron deficiency. Upper row: aspirated bone marrow; middle row: peripheral blood, erythrocytes; lower row: urinary excretion. The hatched areas indicate the normal values

excretion are variable. No rise occurs in the urinary excretion of protoporphyrin – a finding which seems quite understandable in view of the fact that this porphyrin does not pass readily through the kidneys and is mainly excreted in the bile. That there is a close connection between these findings and the presence of iron deficiency is borne out by the results of studies before and after treatment with iron. If the iron deficiency is abolished, the urinary excretion of δ-A.L.A. and P.B.G. reverts to normal; elevated coproporphyrin excretion levels likewise return to normal.

How can these findings be explained? An increase in protoporphyrin might be the consequence of accelerated synthesis. But, judging from the evidence of *in vitro* experiments, synthesis is not accelerated. Fig. 8 shows the results obtained in an *in vitro* test with healthy blood and with blood from a patient with iron-deficiency anaemia. It can be seen that the synthesis of P.B.G., uroporphyrin, and coproporphyrin takes place much more slowly in the blood from the iron-deficient patient than in the blood from a healthy subject. Whereas the latter produces 8.63 mg. of higher synthesis products – equivalent to 12.4 mg. δ-A.L.A. – after addition of 16.5 mg. δ-A.L.A. (i.e. an amount corresponding to 75% of the added δ-A.L.A.), the erythrocytes from the patient with iron-deficiency anaemia produce only 1.7 mg. of higher synthesis products (equivalent to 2.4. mg. δ-A.L.A. = a mere 14%). Porphyrin synthesis takes place five times more slowly in iron-

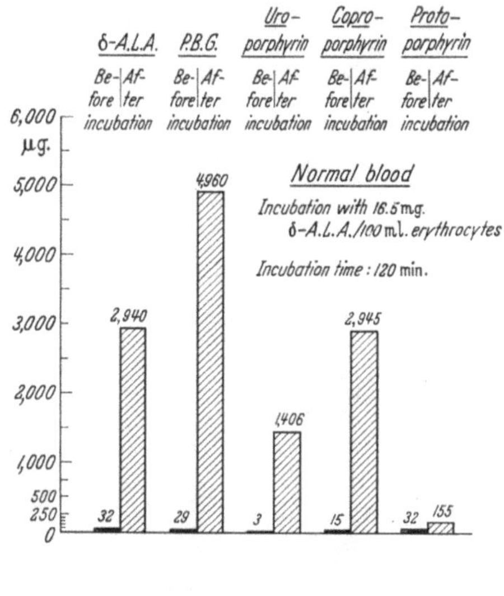

Fig. 8. Porphyrin synthesis in red-cell haemolysate during incubation with δ-A.L.A. (38° C.; pH 7.4; 2 hours)

deficient erythrocytes than in healthy erythrocytes. We investigated this problem further and were able to show that the inhibition of synthesis is probably brought about by the increase in protoporphyrin; for, if a corresponding amount of protoporphyrin is added to *healthy* blood, the rate of synthesis slows down in the same way as in iron-deficient blood (Fig. 9). It will be seen from

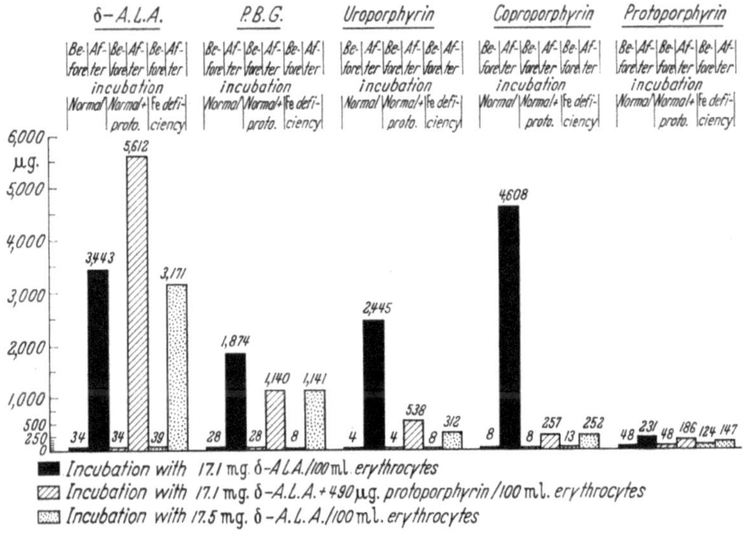

Fig. 9. Porphyrin synthesis in red-cell haemolysate during incubation with δ-A.L.A. Black columns: normal red-cell haemolysate; hatched columns: normal red-cell haemolysate with protoporphyrin added (490 μg./100 ml.); dotted columns: iron-deficient red-cell haemolysate

these experiments that, in iron-deficiency states with a decreased iron supply for haem synthesis, mechanisms exist which consecutively inhibit porphyrin synthesis. The significance of this seems to lie in the fact that the organism would otherwise be overloaded with the toxic porphyrins. Thus, the problem of iron metabolism in iron-deficiency anaemias involves still further metabolic problems. This illustrates once again that a single metabolic disorder is likely to cause many other alterations in metabolism, which will only be detected if the investigator's attention is not too closely fixed on one process alone.

Summary

There are three main circumstances which lead to a decrease in plasma iron in man:

1. An increased outflow of iron from the plasma as compared with the inflow.

2. A delayed release of iron into the plasma.
3. A general deficiency of iron in the organism as a whole.

1. An increased outflow occurs if haemoglobin synthesis is markedly accelerated. This is the case in acute blood loss, in pernicious anaemia under treatment with vitamin B_{12}, during the treatment of B_6-responsive anaemias with vitamin B_6, and also in some haemolytic anaemias if haemoglobin synthesis is greater than the rate of destruction.

An increased outflow is also encountered in anaemias associated with infectious diseases; this is due partly to an acceleration of erythropoiesis and partly to an increase in the iron uptake into the reticulo-endothelial system and into areas of inflammation.

A strong increase in the outflow of iron, together with marked hyposideraemia, also occurs if the transporting protein, transferrin, is greatly diminished or absent altogether. A classic example of this condition is the clinical picture of *congenital atransferrinaemia.*

2. A delayed release of iron into the plasma is met with in infections, in rheumatic diseases, and in cancer. The changes in iron metabolism occurring in such states are described in detail.

3. The most frequent and severest form of hyposideraemia is that associated with *states of general iron deficiency.* Here, all the iron deposits are depleted, as can clearly be seen, for example, in the case of the bone marrow (lack of sideroblasts and of iron-storing reticular cells).

One problem of iron deficiency only recently studied by us concerns porphyrin metabolism. There is an increase in the protoporphyrin and coproporphyrin content of the erythrocytes and an increase in the excretion of δ-aminolaevulinic acid and coproporphyrin in the urine, whereas the excretion of porphobilinogen diminishes. Incubation tests *in vitro* have shown that porphyrin synthesis is decreased in haemolysates of iron-deficient erythrocytes. Model experiments have revealed that the rise in the protoporphyrin concentration is capable of inhibiting porphyrin synthesis. This finding suggests the existence of a mechanism designed to inhibit inundation of the organism with porphyrins.

Zusammenfassung

Grundsätzlich gibt es drei Wege, welche beim Menschen zu einer Verminderung des Plasmaeisens führen:

1. ein im Vergleich zum Zustrom vermehrter Abstrom von Eisen aus dem Plasma,
2. eine verzögerte Abgabe von Eisen in das Plasma und
3. ein allgemeiner Mangel an Eisen im Gesamtorganismus.

zu 1. Ein gesteigerter Abstrom tritt auf, wenn die Haemoglobinsynthese stark zunimmt. Dies ist der Fall bei akuten Blutverlusten, bei der Behandlung der perniziösen Anaemie mit Vitamin B_{12}, bei der Behandlung von B_6-empfindlichen Anaemien mit diesem Vitamin, sowie bei gewissen haemolytischen Anaemien, bei denen die Haemoglobinsynthese größer ist als der Zerfall.

Ein gesteigerter Abstrom kann auch bei Infektanaemien auftreten, entweder infolge Steigerung der Erythropoese oder infolge vermehrter Aufnahme in das R.E.S. oder in Entzündungsgebiete.

Ein hochgradig gesteigerter Abstrom von Eisen mit starker Hyposideraemie findet sich, wenn Transferrin stark vermindert ist oder fehlt. Ein klassisches Beispiel dafür ist das Krankheitsbild der *kongenitalen Atransferrinaemie*, das kurz geschildert wird.

zu 2. Eine verzögerte Abgabe von Eisen an das Plasma liegt bei infektiösen oder bei rheumatischen Erkrankungen und bei Tumoren vor. Die im Eisenstoffwechsel auftretende Umschaltung bei diesen Zuständen wird geschildert.

zu 3. Die häufigste und schwerste Form der Hyposideraemie tritt im *Zustand des Eisenmangels* auf. Er ist durch Erschöpfung aller Eisendepots gekennzeichnet und ist im Knochenmark am Fehlen der Sideroblasten und der eisenhaltigen Retikulumzellen zu erkennen.

Ein erst neuerdings untersuchtes Problem des Eisenmangels betrifft die sich dabei ergebenden Veränderungen im Porphyrinstoffwechsel. Es kommt sowohl zur Vermehrung von Proto- und Koproporphyrin in den Erythrozyten als auch zu gesteigerter Ausscheidung von δ-Aminolaevulinsäure und Koproporphyrin im Harn, während die Ausscheidung von Porphobilinogen vermindert ist. Inkubationsversuche *in vitro* haben ergeben, daß die Porphyrinsynthese im Haemolysat von Erythrozyten bei Eisenmangel vermindert ist. Modellversuche zeigten weiterhin, daß eine Erhöhung der Protoporphyrinkonzentration imstande ist, die Porphyrinsynthese zu hemmen. Dies kann als ein zweckmäßiger Mechanismus gedeutet werden, durch den die Überflutung des Organismus mit Porphyrinen verhindert wird.

Résumé

Trois conditions principales peuvent conduire à une diminution du fer sérique chez l'homme:

1. une fuite du fer hors du plasma plus élevée que les entrées dans le plasma;
2. une libération retardée du fer vers le plasma;
3. une carence générale de l'organisme entier en fer.

1. Une fuite augmentée du fer hors du plasma se produit quand la synthèse de l'hémoglobine est notablement accélérée. C'est le cas dans l'hémorragie aiguë, l'anémie de Biermer traitée à la vitamine B_{12}, les anémies sensibles à la vitamine B_6 traitées par cette vitamine, et aussi quelques anémies hémolytiques dans lesquelles la synthèse de l'hémoglobine est plus intense que sa destruction.

Une fuite augmentée du fer du plasma se rencontre aussi dans les anémies des maladies infectieuses, ce fait étant lié en partie à une accélération de l'érythropoïèse, en partie à une fixation accrue du fer dans le système réticulo-endothélial et les zones d'inflammation.

Une forte augmentation de la fuite de fer, associée à une hyposidérémie marquée se produit également quand la protéine de transport, la transferrine, est très diminuée, voire absente. Un exemple classique en est le tableau clinique de *l'atransferrinémie congénitale*.

2. Une libération retardée du fer vers le plasma se rencontre dans les infections, les maladies rhumatismales, le cancer. Les modifications du métabolisme du fer dans ces états sont décrites en détails.

3. La forme la plus fréquente et la plus grave d'hyposidérémie est celle associée aux *états de carence générale en fer*. Ici, tous les dépôts de fer sont épuisés, comme on le voit clairement dans la moelle osseuse par exemple (manque de sidéroblastes et de cellules réticulaires chargées de fer).

Un problème de carence en fer que nous n'avons que récemment étudié concerne le métabolisme des porphyrines. Il y a une augmentation du taux de la protoporphyrine et de la coproporphyrine dans les hématies, une augmentation de l'excrétion de l'acide δ-aminolévulinique et de la coproporphyrine dans l'urine, tandis que l'excrétion de porphobilinogène diminue. Des tests d'incubation *in vitro* ont montré que la synthèse des porphyrines est diminuée dans les hémolysats d'hématies hyposidérosiques. Des expériences types ont montré que l'élévation de la concentration en protoporphyrine est capable d'inhiber la synthèse des porphyrines. Cette constatation évoque l'existence d'un mécanisme destiné à empêcher l'inondation de l'organisme par les porphyrines.

References

HEILMEYER, L.: Der Eisenstoffwechsel. Handbuch der gesamten Haematologie. Vol. 2/1. Urban und Schwarzenberg, Munich/Berlin, 1959, p. 123. — HEILMEYER, L.: Münch. med. Wschr. **105**, 277 (1963). — HEILMEYER, L.: Disturbances of Blood Heme Synthesis. Charles Thomas, Florida (in press). — HEILMEYER, L., W. KEIDERLING, and F. WÖHLER: Dtsch. med. Wschr. **83**, 1965 (1958). — HEILMEYER, L., W. KELLER, O. VIVELL, W. KEIDERLING, K. BETKE, F. WÖHLER, and H. E. SCHULTZE: Dtsch. med. Wschr. **86**, 1745 (1961). — SEGGEL, K. A.: Fol. haemat. (G.) **52**, 250 (1934). — WATSON, C. F.: Arch. Int. Med. (U.S.A.) **86**, 797 (1950).

Discussion

Undritz: I should like to ask Dr. Morgan what was the sex of the rats he used. Iron metabolism, as well as the formation of haemoglobin and erythrocytes, differs considerably from one sex to the other, as we pointed out some time ago[1,2]. Admittedly, the haemoglobin and absolute erythrocyte levels in normal male and female rats of the same age do not differ to any significant degree — except that the haematocrit is a little higher in the males — but the iron stores are considerably lower in the males than in the females. There is also a "dynamic" difference, i.e. when anaemia is induced by administering a diet of cow's milk, for example, the haemoglobin falls much more markedly in the males than in the females. Moreover, in response to treatment for the anaemia, normal levels are restored more quickly in the males than in the females. In normal rats treated with cobalt, too, the rise in haemoglobin is more marked in the males than in the females. This more intensive reaction on the part of the males is attributable to the presence of testosterone, because the male type of reaction also occurs in castrated males, and in non-castrated or castrated females, if they are given testosterone. In non-treated castrated males the female type of reaction is seen. This difference between the sexes must be taken into account when studying anti-anaemic treatment in rats. We use only female rats when we wish to assess the amount of iron in the iron stores, and only males when we are testing any form of anti-anaemic treatment, e.g. with iron, copper, or cobalt. Both males and females can be used in such tests, but if they are, the results should be recorded separately for each sex.

Morgan: Our rats exhibit the same sex differences that you have referred to. Naturally, the experiments in pregnant animals were performed on female rats, while the other experiments were performed on rats of both sexes. The results presented today were only those from the male rats. The results with females were similar, differing only in the quantities of storage iron involved.

Witts: I was much interested in Dr. Morgan's work, because it is on similar lines to ours in Oxford. In the study of the metabolism of iron, as of vitamin B_{12}, we have moved into what Castle[3] has called the era of the rat. I think Dr. Morgan would agree that there is a general correspondence between the total body content of iron and certain parameters like the plasma iron, the mean haemoglobin concentration, and the iron available for tissue growth and haemoglobin formation, but we can alter this in various ways, as he has shown by partial hepatectomy. With cobalt you increase the competitive power of the erythron for taking up iron for the manufacture of haemoglobin at the expense of the tissues. I wonder if Dr. Morgan has any observations on the effect of cobalt on the transferrin values? In parenthesis

---

[1] von Bidder, H., and E. Undritz: Helvet. physiol. pharmacol. acta **6**, 765 (1948).

[2] Undritz, E.: Proceedings of the 7th Congress of the International Society for Haematology, Rome, 1958.

[3] Castle, W. B.: Gastroenterology (U.S.A.) **37**, 377 (1959).

I might add that the so-called ineffective erythropoiesis which we were discussing yesterday is another way of increasing the competitive power of the marrow in obtaining the available iron, if one can speak in teleological terms. Similarly, the increased absorption of iron in iron deficiency seems to be due, in part at any rate, to a local change in the mucosa of the small intestine — an increased avidity for iron.

I was not sure what Dr. MORGAN had in mind when he referred to the effects of iron in pregnancy. In the rat it is possible to abolish anaemia in infancy and pregnancy by supplementing the diet with iron. The same thing can be done in the human being, though Miss WIDDOWSON[1] showed many years ago that the effect is temporary, and if you interrupt iron administration during pregnancy the haemoglobin level begins to fall again.

MORGAN: Cobalt produces an increase in the total iron-binding capacity in rats and rabbits. As for pregnancy anaemia in rats, I can only say that MITCHELL and MILLER[2] and VAN DONK et al.[3] found that the feeding of extra iron during pregnancy did not prevent the fall in haemoglobin. We obtained similar results in rats whose iron stores were increased by feeding extra dietary iron from the time of weaning until they were mated at the age of 4 months.

EICHHORN: I should like to ask Dr. HEILMEYER a question about the transferrin of the parents of the child with atransferrinaemia. I believe you said that the parents exhibited only half the normal quantity of transferrin. I wonder if you have any information about the amount of iron, on the average, per molecule of transferrin of these parents, in comparison with the amount of iron, on the average, per molecule of transferrin in normal people.

HEILMEYER: The question Dr. EICHHORN has raised involves a fundamental problem concerning the binding of iron by transferrin; namely, is the reason why transferrin is normally saturated to the extent of 33% due to the fact that all transferrin molecules are capable of taking up only one-third of the iron or that only one-third of the transferrin molecules are saturated with iron and the other two-thirds devoid of iron? The latter is usually accepted as the correct explanation, but this is a question which cannot be answered with certainty until such time as we have a more exact knowledge of the chemical structure of the transferrin molecule.

GAJDOS: I'd like to make some remarks on the findings of Dr. HEILMEYER concerning the metabolic disturbances affecting the porphyrins in hyposideraemic anaemia.

We have very frequently found high levels of free protoporphyrin in the red blood cells. This has become a well-known finding since the observations made by CARTWRIGHT et al.[4] some fifteen years ago. We have also noted that there is no simple mathematical correlation between the degree of hyposideraemia and the increase in the free protoporphyrin concentration in the red blood cells. In some cases of pronounced hyposideraemia, even normal erythrocyte protoporphyrin levels may be observed. On the other hand, we have not been able to confirm the observations of Dr. HEILMEYER concerning

---

[1] WIDDOWSON, E. M.: Lancet (G.B.) **1939**/II, 640.

[2] MITCHELL, H. S., and L. MILLER: Amer. J. Physiol. **98**, 311 (1931).

[3] VAN DONK, E. C., H. FELDMAN, and H. STEENBOCK: Amer. J. Physiol. **107**, 616 (1934).

[4] CARTWRIGHT, C. E., C. M. HUGULAY, Jr., H. ASHENBRUCKER, J. FAY, and M. M. WINTROBE: Blood (U.S.A.) **3**, 501 (1948).

the increase in the urinary excretion of coproporphyrin, amino-laevulinic acid, and porphobilinogen in subjects with hyposideraemic anaemia. In our cases, high coproporphyrinuria was not a consistent finding, and an increase in amino-laevulinic acid excretion was exceptional. I do not understand how Dr. HEILMEYER came to observe a decreased renal excretion of porphobilinogen. In 50 normal subjects we found that the amount of this compound present in the 24-hour urine varied from 0 to 2 mg. I should therefore like to ask Dr. HEILMEYER to give us some information about the method he employed for the quantitative determination of porphobilinogen. I was also a little puzzled by the fact that he found uroporphyrin in normal red blood cells, since this is something which we have never detected.

I agree with Dr. HEILMEYER's assumption that excessive protoporphyrin formation may inhibit porphyrin synthesis, probably by a feed-back mechanism, but this latter point has not yet been demonstrated with certainty.

HEILMEYER: The methods for determining porphobilinogen in the urine have lately been very much improved. To determine the porphobilinogen, we employed a method which my colleague, Dr. CLOTTEN, has adapted from that of MAUZERALL and GRANICK. With this method we were able to detect minimum concentrations of 5 μg./ml. When this method was used, 30 healthy subjects were found to excrete an average of 1,513 μg. porphobilinogen daily; the 2 σ value worked out at 444. The lowest excretion level found by us in healthy subjects was 1,100 μg. We are in full agreement with STICH[1] that every healthy individual excretes porphobilinogen. We have not yet encountered a single case in which none was excreted. In many cases of iron deficiency, however, the porphobilinogen excretion drops well beneath the lower 2 σ limit. Incidentally, it is only since CLOTTEN elaborated a more refined technique for this purpose that it has become possible to measure the uroporphyrin content of the erythrocytes. In healthy subjects, we have admittedly only found minute traces, i.e. 0—4 μg./100 ml. of erythrocytes. But in some cases of iron-deficiency anaemia the concentrations are considerably higher. The methods of determination to which I have just referred are to be described in detail in a monograph entitled "Disturbances of Blood Heme Synthesis" to be published shortly by Charles C. Thomas.

HALLBERG: Dr. MORGAN suggested that in pregnant animals the increased absorption was related to a decrease in the iron stores. In humans, Dr. RYBO and I found that this is not the case. We measured the absorption of iron at two stages of pregnancy — at 10 and at 35 weeks — using the double radio-iron technique of SAYLOR and FINCH[2]. Between these two occasions we gave 1,500 mg. iron parenterally, which is more than is needed for the foetus and the placenta and for the increase in the mother's haemoglobin mass. In spite of the fact that more iron was present in the stores at 35 weeks, the absorption was roughly doubled.

We have interpreted these data on the assumption that the rate of mobilisation of storage iron was lower than the need, per unit time, of the mother and child. I should like to ask Dr. MORGAN if he has made any measurements of the absorption in relation to the magnitude of the iron stores in pregnant animals.

Regarding the child with atransferrinaemia referred to by Dr. HEILMEYER, the fact that the total iron-binding capacity of the serum was

---

[1] STICH, W.: Klin. Wschr. (G.) **19**, 338 (1961).

[2] SAYLOR, L., and C. A. FINCH: Amer. J. Physiol. **172**, 372 (1953).

reduced to one-half in both parents raises the question as to whether the parents were related. Were other relatives of this child also studied?

MORGAN: The answer to Dr. HALLBERG's question is that we have made no direct measurements of iron absorption.

HEILMEYER: We were unable to discover any blood relationship between the parents of the child with atransferrinaemia. On the other hand, perhaps this was a case of a purely coincidental union between two heterozygotes.

BEUTLER: Dr. MORGAN has made a very interesting suggestion that the iron-binding capacity may be regulated by the relationship between oxygen supply and demand. He has been quite careful to point out that his observations are limited to rats and to rabbits. In man, the iron-binding capacity has been quite extensively studied clinically by LAURELL[1] and later by many other investigators, and there are really only three conditions in which the iron-binding capacity is considerably increased. One is iron deficiency, the second is a phase occurring during infectious hepatitis, and the third is found during pregnancy, but this may, in point of fact, merely be due to iron deficiency. In other forms of anaemia the iron-binding capacity in man is not, to my knowledge, increased. Therefore there seems to be a discrepancy between the data found in the experimental animals that Dr. MORGAN has studied and in man. I think this might be worth some further comment. I wonder whether Dr. MORGAN has any explanation for this difference between man and the experimental animal.

MORGAN: The experiments we have performed in rats and rabbits suggest that the serum transferrin concentration is affected mainly by two mechanisms. The first appears to be specific for transferrin and depends on the balance between oxygen supply and demand in the tissues. The second is a non-specific alteration in the transferrin concentration, accompanying general changes in the serum protein pattern. It is at present impossible to say definitely whether the first of these mechanisms operates or has any importance in humans.

FINCH: I have just two comments to make concerning the interesting data presented by Dr. HEILMEYER. The first relates to the significance of the absence of iron in the marrow of the patient with atransferrinaemia. Some have come to feel that there is stronger evidence to the effect that iron is supplied directly from transferrin to the developing red cells of the marrow. For example, the levels of plasma iron and transferrin (% saturation) correlate with sideroblast iron and do not correlate with reticulo-endothelial iron. On the other hand, the reticulo-endothelial cells appear, at least from indirect evidence, to be unable to accept iron from transferrin, but rather to get their iron from broken-down red cells. Now if this is true, one would have expected the reticulo-endothelial cells of the marrow in this patient to have iron from broken-down red cells. This case does not appear to support the preceding hypothesis. Further observations are needed to settle the question as to which way the iron goes.

My second comment concerns the problem of haemoglobin-block anaemias. I think Dr. HEILMEYER is faced here with an iceberg of a problem in the sense that the number of laboratory observations which one would like to make to fully characterise such anaemias is far greater than first

[1] LAURELL, C. B.: Acta physiol. Scand. **14**, Suppl. 46, 1 (1947).

appears on the surface. We have been interested in one aspect of this problem and during the past year Dr. WINTERHALTER and Dr. HUEHNS[1] have measured free globin within the red cells. It is important to put all of these measurements together, including the various porphyrin complexes, the amount of iron and its form, and the amount of free globin. Only then will one be able to completely understand the *in vivo* chemistry of these abnormalities of haemoglobin synthesis.

HEILMEYER: I quite agree with you, Dr. FINCH: sideroachrestic anaemias really are like an iceberg, with only a portion of the problems being at present visible. Even so, we should be pleased if only we could find solutions to those problems that are visible.

MOURIQUAND: I should like to ask Dr. HEILMEYER to discuss bone-marrow iron in inflammatory diseases; I should be particularly interested to know whether, in Prussian blue stained smears, he has noticed a consistent relationship between the erythroblasts and the iron-loaded reticular cells of the bone marrow. This brings us back to the same question as was discussed yesterday by Dr. KATZ and again today by Dr. FINCH, namely the relationship between reticular-cell iron, transferrin iron, and erythroblast iron, or rather the role of the reticular-cell "pathway" in the delivery of iron to the erythrocyte precursors.

HEILMEYER: In infectious diseases we find a marked discrepancy between the iron overloading of the reticulo-endothelial cells and the iron content of the erythroblasts. The reticulo-endothelial cells show a pronounced reaction when stained for iron, whereas the erythroblasts have a reduced content of free iron. In the presence of infection, the reticulo-endothelial cells release less iron to the transferrin. This is probably the reason for the reduced plasma iron concentrations observed in patients suffering from infection.

---

[1] WINTERHALTER, K. H., and E. R. HUEHNS: J. Clin. Invest. (U.S.A.) **42**, 995 (1963).

Some aspects of iron-deficiency anaemia in India

By

J. B. CHATTERJEA

Iron deficiency is the most frequent cause of anaemia in India. Factors contributing to the causation of iron deficiency include dietary inadequacy, loss of blood, and malabsorption. Dietary inadequacy manifests itself especially during certain periods of life when iron requirements are increased, e.g. in growing children and child-bearing women. One very important cause of blood loss, particularly operative in certain regions of India, is heavy hookworm infection. An additional factor liable to affect the iron balance is the presence of a considerable amount of phytates and phosphates in the diet, exerting an inhibitory influence on the absorption of iron (MCCANCE et al., 1943; HUSSAIN and PATWARDHAN, 1959). The question of a probable loss of iron due to excessive sweating has also been raised (FOY and KONDI, 1956; HUSSAIN, PATWARDHAN, and SRIRAMACHARI, 1960).

The values for haemoglobin, red cells, and haematocrit in normal Indians, as reported from different parts of the country, vary to a certain extent according to data summarised by NAPIER and DAS GUPTA (1945). This variation is in general explainable by reference to the socio-economic status and dietary habits of the population concerned. The values for male Indians of good socio-economic status partaking of a balanced diet were found to be similar to values reported from other countries. Low haemoglobin values (12.0 g./100 ml. or less) recorded in poor or middle-class Indian women and in poor labourers would appear to be mainly an expression of iron deficiency. Iron therapy improves the haemoglobin level significantly, and normal values are easily obtainable in this way. While treating overt anaemia in this group of subjects, we have found that continuation of iron therapy raises the values to levels which are definitely higher than what is held to be normal in the population concerned. This erythropoietic response to iron therapy is presumably physiological and not pharmacological.

In the present communication an attempt will be made to describe certain aspects of iron-deficiency anaemia in India. In selecting the points to be discussed, emphasis has been placed on material particularly common in India and on problems in which existing knowledge appears to be incomplete. Hereditary disorders of haemoglobin synthesis are common in the population from which the present material has been drawn. There has been a suggestion that the thalassaemia trait may offer resistance to the development of iron deficiency (HALDANE, 1949). Relevant data obtained from a study undertaken to investigate the possibility of an interrelationship between haemoglobinopathy and iron deficiency have been incorporated.

Material and methods

The data in the present series were taken from a study of 120 cases of iron-deficiency anaemia investigated at the School of Tropical Medicine in Calcutta. The ages of the patients (78 males and 42 females) ranged from 2 to 54 years. The initial haemoglobin level varied from 1.8 to 7.2 g./100 ml. The series consisted only of patients suffering from a pure deficiency of iron. Cases with associated deficiencies of vitamin B_{12} and/or folic acid were excluded, but those with associated protein deficiency were included. In addition to standard clinical and laboratory examinations to assess the degree, nature, and cause of the anaemia, the following were also determined:

a) Serum iron, using POWELL's modification of HEILMEYER's method (1944).

b) Iron-binding capacity of the serum, using the method of SCHADE and CAROLINE as modified by CARTWRIGHT and WINTROBE (1949).

c) Semiquantitative estimation of bone-marrow haemosiderin, by the method of RATH and FINCH (1948).

d) Alkaline phosphatase activity of bone-marrow aspirate, estimated by GOMORI's revised technique (GLICK, 1949).

e) Serum vitamin B_{12} content, estimated using a microbiological method of ROSS (1952) with *Euglena gracilis* var. *bacillaris* as the test organism.

f) Alkali-resistant fraction of haemoglobin, estimated by the method of SINGER et al. (1951). Electrophoretic analysis of haemoglobin samples was done according to a technique described elsewhere (CHATTERJEA et al., 1960).

g) Glucose-6-phosphate dehydrogenase activity of red cells, measured by the method of KORNBERG and HORECKER (1955) as modified by MARKS (1958).

Outlines of other methods are given in the relevant sections. Follow-up data on serial studies were collected in order to determine how the disease evolved.

The relevant data on iron deficiency were compared, as and when necessary, with those on dimorphic anaemia (CHATTERJEA and DAS GUPTA, 1953), kwashiorkor, and nutritional macrocytic anaemia (CHATTERJEA, 1958; CHATTERJEA, 1960).

Aetiological factors

In the 120 cases of pure iron-deficiency anaemia without associated deficiency of vitamin B_{12} and/or folic acid, the main factor or factors that appeared to be responsible for causing the anaemia could be grouped as follows:

Nutritional (25)

This group consisted mainly of women and children whose requirements were high.

Hookworm infection (52)

Hookworm infection was the predominating cause operative through blood loss. The role of any associated or predisposing factors will be discussed later.

Haemorrhages (39)

The sites of bleeding and the numbers for each category were as follows:

Uterus	22
Haemorrhoids	8
Duodenum	8
Nose	1

Hookworm plus other causes of haemorrhage (4)

Hookworm infection was associated with haemorrhoids in 3 cases and with duodenal ulcer in 1.

It should be pointed out that the relative frequency of the various causes as indicated above does not denote a constant state of affairs obtainable all over India. Depending upon the types of population (urban or rural, rich or poor) and upon their iron requirements, the relative incidence will vary widely.

In the present series, which includes only iron deficiency, there was no case of malabsorption. This is due to the fact that, in malabsorption, the deficiency is more often mixed. In a series of patients suffering from mixed deficiency (involving iron plus folic acid and/or vitamin B_{12}), the incidence of iron deficiency on the basis of dietary inadequacy and/or malabsorption would be higher.

Some clinical features

The essential clinical features were in general similar to those detailed by WITTS (1931) and WINTROBE and BEEBE (1933). Only a few points of particular interest will therefore be discussed here.

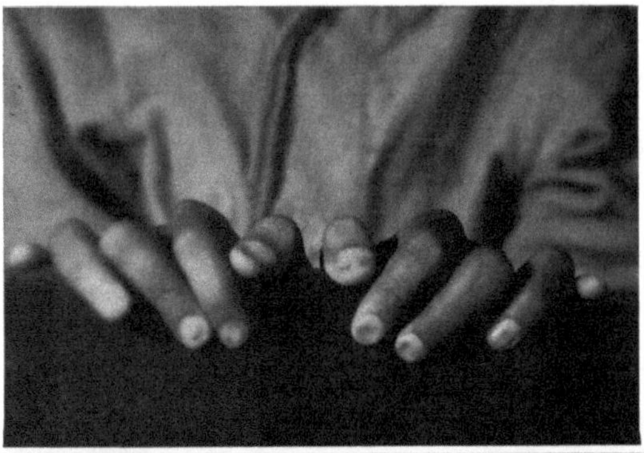

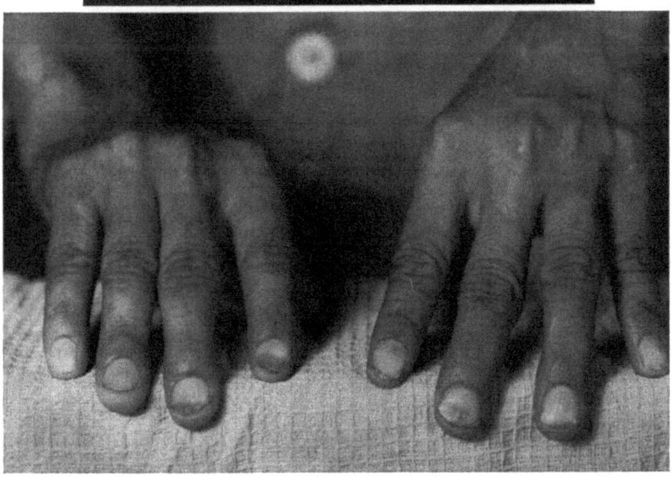

Figs 1 and 2. Changes of the finger-nails and toe-nails

Spleen. Enlarged in 45 cases. The splenic enlargement was usually slight, varying from 1 to 3 cm. below the costal arch. In 6 cases, the enlargement was greater, i.e. between 5 and 8 cm.

Liver. Enlarged in 64 cases, the degree of enlargement varying usually from 1.5 to 3 cm. below the costal arch.

Enlargement of spleen and liver usually regressed along with the improvement in the blood picture, although sometimes the regression was slower.

Nails. Typical koilonychia was noted in 7 cases, and significant thinning of the nails was seen in 12 cases. In 1 case, there were

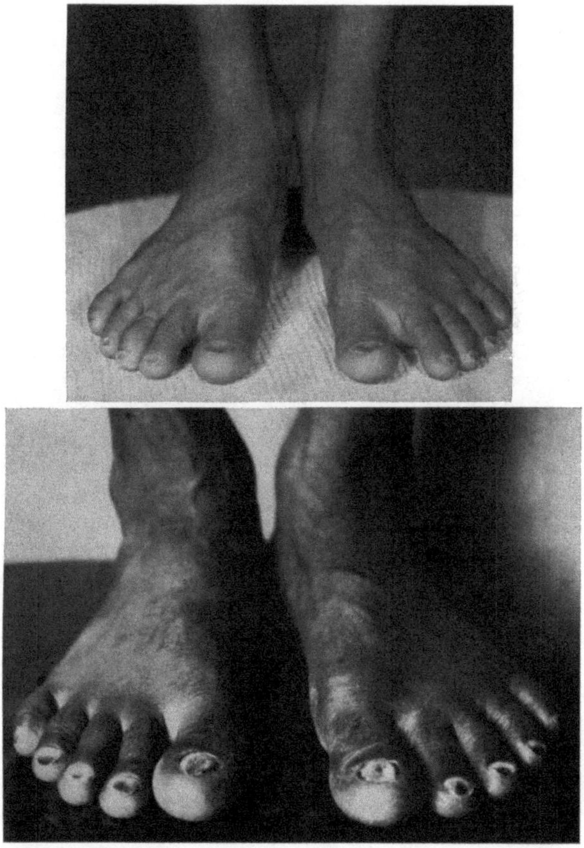

in patients with iron-deficiency anaemia

longitudinal ridges. Sometimes koilonychia was more prominent in the toe-nails (Figs 1 and 2).

Parotid. In 38 cases there was significant enlargement of the parotid glands (Fig. 3). The importance of this finding will be discussed.

Glossitis was present in 17 cases and *angular stomatitis* in 5.

Pigmentation of the skin was observed in 11 cases and *oedema* of face and extremities in 7.

Depigmented patches (leucoderma) were seen in 4 cases.

Not included in the present series were two instances of dwarfism and infantilism in association with iron-deficiency anaemia. In these 2 cases, iron deficiency (dietary), dating from early childhood, appears to have affected both somatic and sexual growth.

Observations on parotid enlargement

Painless enlargement of the parotid glands is regarded as a sign of undernutrition. EHRLICH observed parotid enlargement in many Polish children of both sexes examined during the period of wartime scarcity in 1916–17. By 1918, however, the number was already decreasing, and with the return of plenty this parotid enlargement disappeared completely. Chronic enlargement of the parotid, and sometimes of the submaxillary gland, was not uncommon among poor agricultural workers in Egypt. It was predominantly encountered in male subjects and was due to non-inflammatory hypertrophy. Enlarged parotids have also frequently been noted in malnourished Africans (GILLMAN and GILLMAN, 1947). Parotid enlargement occurring in Germans while they were putting on weight after their repatriation from Russia appears to have been part of a much more general syndrome affecting both sexes. According to McCANCE, DEAN, and BARRETT (1951), who reviewed the relevant literature and recorded the results of investigations on parotid enlargement in Germans repatriated from Russia during the years 1947 and 1948, the enlargement was painless, non-inflammatory, and usually bilateral, and was due partly to enlargement of individual acini. It was not associated with gynaecomastia. In this context, mention must be made of liver disease, in which parotid enlargement has also been known to occur, sometimes associated with enlargement of the breasts; this syndrome has been explained on the basis of an endocrine imbalance due to inactivation of steroids.

A review of the available literature suggests that the precise factor involved in parotid enlargement is not known. In the forms of nutritional anaemia which we see in India, enlargement of the parotid gland is by no means uncommon. In the present series of 120 patients, it was encountered in no less than 38 cases. The enlargement was painless and usually, but not invariably, affected both parotid glands. The data relating to these 38 subjects were compared with those for the other cases of iron deficiency showing no parotid enlargement. Similar parotid enlargement was also found in a miscellaneous group of subjects presenting no obvious evidence of iron deficiency (see Table 1).

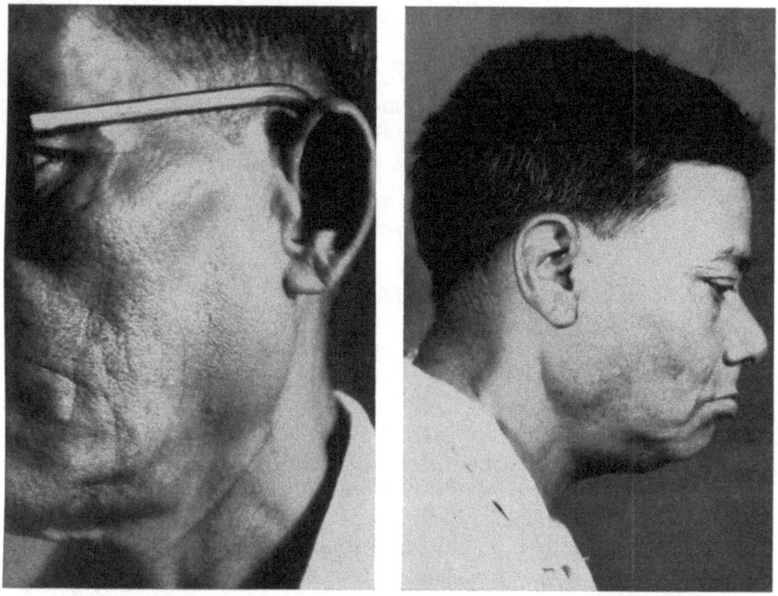

Fig. 3. Enlargement of the parotid glands in iron-deficiency anaemia

Table 1. *Cases showing parotid enlargement*

Disease	No. of cases
Iron-deficiency anaemia	38
Dimorphic anaemia	20
Nutritional macrocytic anaemia	3
Miscellaneous group	22
(haemolytic anaemia, hypoplastic anaemia, cirrhosis of the liver, myxoedema, etc.)	

Comments

Of the 38 patients with parotid enlargement in the iron-deficiency group, 31 were males and 7 females. Compared with the remaining 82 patients showing no enlargement of the parotid, they presented no differences with reference to the following:

socio-economic status, degree of anaemia, glossitis, enlargement of spleen and liver, pigmentation, nail changes, serum protein, or the basic cause of anaemia.

In those cases which it was possible to follow up over a prolonged period, the parotid enlargement decreased in response to iron therapy. No biopsy examinations of the parotid glands have so far been made.

From examination and follow-up of all patients with parotid enlargement it would appear that the latter is in some way related to the iron deficiency, although details of a possible interrelationship between the two have yet to be established. Knowledge to date obviously does not exclude the possibility that other factors – about which, once again, little if anything is known – may be involved.

Eye changes

46 cases of nutritional anaemia, comprising 20 cases of iron-deficiency anaemia, 17 of dimorphic anaemia, and 9 of nutritional macrocytic anaemia, were examined for changes in the eyegrounds. The first examination was carried out immediately after admission to hospital and before the institution of any anti-anaemic therapy. Repeat examinations were undertaken after the conclusion of anti-anaemic therapy.

The series of patients with iron-deficiency anaemia consisted of 16 males and 4 females varying in age from 10 to 45 years. The haemoglobin level before treatment varied from 2.62 to 6.52 g./100 ml.

Ophthalmoscopic examination yielded normal findings in 5 cases. The remaining 15 cases presented the following findings:

Disc – Normal appearance in 4 cases, pallor in 10, and slight blurring of the margin in 1. After therapy, the pallor had disappeared in all 10 cases; the margin had become normal in the case which had initially shown blurring.

Veins – Normal appearance in 5 cases and slight to moderate engorgement in 10. After therapy, the venous engorgement had disappeared in all 10 cases.

Retina – Normal appearance in 10 cases, slight oedema in 2, thin exudate in 2, and slight flame-shaped haemorrhage in 1. After therapy, the oedema had disappeared in the 2 cases in question, and the thin exudate and haemorrhage had subsided in 1 case.

Choroid – Normal in 13 cases, moderate choroidal atrophy in 1, and marked atrophy in another. Upon re-examination after therapy, the choroidal changes of moderate degree seen in 1 case had become normal, whereas the patient with marked choroidal degeneration showed no improvement after therapy, even when the blood picture had become normal.

Other features – Associated cataract of one eye was present in 1 case.

Similar changes were seen in dimorphic anaemia and nutritional macrocytic anaemia. A comparative summary of the relevant findings in different types of nutritional anaemia is given in Table 2.

Table 2. *Summary of eye changes in nutritional anaemia*

Disease (No. of cases)	Abnormal findings in	No. of patients with abnormalities in		
		Disc	Veins	Retina
Iron deficiency (20).	15	10	10	5
Dimorphic (17).	14	10	8	7
Nutritional macrocytic (9). .	6	4	6	4

Comments

Pallor of the optic disc, varying degrees of venous engorgement, retinal exudates, and haemorrhage as seen in some cases of iron deficiency appeared to be reversible changes, which usually cleared up with the improvement of the blood picture following iron therapy. None of the patients showed evidence of papilloedema (Das Gupta, Chatterjea, Ray, and Ghose, 1955). It is possible that an uncorrected iron deficiency, if persisting for a longer period, may give rise to increasing venous engorgement and ultimately to papilloedema as reported by Schwaber and Blumberg (1961) and as reviewed by Beutler (1962). But on the whole this must be a rare occurrence.

Bone-marrow changes

The bone marrow was usually hypercellular with normoblastic hyperplasia. The degree of normoblastic hyperplasia could not always be correlated with the degree of anaemia. The normoblasts showed typical qualitative changes characterised by the smallness of their size and by a poorly developed, ragged cytoplasm with deficient haemoglobinisation. Occasionally, P.A.S.-positive material was found in the cytoplasm of the normoblasts. Haemosiderin and sideroblasts were virtually absent.

In general, there were no significant changes in granulopoiesis. We have the impression that qualitative changes in granulopoiesis (presence of giant metamyelocytes and/or macropolycytes) of any significant degree are usually indicative of an associated deficiency of folic acid and/or vitamin B_{12}. In a few instances of dimorphic anaemia, such changes were seen only after a course of iron therapy, indicating that where iron deficiency is the predominant factor this may mask the granulopoietic changes occurring in the presence of deficiencies of folic acid and/or vitamin B_{12}. As a rule, when iron therapy was given along with a good diet, which contained substantial amounts of vitamin B_{12} and folic acid, the granular changes disappeared in response to correction of the relevant deficiencies.

In average cases, the megakaryocytic changes did not display any significant variation from the normal pattern. The alkaline phosphatase activity of the cytoplasm showed no evidence of inactivation as seen in thrombocytopenic states (CHATTERJEA et al., 1958). The P.A.S. reaction also appeared to be normal.

Observations on serum iron and the iron-binding capacity of the serum

In iron-deficiency anaemia, the serum iron was low, the iron-binding capacity of the serum elevated, and bone-marrow haemosiderin virtually absent. Following iron therapy, the blood picture quickly improved. In a series of 70 patients with iron deficiency, after 4–6 weeks of oral iron therapy the peripheral blood picture reached almost normal levels, but the haemosiderin deposits in the bone marrow showed no significant increase. At this stage, the serum iron level, though still below normal, showed a slight increase. Before therapy, the mean serum iron worked out at 19 μg. % with a range of 5–30 μg. %; after therapy, the mean was 40 μg. % and the range 10–60 μg. %. The unsaturated iron-binding capacity did not become normal in all cases; before therapy, the mean level was 406 μg. % with a range of 350–500 μg. %; after therapy, the mean was 355 μg. % with a range of 260 to 447 μg. %. Continuation of iron therapy was necessary to normalise the serum iron and iron-binding capacity. The relevant changes are illustrated in Fig. 4.

In nutritional macrocytic anaemia involving deficiencies of folic acid and/or vitamin B_{12}, the serum iron was normal or high, the iron-binding capacity decreased, and the bone-marrow haemosiderin increased. Following successful treatment, the serum iron usually dropped precipitously to low levels (CHATTERJEA et al., 1957; CHATTERJEA, 1958). In a series of 32 patients, the mean serum iron before therapy was 135 μg. %, the range varying from 80 to 245 μg. %; the mean value for the unsaturated iron-binding capacity of the serum was 140 μg. %, the range varying from 0 to 200 μg. %. A significant drop in the serum iron level was regularly observed in all patients showing a satisfactory erythropoietic response. A fall in the serum iron level to a mean value of 31.0 μg. % (range 10.0—70.0 μg. %) was observed between 24 and

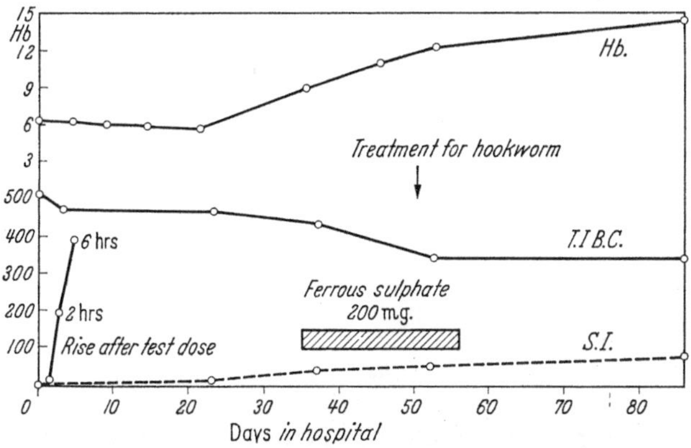

Fig. 4. S. T., male, 22 years of age; iron-deficiency anaemia, ancylostomiasis 2,700 ova/g. faeces. Serum vitamin B_{12} 170 μμg./ml., hypochlorhydria, glucose tolerance test normal. Changes in serum iron (S.I.) and in the total iron-binding capacity of the serum (T.I.B.C.) are shown. After a test dose of iron, there was a sharp rise in serum iron. Following iron therapy, serum iron and the iron-binding capacity of the serum gradually attained normal values

96 hours after institution of therapy. The serum iron level generally showed a decrease before there was any significant degree of reticulocytosis; this early fall in serum iron was not accompanied by any significant change in the iron-binding capacity. Later, the serum iron gradually became normal. The iron-binding capacity slowly improved, usually reverting to normal by the time that the serum iron and haemoglobin had become normal (Fig. 5). These changes which we observed in nutritional macrocytic anaemia were identical with those reported by Moore (1961) in pernicious anaemia. In certain of our patients initially diagnosed as suffering from nutritional macrocytic anaemia, the trend of events was somewhat different. In these subjects, as exemplified in Fig. 6, the serum iron level, having fallen, remained low and did not rise again. Here, persistence of hypoferraemia was associated with cessation of improvement in the haemoglobin level and iron-binding capacity of the serum. There was little or no haemosiderin in the bone marrow at this stage, and the peripheral blood showed hypochromia. The composite pattern indicated iron deficiency, and the blood

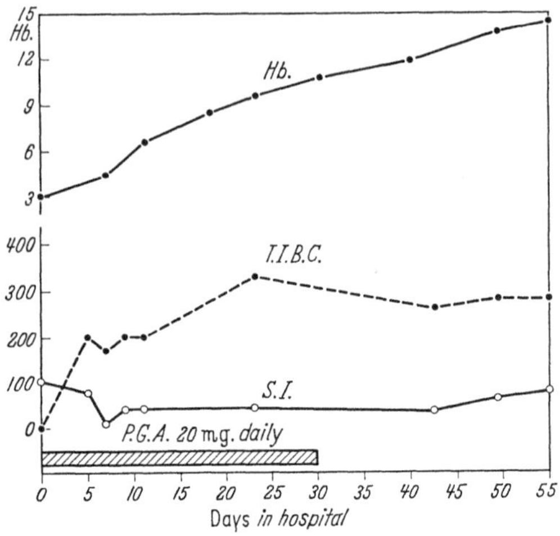

Fig. 5. B. B. D., male, 36 years of age; nutritional macrocytic anaemia (deficiency of vitamin B_{12} and folic acid), megaloblastic. Serum B_{12} 30 $\mu\mu$g., absolute achlorhydria, pteroylglutamic acid (P.G.A.) excretion 1.0 mg. Changes in serum iron (S.I.) and in the total iron-binding capacity of the serum (T.I.B.C.) are shown. Shortly after the initiation of folic acid therapy, the serum iron dropped precipitously to hypoferraemic levels. Thereafter, it gradually attained normal values along with normalisation of Hb. and T.I.B.C.

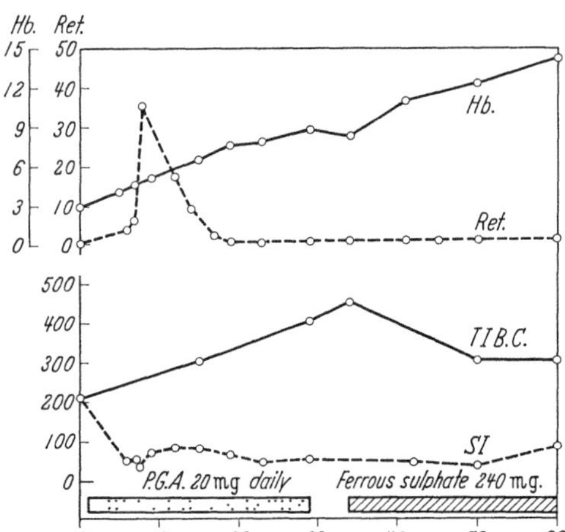

Fig. 6. L. B., female, 30 years of age; megaloblastic anaemia (deficiency of folic acid and iron). 8th pregnancy, last pregnancy 2 years ago. Serum vitamin B_{12} 200 $\mu\mu$g./ml. Changes in serum iron (S.I.) and in the total iron-binding capacity of the serum (T.I.B.C.) are shown. The drop in serum iron following folic acid persisted with significant elevation of T.I.B.C. These changes and the Hb. level could not be normalised without iron therapy. Further details are given in the text

picture did not improve unless iron was administered. These patients were obviously suffering from mixed deficiencies. Administration of folic acid and/or vitamin B_{12} corrected the megaloblastosis, but produced only a partial improvement in the blood values. The amount of iron available in the system was evidently not sufficient to normalise the blood values. Initially there was no overt evidence of iron deficiency in such cases, the iron deficiency being masked by the overriding deficiency of folic acid and/or vitamin B_{12}. In some instances of mixed deficiency, however, there was from the very beginning evidence both of iron deficiency as well as of vitamin B_{12} and /or folic acid deficiency.

Some laboratory data

Serum vitamin B_{12}

The mean value for total serum vitamin B_{12}, as measured with *Euglena gracilis*, was 283, with a range varying from 94 to 820 micromicrogrammes per ml. of serum (normal values: mean 282 $\mu\mu$g./ml.; range 98—940 $\mu\mu$g./ml.).

Serum proteins (23 cases)

The mean values (and range) for the total serum protein, albumin, and globulin were 6.65 (range 4.1—8.2), 3.36 (1.7—4.37), and 3.26 (range 1.88—4.7) g./100 ml., respectively. Total protein levels below 6.0 g. were found in 4 instances, the values being 5.8, 5.3, 4.9, and 4.1 g./100 ml. Albumin levels below 3.0 g. were recorded in 7 instances, the respective values being 2.8, 2.8, 2.8, 2.7, 2.4, 2.2, and 1.7 g./100 ml.

Cholesterol

The mean value for total cholesterol in the blood was 153, the range varying from 108 to 195 mg./100 ml.

Glucose tolerance test

No significant abnormalities were detected.

Gastric acidity

The pattern of gastric acidity was variable. In a series of 49 patients, the range of acidity was as follows: hyperchlorhydria 2, normal 10, hypochlorhydria 17, pseudo-achlorhydria 9, and absolute achlorhydria 11. Following amelioration of the blood picture, acid secretion improved in the majority of cases in which it had originally been deficient. In hookworm infestation, gastric acidity was more often normal or increased.

Hookworm anaemia

In hookworm disease, the anaemia was predominantly of the iron-deficiency type. The red-cell morphology, serum iron level, iron-binding capacity of the serum, erythropoiesis, haemosiderin content of the bone marrow, plasma clearance, erythrocytic uptake of Fe^{59}, and response to oral iron therapy conformed typically to the composite pattern seen in iron deficiency. Oral iron in ferrous form was well absorbed, and a satisfactory erythropoietic response was obtainable without any anthelmintic treatment. In cases of heavy infection, it was possible to speed up the erythropoietic response by administering anthelmintic treatment either before or along with iron therapy.

With iron therapy the blood picture improved satisfactorily, but if the worms were not eliminated, anaemia inevitably recurred, as illustrated in Fig. 7. In a 32-year-old male, the haemoglobin and P.C.V. (packed cell volume) levels improved from 2.7 g. and 11.0% to 11.6 g. and 40.0%, respectively, in the course of 54 days' treatment with iron without any anthelmintic therapy. Upon withdrawal of the iron therapy, the haemoglobin dropped to 4.6 g. and the P.C.V. to 15% over a period of 94 days. Resumption of iron therapy again effected a similar haematological improvement, which could

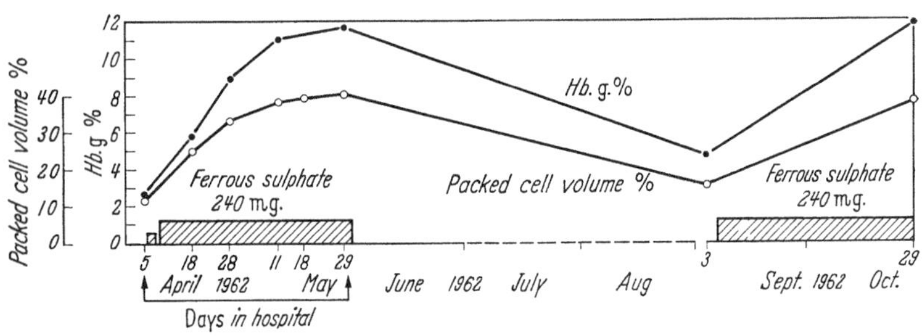

Fig. 7. J. M., male, 32 years of age: ancylostomiasis. Hospital diet. The blood values improved readily in response to oral iron. Without anthelmintic therapy, however, there was an early recurrence of anaemia

not be sustained, however, until specific anthelmintic treatment had been given. An improvement was almost always obtainable without any protein supplement in the diet. In an out-patient receiving his customary home diet, which was usually inadequate, the response was not poorer than that observed in an otherwise similar in-patient receiving a better diet (Fig. 8). To achieve and maintain a satisfactory erythropoietic response in the average case, it is in fact not essential to supplement the diet with protein. This was also confirmed by observations on a group of subjects who were admitted to hospital. These patients were placed on a diet containing 137 g.

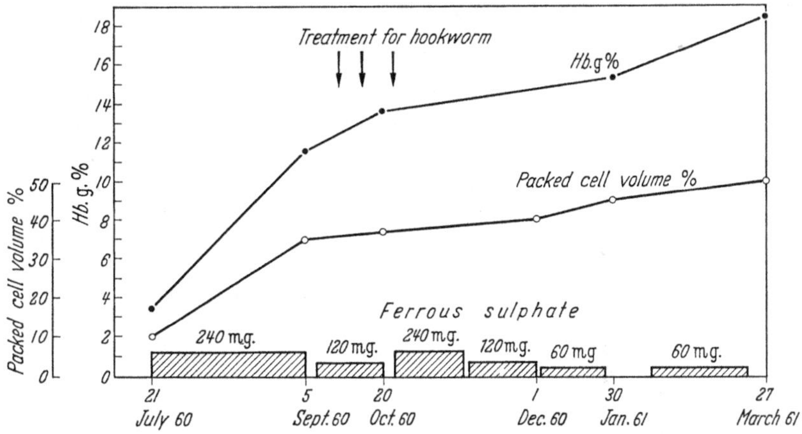

Fig. 8. K. B., male, 40 years of age; ancylostomiasis. Treated in the out-patents' department with his home diet plus adequate anthelmintic treatment (arrows). Glossitis +, parotids +. Blood values became normal in response to oral iron alone. The patient was a poor agricultural labourer and his home diet inadequate in protein. No protein supplement was required to achieve an optimum erythropoietic response

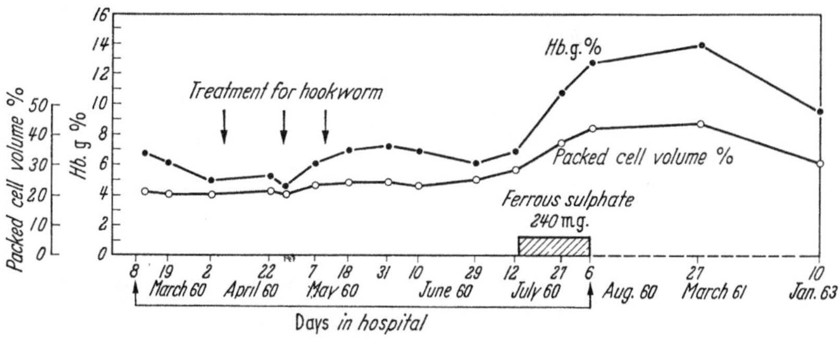

Fig. 9. P. S., male, 16 years of age; ancylostomiasis. Hospital diet plus adequate anthelmintic treatment (arrows). There was no significant improvement in the blood values in this case for as long as 125 days. With oral iron therapy, the Hb. rose steadily from 6.9 to 12.8 g. in 24 days (further details in text)

protein, 80 g. fat, and 400 g. carbohydrate, yielding a total of 2,946 calories. The iron, vitamin B_{12}, and folic acid content of the diet was 36 mg., 26 μg., and 303 μg., respectively. The hookworms were eliminated, but no iron therapy was administered. In one such patient (Fig. 9), the haematological improvement over a period of 125 days was negligible. In response to iron therapy, however, the haemoglobin rose steadily from 6.9 g. to 12.8 g. in the course of 24 days. Without any further treatment and with a home diet, the haemoglobin and haematocrit levels remained normal for the next 8 months. After a further lapse of 10 months, the blood values gradually deteriorated, owing presumably to re-infection in the rural environment in which the patient was living.

Lack of any correlation between the degree of anaemia and the degree of infection has led workers to postulate that hookworms *per se* may not be responsible for the anaemia observed. One important point in the causation of anaemia due to hookworm is the duration of infection, which in an average case is not possible to estimate. In patients in whom the degree of infection is similar, the severity of the anaemia will depend upon the duration of infection or, in other words, upon the duration of blood loss. The pre-existing state of nutrition with respect to the iron stores in the body will certainly be a contributory factor; but in the evolution of anaemia, the total period during which the subject has been losing blood obviously plays a more important role. The erythropoietic response and the nature of the relapse as exemplified in Figs 7, 8, and 9 would appear to provide evidence in favour of the assumption that hookworms cause anaemia due to blood loss. The presence of occult blood in the stools and radiological findings suggesting significant duodenal abnormalities also afford strong evidence of blood loss. The haematological status of these patients is comparable to that of professional blood donors of similar socio-economic status. After a variable number of donations, the latter develop anaemia as a direct consequence of blood loss. Depending on their previous haematological and nutritional status, the evolution of the anaemia may be slow or rapid.

Vitamin B_{12} and folic acid deficiency was not found to be significantly greater than in the general population. Nor did protein deficiency appear to play any definite role in the pathogenesis of anaemia due to hookworm infection. In average cases of hookworm anaemia, there was no evidence of malabsorption of iron, folic acid, vitamin B_{12}, or protein. Glucose tolerance and fat-balance studies yielded normal results. Gastric acidity was somewhat reduced, but not as a rule to the same extent as in iron deficiency due to dietary inadequacy. The depressive effect of iron deficiency on the gastric mucosa appears to have been offset to some extent by the irritant effect of the parasites on the duodenum.

The composite data indicate that blood loss is the major factor responsible for anaemia in the presence of hookworm infestation, although whether the patient develops anaemia at an early or a later stage will depend on his pre-existing nutritional status. Deficiencis of folic acid, vitamin B_{12}, and protein are associated factors related chiefly to dietary inadequacy.

Iron deficiency and kwashiorkor

Kwashiorkor is a classic manifestation of protein deficiency in infants and young children, the patients showing marked hypoproteinaemia and hypo-albuminaemia associated invariably with a certain degree of anaemia. In a series of 38 patients investigated with a view to clarifying the pathogenesis of the anaemia, some degree of iron deficiency – due presumably to dietary inadequacy – was found in the vast majority of cases (BASU, CHATTERJEA, and CHAUDHURI, 1961).

Iron deficiency, haemoglobinopathy, and allied problems

To illustrate the theory of balanced polymorphism as a genetic equilibrator in a population, HALDANE (1949) suggested that the thalassaemia trait may offer resistance to the development of iron deficiency. This theory received support from SIJPESTEIN (1955), who wrote: "It is surmised that mild chronic anaemia that results from thalassaemia minor may give rise to an increased absorption of iron. It is pointed out that this might be of great importance to the women in a community where a high infant mortality rate has to be compensated for by a large number of births". To test the validity of this hypothesis, 120 subjects suffering from varying degrees of iron-deficiency anaemia were examined in order to determine the incidence of the haemoglobinopathic trait in them as compared with the incidence in the general population. The relevant data are shown in Table 3.

Table 3. *Incidence of thalassaemia and Hb.E trait in iron deficiency*

Subjects	Number	Thalassaemia trait %	Hb.E trait %
Iron-deficiency anaemia . . .	120	4.4	5.3
Normal.	700	3.7	3.9

In the general Bengali population, 7.6% had a haemoglobinopathic trait, 3.7% showing a thalassaemia trait and 3.9% an Hb.E trait (CHATTERJEA et al., 1957). In the iron-deficiency group, 9.7% showed a haemoglobinopathic trait, 4.4% having a thalassaemia trait and 5.3% an Hb.E trait. The degree of anaemia did not appear to bear any relationship to the haemoglobinopathic traits. It should also be pointed out that SIJPESTEIN's hypothesis, postulated on the assumption that iron absorption is increased in subjects with a thalassaemia trait, is not borne out by recent studies on iron absorption (ERLANDSON et al., 1962).

Hb.A_2 and Hb.F in iron-deficiency anaemia

91 cases of iron-deficiency anaemia were investigated with a view to discovering whether iron deficiency produces any significant change in the proportion of Hb.A_2 and Hb.F. The results are shown in Table 4. In patients suffering from iron deficiency, there was no significant alteration in either of these components.

Table 4. *Hb.A_2 and Hb.F in iron deficiency*

	Hb.A_2%		Hb.F%	
	Mean	Range	Mean	Range
Normal (20)	3.1	1.5— 5.2	1.9	0 — 3.9
Thalassaemia trait (63) . . .	13.5	3.5—24.2	4.0	0.6—28.7
Iron deficiency (91).	3.6	0.5— 6.0	2.1	0.4— 8.2

Iron deficiency and malaria

It has been suggested that the resistance of the haemoglobinopathic trait to plasmodial infection is related to the abnormal red-cell morphology (LIVINGSTONE, 1961). The red-cell morphology in haemoglobinopathy resembles that in iron-deficiency anaemia. Direct experiments were designed to test the resistance of patients with iron deficiency to induced infection with *Plasmodium vivax*. Two such patients and 11 out of 12 controls were readily infected, whereas 9 out of 11 subjects with Hb.E thalassaemia disease escaped infection (RAY, CHATTERJEA, and CHAUDHURI, 1963). The red-cell morphology *per se* (or iron deficiency) is therefore unlikely to afford any protection against induced malaria.

Glutathione stability and glucose-6-phosphate dehydrogenase (G-6-PD) activity of the red cells

Approximately 4% of the normal population in West Bengal appeared to be suffering from a deficiency of the erythrocytic enzyme G-6-PD (SWARUP et al., 1963). The reduced glutathione was grossly unstable in all enzyme-deficient subjects. The percentage of enzyme deficiency appeared to be slightly higher both in the thalassaemia trait and in the Hb.E trait. Among a group of 20 subjects with iron deficiency, low G-6-PD activity was found only in one instance. The relevant findings are shown in Table 5. Although this was only a small series, the results would appear to suggest that the incidence of G-6-PD deficiency in iron-deficient subjects is no different from that in a normal population.

Table 5. *G-6-PD activity in relation to iron deficiency*

Subjects	Number	G-6-PD activity		
		Low	Intermediate	Normal
Normal	87	3	2	82
Thalassaemia trait	50	7	2	41
Hb. E trait	25	5	—	20
Iron-deficiency anaemia . . .	20	1	—	19

Summary

A series of 120 cases of iron-deficiency anaemia was investigated. Classified according to the main aetiological factor, the cases could be grouped as follows: nutritional 25, hookworm 52, haemorrhage 39, and hookworm plus haemorrhage 4.

The spleen was enlarged in 45 cases, and the liver enlarged in 64 cases. Painless enlargement of the parotid glands was noted in 38 cases, nail changes in 20, glossitis in 17, pigmentation of the skin in 11, oedema in 7, angular stomatitis in 5, and leucoderma in 4. In 15 out of 20 cases, ophthalmoscopic examination revealed abnormalities, including pallor of the optic disc, varying degrees of venous engorgement, retinal exudates, and haemorrhages.

Serial studies of serum iron, the iron-binding capacity of the serum, and bone-marrow haemosiderin indicated differential patterns for iron deficiency, nutritional macrocytic anaemia (vitamin B_{12} and/or folic acid deficiency), and dimorphic anaemia (iron deficiency plus vitamin B_{12} and/or folic acid deficiency).

In hookworm infection, blood loss appeared to be the major factor responsible for anaemia, although whether the patient develops anaemia at an early or a later stage depends upon his pre-existing nutritional status. The duration of infection, which mainly determines the degree of iron depletion, is an unknown factor — which would in many instances explain the lack of correlation between the degree of anaemia observed and the estimated severity of hookworm infestation at any particular moment. Such deficiencies of vitamin B_{12} and folic acid as were found appeared to be associated factors related mostly to dietary inadequacy.

The low haemoglobin levels reported in poorer sections of the Indian population, particularly among women, can be explained chiefly on the basis of iron deficiency. Kwashiorkor, which represents a classic manifestation of protein deficiency in infants and children, is commonly associated with iron deficiency due to dietary inadequacy.

In patients suffering from iron deficiency, the incidence of the haemoglobinopathic trait and of G-6-PD deficiency did not appear to be significantly different from that in the normal population. Iron-deficient red cells did not appear to show any resistance to induced infection with *Plasmodium vivax*.

Zusammenfassung

Es wird über 120 Patienten mit Eisenmangelanaemien berichtet, die sich entsprechend ihrer Aetiologie in folgende Gruppen einteilen lassen: alimentär bedingt 25, durch Hakenwurm 52, durch Haemorrhagie 39 und durch Hakenwurm plus Haemorrhagie 4 hervorgerufen.

Die Milz war in 45, die Leber in 64 Fällen vergrößert. Schmerzlose Vergrößerung der Parotis wurde 38mal beobachtet, Nagelveränderungen 20mal, Glossitis 17mal, Hautpigmentierungen 11mal, Oedeme 7mal, anguläre Stomatitis 5mal und Leukoderm 4mal. Bei 15 von 20 Fällen ergab die ophthalmoskopische Untersuchung Veränderungen wie Abblassung der Papille, verschiedene Grade venöser Stauung, Retinaexsudate und Haemorrhagien.

Reihenuntersuchungen des Serumeisens, der Eisenbindungsfähigkeit, des Serums sowie des Haemosiderins im Knochenmark ergaben verschiedene Muster für Eisenmangel, alimentäre makrozytäre Anaemien (Vitamin B_{12}- und/oder Folsäuremangel) und dimorphe Anaemien (Eisenmangel plus Vitamin B_{12}- und/oder Folsäuremangel).

Bei der Hakenwurminfektion schien hauptsächlich der Blutverlust der der Anaemie zugrunde liegende Faktor zu sein, obwohl der Ernährungszustand weitgehend dafür verantwortlich ist, ob sich die Anaemie zu einem früheren oder späteren Zeitpunkt entwickelt. Die Dauer der Infektion, die weitgehend den Grad der Eisenverarmung bedingt, ist meist unbekannt, woraus sich das Fehlen einer Korrelation zwischen dem Grad der Anaemie und der Schwere des Befalls mit Hakenwürmern erklärt. Zusätzlicher Mangel an Vitamin B_{12} und Folsäure waren meist Folge ungenügender Ernährung.

Die niedrigen Haemoglobinwerte, die bei den ärmeren Schichten der indischen Bevölkerung, besonders bei Frauen, gefunden werden, sind hauptsächlich auf Eisenmangel zurückzuführen. Kwashiorkor als klassischer Ausdruck eines Eiweißmangels bei Kleinkindern und Kindern ist gewöhnlich mit Eisenmangel infolge Unterernährung verbunden.

Bei Patienten mit Eisenmangel scheint die Häufigkeit einer genetischen Prädisposition gegenüber Haemoglobinopathien und Mangel an Glukose-6-phosphatdehydrogenase nicht in signifikanter Weise von der bei einer normalen Population abzuweichen. Erythrozyten mit Eisenmangel zeigten keine Resistenz gegenüber Infektion mit *Plasmodium vivax*.

Résumé

120 cas d'anémie par carence en fer ont été étudiés, pouvant être ainsi répartis, selon le principal facteur étiologique: 25 cas d'origine nutritionnelle, 52 par ankylostomiase, 39 par hémorragie et 4 par ankylostomiase et hémorragie.

La rate était augmentée de volume dans 45 cas et le foie dans 64 cas. Une tuméfaction indolore des parotides a été notée dans 38 cas, des altérations des ongles dans 20 cas, une glossite dans 17 cas, une pigmentation cutanée dans 11 cas, des oedèmes dans 7 cas, une stomatite angulaire dans 5 cas, une leucodermie dans 4 cas. L'examen ophthalmoscopique a montré des anomalies dans 15 cas sur 20: pâleur de la papille, congestion veineuse plus ou moins marquée, exsudats rétiniens, hémorragies.

Des études en série du fer sérique, de la capacité de fixation en fer du sérum, de l'hémosidérine de la moelle osseuse ont permis d'établir des tableaux distinctifs entre les carences en fer, les anémies macrocytaires nutritionnelles (carence en vitamine B_{12} ou en acide folique ou en ces deux facteurs) et les anémies micro-macrocytaires (carence en fer et carence en vitamine B_{12} ou acide folique).

Dans l'infestation à ankylostome, la déperdition sanguine semble être la cause principale de l'anémie encore que le délai d'apparition, plus ou moins long, de l'anémie dépende de l'état de nutrition antérieur. L'ancienneté de l'infestation, principal facteur de l'importance des pertes de fer, est inconnue, ce qui expliquerait dans beaucoup de cas l'absence de corrélation entre le degré de l'anémie et la gravité supposée de l'infestation à un moment donné. De telles carences en vitamine B_{12} et en acide folique semblent être des facteurs associés relevant principalement d'une mauvaise alimentation.

Les taux bas d'hémoglobine rencontrés dans les classes pauvres de la population de l'Inde, en particulier chez les femmes, peuvent s'expliquer surtout par la carence en fer. Le kwashiorkor, manifestation classique d'une carence en protéines chez le petit et le grand enfant, s'accompagne habituellement d'une carence en fer due à la mauvaise alimentation.

L'incidence, chez les malades en carence ferrique, d'une prédisposition génétique aux hémoglobinopathies et de la carence en G-6-PD n'a pas différé de façon significative de celle observée dans la population normale. Les hématies pauvres en fer n'ont pas paru présenter de diminution de résistance à l'infection à *Plasmodium vivax.*

Acknowledgements

Grateful thanks are due to Director Dr. R. N. Chaudhuri, Dr. Sushiela Swarup, Dr. R. N. Ray, Dr. Sandhya Ghose, Mr. S. K. Ghosh, Dr. D. K. Banerjee, Dr. N. Ghosh, Prof. A. B. Chowdhury, Prof. R. L. Nath, Prof. P. C. Sen Gupta, and Dr. S. P. Basu for their kind help in connection with this study. Part of the work was done with a grant-in-aid from the Indian Council of Medical Research.

References

Bannerman, M. A.: Thalassemia. Grune & Stratton, New York, 1961. — Basu, A. K., J. B. Chatterjea, and R. N. Chaudhuri: Bull. Calcutta School Trop. Med. **9**, 22 (1961). — Beutler, E., V. F. Fairbanks, and J. J. Fahey: Clinical Disorders of Iron Metabolism. Grune & Stratton, New York, 1962. — Cartwright, G. E., and M. M. Wintrobe: J. Clin. Invest. (U.S.A.) **28**, 86 (1949). — Chatterjea, J. B.: J. Indian Med. Ass. **31**, 4 (1958). — Chatterjea, J. B.: Bull. Calcutta School Trop. Med. **8**, 9 (1960). — Chatterjea, J. B., A. B. Chowdhury, C. R. Das Gupta, and H. N. Ray: In: Proceedings of the 6th International Congress of the International Society of Haematology. Grune & Stratton, New York, 1958, p. 562. — Chatterjea, J. B., and C. R. Das Gupta: Indian Med. Gaz. **88**, 126 (1953). — Chatterjea, J. B., S. K. Ghosh, R. N. Ray, A. K. Basu, and D. K. Banerjee: Indian J. Med. Sc. **11**, 565 (1957). — Chatterjea, J. B., S. Swarup, and S. K. Ghosh: In: Proceedings of the 7th International Congress of the International Society of Haematology. Il Pensiero Scientifico, Rome, **2**, 448 (1960). — Chatterjea, J. B., S. Swarup, S. K. Ghosh, and R. N. Ray: Bull. Calcutta School Trop. Med. **5**, 159 (1957). — Das Gupta, C. R., J. B. Chatterjea, R. N. Ray, and N. Ghosh: Bull. Calcutta School Trop. Med. **3**, 101 (1955). — Erlandson, M. E., B. Walden,

G. Stern, M. W. Hilgartner, J. Wehman, and C. H. Smith: Blood (U.S.A.) **19**, 359 (1962). — Foy, H., and A. Kondi: J. Trop. Med. Hyg. (G.B.) **60**, 105 (1957). — Gillman, J., G. Christine, and G. Theodore: S. Afr. J. Med. Sc. **12**, 99 (1947). — Gillman, J., and T. Gillman: Nutr. Rev. (U.S.A.) **5**, 353 (1947). — Glick, D.: Techniques of Histo- and Cytochemistry. Interscience Publishers, New York, 1949. — Haldane, J. B. S.: Ricerca sc. (It.) Suppl., p. 75 (1949), quoted by M. A. Bannerman (1961). — Hussain, R., and V. N. Patwardhan: Indian J. Med. Res. **47**, 676 (1959). — Hussain, R., V. N. Patwardhan, and S. Sriramachari: Indian J. Med. Res. **48**, 235 (1960). — Kornberg, A., and B. L. Horecker: In: Methods in Enzymology. Ed. by S. P. Colowick and N. O. Kaplan. Academic Press, New York, **1**, 323 (1955). — Livingstone, F. B.: Human Biol. (U.S.A.) **33**, 205 (1961). — Marks, P. A.: Science (U.S.A.) **127**, 1358 (1958). — McCance, R. A., R. F. A. Dean, and A. M. Barrett: Med. Res. Council, Special Rep. Ser., No. 275. H. M. Stationery Office, London, 1951. — McCance, R. A., C. N. Edgecombe, and E. M. Widdowson: Lancet (G.B.) **1943**/II, 126. — Moore, C. V.: The Harvey Lectures. Academic Press, New York, 1961, p. 67. — Napier, L. E., and C. R. Das Gupta: Haematological Technique. 3rd Ed. U.N. Dhur and Sons, Calcutta, 1945. — Powell, J. F.: Quart. J. Med. (G.B.) **13**, 19 (1944). — Rath, C. E., and C. A. Finch: J. Laborat. Clin. Med. (U.S.A.) **33**, 61 (1948). — Ray, R. N., J. B. Chatterjea, and R. N. Chaudhuri: W. H. O./Mal/395, 17th May, p. 1—9 (1963). — Ross, C. I. W.: J. Clin. Path. (G.B.) **5**, 250 (1952). — Schwaber, J. R., and A. G. Blumberg: Ann. Int. Med. (U.S.A.) **55**, 1004 (1961). — Sijpestein, J. A. K.: Enige vormen van erfelijke nietspherocytaire anaemie bij kinderen. Oppenheim, Groningen, 1955. — Singer, K., A. I. Chernoff, and L. Singer: Blood (U.S.A.) **6**, 413 (1951). — Swarup, S., S. K. Ghosh, and J. B. Chatterjea: Bull. Calcutta School Trop. Med. **11**, 46 (1963). — Wintrobe, M. M., and R. T. Beebe: Medicine (U.S.A.) **12**, 187 (1933). — Witts, L. J.: Brit. Med. J. **1931**/II, 883.

Iron nutrition

By

C. V. Moore

Before the normal dietary requirement for iron can be stated with reasonable accuracy, one must know how much iron is lost or excreted from the body, how much is needed for the special requirements of growth and pregnancy, and how much is absorbed from the diet under a wide variety of physiological circumstances. Information in all three areas is incomplete; moreover, in the case of iron excretion, widely divergent views have been advanced. For instance, my associates and I (*8*, *26*) and Finch (*10*) have estimated the daily loss or turnover of iron to be in the range of 0.5 to 1.0 mg. for adult males and post-menopausal women, whereas other workers believe that dermal loss alone may be 6 or more mg. per day. Until these differences are resolved and more data are accumulated, any evaluation of iron nutrition can hope only to summarize available evidence, focus on the areas of confusion, and suggest values which currently seem reasonable. One thing is evident: in those temperate climates where hygienic conditions are relatively good and parasitic infections are comparatively infrequent, healthy adult men and post-menopausal women without demonstrable blood loss do not become iron-deficient when their diets contain 12 or more mg. of food iron per day. They must, on the average, therefore, absorb enough of the metal to compensate for normal losses. Any formulation of iron requirements should be compatible with this experience.

A. Intake and absorption of dietary iron

Very little precise information about the iron in the diet of different peoples is available. Most of the published figures, obtained from dietary surveys rather than from actual analysis, indicate that the average daily intake is between 10 and 30 mg. (*42*). Estimates for urban populations in the United States suggest that the daily consumption of food iron has increased from an average of 11.8 mg. in 1936 to about 17 mg. in 1955 (Table 1) (*38*). People in the lower income groups and in those parts of the world where food is in short supply get lesser amounts. Survey data, however, are inaccurate, not only because they are obtained by history and calculation, but also because they ignore the iron in drinking fluids

Table 1. *Iron in city diets, U.S.A., in a week in spring*
Average (in mg.) per person per day from food used at home

	All households	Income thirds		
		Lowest	Middle	Highest
1936	11.8	10.2	11.8	14.0
1942	13.6	12.8	13.5	13.8
1948	15.9	15.6	15.8	16.2
1955	17.0	16.4	17.0	17.6

Household Food Consumption Survey. U.S. Dept. of Agriculture, Rep. No. 16, 1955.

(1955 Survey based on approx. 6,000 housekeeping households of 1 or more persons, about 3,000 of which were urban).

or added or lost during food preparation. The high iron content in the diet of the Bantu, derived from the iron utensils used in cooking or for the fermentation of Kaffir beer, is now well known (*39*). MacDonald has recently re-emphasized the fact that ale and wine made in Europe or the United States may have as much as 2 to 16 or more mg. per liter (*20*) (Table 2). The iron in city water supplies

Table 2. *Iron content of various alcoholic beverages*
From R. A. MacDonald: A.M.A. Arch. Int. Med. **112**, 184 (1963)

U.S. beer	0.1 mg./liter
Gin, whiskey, bourbon, scotch	0.6 mg./liter
U.S. (New York) wine	2.3 mg./liter
U.S. (California) wine	2.6 mg./liter
3 U.S. wines popular with Boston alcoholics	4.4 mg./liter
44 French wines, red and white, sold in Boston	6.2 mg./liter
Cider and wine from Rennes, France	10—16 mg./liter

is very low, but amounts greater than 5 mg. per liter may be found in the water from some deep wells or bore-holes (*36*). We do not know the minimum level of dietary iron capable of sustaining a positive iron balance in adults who have no detectable blood loss.

Assessment of adequate intake is further complicated by the meagerness of information about absorption of iron from a wide variety of foods or about the effect on absorption of other foods eaten at the same time. These data have been difficult to obtain. There is a current tendency to deprecate chemical balance studies, because the danger of contamination or inaccuracy is so great, but they have several advantages: observations are made over a long enough period to smooth out variations produced by such influences as differences in intestinal motility, and uptake is measured from a whole diet rather than from one food only. It is true that results cannot be adjusted for iron which may be excreted by way of the gastro-intestinal tract. While no detailed analysis of balance data will be attempted, it is pertinent to remember that in four of the most meticulous studies on adults, the mean absorption from carefully controlled basal diets varied from 11 to 14% (*18, 23, 32, 41*). In two instances, the experimental design was altered so that additions of beef and spinach were made to the basal ration; 21% of the iron in beef and 13% of the iron in spinach were retained.

During the last decade, radio-iron has been used to assay the absorption of iron from foods. Foods have been produced so as to contain the isotope, prepared as they would be in a normal diet, and then fed to fasting subjects. Fig. 1 summarizes the data published by several groups of investigators (*5, 7, 26, 27, 33, 35*). Either the unabsorbed radioactivity recovered in feces or the amount utilized for hemoglobin synthesis, or both, were measured; objection has been made to each of the methods, but the results would seem to provide a reasonable approximation; data may possibly be accumulated more rapidly and with greater accuracy in the near future now that whole-body counters have become available in some laboratories. The absorption by different subjects has varied widely. Iron-deficient patients tend to absorb iron more efficiently from the foods used in these studies than do normal subjects. The absorption from liver, hemoglobin, muscle, and "enriched" bread was better than from eggs or from the available tagged vegetables. Eggs may be a relatively poor source, because the ferric iron they contain is strongly complexed to the phosphate of yolk phosphoproteins. The relatively good assimilation of hemoglobin iron deserves particular attention, since recent evidence suggests that iron in heme complexes may be absorbed as a porphyrin complex without conversion to the free ionized form (*37*). When hemoglobin is digested in the stomach and small intestine, globin may be split off, but the iron not detached from the porphyrin ring. Not included in Fig. 1 are a few values obtained when Fe^{59}-tagged blood, liver, and kidney from a sheep were fed to normal subjects (*40*): 2.5 and 3.7% were absorbed from blood, 8% from liver, and 20.7% from kidney; these results were excluded, because the amounts of iron fed were larger than the 1 to 17 mg. given in the other studies. The over-all average absorption for 133 experiments on normal subjects was 6.5%, and for 58 determinations on iron-deficient subjects

19.6%. The lower two sets of figures are from a study by PIRZIO-BIROLI and his associates (*29*), in which a tracer dose of 50 μc. of $Fe^{59}Cl_3$ was added to a standard meal containing 4.6 mg. iron; the radio-iron was not actually incorporated into the food. Results,

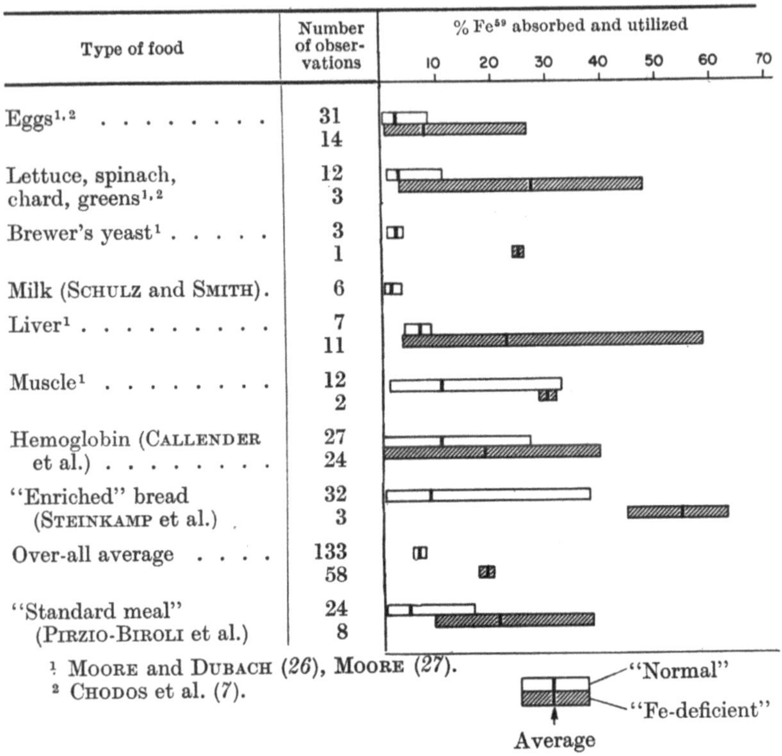

Fig. 1. Radio-iron measurement of the absorption of iron from foods by adult subjects. The length of the bars indicates the variation among different subjects for each food; the heavy vertical line across each bar indicates the average value. The amount of iron in each feeding varied from 1 to 17 mg. Cross-hatched bars: iron-deficient; white bars: normal

however, agree very closely: variation from subject to subject is broad, normal adults retaining an average of 5.3%, while iron-deficient patients retained 21.6%.

Similar data for children are recorded in Fig. 2. Assimilation seems to be better than in adults; there is the same variation and similar increased absorption in iron deficiency.

It is apparent that the number of individual foods studied has been small; no human data are known to me on the assimilation of iron from beans, rice, pulses, and other foodstuffs which form a large part of the diet of many peoples. Except for hemoglobin (*37*), absorption decreases with greater bulk or when the amounts of phosphates and phytates are increased (*34*). The addition of ascorbic acid causes greater absorption of iron from all foods tested (*26, 29*), with the exception of hemoglobin (*37*). The importance

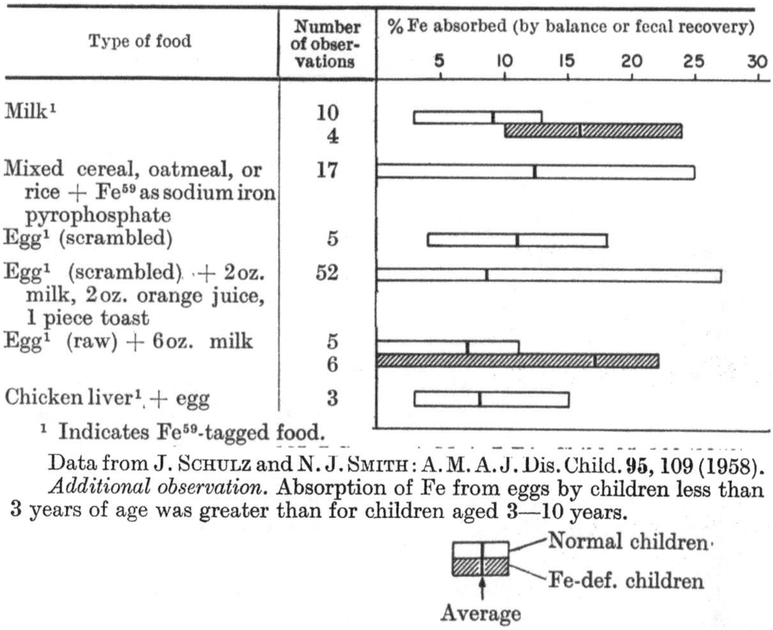

Fig. 2. Absorption of iron by children from foods tagged with Fe^{59}. White bars: normal children; cross-hatched bars: iron-deficient children. The heavy vertical line across each bar indicates the average value. Data from SCHULZ and SMITH (*33*)

of gastric acid is in dispute; most workers have been unable to demonstrate any effect of achlorhydria on the absorption of food iron (*3, 26, 29*), but GOLDBERG et al., using the technic of adding a tracer dose of inorganic iron to a standard meal, have recently presented contrary results (*13*). There is some evidence that the assimilation of food iron is impaired after partial gastrectomy (*2*).

When one tries to make a prediction about the amount of iron our diets should contain, one is faced with absorption data that are most incomplete, with striking variation among subjects and, in some instances, with conflicting evidence. Even so, a few generalizations seem reasonable: a) from a European or North American type of diet, containing 12 to 18 mg. iron per day, approximately 5 to 10% of the metal is probably absorbed to provide a retention of somewhere between 0.6 and 1.8 mg. daily; b) in states of iron deficiency, the efficiency of mean assimilation increases, probably by a factor of 2 or 3, so that retention of 1.2 to 4.8 mg. seems likely. These estimates are probably not far wrong, but percent absorption might differ quite significantly with other types of diet or with grossly different levels of iron intake.

B. Iron loss

Confusion about daily non-hemoglobin iron losses causes even greater uncertainty concerning the amount of iron required to maintain normal nutrition. Excretion of the metal is exceedingly difficult to determine, because contamination is hard to avoid, because no good way exists for differentiating between unabsorbed and excreted iron in the feces, and because radio-iron does not distribute itself equally in the various body pools when isotopic methods are employed.

Urinary iron excretion is small, with mean values of approximately 0.1 mg. or less per day; in patients with proteinuria or iron overload, however, the values may be several times higher because of the iron lost with excreted transferrin or contained within desquamated renal tubular cells (*31*). Fecal iron losses were estimated in one careful balance experiment by feeding three different levels of iron to women volunteers for 8-day periods (*16*). An attempt was made to differentiate between excreted and unabsorbed iron by plotting fecal iron against different levels of dietary iron and extending the fecal iron regression-line to zero. From this plot the increment of iron contributed by losses into the intestinal tract was estimated to be 0.2 mg. per day. DUBACH and her associates measured fecal radioactivity at intervals for 140 days after giving radioactive iron parenterally (*8*). Some radioactivity could be detected in every fecal collection made. The average daily excretion by five healthy young adults varied from 0.008 to 0.015% of the injected dose. Three iron-deficient patients similarly studied excreted considerably smaller amounts; one patient with sickle-cell anemia excreted six times as much as normal subjects. From these data, and the ratio of the injected radio-iron to estimated total body iron, the calculated average fecal excretion by the normal subjects was between 0.3 and 0.5 mg. per day. This calculation suffers from the assumption that the Fe^{59} was equally distributed throughout the total pool of body iron. The study clearly demonstrates that a small amount of iron is lost from the gastro-intestinal tract, but provides no information as to its source: active excretion, unabsorbed iron delivered to the small intestine in bile, iron in desquamated mucosal cells, and/or a small loss of hemoglobin iron [1.2 ± 0.5 ml. whole blood per day (*9*)]. Sweat was collected from three of these normal subjects at different times for as long as 320 days; they wore a plastic suit which covered all of the body except the feet, hands, head, and neck; during $^1/_2$ to $2^1/_2$ hours in a warm room, as much as a liter of sweat was obtained. Small but measurable amounts of tracer iron were found in each collection. Calculations indicated that, at these accelerated rates of sweating, no more than 0.5 to 1 mg. iron would have been lost in 24 hours. The iron removed in nail and hair clippings is nutritionally insignificant (*17*). At the completion of these studies, we suggested that the non-hemoglobin iron loss by adults in urine, feces, and sweat was probably in the range of 0.5 to 1 mg. per day.

Similar conclusions were reached by FINCH in long-term experiments designed to measure the total body iron turnover in normal men and women (*10*). He injected intravenously a tracer dose of Fe^{55} and followed the radioactivity in circulating hemoglobin for a period of 46 to 54 months. An excessive fall in radioactivity was observed during the first year, but the rate of decline seemed to be relatively constant thereafter. The iron turnover of total miscible body iron was 0.61 mg. per day in men, 0.64 mg. per day in non-menstruating women, and 1.22 mg. per day in menstruating women.

The agreement between these results was reassuring, but doubt has been cast from two sources: a) conflicting claims over the magnitude of dermal iron losses; and b) data from whole-body counting which suggest that the daily excretion may be as high as 0.14% of body iron. It is agreed that the greatest dermal loss occurs in desquamated cells, but some iron is found in cell-poor sweat. Some workers have obtained values similar to ours (*19*), whereas others have found as much as 6.5 mg. per day (*1,11,25*). Sweat collected from the forearm of iron-deficient patients has been reported to contain less iron than that from normal subjects and to increase to normal levels after iron therapy (*14, 15*). The importance of resolving this question has been emphasized by the suggestion that the high incidence of iron deficiency in the hot, moist regions of India, Ceylon, and Africa may be attributed to large dermal loss of iron. CHATTERJEA, on the other hand, has told me that: a) there is no correlation in India between the incidence of iron deficiency and the temperature of the climate; and b) in male patients whose occupation causes them to sweat profusely he has never found iron deficiency without significant association with one or more of the conventional causes (*6*). The data and calculations summarized in Table 3 make the claims for high dermal losses difficult to believe.

Table 3. *Estimate of iron in epidermis*

Iron in epidermis stripped from 1 g. of whole skin	Average 1.44 μg./g. Range 0.6—2.9 μg./g.
Skin = ~ 7% of total body-weight or ~ 4,900 g./70 kg. man	
Iron in epidermis which could be stripped from the total skin of 70 kg. man	2.94—14.21 mg.

The epidermis stripped by heat from 1 g. of skin contains about 1.44 μg. iron (0.6 to 2.9 μg./g.). Since about 7% of the total body-weight is skin, there would be about 4,900 g. of skin on a 70 kg. man. The iron in epidermis that could be stripped from the total skin surface, therefore, would be about 3 to 14 mg. The turnover rate would have to be 2 or 3 days, rather than the estimated 2 or 3 weeks, to account for an iron loss of 5 to 7 mg. The issue, however, is still not resolved.

With whole-body counting, BONNET et al. in one case (*4*) and PRICE and his associates in three (*30*) have concluded that radio-iron leaves the body of normal men at a rate of 0.14% per day (Table 4). If one assumes that excretion occurs at the same rate from total body iron (Fig. 3A), then a man with a total body iron load of 5 g. would be excreting 7 mg. per day. PRICE (*30*) has uttered a warning against the fallacy of making this assumption (Fig. 3B), because of the incomplete mixing of radio-iron within the various body compartments; he points out that, if excretion were occurring from a labile pool of 135 mg., then a daily radioactivity loss would be equivalent to an excretion of only 1 mg. To date, therefore, the difficulties

Table 4. *Iron loss during 20—100 days after an oral dose of 0.25 mg. Fe as ferrous citrate*
(Fe^{59} tag; whole-body counting)
From D.C. PRICE, S. H. COHN, and E. P. CRONKITE

Disease	Fe^{59} abs. %	20—100 day loss	
		% per day	Mean
3 Normal	5.9—19.5	0.110—0.182	0.134
2 Aplastic anemia. . .	5.4— 8.2	0.103—0.173	0.138
10 Iron deficiency . . .	20.6—96.9	0—0.044	0.019

of interpreting radio-iron loss by total-body counting technics have kept these data from providing the definitive information about iron excretion that had been anticipated. H. SAITO and co-workers (*31a*) have also studied with a whole-body counter the iron loss in 8 normal male human subjects. These authors concluded that for the first 100 days of the study their subjects lost an average of 1.6 ± 0.3% iron per month from a miscible pool estimated to be 2,990 mg.; the calculated total-body iron loss was 1.5 ± 0.3 mg.

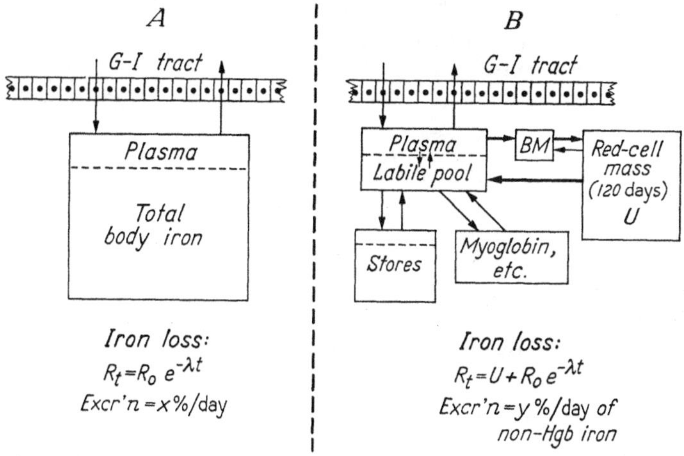

Fig. 3. A: simplified model for Fe^{59} excretion applicable to only long-term studies. B: more complex kinetic model suggested for analysis of Fe^{59} loss during first 100 days after intestinal absorption. From PRICE et al. (*30*)

per day. Discussing the difficulties in interpreting the results – difficulties due partly to the time required for the mixing of radio-iron with all the iron of the body – SAITO suggests that the most accurate way to measure total-body iron loss would be to label a subject as uniformly as possible, by administering the label at intervals for several months, and then to count him for a year or more after completion of labeling.

When discussion of iron excretion is extended to a consideration of normal menstrual loss or the iron "cost" of a normal pregnancy, further difficulty is encountered because of the wide normal variation. The average monthly loss of menstrual iron is about 20 mg. (or 0.7 mg. per day), but values extending from 2.3 to 79 mg. have been reported (*12*). Hemorrhage at the time of delivery has been described as 507 ± 308 ml. for primiparae and 280 ± 293 ml. for multiparae (Table 5) (*28*). The iron contained in the placenta and

Table 5. *Blood loss at time of delivery*
From M. NEWTON et al.: Obstetr. Gynec. (U.S.A.) **17**, 9 (1961)

	26 Primiparae	74 Multiparae
Blood loss on delivery table, ml.	507±308	280±293
Blood loss in 1st hour after removal from delivery table, ml.	16± 17	50± 61
Iron equivalent on basis of 12 g. Hb./100 ml.	209 mg.	132 mg.

cord varies from 34 to 170 mg., with an average of approximately 75 mg. (Table 6) (*22, 24*). If one adds to these values the variable amount of iron contained in a full-term fetus and provided to the baby through milk, the "cost" of a normal pregnancy can be

Table 6. *Iron content of placentas and cord*

	Number	Iron mg.
McCoy, et al.	49 placentas and cord	75.5 (range 34.5—170)
MISCHEL, W..	143 placentas	63.7 } 74.8
	cords	11.1 }

anywhere from 400 to over 900 mg. (Table 7). A woman who normally loses an average of 1 mg. iron per day in menstrual blood and has 15 months of amenorrhea during pregnancy and lactation could end up by not having her iron requirement increased at all

Table 7. *Iron "cost" of a normal pregnancy*

Iron contributed to fetus	201—372 mg.
In placenta and cord	34—170 mg.
In blood loss at delivery	~ 100—250 mg.
In milk, lactation 6 months	~ 100—180 mg.
	435—972 mg.
Conserved by 15 months' amenorrhea	(480—240)mg.
Net cost approximately	0—700 mg.

by the pregnancy, whereas in another normal mother the net cost could be nearly 2 mg. per day. These figures emphasize that average values for the physiological iron losses must be regarded as having wide standard deviations.

I would like to treat the iron required for growth in broad terms, realizing that the need varies with rapidity of growth at different periods of infancy and childhood. If one assumes that the normal infant at birth has 300 mg. total body iron, that the male has 5 g.

when he stops growing at the age of 20 years, and that the normal girl has 4 g. when she stops growing at the age of 15, then the average amount of iron required for growth and development is about 240 mg. per year or about 0.6 mg. per day.

C. Iron requirement and nutritional allowances

The difficulty of estimating the iron required for normal excretory loss, menstruation, pregnancy, and growth has been emphasized sufficiently. However, since iron deficiency is so common throughout the world, there is a moral and practical obligation to arrive at recommendations which now seem reasonable, so that health organizations have guidance. At present, the knowledge that healthy adult men and non-menstruating women do not become iron-deficient while absorbing 5 to 10% of the iron in diets providing 12 to 15 mg. of the metal, affords the most compelling reason for questioning the validity of any claim that excretion is greater than 1 to 1.5 mg. per day. I am inclined not to believe that dermal losses are high and to suggest the values recorded in Table 8

Table 8. *Estimated iron requirement (in mg./day)*

	Urine, sweat, feces	Menses	Pregnancy	Growth	Total
Men and post-menopausal women	0.5—1				0.5—1
Menstruating women	0.5—1	0.5—1			1 —2
Pregnant women	0.5—1		1—2		1.5—2.5
Children (average)	? 0.5			0.6	1
Girls (age 12—15)	0.5—1	0.5—1		0.6	1 —2.5

as acceptable approximations of iron requirements. When these figures are translated into recommended dietary allowances, it is difficult to know what value to use for average percent absorption of food iron. If calculations are made on the basis of 10% absorption – an assumption that seems reasonable to me, since assimilation tends to become more efficient as need increases – then 15 to 18 mg. of food iron should be sufficient for all normal adults, with the possible exception of women during pregnancy. In pregnancy, the recommended dietary allowances might better be 18 to 21 mg. These values are higher then those currently recommended by the Food and Nutrition Board in the United States, but they are attainable in many countries and would provide a greater margin of safety.

Summary

Quantitative information defining the absorption of iron from foods and the non-hemoglobin loss of iron from the body is so incomplete that a precise statement about the nutritional requirement for iron is still not possible. One thing is evident: in those temperate climates where hygienic conditions are relatively good and parasitic infections are comparatively infrequent, healthy adult men and post-menopausal women without detectable blood loss do not become iron-deficient when their diets contain 12 or more mg. food iron per day. They must, on the average, therefore, absorb enough of the metal to compensate for normal losses.

In nearly 150 reported observations in healthy adult human subjects on the absorption of iron from foods produced so as to contain Fe^{59}, the composite average retention of the isotope was 5.6%, with values ranging from less than 1% to more than 30%. When tracer doses of ferric chloride were fed along with a standard meal containing 4.5 mg. food iron, the results were quite similar: average 6.5% (variation from a fraction of 1% to approximately 16%). With meticulously performed balance experiments (instead of isotopic technics), the values have varied from 11% to 20%. Objection has been made to each of the methods used, but the results would seem to provide a reasonable approximation. More serious objections are these: the number of individual foods studied has been very small; the effect which other foods eaten at the same time (e.g. foods with a high phytic acid content) have on iron absorption has hardly been evaluated; no data are available for beans, rice, pulses, and other foodstuffs which form the dietary mainstay in many parts of the world. One can say with reasonable assurance, however, that normal adults eating a European or American type of diet probably absorb from 5% to 10% of food iron; they should retain roughly 0.6 to 1.5 mg. Fe from a daily intake of 12 to 15 mg. Fe. Not included in this estimate is the iron in water, wine, and other beverages.

If the above estimates for healthy subjects in temperate climates represent a close approximation of dietary iron retention, then normal loss of iron must be less than (or not more than) these amounts. Using radio-iron, we have estimated the daily excretion of iron to be from 0.5 to 1 mg.; FINCH and his associates have reported the daily turnover of iron to be 0.61 mg. per day for men and 0.64 mg. per day for non-menstruating women. However, other workers have presented evidence that the daily dermal loss of iron may be as much as 6 mg. per day, particularly in hot, moist climates. The technics and methods of calculation in all these studies are open to question. The hope that whole-body counters might resolve these difficulties has not materialized; the few preliminary reported data suggest that normal subjects during the first 3 or 4 months after administration of a tracer dose of iron lose about 0.14% per day, but the pool from which this excretion occurs has not been identified. At present, the knowledge that adult men and non-menstruating women do not become iron-deficient when they absorb 5% to 10% of the iron in diets providing 12 to 15 mg. of the metal, affords the most compelling reason for questioning the validity of any excretion data greater than 1 to 1.5 mg. per day.

Zusammenfassung

Unsere Kenntnisse über die Resorption von Eisen aus der Nahrung und den Verlust von Eisen — ausgenommen das Haemoglobineisen — sind in quantitativer Hinsicht so unvollständig, daß es noch immer nicht möglich ist, genaue Angaben über den Bedarf an Eisen in der Nahrung zu machen.

Es ist lediglich festzuhalten, daß im gemäßigten Klima, unter guten hygienischen Verhältnissen und vorausgesetzt, daß parasitäre Infektionen nicht häufig sind, gesunde erwachsene Männer oder Frauen in der Menopause ohne erkennbare Blutverluste keinen Eisenmangel zeigen, wenn ihre Nahrung 12 mg. oder mehr Eisen täglich enthält. Sie müssen somit im Durchschnitt genügend Eisen resorbieren, um den üblichen Verlust auszugleichen.

An gesunden Probanden ließ sich in annähernd 150 Beobachtungen über die Resorption von Nahrungsmitteln, die Fe^{59} enthielten, feststellen, daß die durchschnittliche Retention des Isotops 5,6% betrug, mit Schwankungen zwischen weniger als 1% bis zu mehr als 30%. Wenn Spuren von Ferrichlorid zusammen mit einer Standardmahlzeit gegeben wurden, die 4,5 mg. Nahrungseisen enthielt, waren die Resultate ähnlich: durchschnittliche Retention von 6,5% (mit Schwankungen von weniger als 1% bis zu ungefähr 16%). Wurden anstelle der Isotopentechnik genaue Bilanzuntersuchungen vorgenommen, so ergaben sich Werte zwischen 11% und 20%. Beide Methoden sind kritisiert worden, aber die Befunde dürften den tatsächlichen Verhältnissen annähernd entsprechen. Schwerwiegendere Einwände sind, daß die Zahl der untersuchten Nahrungsmittel sehr klein ist, daß der Einfluß gleichzeitig aufgenommener Nahrung (z. B. Nahrungsmittel, die reich an Phytinsäure sind) auf die Resorption kaum geprüft wurde, und daß keine Daten für Reis, Hülsenfrüchte und andere Nahrungsmittel vorliegen, welche in vielen Teilen der Erde die hauptsächliche Nahrung darstellen. Es läßt sich jedoch mit einiger Sicherheit angeben, daß normale Erwachsene, die eine europäische oder amerikanische Durchschnittsnahrung zu sich nehmen, etwa 5—10% des Nahrungseisens resorbieren; dabei sollten bei einer täglichen Aufnahme von 12—15 mg. Eisen etwa 0,6—1,5 mg. zurückgehalten werden, nicht eingeschlossen das Eisen, das in Wasser, Wein und anderen Getränken enthalten ist.

Wenn diese Schätzungen für gesunde Individuen in gemäßigtem Klima zutreffen, so muß der normale tägliche Eisenverlust niedriger oder darf höchstens gleich sein wie diese Mengen. Mit Hilfe von radioaktiv markiertem Eisen haben wir die tägliche Eisenausscheidung zwischen 0,5—1,0 mg. bestimmt; Finch u. Mitarb. geben den täglichen Eisenumsatz mit 0,61 mg. für den Mann und mit 0,64 mg. für die nicht menstruierende Frau an. Andere Untersucher haben allerdings festgestellt, daß der tägliche Eisenverlust durch die Haut bis zu 6 mg. beträgt, besonders in heißem, feuchtem Klima. Die angewendete Technik und die Berechnungsmethoden sind jedoch fraglich. Die Hoffnung, daß Zählungen der Impulse am Gesamtorganismus diese Schwierigkeiten lösen würden, hat sich nicht erfüllt; die wenigen mitgeteilten präliminären Befunde sprechen dafür, daß normale Personen während 3 bis 4 Monaten nach Gabe einer Dosis von radioaktiv markiertem Eisen etwa 0,14% pro Tag verlieren, daß aber der Vorrat, von dem diese Ausscheidung erfolgt, nicht identifiziert ist. Vorläufig ist die Kenntnis, daß erwachsene Männer und nicht menstruierende Frauen keinen Eisenmangel entwickeln, wenn sie 5—10% des Nahrungseisens in einer Diät, die 12—15 mg. enthält, resorbieren, der überzeugendste Befund dafür, daß die Ausscheidung zwischen 1 und 1,5 mg. pro Tag liegt.

Résumé

Les renseignements d'ordre quantitatif sur l'absorption du fer alimentaire et sur les pertes de fer non hémoglobinique par l'organisme sont si incomplets que toute affirmation précise sur les besoins en fer est encore impossible. Une chose est sûre: dans les régions tempérées, où les conditions d'hygiène sont satisfaisantes et l'infestation parasitaire relativement peu fréquente, les hommes adultes normaux et les femmes ménopausées ne présentant pas de pertes de sang décelables, ne font pas d'hyposidérose si leur régime contient au moins 12 mg. de fer par jour. C'est donc qu'ils doivent absorber en moyenne une quantité de ce métal suffisante pour compenser les pertes normales.

Dans près de 150 observations, chez des sujets adultes normaux, sur l'absorption du fer d'aliments préparés de façon à ce qu'ils contiennent du Fe^{59}, la rétention moyenne de l'isotope a été de 5,6% avec des valeurs extrêmes de moins de 1% et de plus de 30%. Quand des doses traçantes de chlorure ferrique ont été additionnées à un repas standard renfermant 4,5 mg. de fer, les résultats ont été tout à fait semblables: moyenne de 6,5% (variation de moins de 1% à environ 16%). Avec des études de bilans très soigneuses (au lieu de techniques isotopiques), les valeurs ont varié de 11 à 20%. Des objections ont été faites à chacune de ces méthodes, mais les résultats semblent réaliser une approximation raisonnable. Plus sérieuses sont les objections suivantes: le nombre des différents aliments étudiés a été très petit; l'influence de la consommation simultanée d'autres aliments (par exemple aliments riches en acide phytique) a été à peine évaluée; il n'existe aucune donnée pour le riz, les légumineuses et autres aliments qui constituent la base de l'alimentation dans de nombreuses parties du monde. On peut néanmoins dire avec beaucoup de vraisemblance qu'un adulte normal soumis à un régime de type européen ou américain absorbe probablement 5 à 10% du fer de l'alimentation; il doit donc en gros retenir 0,6 à 1,5 mg. de fer d'un apport quotidien de 12 à 15 mg. Il n'est pas tenu compte dans cette estimation du fer contenu dans l'eau, le vin et autres boissons.

Si l'on admet que les estimations précédentes chez des sujets normaux dans des climats tempérés représentent une approximation assez précise de l'absorption du fer alimentaire, la perte normale de fer doit donc être inférieure ou au plus égale à ces quantités. Nous avons estimé à l'aide de fer radioactif que l'excrétion journalière de fer est de 0,5 à 1 mg.; FINCH et coll. ont rapporté que le *turnover* du fer est de 0,61 mg. par jour chez l'homme et de 0,64 mg. par jour chez la femme en dehors de la période d'activité génitale. Cependant, d'autres chercheurs ont montré que la perte de fer par la peau peut atteindre 6 mg. par jour, en particulier dans les climats chauds et humides. Les techniques et méthodes de calcul prêtent encore à discussion. L'existence de compteurs pour l'organisme entier, qui pourraient résoudre ces difficultés, n'est encore qu'un espoir; les quelques données préliminaires rapportées laissent à penser que le sujet normal perd environ 0,14% par jour de la dose traçante de fer au cours des 3 ou 4 premiers mois suivant son administration, mais le *pool* d'où provient cette excrétion n'a pas été identifié. Actuellement, le fait de savoir que les hommes normaux adultes et les femmes en dehors de la période d'activité génitale ne deviennent pas carencés en fer s'ils absorbent 5 à 10% d'un régime réalisant un apport de 12 à 15 mg. de ce métal, constitue une raison impérative pour mettre en doute la validité de tout chiffre d'excrétion supérieur à 1 ou 1,5 mg. par jour.

Acknowledgement

The investigations by the author and his associates which are described here were supported in part by U.S.P.H.S. research grant H22 from the National Heart Institute.

References

1. ADAMS, W. S., A. LESLIE, and M. H. LEVIN: Proc. Soc. Exper. Biol. Med. (U.S.A.) **74**, 46 (1950). — 2. BAIRD, I. McL., and G. M. WILSON:

Quart. J. Med. (G.B.) **28**, 35 (1959). — 3. Bigg, J. C., R. M. Bannerman, and S. T. Callender: Proceedings of the 8th Congress of the European Society of Haematology, Basle, 1961. — 4. Bonnet, J. D., A. L. Orvis, A. B. Hagedorn, and C. A. Owen: Amer. J. Physiol. **198**, 784 (1960). — 5. Callender, S. T., B. J. Mallet, and M. D. Smith: Brit. J. Haemat. **3**, 186 (1957). — 6. Chatterjea, J. B.: Personal communication. — 7. Chodos, R. B., J. F. Ross, L. Apt, M. Pollycove, and J. A. E. Halkett: J. Clin. Invest. (U.S.A.) **36**, 314 (1957). — 8. Dubach, R., C. V. Moore, and S. Callender: J. Laborat. Clin. Med. (U.S.A.) **45**, 599 (1955). — 9. Ebaugh, F. G. Jr., T. Clemens Jr., G. Rodman, and R. E. Peterson: Amer. J. Med. **25**, 169 (1958). — 10. Finch, C. A.: J. Clin. Invest. (U.S.A.) **38**, 392 (1959). — 11. Foy, H., and A. Kondi: J. Trop. Med. Hyg. (G.B.) **60**, 105 (1957). — 12. Frenchman, R., and F. A. Johnston: J. Amer. Diet. Ass. **25**, 217 (1949). — 13. Goldberg, A., A. C. Lochhead, and J. H. Dagg: Lancet (G.B.) **1963/I**, 848. — 14. Hussain, R., and V. N. Patwardhan: Lancet (G.B.) **1959/I**, 1073. — 15. Hussain, R., V. N. Patwardhan, and S. Sriramachari: Indian J. Med. Res. **48**, 235 (1960). — 16. Ingalls, R. L., and F. A. Johnston: J. Nutrit. (U.S.A.) **53**, 351 (1954). — 17. Johnston, F. A.: Amer. J. Clin. Nutrit. **6**, 136 (1958). — 18. Johnston, F. A., R. Frenchman, and E. D. Buroughs: J. Nutrit. (U.S.A.) **35**, 453 (1948). — 19. Johnston, F. A., T. J. McMillan, and E. R. Evans: J. Nutrit. (U.S.A.) **42**, 285 (1950). — 20. MacDonald, R. A.: A.M.A. Arch. Int. Med. **112**, 184 (1963) — 21. McCance, R. A., C. N. Edgecombe, and E. M. Widdowson: Lancet (G.B.) **1943/II**, 126. — 22. McCoy,B. A., R. E. Beiler, and M. A. Ohlson: Amer. J. Clin. Nutrit. **9**, 613 (1961). — 23. McMillan, T. J., and F. A. Johnston: J. Nutrit. (U.S.A.) **44**, 383 (1951). — 24. Mischel, W.: Arch. Gynäk. (G.) **190**, 638 (1958). — 25. Mitchell, H. H., and T. S. Hamilton: J. Biol. Chem. (U.S.A.) **178**, 345 (1949). — 26. Moore, C. V., and R. Dubach: J. Amer. Med. Ass. **162**, 197 (1956). — 27. Moore, C. V.: Harvey Lect. (U.S.A). **55**, 67 (1961). — 28. Newton, M., L. M. Mosey, G. E. Egli, W. B. Gifford, and C. T. Hull: Obstetr. Gynec. (U.S.A.) **17**, 9 (1961). — 29. Pirzio-Biroli, G., T. H. Bothwell, and C. A. Finch: J. Laborat. Clin. Med. (U.S.A.) **51**, 37 (1958). — 30. Price, D. C., S. H. Cohn, and E. P. Cronkite: In: Second Symposium on Radioactivity in Man. Ed. by G. Meneely. Thomas, Springfield, Ill. (in press). — 31. Rifkind, D., H. M. Kravetz, V. Knight, and A. L. Schade: N. England J. Med. **265**, 118 (1961). — 31 a. Saito, H., T. Sargent III, H. G. Parker, and J. H. Lawrence: Semiannual Report of the Donner Laboratory, Lawrence Radiation Laboratory, University of California, Dec. 1962, p. 32. — 32. Schlaphoff, D. M., and F. A. Johnston: J. Nutrit. (U.S.A.) **39**, 67 (1949). — 33. Schulz, J., and N. J. Smith: A.M.A. J. Dis. Child. **95**, 109 (1958). — 34. Sharpe, L. M., W. C. Peacock, R. Cooke, and R. S. Harris: J. Nutrit. (U.S.A.) **41**, 433 (1950). — 35. Steinkamp, R., R. Dubach, and C. V. Moore: A.M.A. Arch. Int. Med. **95**, 181 (1955). — 36. Taylor, E. W.: The Examination of Water and Water Supplies (Thresh, Beale, and Suckling). 7th Ed. Little, Brown & Co., Boston, 1958, p. 699. — 37. Turnbull, A., F. Cleton, and C. A. Finch: J. Clin. Invest. (U.S.A.) **41**, 1897 (1962). — 38. U.S. Dept. of Agriculture, Report No. 16. U.S. Printing Office, Washington, D.C., 1955. — 39. Walker, A. R. P., and U. B. Arvidsson: Transact. Roy. Soc. Trop. Med. (G.B.) **47**, 536 (1953). — 40. Walsh, R. J., J. Kaldor, I. Brading, and E. P. George: Australas. Ann. Med. **4**, 272 (1955). — 41. Widdowson, E. M., and R. A. McCance: Lancet (G.B.) **1942/I**, 588. — 42. World Health Organisation, Study Group on Anaemia, Working Paper No. 10 (Sept. 5, 1958).

Tissue effects of iron deficiency

By

E. Beutler

Since iron plays a central role in the formation of red blood cells, it is not surprising that iron deficiency leads to marked hematologic abnormalities. Because of this, and because blood represents the tissue which is most readily sampled in the clinical laboratory, iron deficiency is generally regarded as a hematologic disorder. Yet, for many years, perceptive clinicians and veterinarians have noted that iron-deficiency anemia is commonly associated with certain tissue changes. These changes are not the result of the anemia, since, in patients and in animals with other types of anemia, the same tissue effects are not seen. An analogous situation occurs in pernicious anemia and vitamin B_{12} deficiency. Here, too, is a disorder which is generally considered a hematologic disease, but it involves a number of tissue changes which are quite distinct from those found in other anemias. The most prominent and clinically important of these changes are those found in the nervous system. The crippling effects of vitamin B_{12} deficiency are not due to the anemia. They result from the effects of vitamin B_{12} deficiency on the nervous tissues. Similarly, the tissue changes found in iron deficiency, and very possibly much of the symptomatology, may be a result of effects produced by the lack of iron on the tissues. Today, I should like to review the nature of the tissue manifestations of iron deficiency and how they may come about.

Iron deficiency in plants

If anyone doubts that iron deficiency can cause changes in living tissues which are not related to anemia, he need look no further than his own garden or the garden of a friend. Iron deficiency is a widespread affliction among plants. The fact that these bloodless forms of life develop changes due to iron deficiency clearly demonstrates that iron deficiency affects tissues other than the blood. It is also interesting that the gardener and the botanist have chosen the term "chlorosis" to describe this affliction among their patients.

Iron deficiency in animals

Iron deficiency is also well known to the veterinarian, and some findings have been described which are clearly not due to anemia *per se*. It has been shown that iron-deficient New Hampshire chicks have white feathers instead of their normally reddish-brown plumage (Davis et al., 1962). The iron-deficient rat has been found to lose the deep orange pigment of its incisors, which become white (Ratner, 1935; Valberg et al., 1961). Some decrease in gastric acid secretion and an increase in the size of the caecum (McCall et al., 1962a; Valberg et al., 1961) have been found in rats given an iron-poor diet. A decrease in the ability of iron-deficient rats to absorb vitamin B_{12} has also been described (Yeh et al., 1961), and this decrease seems to be due to defective intrinsic factor secretion (Biggs et al., 1962).

Tissue changes in iron-deficient humans

The tissue changes in patients with iron-deficiency anemia have been extensively documented. Alterations have been described in the mucosa of much of the alimentary tract. Jacobs (1960) has found that the oral mucosal epithelium of some patients with iron deficiency was abnormally thin. Mitoses in the prickle-cell layer were seen more frequently in iron-deficient than in normal subjects. Fewer biopsy specimens from iron-deficient subjects contained melanin than is normally the case, but an increased number had subepithelial inflammation. Mature keratin was seen in some biopsies from iron-deficient subjects, but not in normal biopsies. It has also been reported (Boddington, 1959; Dabski, 1960) that the cytoplasmic diameter of buccal cells in patients with iron-deficiency anemia tended to be smaller than normal. Serial biopsies of the tongue before and after iron treatment showed that these histopathologic abnormalities were reversed after one to two weeks of iron therapy.

Changes in the esophagus of iron-deficient patients give rise to "sideropenic dysphagia". Constrictions or webs of the hypopharynx or esophagus result in inability to swallow solid food (Kelly, 1919; Paterson, 1919; Vinson, 1922; Suzman, 1933). Histopathologic findings have included keratinization of the lingual epithelium and leukocytic infiltration of the submucosa. Atrophy, hyperkeratinization, and changes resembling leukoplakia have been described in the esophageal mucosa. It has been suggested that the esophageal lesions of iron deficiency may be pre-cancerous (Ahlbom, 1936).

One of the tissue changes most frequently investigated in iron deficiency is the gastric atrophy and achlorhydria which are so commonly associated with this disorder. Here, changes varying from superficial gastritis and interstitial gastritis to atrophic gastritis have been reported (MORRISON et al., 1937; JOSKE et al., 1955; COGHILL and WILLIAMS, 1955; DAVIDSON and MARKSON 1955; BADENOCH et al., 1957; CHELI et al., 1959; LEES and ROSENTHAL, 1958). It is not entirely clear whether these abnormalities are a result of the iron-deficiency state or whether they are of etiologic significance in the development of iron deficiency. Indeed, iron therapy often fails to reverse gastric changes in iron-deficiency anemia (LEES and ROSENTHAL, 1958). It is possible, however, that the gastric changes are a result of iron deficiency, but have reached an irreversible stage by the time therapy is initiated. Even in the blood itself, not all of the changes found in iron deficiency can be attributed to decreased hemoglobin synthesis. Decreased white blood counts and platelet counts are sometimes seen in severe cases (WINTROBE, 1961), and a poorly defined bleeding tendency has also been observed (STAFFORD, 1961).

Generally the tissue effects of iron deficiency are found in patients suffering from iron-deficiency anemia, but they have also been described in individuals whose blood appeared to be normal (WALDENSTRÖM, 1938, 1946; RUSTUNG, 1949) and even in patients with polycythemia (GLAZEBROOK, 1944; WASSERMAN, 1955). This constitutes additional evidence that the tissue changes in iron deficiency are not a result of prolonged anemia, but rather represent manifestations of tissue iron deprivation. It is of interest that the tissue changes which have been described in iron deficiency occur only in a minority of patients with this disorder. The reason for this is unclear. It has been suggested that tissue changes are evidence of the chronicity of the iron-deficiency state (STEVENS, 1956). This is possible, but remains unproven. It may also be that other deficiencies in addition to the deficiency of iron must be present for some tissue changes of iron deficiency to manifest themselves. The defective B_{12} absorption, which has been found in iron-deficient subjects, may be of significance in this regard (BADENOCH et al., 1957). Dwarfism and geophagia with severe iron deficiency have been observed in Turkey, Iran, and Egypt. Here, an associated zinc deficiency seems to play a significant role (PRASAD et al., 1963). Changes in the fingernails, i.e. spoon-nails, are a typical finding (STAFFURTH, 1951). It has been suggested that a dietary cystine deficiency may be important in the development of this abnormality (JALILI and AL-KASSAB, 1959). In Africa the edematous depigmentation syndrome, or "*diboba*", is believed to be a consequence of iron deficiency (PIERAERTS, 1942), but here, too, other dietary deficiencies — possibly protein deprivation — may play a contributory role.

There is no doubt, then, that well-defined tissue changes occur in iron-deficient plants, in experimental animals, and in some iron-deficient human subjects. The origin of the more common but less easily measured symptoms of iron deficiency — fatigue, lassitude, headaches, and paresthesias — is much more difficult to define. All these symptoms may occur in subjects who have anemia from any cause. When they appear in a subject with iron-deficiency anemia, it is impossible to determine whether they are due to the anemia or to more subtle tissue changes which are the consequence of iron deprivation.

There are several clinical observations which would lead one to believe that symptoms in the iron-deficient patient arise from effects of iron deficiency other than hemoglobin depletion. First of all, there seems to be little relationship between the severity of anemia and the severity of symptoms. It is not unusual for patients with mild anemia to have marked symptoms; conversely, severely anemic patients may feel remarkably well. A second suggestive observation is that the clinical response to treatment for iron deficiency often precedes any change in the hemoglobin level of the patient's blood (HEILMEYER and PLÖTNER, 1937; BROWN and MOORE, 1956; BROWN et al., 1950; SLACK and WILKINSON, 1949; GOVAN and SCOTT, 1949). It is possible, of course, that this rapid symptomatic improvement is due entirely to suggestion. However, pediatricians treating iron-deficient infants have observed a marked decrease in irritability, coupled with an increase in the appetite of such babies, within one or two days of initiating iron therapy (YU et al., 1959; ROSS, 1962). It is unlikely, in this situation, that psychogenic factors are of much importance.

Finally, it has been suggested that iron deficiency may give rise to symptoms even when the blood count is entirely normal. If this suggestion is correct, then the symptoms of iron deficiency cannot be due entirely to a lowering of blood hemoglobin levels.

As early as 1844, BECQUEREL and RODIER commented that chlorosis could be found in some patients in whom the gross appearance of the blood was normal. Using more quantitative methods, such eminent clinicians of the past as LAACHE (1883), SAHLI (1908), NAEGELI (1908), and MORAWITZ (1910) all taught that the symptoms of chlorosis could occur in non-anemic subjects. Indeed, in 1910 MORAWITZ wrote, perhaps with surprising insight:

"There are definite cases of chlorosis with normal or near-normal blood findings. These cases are not rare. They are benefited by iron in the same way as chlorosis with marked anemia. Anemia, therefore, is not the cardinal symptom of chlorosis which governs all else, but rather a symptom among others. Menstrual disturbances, the venous hum, and water retention in chlorosis are not always dependent on the anemia; equally little the majority of the subjective symptoms. ... the point of attack of iron in chlorosis is not alone on the blood-building organs, but rather in the as yet unknown root of the entire clinical picture of chlorosis".

The idea that iron deficiency could give rise to symptoms in the absence of anemia has received support in the past 15 years from the clinical observations of JASINSKI and ROTH (1954), THEDERING (1955), UNDRITZ (1956), VERLOOP et al. (1958), and GOLDECK et al. (1954). However, the symptoms of which such patients complain are so common among women and are so readily influenced by the suggestibility of the subject that the notion that iron deficiency may give rise to symptoms in non-anemic patients has generally been regarded with considerable skepticism (WINTROBE, 1961).

We have attempted to explore this problem further in a double-blind study (BEUTLER et al., 1960a). Thirty-five women participated in this investigation. All of them were in good general health, without any detectable organic disease, and had hemoglobin levels in excess of 12.0 g. %. All of the patients complained of chronic fatigue, which persisted during a base-line period of observation. In each case, a plasma iron and unsaturated iron-binding capacity determination was carried out, and a sternal bone-marrow aspiration was done. The results of these studies were, however, unknown to the physicians who evaluated the response of the patient to medication. Each patient was given two courses of therapy, one of iron and the other of a bismuth subcarbonate placebo. Most patients were unaware that a placebo was being used and thought that two iron preparations were being compared. The order of presentation of iron and placebo was varied at random, and neither physician nor patient had any knowledge of which medication was being given. Hemoglobin determinations were made at monthly intervals, and the patients' subjective symptoms were recorded. At the conclusion of the study, an evaluation was made of whether the patient had improved and, if so, whether maximum improvement had taken place during the first or the second period of drug administration. Finally, the "code" was broken, and a correlation was made between the state of the patients' iron stores and the period of drug therapy which had proved most helpful.

It is of interest, first of all, that all but two of the patients improved in the course of this study. This merely attests again to the powerful influence which the physician's suggestion may have on a patient, whether or not the symptoms are of organic origin. Secondly, it was found that in the groups in which iron depletion was demonstrated, more patients experienced improvement during iron therapy than during placebo therapy, while the reverse was true in patients without iron depletion. These differences were significant, with P values ranging from 0.02 to 0.16, depending on the criterion used in dividing the patients into iron-depleted and non-iron-depleted groups and on the method of statistical analysis. It was also interesting that, although the hemoglobin values of all patients were normal at the outset of the study, there was a relatively small, but undoubtedly highly statistically significant rise in the hemoglobin concentration in the blood of iron-depleted patients during iron administration, but under no other circumstances. It is apparent, therefore, that, although a patient's hemoglobin may be within the population norm, it may be below his or her individual norm and may respond to iron therapy. While we cannot regard these results as giving conclusive evidence that symptoms of iron deficiency may arise without changes in the hemoglobin, we do feel that they are suggestive and that further studies of this type are needed.

Biochemical abnormalities

I have reviewed some of the changes which occur in the tissues of iron-deficient subjects. Clearly, they are not the result of hemoglobin deprivation. How, then, do they come about? Clinicians in the early 1930's suggested that the tissue changes which they observed in their iron-deficient patients might be due to depletion of tissue iron (Heath et al., 1932; Dameshek, 1933). Although Cohen and Elvehjem, in 1934, and Vannotti, in 1949, had noted a decrease in the cytochrome C content of tissues of iron-deficient animals, it was generally held, even by very eminent authorities, that iron enzymes were protected at all costs, even when iron deficiency was very severe (Hahn, 1948; Theorell et al., 1951; Paul, 1951; Goodman and Gilman, 1955). This belief arose as a result of an experiment done by Hahn and Whipple in 1936, in which the tissues of a single dog were perfused free of blood, and tissue iron analyses were carried out. Although no actual enzymes were studied in these investigations, the problem of the fate of tissue enzymes in iron deficiency was generally ignored until the late 1950's, with the exception of isolated inconclusive observations which have been reviewed elsewhere (BEUTLER, 1961; BEUTLER et al., 1963). In 1957, we undertook investigations of iron

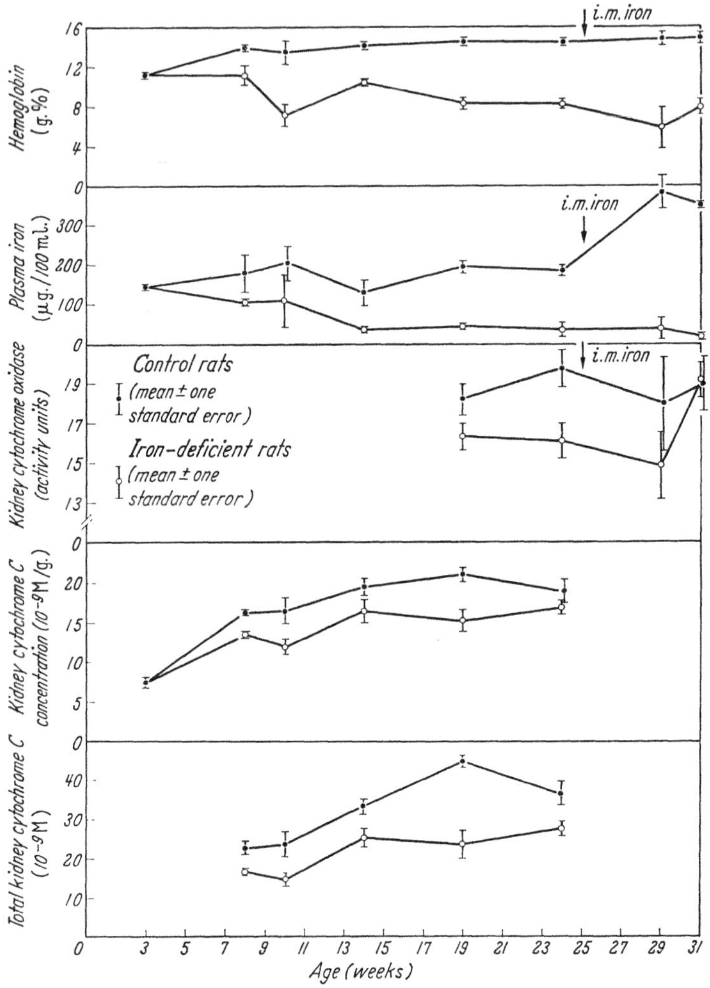

Fig. 1. The hemoglobin values, plasma iron, and kidney cytochrome oxidase and cytochrome C of young rats fed a normal or an iron-deficient diet. A statistically significant decrease in cytochrome-oxidase activity and cytochrome C level was observed in the iron-deficient animals (based on data of BEUTLER and BLAISDELL, 1958b)

enzymes in iron-deficient rats. We soon learned that not all iron enzymes were affected in the same way by iron deficiency. Furthermore, it became apparent that the same enzyme sometimes behaved in a different fashion in different tissues.

For example, it was possible to demonstrate a statistically significant difference in the cytochrome-oxidase content of the kidneys of rats placed on an iron-deficient diet and iron-supplemented controls (Fig. 1), but no such difference could be demonstrated when the hearts of the same animals were examined. Indeed, the cytochrome-oxidase activity of the hearts of iron-deficient animals was somewhat greater than that of the hearts of the control animals (BEUTLER, 1959a).

We also demonstrated a decrease in the cytochrome C content of the kidneys of iron-deficient rats (BEUTLER, 1957; BEUTLER and BLAISDELL, 1958b), and GUBLER et al. (1957) independently found a decrease in the concentration of cytochrome C in the kidneys and hearts of three iron-deficient piglets. These findings have been confirmed by others (KAMPSCHMIDT et al., 1959; SALMON, 1962; McCALL et al., 1962b). McCALL et al., in a careful examination of this problem, pointed out that in their studies and in some of those previously reported there had not been a true decrease in cytochrome C, but that the amount of the enzyme had simply failed to increase normally in the growing animal as the organ involved increased in size. In the heart, an increase in cytochrome C was actually found as this organ hypertrophied greatly in response to the anemia.

We have examined the catalase content of the red cells and liver of iron-deficient rats and have found these to be normal (BEUTLER and BLAISDELL, 1958b). Indeed, if catalase activity in iron-deficient animals is expressed as activity/g. hemoglobin, the catalase content of erythrocytes appears to be increased: the levels of the enzyme are maintained even as the red cells become hypochromic and no longer contain normal amounts of hemoglobin.

Subsequently, we examined succinic dehydrogenase activity. Succinic dehydrogenase is an enzyme which appears to contain non-heme iron. Here again we noted differences in the susceptibility of the enzyme to depletion in different tissues (BEUTLER and BLAISDELL, 1960). Heart and kidney consistently show mild enzyme deficiency, but liver succinic dehydrogenase seems unaffected.

Another enzyme of interest was aconitase. Although it does not, to our knowledge, contain iron, it appears to require iron as a co-factor for its activity (DICKMAN and CLOUTIER, 1950). Dilute tissue homogenates rapidly lose their aconitase activity at 37° C. The addition of iron and ascorbic acid rapidly reactivated aconitase activity (Fig. 2). Iron or ascorbic acid alone did not have such an effect (BEUTLER, 1959b). We have studied the tissues of rats rendered iron-deficient by the administration of an iron-poor diet and those of control rats receiving the same diet plus an injection of iron dextran. Enzyme assays were carried out in iron-deficient and control animals 10 days and 26 days after the beginning of the study. Consistent depletion of kidney aconitase was found to

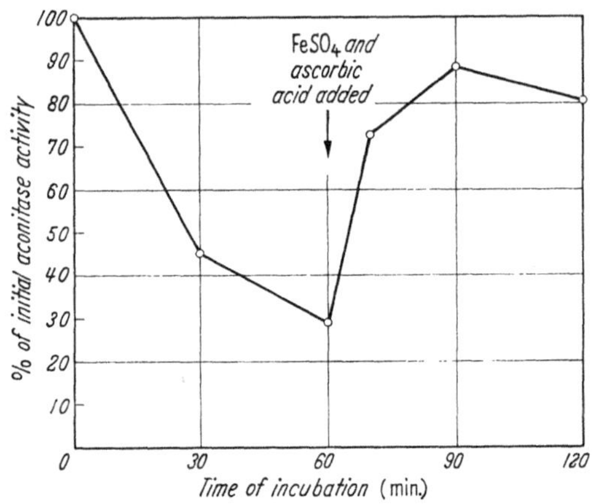

Fig. 2. The reactivation of aconitase by iron and ascorbic acid. After 60 min. incubation of a dilute solution at 37° C., approximately 70% of the aconitase activity had disappeared. The addition of iron and ascorbic acid, to give a final concentration of 0.003 M each, resulted in almost complete reactivation of aconitase

occur (Fig. 3), but no significant decrease in the aconitase content of the heart, liver, or brain was observed. In order to determine whether the decrease in kidney aconitase was due merely to the absence of sufficient ionic ion to "activate" pre-formed apo-enzyme, iron and ascorbic acid were added *in vitro* to the kidney homogenates from iron-deficient and control animals (Fig. 4). No reactivation took place. Apparently, in the absence of the co-factor, iron, there was inadequate synthesis of the apo-enzyme. On the other hand, when iron-deficient rats were fed iron, the kidney aconitase activity returned to normal (Fig. 5). It was also possible to demonstrate that the decrease in kidney aconitase in iron-deficient animals was not the result of anemia. Rats were divided into four groups: control animals, animals that were bled but were given iron supplements, rats that were bled and allowed to become iron-deficient, and, finally, rats treated with phenylhydrazine to produce a comparable degree of anemia. Only the kidneys of the animals that were bled without being given iron supplements, namely the iron-deficient group, became depleted of aconitase activity.

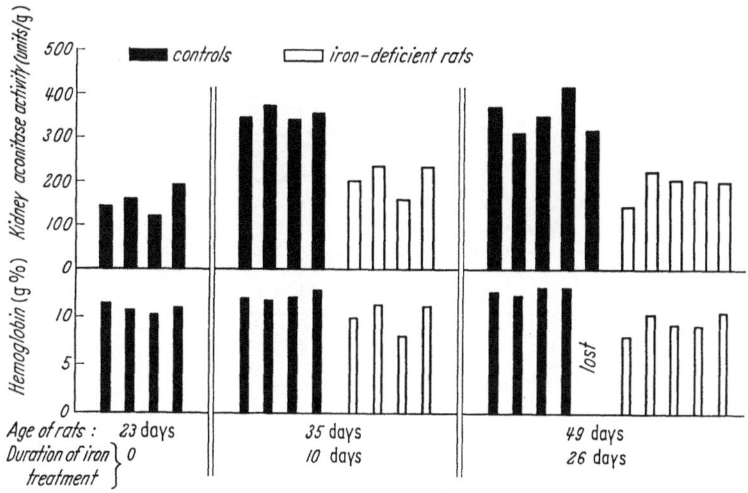

Fig. 3. The kidney aconitase activity and hemoglobin levels of young rats placed on an iron-poor diet. The control animals were given 25 mg. iron dextran in two divided doses, one at the beginning of the experiment, the other two weeks later. The aconitase activity of the kidneys of the iron-treated rats increased rapidly, while aconitase activity of the iron-deficient animals remained at relatively low levels (based on data of BEUTLER, 1959b)

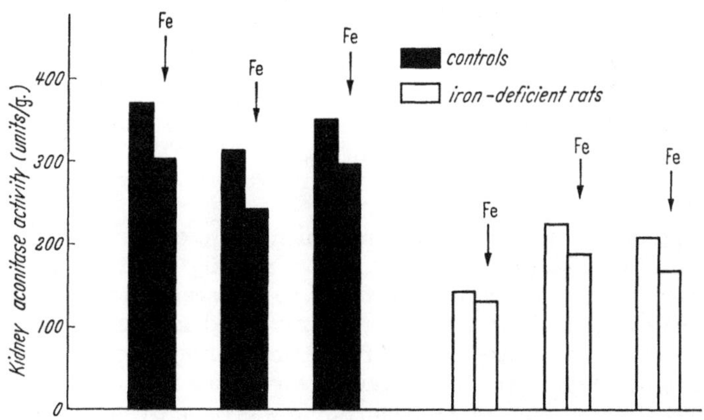

Fig. 4. The failure of iron and ascorbate (arrows) to "reactivate" aconitase from normal and iron-deficient rat kidneys. The columns under the arrows represent aconitase activity of homogenates that have been incubated for one-half hour with ascorbate and ferrous sulfate, both in final concentrations of 0.003 M (by courtesy of the J. Clin. Invest., from BEUTLER, 1959b)

Much less data are available regarding the fate of iron enzymes in the tissues of human iron-deficient subjects than is the case with iron-deficient animals. This is because tissues suitable for the study of iron enzymes are not readily available clinically. An

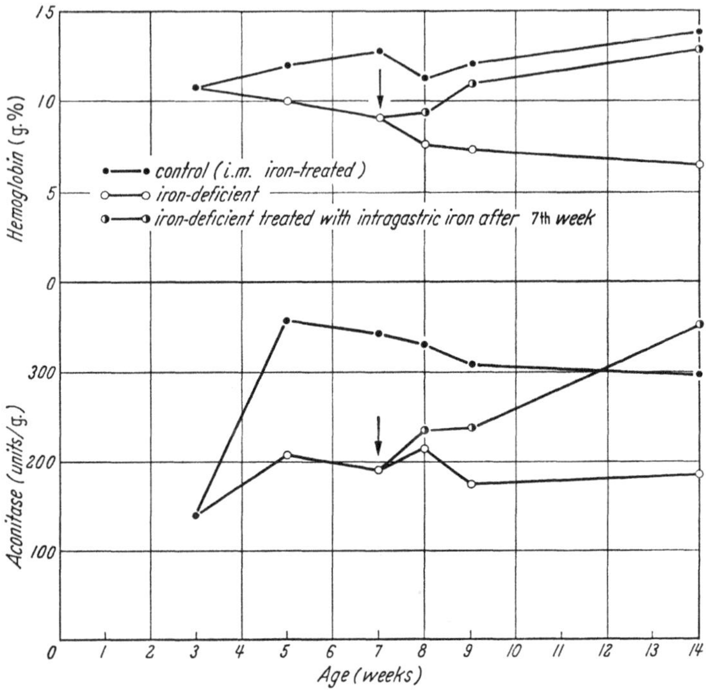

Fig. 5. The effect of iron feeding on the aconitase activity and hemoglobin levels of iron-deficient rat kidneys. Rats were placed on an iron-poor diet, and control animals were given iron dextran injections. The daily administration of iron by the intragastric route (at arrow) resulted in the return of both hemoglobin levels and aconitase activity to normal

exception is catalase, an enzyme which is present in high concentration in human erythrocytes. Unfortunately from a diagnostic point of view, this enzyme was found to be normal in iron-deficient subjects, just as it was in rats (BEUTLER and BLAISDELL, 1958a). The activity of this enzyme per unit volume of red cells was unaltered (Fig. 6), even in very severe iron-deficiency anemia. The enzyme activity per g. hemoglobin was actually increased, as it was in rats. Apparently, catalase activity is preserved, even when there is a marked decrease in hemoglobin synthesis. From a teleological aspect, this is particularly difficult to understand, since congenital absence of catalase from erythrocytes does not result in any serious disturbance of red-cell function (TAKAHARA, 1960).

Attempts to measure the cytochrome C content of human leukocytes were entirely unsuccessful. Although not completely satisfactory, efforts to measure the cytochrome-oxidase content of sonated human leukocytes have been somewhat more rewarding (BEUTLER, 1959c, 1960): there seemed to be a moderate decrease in the average cytochrome-oxidase content of leukocytes obtained from iron-deficient subjects (Fig. 7). We have attempted to study leukocyte cytochrome oxidase by histochemical means: these studies have been frustrated by technical difficulties. It has been possible to assay the aconitase activity of leukocytes of iron-deficient subjects. No abnormality was detected (BEUTLER and YEH, 1959; TANAKA and VALENTINE, 1961).

Perhaps the most meaningful observations regarding the fate of iron enzymes in the human subject come from the histochemical investigations of JACOBS (1961) in buccal mucosal biopsies. Absence of cytochrome-oxidase activity was demonstrated in the mucosas of

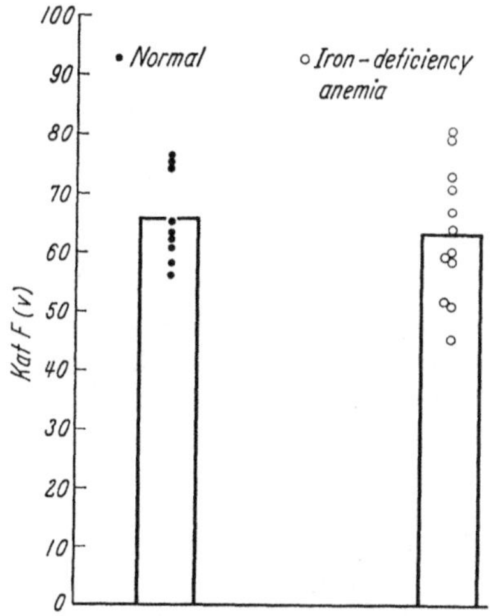

Fig. 6. The effect of iron-deficiency anemia on the catalase activity per unit volume [Kat F (v)] of human erythrocytes. No depletion of catalase was observed (based on the data of BEUTLER and BLAISDELL, 1958a)

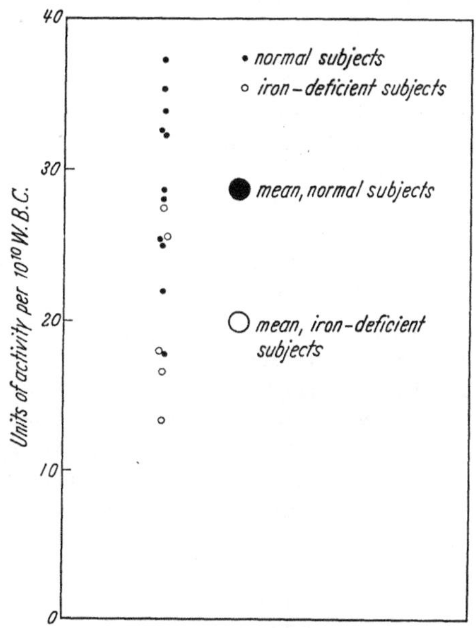

Fig. 7. The effect of iron deficiency on human leukocyte cytochrome-oxidase activity

some iron-deficient subjects. Enzyme activity returned to normal after iron therapy. It is interesting to note that enzyme depletion was observed in one patient whose hemoglobin was nearly normal. In contrast, no depletion of the succinic dehydrogenase system could be demonstrated.

The fragmentary evidence of enzyme depletion derived from patients is supplemented by the finding that the iron content of sweat (HUSSAIN and PATWARDHAN, 1959) and of urine (DUBACH et al., 1955) is diminished in iron deficiency and possibly that there may be a decrease in the iron content of the fingernails in anemic subjects (JACOBS and JENKINS, 1960). Clearly, these changes cannot be a direct reflection of the loss of storage iron or of hemoglobin iron, but rather represent a manifestation of enzyme loss in human subjects. Hair iron, on the other hand, does not seem to be affected by iron deficiency (GREEN and DUFFIELD, 1956), possibly because of the large variability produced by inherited differences in the quantities of iron-containing pigments which may be present (DUTCHER and ROTHMAN, 1951).

These studies clearly demonstrate that the long-accepted concept that iron enzymes are not affected in iron-deficiency anemia, no matter how severe the degree of iron deprivation, is incorrect. Rather it seems that, after the loss of storage iron, competition for the little iron available leads to decreased synthesis not only of hemoglobin but also of various enzymes (Fig. 8). Some enzymes, such as aconitase and cytochrome C, seem to be affected quite readily, at least in certain tissues. Other enzymes, such as catalase, may behave in the "inviolate" fashion which HAHN and WHIPPLE had postulated to describe the behavior of all iron enzymes in iron deficiency.

Although there is no doubt that certain enzymes, notably cytochrome C, cytochrome oxidase, succinic dehydrogenase, and aconitase, are present in smaller than normal quantities in some tissues of iron-deficient subjects or experimental animals, we should not like to imply that it is necessarily a deficiency of *these* enzymes which results in either the tissue changes or the symptomatology of iron-deficiency anemia. It is quite possible that the degree of depletion of these enzymes which occurs may not be sufficient to cause any functional impairment. Indeed, efforts in our laboratory to demonstrate an increased oxygen debt in iron-deficient subjects during exercise yielded entirely negative results (BEUTLER et al., 1960b). Efforts to demonstrate abnormalities in the metabolism of exogenously administered citrate were also unsuccessful (BEUTLER, 1959b). Yet it must be emphasized that the enzymes which have been studied represent only a few of many biologically important iron compounds which occur in the body. It is quite likely that the Achilles heel of the patient who becomes iron-depleted is not one of the cytochromes or aconitase but some, as yet unstudied or even

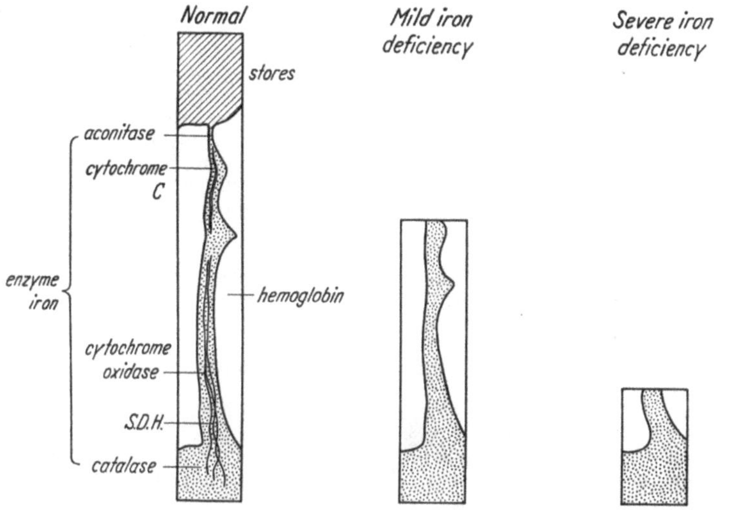

Fig. 8. Schematic representation of stages of iron depletion. It is suggested that there is a concurrent loss of hemoglobin and enzyme iron, with different enzymes varying in their susceptibility to depletion (by courtesy of Grune & Stratton, from BEUTLER et al., 1963)

undiscovered, iron-requiring biological substance. The elucidation of the biochemical pathogenesis of tissue changes in iron deficiency remains a task for the future.

Summary

Iron deficiency is a disorder which gives rise not only to changes in the blood hemoglobin level, but also to well-defined tissue changes. These abnormalities can be observed both in experimental animals and in man. In man, the gastro-intestinal tract is most commonly affected. Other tissue changes have also been seen, however, and some of these may be related to other associated nutritional deficiencies.

It is also possible that the symptoms of iron-deficiency anemia, commonly attributed to the lowering of blood hemoglobin levels, are due to subtle disorders in tissue metabolism. Evidence which suggests that this may be the case includes the dissociation between the severity of anemia and the severity of symptoms, the finding that the symptomatic response to iron therapy precedes the hemoglobin response, and possibly that iron deficiency may be symptomatic even in patients in whom the hemoglobin level is normal. Studies of various enzymes in iron-deficient experimental animals and man have shown that different iron enzymes behave differently and that there are also tissue-to-tissue differences. Cytochrome C, cytochrome oxidase, aconitase, and succinic dehydrogenase appear to be susceptible to depletion. Catalase appears to be resistant to depletion. It is emphasized that the demonstration that the concentration of these enzymes is diminished in iron deficiency does not prove that a decrease in the concentration of these enzymes results in either symptoms or tissue changes.

Zusammenfassung

Eisenmangel ist eine Störung, die nicht nur den Haemoglobingehalt des Blutes beeinträchtigt, sondern auch zu gut definierten Gewebsveränderungen führt. Diese Abweichungen können sowohl am Versuchstier als auch beim Menschen beobachtet werden. Beim Menschen ist im allgemeinen der Magen-Darmtrakt befallen, jedoch treten auch Gewebsveränderungen auf, die zum Teil zu anderen, gleichzeitig vorhandenen Ernährungsstörungen in Beziehung stehen können.

Es ist durchaus möglich, daß den Symptomen der Eisenmangelanaemie, die allgemein auf die Verminderung der Haemoglobinkonzentration im Blut zurückgeführt werden, diskretere Störungen im Gewebsstoffwechsel zugrunde liegen. Dafür sprechen Hinweise über die Unterschiede zwischen dem Schweregrad der Anaemie und der dadurch bedingten Symptome sowie die Beobachtung, daß ein Ansprechen auf Eisenbehandlung dem Einfluß auf die Haemoglobinkonzentration vorangeht, und daß Eisenmangel sogar bei Patienten mit normalen Haemoglobinwerten Symptome hervorrufen kann. Untersuchungen bei Tieren mit experimentellem Eisenmangel und am Menschen haben ergeben, daß sich einzelne eisenhaltige Fermente verschieden verhalten, und daß auch Abweichungen zwischen einzelnen Geweben bestehen. Cytochrom C, Cytochromoxydase, Akonitase und Succindehydrogenase scheinen durch Eisenmangel beeinflußt zu werden, während Katalase resistent ist. Es wird hervorgehoben, daß der Nachweis einer verminderten Konzentration dieser Fermente beim Eisenmangel noch kein Beweis dafür ist, daß ihre Abnahme entweder zu Symptomen führt oder Gewebsveränderungen hervorruft.

Résumé

L'hyposidérose est un trouble qui donne lieu non seulement à des modifications du taux d'hémoglobine dans le sang, mais aussi à des modifications tissulaires bien définies. Ces anomalies s'observent aussi bien chez l'animal d'expérience que chez l'homme. Chez l'homme, c'est le tube digestif qui est le plus souvent touché. D'autres modifications tissulaires cependant peuvent se voir, dont certaines peuvent relever d'autres carences nutritionnelles associées.

Il est aussi possible que les signes de l'anémie ferriprive, habituellement attribués à l'abaissement de l'hémoglobine, soient dus à de fines perturbations du métabolisme tissulaire. Seraient en faveur de cette hypothèse: l'absence de parallélisme entre la gravité de l'anémie et l'intensité des symptômes, la précession de l'amélioration symptomatique sur l'amélioration des chiffres d'hémoglobine au cours de la thérapeutique martiale, peut-être aussi l'existence de signes d'hyposidérose chez certains malades présentant des taux d'hémoglobine normaux. L'étude de différents enzymes au cours des hyposidéroses expérimentales et chez l'homme a montré que les différents enzymes contenant du fer se comportent différemment; il existe aussi des différences d'un tissu à l'autre. Le cytochrome *C*, la cytochrome-oxydase, l'aconitase, la déhydrogénase succinique semblent sensibles à la déperdition de fer, tandis que la catalase semble plus résistante. On souligne que le fait de démontrer la baisse de concentration de ces enzymes dans l'hyposidérose ne prouve pas que ce soit là la cause ni des symptômes ni des modifications tissulaires.

Acknowledgement

This work was supported in part by the National Institutes of Health, P.H.S. Grant HE 07449-01.

References

AHLBOM, H. E.: Brit. Med. J., **1936**/II, 331. — BADENOCH, J., J. R. EVANS, and W. C. D. RICHARDS: Brit. J. Haemat. **3**, 175 (1957). — BECQUEREL, A., and A. RODIER: Gaz. méd. Paris **12**, 751 (1844). Quoted by UNDRITZ, E.: Schweiz. med. Wschr. **85**, 936 (1955). — BEUTLER, E.: Amer. J. Med. Sc. **234**, 517 (1957). — BEUTLER, E., and R. K. BLAISDELL: J. Clin. Invest. (U.S.A.) **37**, 833 (1958a). — BEUTLER, E., and R. K. BLAISDELL: J. Laborat. Clin. Med. (U.S.A.) **52**, 694 (1958b). — BEUTLER, E.: Acta haemat. (Switz). **21**, 371 (1959a). — BEUTLER, E.: J. Clin. Invest. (U.S.A.) **38**, 1605 (1959b). — BEUTLER, E.: Illinois Med. J. **116**, 16 (1959c). — BEUTLER, E., and M. YEH: J. Laborat. Clin. Med. (U.S.A.) **54**, 456 (1959). — BEUTLER, E.: Blut (G.) **6**, 130 (1960). — BEUTLER, E., and R. K. BLAISDELL: Blood (U.S.A.) **15**, 30 (1960). — BEUTLER, E., S. E. LARSH, and C. W. GURNEY: Ann. Int. Med. (U.S.A.) **52**, 378 (1960a). — BEUTLER, E., S. LARSH, and F. TANZI: Amer. J. Med. Sc. **239**, 759 (1960b). — BEUTLER, E.: Ann. Rev. Med. (U.S.A.) **12**, 195 (1961). — BEUTLER, E., V. F. FAIRBANKS, and J. L. FAHEY: Clinical Disorders of Iron Metabolism. Grune & Stratton, New York, 1963. — BIGGS, J. C., K. B. TAYLOR, L. S. VALBERG, and M. A. WITTS: Gastroenterology (U.S.A.) **43**, 430 (1962). — BODDINGTON, M. M.: J. Clin. Path. (G.B.) **12**, 222 (1959). — BROWN, E. B., C. V. MOORE, C. REYNAFARJE, and D. E. SMITH: J. Amer. Med. Ass. **144**, 1084 (1950). — BROWN, E. B., and C. V. MOORE: In: Progress in Hematology. Ed. by L. TOCANTINES. Grune & Stratton, New York, 1956, p. 22—46. — CHELI, R., M. DODERO, G. CELLE, and M. VASSALOTTI: Acta haemat. (Switz.) **22**, 1 (1959). — COGHILL, N. F., and A. W. WILLIAMS: Gastroenterology (U.S.A.) **83**, 60 (1955). — COHEN, E., and C. A. ELVEHJEM: J. Biol. Chem. (U.S.A.) **107**, 97 (1934). — DABSKI, H.: Polski tygodn. lek. **15**, 942, abstracted in: Blood (U.S.A.) **16**, 1659 (1960). — DAMESHEK, W.: J. Amer. Med. Ass. **100**, 540 (1933). — DAVIDSON, W. M. B., and J. L. MARKSON: Lancet (G.B.) **269**, 639 (1955). — DAVIS, P. N., L. C. NORRIS, and F. H. KRATZER: J. Nutrit. (U.S.A.) **78**, 445 (1962). — DICKMAN, S. R., and A. A. CLOUTIER: Arch. Biochem. (U.S.A.) **25**, 229 (1950). — DUBACH, R., C. V. MOORE, and S. T. CALLENDER: J. Laborat. Clin. Med. (U.S.A.) **45**, 599 (1955). — DUTCHER, T. F., and S. ROTHMAN: J. Invest. Dermat. (U.S.A.) **17**, 65 (1951). — GLAZEBROOK, A. J.: Edinburgh Med. J. **51**, 65 (1944). — GOLDECK, H., D. REMY, and H. LABHARD: Dtsch. med. Wschr. **79**, 211 (1954). — GOODMAN, L. S., and A. GILMAN: The Pharmacologic Basis of Therapeutics. 2nd Ed. Macmillan, New York, 1955. — GOVAN, A. D. T., and J. J. SCOTT: Lancet (G.B.) **1949**/I, 14. — GREEN, P. T., and J. DUFFIELD: Canad. Serv. Med. J. **12**, 987 (1956). — GUBLER, C. J., G. E. CARTWRIGHT, and M. M. WINTROBE: J. Biol. Chem. (U.S.A.) **224**, 533 (1957). — HAHN, P. F.: Fed. Proc. (U.S.A.) **7**, 493 (1948). — HAHN, P. F., and G. H. WHIPPLE:

Amer. J. Med. Sc. **191**, 24 (1936). — HEATH, C. W., M. B. STRAUSS, and W. B. CASTLE: J. Clin. Invest. (U.S.A.) **11**, 1293 (1932). — HEILMEYER, L., and K. PLÖTNER: Das Serumeisen und die Eisenmangelkrankheit. Fischer, Jena, 1937. — HUSSAIN, R., and V. N. PATWARDHAN: Lancet (G.B.) **1959**/I, 1073. — JACOBS, A.: J. Clin. Path. (G.B.) **13**, 463 (1960). — JACOBS, A., and D. J. JENKINS: Brit. J. Dermat. **72**, 145 (1960). — JACOBS, A.: Lancet (G.B.) **1961**/II, 1331. — JALILI, M. A., and S. AL-KASSAB: Lancet (G.B.) **1959**/II, 108. — JASINSKI, B., and O. ROTH: Larvierte Eisenmangelkrankheit. Benno Schwabe & Co., Basle, 1954. — JOSKE, R. A., E. S. FINCKH, and I. J. WOOD: Quart. J. Med. (G.B.) **24**, 269 (1955). — KAMPSCHMIDT, R. F., M. E. ADAMS, and W. L. GOODWIN: Arch. Biochem. Biophys. (U.S.A.) **82**, 42 (1959). — KELLY, A. B.: J. Laryng. Rhinol. Otol. (G.B.) **34**, 285 (1919). — LAACHE, S.: Die Anämie. Walling, Christiania, 1883. — LEES, F., and F. D. ROSENTHAL: Quart. J. Med. (G.B.) **27**, 19 (1958). — MCCALL, M. G., G. E. NEWMAN, and L. S. VALBERG: Brit. J. Nutrit. **16**, 333 (1962 a). — MCCALL, M. G., G. E. NEWMAN, J. R. P. O'BRIEN, and L. J. WITTS: Brit. J. Nutrit. **16**, 305 (1962). — MORAWITZ, P.: Münch. med. Wschr. **57**, 1425 (1910). — MORRISON, L. M., W. A. SWALM, and C. L. JACKSON: J. Amer. Med. Ass. **109**, 108 (1937). — NAEGELI, O.: In: Blutkrankheiten und Blutdiagnostik. Von Veit & Company, Leipzig, 1908, p. 237. — PATERSON, D. R.: J. Laryng. Rhinol. Otol. (G.B.) **34**, 289 (1919). — PAUL, K. G.: In: The Enzymes. Vol. 2. Academic Press, New York, 1951, p. 357. — PIERAERTS, G.: Recueil sc. méd. Congo **1**, 104 (1942). — PRASAD, A. S., A. MIALE Jr., Z. FARID, H. H. SANDSTEAD, A. R. SCHULER, and W. J. DARBY: Arch. Int. Med. (U.S.A.) **111**, 407 (1963). — RATNER, S.: J. Dent. Res. (U.S.A.) **15**, 89 (1935). — ROSS, J. D.: N. England J. Med. **266**, 1372 (1962). — RUSTUNG, E.: Acta dermat.-venereol. (Sweden) **29**, 1 (1949). — SAHLI, H.: In: Lehrbuch der Klinischen Untersuchungs-Methoden. Franz Deuticke, Leipzig/Vienna, 1908, p. 993. — SALMON, H. A.: J. Physiol. (G.B.) **164**, 17 (1962). — SLACK, H. G. B., and J. R. WILKINSON: Lancet (G.B.) **1949**/I, 11. — STAFFORD, J. J.: Proc. Roy. Soc. Med. (G.B.) **54**, 1000 (1961). — STAFFURTH, J. S.: St. Thomas's Hosp. Rep. (G.B.) **7**, 103 (1951). — STEVENS, A. R.: A. M. A. Arch. Int. Med. **96**, 550 (1956). — SUZMAN, M. M.: Arch. Int. Med. (U.S.A.) **51**, 1 (1933). — TAKAHARA, S.: In: Proceedings of the 8th International Congress of Haematology. Pan-Pacific Press, Tokyo, 1960, p. 286. — TANAKA, K. R., and W. N. VALENTINE: Acta haemat. (Switz.) **26**, 12 (1961). — THEDERING, F.: Med. Klin. (G.) **50**, 1463 (1955). — THEORELL, H., M. BEZNAK, R. BONNICHSEN, K. G. PAUL, and A. AKESON: Acta chem. Scand. **5**, 445 (1951). — UNDRITZ, E.: Verh. Schweiz. Naturforsch. Ges. **136**, 169 (1956). — VALBERG, L. S., K. B. TAYLOR, and L. J. WITTS: Brit. J. Nutrit. **15**, 473 (1961). — VANNOTTI, A.: Schweiz. med. Wschr. **79**, 261 (1949). — VERLOOP, M. C., J. E. MEEUWISSEN, and E. W. BLOKHUIS: Brit. J. Haemat. **4**, 70 (1958). — VINSON, P. P.: Minnesota Med. **5**, 107 (1922). — WALDENSTRÖM, J.: Acta med. Scand. **90**, 380 (1938). — WALDENSTRÖM, J.: Acta med. Scand. **170**, 252 (1946). — WASSERMAN, L. R.: Blood (U.S.A.) **10**, 655 (1955). — WINTROBE, M. M.: Clinical Hematology. Lea & Febiger, Philadelphia, 1961. — YEH, S. D. J., A. R. GABRIEL, and B. F. CHOW: Fed. Proc. (U.S.A.) **20**, 451 (1961). — YU, W. L., K. MANONMANI, and R. J. WATSON: J. Pediatr. (U.S.A.) **54**, 50 (1959).

Discussion

Schapira: As I understand it, the purpose of Dr. Beutler's paper was twofold: firstly, to investigate iron-enzyme changes occurring in the tissues in the presence of iron deficiency and, secondly, to explain some of the subjective symptoms encountered, such as fatigue. If I understood you correctly, you regard the kidney as the centre of the fatigue.

Beutler: I have a strong suspicion that the centre of fatigue is identical with the seat of the soul, and when you tell me where the seat of the soul is, then perhaps I can tell you where the centre of fatigue is. This question, however, re-emphasises an important point: that the results of our enzyme studies in animals cannot be extrapolated to man and used as evidence that iron deficiency produces fatigue in man or in woman because of the depletion of one or another enzyme which we have specifically studied.

Hallberg: As a comment on Dr. Moore's paper I should like to add some recent observations of ours on the incidence of iron deficiency in women and its relation to the menstrual blood loss.

I should perhaps first mention that we have found the menstrual blood loss to be very constant from period to period and from one year to another. This means that, if you have data on the distribution of the menstrual blood loss in a population, you also have data which make it possible to estimate the distribution of the iron need in a population where the menstrual blood loss is the main variable determining the iron need in women.

In 137 women selected at random from among workers in a large industry in Göteborg, Dr. Nilsson and I[1] found that, in those women having a blood loss of more than 60 ml., the total iron-binding capacity of the serum was increased, the increase being roughly related to the magnitude of the blood loss. Similarly, the plasma iron was decreased in women with a blood loss of more than 100 ml. All in all, about 13% of the women had a blood loss of more than 60 ml. Only 5% had a haemoglobin level below 11.5 g./100 ml. These findings prompted a larger study of women from the general population of Göteborg in which 1,000 women were selected at random from among certain age groups. The results of this latter study showed, firstly, that the average menstrual blood loss was larger, 25% of the women having a loss of more than 60 ml. per period, and, secondly, that the frequency of anaemia as defined previously was higher, the highest rate occurring at 30 years, 25% of the women in this age group showing haemoglobin levels of less than 11.5 g./100 ml.

Without going into further details I would say that, in a great proportion of menstruating women, the average diet consumed is inadequate.

Najean: From a clinical point of view, I should like to ask Dr. Chatterjea whether the adult subjects suffering from chronic undernutrition (cirrhosis and thalassaemia excluded) do or do not have an enlarged spleen. I also have another question. Dr. Beutler said that rats with iron deficiency show

[1] Hallberg, L., and L. Nilsson: To be published.

a decreased intrinsic-factor activity in their gastric juice. Is the same thing likewise observed in human beings, and if so, does this deficiency disappear after iron treatment has been given to correct the hyposideraemia?

CHATTERJEA: In reply to Dr. NAJEAN's question, I should like to emphasise that in my series I took particular care to exclude thalassaemia trait and cirrhosis of the liver. Approximately 37% of the patients with iron-deficiency anaemia showed splenic enlargement, which usually regressed when the iron deficiency was corrected. Dr. POLLYCOVE in his paper presented evidence of haemolysis in some cases of iron-deficiency anaemia (p. 165). The splenic enlargement is possibly related to this haemolysis.

BEUTLER: Regarding the question about intrinsic-factor secretion by iron-deficient subjects, I would point out that in 1961 YEH and associates[1] showed a decrease in iron absorption in rats and that BIGGS and associates[2] demonstrated a decrease in intrinsic-factor secretion by the stomach in iron-deficient rats. In man, however, BADENOCH and associates[3] had shown as early as 1957 that a decrease occurred in intrinsic-factor secretion.

BRICK: With reference to Dr. CHATTERJEA's paper, the finding of frequent hepatosplenomegaly in many of these cases raises the question as to how many of these patients had cirrhosis. Were liver biopsies done in any of these patients? Italian workers[4] reported, some years before this appeared in the English literature, that parotid enlargement occurred in cirrhosis in the background of alcoholism. About 6 years ago, three different groups in the United States reported cases of cirrhosis and parotid enlargement[5]. In our report the patients were alcoholics, but other patients have been seen with post-necrotic cirrhosis or haemochromatosis and with parotid enlargement. Interestingly enough, nutritional surveys were done among the Indians in America by the Public Health Service, and in Indians who were not nutritionally deficient a high percentage of patients with parotid enlargement were found as compared with the normal Caucasian population. Studies in the Philippine Islands and in China have also revealed a fair number of patients with parotid enlargement. It must be pointed out that, as a clinical sign, parotid enlargement is often missed, because it is not carefully searched for in the way that I am sure Dr. CHATTERJEA searched for it. The question of the histology of this painless parotid enlargement is also interesting. We did punch biopsies in two cases, and the histology was completely normal. There has been some dispute as to why this parotid enlargement occurs. British workers, studying a starved group in Wuppertal, Germany, after the war, found that on refeeding these patients, parotid enlargement occurred in somewhat the same manner as the refeeding gynaecomastia observed in our

---

[1] YEH, S. D. J., A. R. GABRIEL, and B. F. CHOW: Fed. Proc. (U.S.A.) **20**, 451 (1961) (abstract).

[2] BIGGS, J. C., K. B. TAYLOR, L. S. VALBERG, and M. A. WITTS: Gastroenterology (U.S.A.) **43**, 430 (1962).

[3] BADENOCH, J., J. R. EVANS, and W. C. D. RICHARDS: Brit. J. Haemat. **3**, 175 (1957).

[4] SPOSITO, M.: Riforma med. (It.) **58**, 1311 (1942); SPOSITO, M., and R. CHELI: Riforma med. (It.) **65**, 1250 (1951).

[5] WOLFE, S. J., W. H. J. SUMMERSKILL, and C. S. DAVIDSON: N. England J. Med. **256**, 491 (1957); ROTHBELL, E. N., and J. J. DUGGAN: Amer. J. Med. **22**, 367 (1957); BRICK, I. B.: Ann. Int. Med. (U.S.A.) **49**, 439 (1958).

repatriated Japanese prisoners of war. I should be pleased to hear Dr. CHATTERJEA's explanation for the occurrence of parotid enlargement and its frequency in iron-deficiency anaemia.

CHATTERJEA: Not all the patients with iron deficiency who showed enlargement of the parotids had hepatosplenomegaly. None had gynaecomastia. We were convinced that parotid enlargement in our series was unrelated to any affection of the liver. Of course, we did find parotid enlargement in hepatic cirrhosis, as listed in the miscellaneous group included in Table 1 of my paper (p. 225). Parotid enlargement in hepatic cirrhosis is a well-known phenomenon, but here again the precise cause that leads to such an enlargement is unknown. The role which inactivation of oestrogens is alleged to play may be a contributory factor. But is it the only factor? Can we definitely exclude the possibility that some deficiency factor also plays a causative role?

The syndrome of parotid enlargement recorded in prisoners of war as reviewed by MCCANCE, DEAN, and BARRETT[1], to which I had referred in my paper, is perhaps a different phenomenon and one which should not be confused with the enlargement seen in the states of undernutrition we are discussing at present. Overfeeding with a high calorie diet following a long period of grossly inadequate nutrition possibly leads to overactivity on the part of the parotids.

I wanted to record that parotid enlargement could be found in chronic iron-deficiency states if only one looked carefully for this sign. This painless enlargement causes the patient no discomfort and is therefore liable to be overlooked. I never meant to attribute any particularly specific significance to this sign, especially since I have found the same type of enlargement in other conditions as well.

VENTURA: I was very pleased to have received from Dr. CHATTERJEA fresh confirmation for the results of the first clinical trial by CRUZ[2] in 1932 and of the more recent biochemical and clinical investigations which LARIZZA and I[3] undertook in 1950, i.e. that iron therapy by itself is capable of curing hookworm anaemia, whereas mere eradication of the parasites is not. May I now ask Dr. CHATTERJEA what he thinks about the pathogenesis of hookworm anaemia? Is it simply a form of anaemia due to haemorrhage or is there more to it than that? Secondly, has he done any ferrokinetic determinations in his cases of iron-deficiency anaemia with protein, vitamin B_{12}, and folic acid deficiency? I should be interested to know whether any modifications occur in the pure iron-deficiency pattern and, if so, what they are; and I should like to know if Dr. POLLYCOVE has had any experience in this connection.

I should also like Dr. MOORE to give us his opinion as to the character of the processes of iron absorption in partially gastrectomised patients.

Finally, what, in Dr. BEUTLER's view, is the best test to use for diagnosing iron deficiency in the stage at which the haemoglobin content is normal?

CHATTERJEA: In reply to Dr. VENTURA, may I point out that the fact that iron therapy alone, without any anthelmintic treatment, will improve the blood picture in hookworm anaemia is now a well-known phenomenon

[1] MCCANCE, R. A., R. F. A. DEAN, and A. M. BARRETT: Med. Res. Council, Special Rep. Ser. No. 275, H. M. Stationery Offiice, London, 1951.

[2] CRUZ, W. O.: Compt. rend. Soc. biol. (Fr.) **91**, 483 (1932).

[3] LARIZZA, P., and S. VENTURA: L'anemia da anchilostoma. Studio patogenetico. Tipografia Libro, Pavia, 1950.

which was clearly demonstrated by my predecessors at the School of Tropical Medicine 22 years ago[1].

I firmly believe that haemorrhage is the predominant, if not the only factor, in the causation of anaemia in hookworm disease. Deficiencies of folic acid and vitamin B_{12} are associated events related to the consumption of an inadequate diet.

BEUTLER: In answer to Dr. VENTURA's question I feel that the best test for the detection of iron deficiency in the non-anaemic subject is examination of the bone marrow for stainable iron; and this, in conjunction with the plasma iron and iron-binding capacity, are the criteria we use in the studies which I briefly described here for the classification of patients with regard to varying degrees of iron depletion.

POLLYCOVE: With respect to Dr. BEUTLER's paper I should like to point out that his data are in agreement with the excellent work of GUBLER, CARTWRIGHT, and WINTROBE[2], who in 1957 published their measurements of various tissue concentrations of cytochrome C, catalase, and cytochrome oxidase in iron-deficient and copper-deficient pigs with severe anaemia. Despite the severe anaemia of 3 g./100 ml., they also found only a moderate reduction to not less than half of the normal concentration of cytochrome C; the concentrations of cytochrome oxidase and catalase in severe iron-deficiency anaemia were normal. Since it is probable that the normal enzyme concentration is not a rate-limiting concentration, a moderate reduction probably does not give rise to symptoms. Severe cases of iron deficiency occur frequently in various parts of the world where heavy labour is performed for many years by anaemic individuals at haemoglobin levels of 4—6 g./100 ml. We have studied a patient with an iron-deficiency anaemia of 2 g. haemoglobin/100 ml. who was working a 40-hour week as a building inspector and was able to walk up a flight of stairs without pausing. Consequently, it is difficult to believe that, in the absence of significant anaemia, loss of storage iron and a mild reduction in the plasma iron concentration would give rise to significant symptoms.

With regard to the question asked by Dr. VENTURA, we have studied various patients with vitamin B_{12} deficiency and simultaneous iron deficiency. The vitamin B_{12} deficiency was predominant, so that the patients had a megaloblastic anaemia, and the iron-kinetic study performed at that time was typical of pernicious anaemia. In response to vitamin B_{12} therapy the haemoglobin concentration increased by 2 g./100 ml. At that level another iron-kinetic study yielded findings characteristic of iron-deficiency anaemia. So I think that the deficiency which predominates and results in the existing level of anaemia will produce its characteristic disturbance of the erythropoietic system corresponding to that degree of anaemia. Coexisting deficiencies will not affect erythropoiesis characteristically until they become limiting factors in erythropoiesis.

CHATTERJEA: The observations of Dr. POLLYCOVE concerning his ferrokinetic studies in mixed deficiency states (iron plus vitamin B_{12}) are, I am happy to note, in complete agreement with what we had reported in 1953[3].

[1] NAPIER, L. E., C. R. DAS GUPTA, and D. N. MAJUMDAR: Indian Med. Gaz. **76**, 1 (1941).

[2] GUBLER, C. J., G. E. CARTWRIGHT, and M. M. WINTROBE: J. Biol. Chem. (U.S.A.) **224**, 533 (1957).

[3] CHATTERJEA, J. B., and C. R. DAS GUPTA: Indian Med. Gaz. 88, 126 (1953).

Evidence for the presence of masked deficiency could be satisfactorily demonstrated only after the major deficiency had been corrected by appropriate therapy.

Beutler: Dr. Pollycove has cited some work by Cartwright on iron enzymes. I have undoubtedly left unmentioned the important contribution made by many authors in this field. However, I should like to quote briefly from my paper: "We also demonstrated a decrease in the cytochrome C content of the kidneys of iron-deficient rats, and Gubler[1] and associates independently found a decrease in the concentration of cytochrome C in the kidneys and hearts of three iron-deficient piglets."

With regard to the mild decrease in cytochrome C which we have reported and its possible effect on the symptoms, I've tried to emphasise that we do not regard these changes as necessarily being the cause of symptoms or of tissue changes in the patient with iron deficiency. Certainly we have not been able to demonstrate any abnormality in oxygen transport in iron-deficient patients. However, it should be emphasised that in any series of enzymatic reactions, there is at least one reaction which is "limiting", and the decrease in the concentration of the enzyme concerned will slow down the series of reactions. There are many iron enzymes which we have not studied; there are probably many iron enzymes which are not even known to be iron enzymes, and these may be important in the origin of tissue changes in iron deficiency.

As for the relationship of the haemoglobin levels to the symptoms, which Dr. Pollycove also mentioned, his observations are in precise agreement with ours. There is poor relationship between haemoglobin levels and the symptoms displayed by iron-deficient patients, and this is one of the things which makes us feel that it is not primarily the haemoglobin level of the blood which determines the symptoms in such patients. In the final analysis, the question whether non-anaemic patients may have symptoms due to iron deficiency or not cannot be settled by conjectures about whether decreases in various iron enzymes are great enough to produce symptoms, but by carefully controlled clinical studies of the effect of iron administration and placebo administration in such patients. It is my understanding that additional studies along these lines are now in progress, and I hope that some members participating in this Symposium will also carry out further investigations of this kind.

Moeschlin: I should just like to ask Dr. Moore a question. Do you think it advisable to give regular doses of hydrochloric acid to the gastrectomised patient? In our clinical experience, we have been impressed by the fact that such patients usually develop less anaemia if we do this.

Tubiana: A few years ago we studied iron excretion after intravenous injection of radio-iron in mice[2]. We found that the iron was excreted all along the gastro-intestinal tract, but chiefly in the small intestine. Most probably part of this iron was reabsorbed. I should like to ask Dr. Moore and Dr. Chatterjea if they think that excessive excretion or lack of re-absorption could cause iron deficiency.

---

[1] Gubler, C. J., G. E. Cartwright, and M. M. Wintrobe: J. Biol. Chem. (U.S.A.) **224**, 533 (1957).

[2] Tubiana, M., and E. Frindel: Rev. fr. études clin. biol. **6**, 276 (1961).

MOORE: Dr. VENTURA asked about the nature of the processes of iron absorption in partially gastrectomised patients. I am sorry, but we have done no systematic studies of iron absorption in this type of patient. BAIRD and his associates[1] and STEVENS and FINCH[2], however, have reported that such individuals: a) absorb inorganic iron normally; b) retain less than normal amounts of food iron; and c) fail to absorb iron more efficiently as they become iron deficient. The few observations we have made are in agreement with those findings. To answer Dr. MOESCHLIN's question, it is difficult for me to believe that therapeutic doses of hydrochloric acid could influence these changes. We have never been able to influence the absorption of food iron in patients with achlorhydria by the simultaneous administration of hydrochloric acid.

Whatever iron is lost into the gut is almost certainly partially re-absorbed depending on its form and on the site of its addition to the intestinal tract. No quantitative data, however, can be quoted, so I do not know how to answer Dr. TUBIANA's question.

CALLENDER: Dr. MOORE, your figures on the dietary iron intake in America seem to me extraordinarily high, and I'm sure they would not apply in England. I feel there is a need for investigating, by actual iron estimation, the dietary intake in different parts of the world. Recently we were trying to devise a standard diet for some of our experiments, and the hospital dietician prepared what she thought was an adequate day's intake as calculated from tables. In fact, when we estimated the daily iron content chemically, we found the value to be only something like 6 to 7 mg. I'm quite sure that, although people may be able to afford a high iron diet, personal habits and preferences may reduce the intake very considerably.

MOORE: Your statement about dietary iron in England reinforces my argument that we need more precise information about the dietary intakes of different population groups. I have the impression from talking with Dr. CALLENDER and various of my other British friends that iron-deficiency anaemia is considerably more common in England than it is in the United States. Perhaps the difference in dietary intake is responsible. If a large percentage of the English population does indeed exist on food containing less than 10 mg. iron per day, then it is even more difficult to believe that dermal losses can be more than a fraction of a milligramme.

SALERA: Dr. BEUTLER, have you any information on the cytochrome activity of the heart in experimental iron-deficiency states? I mention this because in clinical experience we find some alterations in the electrocardiogram in iron-deficiency anaemia, and I don't know whether these alterations are due to the iron deficiency of the tissues or to the low blood level of haemoglobin.

BEUTLER: We have not done any studies on cytochrome C activity in the heart. GUBLER and associates[3] found an increase in the cytochrome C activity in the heart, whereas McCALL and his associates[4] report a

[1] BAIRD, I. McL., and G. M. WILSON: Quart. J. Med. (G.B.) **28**, 35 (1959).

[2] STEVENS, A. R. Jr., G. PIRZIO-BIROLI, H. N. HARKINS, L. M. NYHUS, and C. A. FINCH: Ann. Surg. (U.S.A.) **149**, 534 (1959).

[3] GUBLER, C. J., G. E. CARTWRIGHT, and M. M. WINTROBE: J. Biol. Chem. (U.S.A.) **224**, 533 (1957).

[4] McCALL, M. G., G. E. NEWMAN, J. R. P. O'BRIEN, and L. J. WITTS: Brit. J. Nutr. **16**, 305 (1962).

decrease. I'm sure there are many iron enzymes in the heart, and perhaps some of them are more severely affected than cytochrome C.

Hallberg: I should like to comment on Dr. Beutler's paper. I have the impression that the clinical picture in patients with iron deficiency due to a low intake of iron is different from the clinical picture in those with iron deficiency due to a high output of iron. The reason for this may be that, if the patient has a low intake of iron, he also has a low intake of, for instance, zinc. We all know that if we rear animals on a zinc-free diet they develop changes such as hyperkeratosis of the hypopharynx and also abnormalities affecting the claws. These are quite similar to the changes we may see in iron deficiency. You may say that this is not consistent with the observation that, when we give iron to patients with these nail changes, the nails become quite normal. However, all iron preparations, including even the parenteral ones, contain sufficient amounts of zinc.

Beutler: Dr. Hallberg's concept of the low intake or high output causing different clinical pictures in iron deficiency is certainly an interesting one and may very well be entirely correct, and I should like to thank him for his contribution.

Neuro-endocrine control of iron metabolism

By

K. H. Schäfer

It is usually accepted that there are definite pathways for the control of iron metabolism. The following are two examples of a typical and an apparently pre-planned reaction involving iron metabolism as a whole:

1. The characteristic development of hyposideraemia following stress of any sort.
2. The equally characteristic diurnal and nocturnal rhythm of the serum iron level.

Both examples can be taken as test situations which are relevant to the ensuing discussion on the *intermediary* steps in iron metabolism. In this context, however, I do not propose to deal with the *metabolism of exogenous iron*, which involves the still hypothetical concept of extra-enteral control of iron absorption from the gastro-intestinal tract.

The reticulo-endothelial system, since it takes up, stores, and releases iron, is generally regarded as one of the most decisive factors in intermediary iron metabolism. This was already postulated 25 years ago by Heilmeyer and Plötner and has been confirmed by the following experiments and facts:

1. A single stimulus applied to the R.E.S., e.g. an intravenous injection of a storable substance (in our experiments we used colloidal silver), results in changes in intermediary iron metabolism similar to those seen after an infection or some comparable process, such as an allergic antibody-antigen reaction, histamine injection, etc. A fall occurs in the serum iron level, and the R.E.S. takes up iron.
2. When such injections are repeated frequently, the R.E.S. eventually becomes unresponsive to further stimuli, e.g. to a renewed injection of the same storable substance or to an infection. This "blockade" of the R.E.S. is reversible, provided storage has been intermittent and not of excessive duration. On the other hand, however, it may become more or less irreversible if storage has occurred over a prolonged period, as for example in cases of severe transfusion haemosiderosis. I shall later be giving examples of both

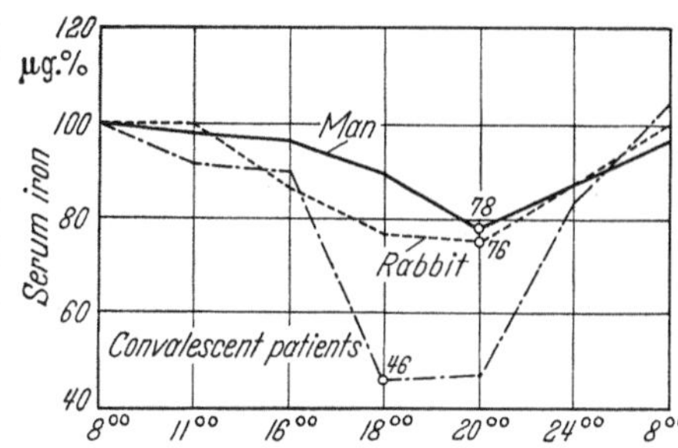

Fig. 1. The 24-hour rhythm of the serum iron levels in man and rabbit (SCHÄFER and BOENECKE)

these situations. *It is therefore not surprising that prior blockade of the R.E.S. will inhibit, or at least reduce, the hyposideraemia usually resulting from stress.*

3. The same also applies to the *diurnal rhythm of the serum iron level*. This rhythm is similar in animals and in man and takes the form of a sinusoid curve over 24 hours. The highest values are reached during the morning and the lowest in the late afternoon and early evening (Fig. 1).

In man, the difference between the values in the morning and in the evening averages between approximately 20 and 40 μg./100 ml. In the rabbit, the range tends to be wider. The degree of rhythm depends on the level of the initial morning values, and this corresponds to WILDER's so-called "law of initial levels"; in other words, one can only expect a clear-cut variation in the diurnal rhythm when the initial levels are medium or high, and not when they are low.

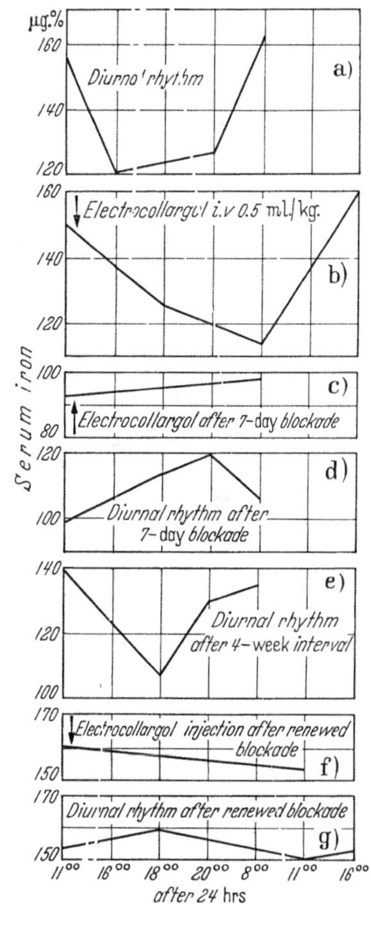

Fig. 2. Suppression of the normal 24-hour serum iron rhythm by repeated injections of a storable substance, Electrocollargol (a colloidal silver preparation), in the rabbit: a) Spontaneous 24-hour rhythm; b) A single injection of the storable substance leads to marked hyposideraemia; c) After daily injection of Electrocollargol for 7 days, blockade occurs, and the serum iron level no longer responds to an injection of this substance; d) The spontaneous 24-hour rhythm is also suppressed; e) After an interval of 4 weeks the normal diurnal rhythm is restored; f) and g) Repetition of the blocking process (SCHÄFER and BOENECKE)

For the purposes of our discussion, it is interesting to note that this diurnal rhythm can be abolished experimentally by blocking the R.E.S. (Fig. 2). Under certain circumstances, the diurnal rhythm may also disappear spontaneously, as illustrated in Fig. 3. Here, the transfusion haemosiderosis was obviously responsible for blockade of the R.E.S. A single injection of a corticosteroid (Medrol) had no effect.

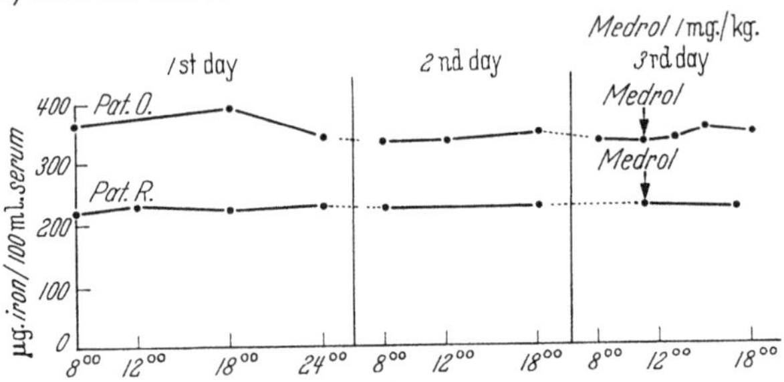

Fig. 3. Absence of 24-hour serum iron rhythm in 2 children with aplastic anaemia and severe transfusion haemosiderosis. No hyposideraemic response to an injection of Medrol

From this it appears that the R.E.S. has a decisive influence on intermediary iron metabolism and that higher regulatory mechanisms, if indeed they exist at all, probably end here.

Table 1. *Factors responsible for hyposideraemia*

I. *Intravenous injection of storable substances:* e.g. colloidal silver

II. *Stress situations:*
e.g. Infections
Bacterial intoxication, e.g. diphtheria, tetanus
Pyrogens, e.g. the colitoxin preparation Pyrifer or the lipopolysaccharide Pyrexal
Turpentine abscesses
Abacterial antibody-antigen reaction, e.g. serum sickness, anaphylactic shock, reverse passive anaphylaxis
Hyperthermia due to overheating
Severe physical exertion
Delivery for the mother, and birth for the baby (see also IV)

III. *Hormones:*
e.g. Cortisol and cortisol derivatives
A.C.T.H. (effect uncertain)
Adrenaline (acetylcholine and physostigmine have no action)
Hormones produced in the tissues, e.g. histamine, serotonin (?)

IV. *Cerebral stimuli* (partly via the stress reaction):
e.g. Intravenous aminophenazone
Short-wave irradiation of the brain-stem
Lumbar puncture, pneumo-encephalography
Intraventricular bleeding
Birth (see also II)

This brings us to the question whether the R.E.S. is subordinated to *higher regulatory controls* influencing the iron uptake, and if so, what is the nature of these controls. Listed in Table 1 are the various substances and other miscellaneous causes which lead to hyposideraemia in man as well as in animals.

Before attempting – by reference to the factors listed in this table – to answer the question as to the existence of higher regulatory controls, I should first like to discuss a few examples of the development of hyposideraemia. In the case of the cerebral stimuli listed, it is apparent that hyposideraemia occurs within 15 minutes following the stimulus. For a stress reaction this appears to be too short; in a naturally occurring stress reaction, several hours are needed before hyposideraemia develops. The same applies to the hyposideraemic response to cortisone and particularly to A.C.T.H., which, incidentally, does not always induce hyposideraemia. These findings suggest that there may be an area in the brain – probably the hypothalamus – which, when stimulated, in turn stimulates the R.E.S. to take up iron. How this occurs is unknown. In this connection it is of interest to note that, of all the hormones and so-called autonomic poisons, adrenaline is the only one leading to the rapid development of hyposideraemia within one hour, or, at the latest, within 3 hours.

It is tempting to assume that stimulation of the R.E.S. by the hypothalamus is mediated via the autonomic nervous system. Though this may indeed be the case, it has so far not been proven. The very rapid response observed would certainly seem to suggest that a neurogenic pathway of this kind is involved.

This hypothesis, which I advance with all due caution, does not exclude the possibility that humoral pathways exist as well. It is quite conceivable, for example, that the pituitary-adrenocortical axis acts as a pathway, as has been postulated in the case of the stress reaction. A schematic representation of the stress reaction would show an interaction between the pituitary-adrenocortical axis and the sympathetic-adrenomedullary axis. Both are under the influence of the hypothalamus. The substances released at the other end of the reaction, i.e. cortisol and adrenaline, lead, as shown, to hyposideraemia.

The R.E.S. can be stimulated via a humoral pathway in response to stress, as a result of which an increase in the iron uptake occurs. We were able to demonstrate the presence of a humoral pathway in the following way:

The spleens of mice were autotransplanted under the skin of the neck. Most of the splenic tissue survived – a fact which could be demonstrated histologically. That it also continued to function normally was confirmed by means of tests with radioactive iron and with red cells. When haemolytic anaemia was induced in intact control animals, the spleen-liver quotient rose to 4.5, whereas in the operated animals the autotransplant-liver quotient rose to 3.5. This showed that function of the autotransplant, though somewhat reduced, was still maintained. The transplanted splenic tissue is, in fact, able to take up radioactive iron and to phagocytose labelled erythrocytes. When a turpentine abscess was

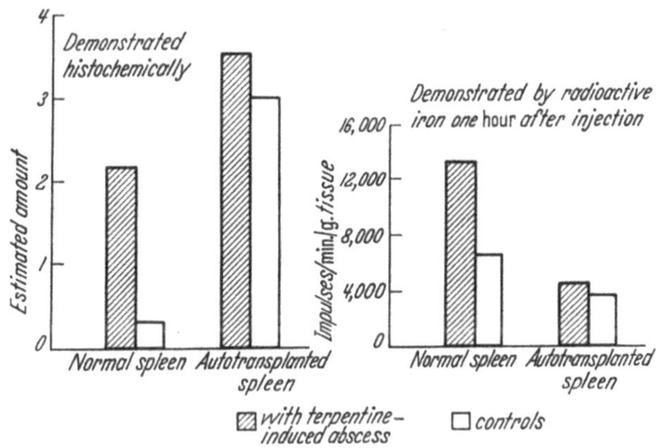

Fig. 4. Demonstration of the storage of iron by the normal and autotransplanted spleen in mice with turpentine abscesses and in controls (mice without turpentine abscesses) (in collaboration with H. HENKE, Univ.-Frauenklinik, Hamburg)

induced in the operated and in the control animals, an increased uptake of iron could be demonstrated by means of radioactive iron, both in the normal spleen as well as in the autotransplanted spleen, although in the case of the latter the increase was less marked (Fig. 4).

By these means it has been demonstrated that, in response to stress, the R.E.S. of the spleen is stimulated to store iron even though denervated; hence a humoral pathway must be involved.

Our attempts to identify in the tissue a specific factor responsible for the humoral action – possibly cortisone – have so far not yielded consistently reproducible results. However, these experiments are being continued.

It is important to determine to what extent the neuro-endocrine regulatory mechanisms discussed depend on the presence of an intact organism. Adrenalectomy, suppression of pituitary function, section of the cervical cord, and even decapitation inhibit stress-induced hyposideraemia and spontaneous rhythm to a greater or lesser degree, but do not abolish it. Shown in Fig. 5 is an example of an experiment on the decapitated cat. It is clear that after decapitation the cat displays practically the same marked hyposideraemic response to overheating as before decapitation.

From this it follows that, even in the absence of a higher regulatory mechanism, iron storage and hyposideraemia still occur. In this instance, the R.E.S. probably reacts just as directly, i.e. with no intermediary regulation, as it does following intravenous injection of colloidal silver. *This implies that, although the R.E.S. may obey the control of a higher regulatory mechanism, it does not depend exclusively upon such a mechanism in order to react in a reasonably physiological fashion.*

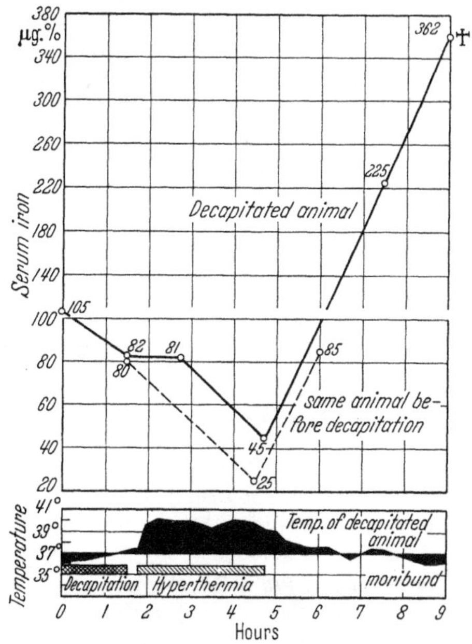

Fig. 5. Serum iron curves in a cat in response to overheating before and after decapitation. Note that after decapitation the cat displays marked hyposideraemia following overheating in the same way as before decapitation (SCHÄFER and BOENECKE)

Similar arguments are now thought to apply to the daily rhythm of biological functions. These, too, do not seem to be under central control, as was formerly believed, but appear to be dependent on mechanisms inherent in the cell itself. It is impossible to explain in any other way the rhythmic variation observed in tissue cultures over a period of 24 hours. The same evidently applies to the observation that the daily rhythm is very rapidly restored in a decapitated animal. Similarly, in a patient with practically no anterior-pituitary function, the serum iron level still shows a marked daily rhythm. Fig. 6 illustrates the pronounced daily rhythm of the serum iron level in two children in whom anterior-pituitary function was almost completely absent.

Such patients also display hyposideraemia as a reaction to stress. It has already been mentioned that stress-induced hyposideraemia can still be observed following adrenalectomy. *From all this it follows that, even in the absence of higher regulatory centres, including absence of the hypothalamus, the sympathetic-adrenomedullary axis, and the pituitary-adrenocortical axis, the organism's iron metabolism is still capable of reacting in a reasonably physiological manner.*

It is interesting to note that, in people who work on nightshifts, e.g. night-nurses, the diurnal serum iron rhythm also becomes reversed. This takes place after a varying interval of time, during

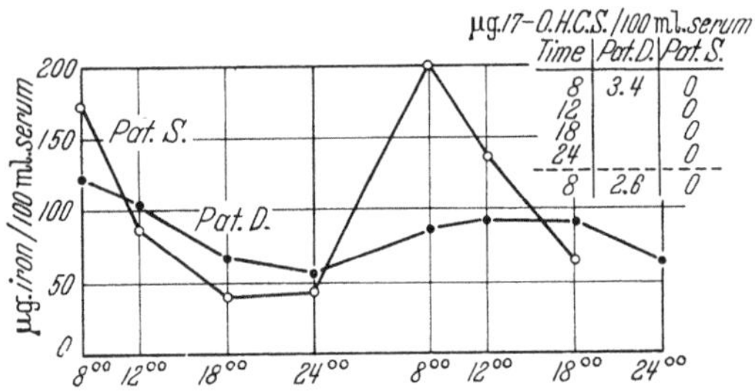

Fig. 6. Diurnal serum iron rhythm in two patients with severe pituitary insufficiency. Note that, although anterior-pituitary function was almost completely absent, there is still a pronounced 24-hour rhythm

which the serum iron level undergoes irregular fluctuations; ultimately, however, the serum iron level in such persons becomes characterised by peak levels in the afternoon and minimum levels at night. *This phenomenon illustrates how the normal rhythmic variation between night and day can be influenced by changes in the subject's way of life with the result that the endogenous rhythm is thereby suppressed.* Nothing is known, however, about the nature of the stimuli which produce such an alteration in rhythm or about the pathways via which they operate.

Finally, it should perhaps be added that a similar process is observed in the premature and newborn infant. In the newborn infant, the serum iron level establishes a day-and-night rhythm after the first few days, whereas in premature infants this process takes longer and requires more time the greater the degree of prematurity. It is not known whether in this connection the factor of prematurity influences the R.E.S. itself or higher regulatory centres. The fact that transient hyposideraemia occurs both in response to the stress of birth (the well-known phenomenon of post-natal hyposideraemia) as well as in response to the administration of cortisone would seem to suggest that higher regulatory centres are involved.

Summary

Neuro-endocrine control of iron metabolism is discussed with reference to the role of the reticulo-endothelial system, but without reference to that of haemopoiesis or of the liver. The following conclusions are drawn:

1. Of those agents not directly connected with haemopoiesis, it is the R.E.S. which reacts upon intermediary iron metabolism. Typical reactions include particularly stress-induced hyposideraemia and the day-and-night rhythm of the serum iron level.

2. The R.E.S. can be stimulated by a single injection of a storable substance, the result being a fall in the serum iron level. Repeated injections of the same substance lead to blockade of the R.E.S.; stress then no longer results in hyposideraemia, and the spontaneous daily rhythm disappears.

3. The hyposideraemia induced by stress is brought about via a humoral pathway, but the humoral agent has not been identified. Although adrenaline and cortisone both have a similar hyposideraemic action, this does not prove that they are the agents normally responsible for influencing the serum iron levels.

4. Cerebral stimuli lead to hyposideraemia within 15 minutes. Probably certain areas of the hypothalamus are stimulated and in turn emit stimuli to the periphery. The pathway of these stimuli is still uncertain. There is evidence to suggest that the sympathetic-adrenomedullary axis and the pituitary-adrenocortical axis are involved.

5. Though the R.E.S. is probably subject to control from these higher regulatory mechanisms, it also has its own independent mode of action. However, our knowledge concerning the regulation of intermediary iron metabolism at these lower levels is still very limited.

Zusammenfassung

Die neuroendokrine Kontrolle des Eisenstoffwechsels wird im Hinblick auf die Rolle, die das retikulo-endotheliale System dabei spielt, besprochen, jedoch ohne Berücksichtigung der Haematopoese und der Leber. Die Schlußfolgerungen sind:

1. Von den nicht direkt mit der Haematopoese in Beziehung stehenden Faktoren beeinflußt das R.E.S. den intermediären Eisenstoffwechsel. Typischer Ausdruck dafür sind besonders die durch Stress hervorgerufene Hyposideraemie und der Tag-Nacht-Rhythmus der Serumeisenkonzentration.

2. Das R.E.S. kann durch eine einzelne Injektion einer speicherfähigen Substanz so angeregt werden, daß es zum Abfall der Serumeisenkonzentration kommt. Wiederholte Injektionen der gleichen Substanz blockieren das R.E.S., so daß Stress in der Folge nicht mehr zu Hyposideraemie führt und der spontane Tagesrhythmus verschwindet.

3. Die durch Stress ausgelöste Hyposideraemie wird auf humoralem Wege vermittelt, jedoch ist der dafür verantwortliche Faktor bisher nicht bekannt. Obwohl Adrenalin und Cortison eine ähnliche hyposideraemische Wirkung besitzen, kann daraus noch nicht geschlossen werden, daß diese beiden Stoffe normalerweise die Serumeisenkonzentration beeinflussen.

4. Zerebrale Reize rufen innerhalb von 15 Minuten eine Hyposideraemie hervor. Wahrscheinlich werden dabei bestimmte Gebiete des Hypothalamus stimuliert, von denen aus dann Reize in die Peripherie gehen. Die Bahnen dafür sind zwar noch unbekannt, jedoch liegen Hinweise dafür vor, daß das System Sympathikus-Nebennierenmark sowie das Hypophysen-Nebennierenrinden-System daran beteiligt sind.

5. Obwohl das R.E.S. wahrscheinlich durch diese übergeordneten Mechanismen kontrolliert wird, besitzt es auch davon unabhängige Wirkungen. Unsere Kenntnisse über die Regulation des intermediären Eisenstoffwechsels auf dieser peripheren Ebene sind jedoch noch sehr begrenzt.

Résumé

La régulation neuro-endocrinienne du métabolisme du fer est envisagée en ce qui concerne le rôle du système réticulo-endothélial, à l'exclusion de celui de l'hématopoïèse et du foie. Les conclusions suivantes peuvent être tirées:

1. Parmi les facteurs qui ne sont pas en relation directe avec l'hématopoïèse, c'est le système réticulo-endothélial qui agit sur le métabolisme intermédiaire du fer. Typiques à ce point de vue sont en particulier l'hyposidérémie provoquée par le *stress*, et la variation diurne et nocturne du fer sérique.

2. La stimulation du système réticulo-endothélial par une injection unique d'une substance qu'il peut fixer provoque une chute du taux du fer sérique. Des injections répétées de la même substance conduisent à un blocage du système réticulo-endothélial; alors un *stress* ne provoque plus d'hyposidérémie et le rythme spontané nycthéméral de la sidérémie disparaît.

3. Une hyposidérémie provoquée par le *stress* relève d'un mécanisme humoral, mais le facteur humoral en cause n'a pas été identifié. Bien que l'adrénaline et la cortisone aient toutes deux une action similaire hyposidérémiante, il n'est pas prouvé que ce sont les agents normalement responsables des modifications du taux du fer sérique.

4. La stimulation cérébrale provoque une hyposidérémie en 15 minutes. Il est probable que certaines aires de l'hypothalamus sont stimulées et émettent à leur tour des stimulations vers la périphérie. Les voies de conduction de ces stimulations sont encore mal connues. Certains faits conduisent à penser que le système sympathique et la médullaire de la surrénale ainsi que l'axe hypophyso-surrénal interviennent.

5. Bien que le système réticulo-endothélial soit probablement soumis au contrôle de ces mécanismes régulateurs supérieurs, il a également son propre mode d'action indépendant. Cependant, nos connaissances sur la régulation du métabolisme intermédiaire du fer à ces niveaux inférieurs sont encore très limitées.

References

Heilmeyer, L., and K. Plötner: Das Serumeisen und die Eisenmangelkrankheit. Jena, 1937. — Schäfer, K. H., and I. Boenecke: Naunyn-Schmiedebergs Arch. exper. Path. (G.) **207**, 666 (1949). — Wilder, J.: Klin. Wschr. (G.) **10**, 1889 (1931).

Discussion

SCHAPIRA: I am interested in the question of fatigue. To what extent can muscular fatigue account for diurnal variations in serum iron?

SCHÄFER: Muscular exercise induced a fall in serum iron as shown in Fig. 1 (p. 281), but more than that I am afraid I cannot say.

KATZ: I should like to ask Dr. SCHÄFER if he believes that the decrease in serum iron in response to reticulo-endothelial stimulation is due to an abstraction of iron from plasma or that it is due, on the other hand, to a decrease in the release of the iron derived from newly broken-down haemoglobin found in the reticulo-endothelial cells.

SCHÄFER: I think that the decrease in serum iron which is observed in the daily rhythm is due to the uptake of iron into the reticulo-endothelial system rather than to a decrease in the release of iron from the reticulo-endothelial system. My reason for believing this is that, if one analyses the body tissues, including especially those of organs containing an abundance of reticulo-endothelial cells, e.g. the spleen and liver, one finds that the amount of iron in them invariably increases. There are several grounds for assuming that the very prompt reaction which occurs within a few minutes in the organism with haemosiderosis is probably due to an active rather than a passive process in the reticulo-endothelial system.

SAADI: I should like you to repeat, if possible, your statement about the question of tissue cultures. I am not quite sure if I understood you correctly, Dr. SCHÄFER, but I believe you said that in tissue cultures there was a diurnal variation in the uptake of iron into the cells from the surrounding fluid.

SCHÄFER: I am glad you raised that point, because there is a difference between what is written in the abstract of my paper which you have before you and what I have just said in my talk to you today. When I prepared the abstract some months ago, I had seen a series of experiments which seemed to show that the macrophages in the tissue culture were able to store iron under the influence of cortisol; but when I continued these experiments, I found that this is not quite so, and I therefore decided not to refer to this in my paper.

Introduction to the General Discussion

By

A. Vannotti

In opening the general discussion on this important problem of iron deficiency, I should like to recapitulate just a few of the points in particular that have already been raised today. First of all, I am sure we are all grateful to Dr. Moore for having given us some very interesting data on the normal iron content of food and on the absorption and excretion of iron in normal subjects. This is extremely important because, although the results of Dr. Moore appear to confirm what we know about the body's iron requirements, we still find in some papers that certain of the values quoted for the absorption and excretion of iron differ from author to author.

Reference has been made today to geographic differences in the iron content of staple diets. On the other hand, Dr. Chatterjea has told us that the distribution of the various forms of iron-deficiency anaemia in India is different from what, on the basis of our clinical observations, we are accustomed to in Europe. Whereas acute or chronic haemorrhage occurs in 80 to 90% of our patients suffering from iron deficiency, the statistics for India show hookworm in 52% of cases, haemorrhages in 39%, and malnutrition in 25%.

Dr. Heilmeyer mentioned that intense iron utilisation was observed by him in patients with anaemia recovering from acute and chronic infectious diseases, as well as in pregnancy and in lactation. We, too, have observed the same phenomenon; in this connection, however, we must not forget the intense iron utilisation which also occurs during the process of tissue regeneration. This can be seen in liver-regeneration experiments after subtotal hepatectomy, in which there is an intense increase in cytochrome C and a high concentration of iron *in situ*.

With regard to the question of iron excretion, it was interesting to learn from Dr. Moore that, although – as we all know – urinary iron excretion is normally very low, iron can also leave the body through the skin. We have been told that the daily cutaneous loss of iron can amount to as much as 3 – 6 mg., especially in hot climates. Is it possible that this may partly account for the iron deficiency observed in India? I should also like to know whether or not the cutaneous loss of iron is important in febrile and infectious diseases. Conversely, it would be interesting to discover whether, in cases involving destruction of very large areas of skin by burns, the excretion of iron is correspondingly reduced.

As for the problem of iron absorption, this still does not seem to have been completely solved. In human pathology, there are still some cases in which one finds it difficult to reconcile one's observations with GRANICK's theory of the ferritin mechanism regulating iron absorption in the intestinal mucosa. In recent years, many authors have demonstrated that iron can be absorbed not only via the ferritin system, but also in the form of various chelates. The iron seems to form chelates with a variety of substances, such as organic acids, amino acids, sugars, and other biological substances, which are either produced by intestinal secretion or contained in the food. This possibility would explain the absorption of iron through the intestine without the intermediary activity of the ferritin system. I should like to ask if there is any confirmatory evidence on this point, since the whole problem is an extremely important one as regards human pathology. In this connection, I am thinking particularly of the increased iron absorption encountered in haemochromatosis or in the presence of liver damage, as well as in pancreatitis or following pancreatectomy.

Another interesting point concerns hyposiderosis; here it should be noted that a low iron level in the blood, i.e. hyposideraemia, is not necessarily a sign of iron deficiency. This is the case, for instance, in infectious anaemia, in uraemia, and in patients with cancer. It must therefore be concluded that, besides the blood and tissue compartments of the iron pool, there must be some other compartments – especially in the reticulo-endothelial and possibly other tissues – which can modify the distribution of iron and its intermediary metabolism. Dr. MORGAN has suggested that the iron reserves in tissues such as muscle and connective tissue may be less easily mobilised than in certain other tissues, e.g. those of the liver and spleen. This might also account for one of our own observations with regard to iron mobilisation by means of chelating agents, such as desferrioxamine, in liver cirrhosis. We found that, whereas it is very easy to mobilise iron from the normal liver or from the livers of patients with haemochromatosis, it is most difficult to mobilise it from a cirrhotic liver, in other words, from a liver in which fibrotic infiltration has occurred.

Dr. MORGAN also drew attention to a very significant observation concerning the increase in plasma transferrin in the presence of iron-deficiency anaemia. This increase, which has not only been noted in animals, but has also been observed by LAURELL and ourselves in human beings, cannot be satisfactorily explained for the moment. Dr. MORGAN thinks that the increased transferrin level might be due to the fall in the blood haemoglobin concentration. It is possible, however, that this mechanism may be more complicated than Dr. MORGAN supposes and may conceivably be related to hepatic function. In this connection, it may be recalled that transferrin levels are decreased in liver diseases and that LAURELL has pointed to a correlation between the concentration of albumin and transferrin in the plasma and the activity of the liver. A relationship between liver and transferrin has also been reported by Dr. MORGAN on the basis of findings following hepatectomy. It is possible that, in iron deficiency, the production of transferrin may be increased in response to hepatic and hormonal influences. We ourselves also found a high level of transferrin in pregnancy, and in this instance it is interesting to observe that not only the transferrin, but also the T.B.P. (the specific carrier of thyroxine) is increased. The hormonal influence emanating from the protein synthesis of active plasma proteins such as transferrin, transcortin, and T.B.P. has been observed during recent years in various conditions, especially in the presence of liver damage – a fact which underlines the very important role which the different plasma protein fractions play in the transport of active substances.

Finally, I should like to revert once again to the problem of hyposiderosis. It has often been pointed out that the turnover of tissue iron is very low. It is true that the life-span of myoglobin is extremely long (more than one month), but the life-span of cytochrome C is shorter (2—4 weeks), and that of the catalase is only 10 days. It is clear that in chronic anaemia the myoglobin level shows no marked change; on the other hand, as Dr. BEUTLER has noted, in chronic iron deficiency a reduction occurs in the levels of cytochrome C and catalase in the tissues. There are a variety of conditions in which cytochrome C undergoes very significant quantitative alterations. It is well known, for example, that in hyperthyroidism the cytochrome C levels increase in the muscles and in the liver, as observed by DRABKIN, TISSIÈRES, and ourselves. We also found that an increase in cytochrome C occurs in response to chronic hypoxaemia and to starvation, during which the oxygen consumption of the liver rises. In this context, it is interesting to note Dr. BEUTLER's finding concerning the decrease in oxidase in the case of leucocytes in iron deficiency.

Quite apart from all the clinical signs and symptoms of iron deficiency, the iron content of the tissues has a very important bearing on local oxygen consumption, as illustrated by an interesting case of ours which I should like briefly to describe. This case, which dates back to 1942, was that of an 18-year-old girl suffering from hyperthyroidism and chronic anaemia with a haemoglobin level of 38%. Prior to treatment, her serum iron was 10 μg.% and she presented classic symptoms of hyperthyroidism, although her metabolic rate was relatively low (+9.6% — +19%). After oral treatment with iron and after iron injections, the serum iron level rose to 80 μg.%. The haemoglobin remained low (42%), but the metabolic rate increased to +24% – +34%, and the patient then developed very severe hyperthyroidism.

This case seems to indicate that a lack of tissue iron in a patient with hyperthyroidism may well lead to a diminution in the rate of cellular combustion. It is also interesting to note that, judging from this case, treatment with iron appears to offset primarily the deficiency of tissue iron and only secondarily, and to a less significant degree, the deficiency of iron for erythropoiesis. This is very intriguing, because as a general rule iron metabolism seems to be concentrated upon the task of maintaining normal erythropoiesis, whereas the rate of iron metabolism in the tissues is very low.

Last year we had an opportunity of studying thyroid function with radioactive iodine in a similar case. We were able to confirm our previous observation that, in cases of iron-deficiency anaemia associated at the same time with hyperthyroidism, treatment with iron stimulates the B.M.R. Incidentally, another finding encountered in response to iron treatment in cases of severe iron deficiency is an increase in hydrochloric-acid secretion by the gastric mucosa.

I hope that these few points I have raised will pave the way for a fruitful discussion. That we shall have much to discuss, I feel sure, because it seems to me that the problem of iron deficiency is still far from having been solved.

References

DRABKIN, D. L.: Physiol. Rev. (U.S.A.) **31**, 435 (1951). — LAURELL, C. B.: In: F. W. PUTNAM: The Plasma Proteins, Vol. I. Academic Press, New York, 1960, p. 351. — TISSIÈRES, A.: Arch. internat. physiol. (Belg.) **54**, 305 (1946). — VANNOTTI, A.: In: W. KEIDERLING: Eisenstoffwechsel. Georg Thieme, Stuttgart, 1959.

General Discussion

SCHAPIRA: We have to remember the importance of GRANICK's[1] theory in his time. It gave impetus to many studies, and I think we are still waiting for someone to come up with a better theory.

I feel there is another point that should also be emphasised. The induction of the synthesis of apoferritin by iron is one of the first examples of the adaptational synthesis of a protein in mammalian cells. The synthesis of this protein in a cell-free system has still to be demonstrated. Dr. SAADI in our laboratory is carrying out experiments along these lines.

POLLYCOVE: With reference to Dr. KATZ's question regarding Dr. SCHÄFER's paper, I have one comment on the question as to how the plasma iron level decreases in response to stress. We have studied several individuals who were placed in a high-altitude chamber at 15,000—17,000 feet. While they were under this stress, a series of iron turnover studies were performed. Though the plasma iron concentration decreased from an average of 125 μg./100 ml. to 80 μg./100 ml. within 2 hours, the removal of iron from the plasma remained constant. These data indicate that an increase in the uptake of plasma iron by the reticulo-endothelial cells did not occur and that, in response to the stress of hypoxia, there was a decrease in the reticulo-endothelial release into the plasma of iron derived from erythrophagocytosis, which resulted in a diminution of plasma iron. The reduced plasma iron concentration shifts the equilibrium of iron between the plasma and the reticulo-endothelial cells toward the plasma. Finally, the reticulo-endothelial cells, though they are more retentive of iron, at an appropriately low concentration of plasma iron now release the amount of iron that is required for haemoglobin synthesis. Similarly, when the stress abates, the reticulo-endothelial cells then release iron more rapidly, thereby increasing the plasma iron concentration until a new equilibrium is established at a higher normal level.

CHATTERJEA: Dr. VANNOTTI was wondering why the incidence of iron deficiency due to haemorrhage was so small in my series in contrast to his experience in Switzerland. The anaemia in hookworm infestation is obviously due to haemorrhage. Thus, in my series of 120 cases, haemorrhage was the cause of anaemia not in 39 cases only, but in as many as 95 cases. For various reasons discussed in my paper, I had placed the hookworm group in a separate category. Aetiologically, the hookworm group should belong to the haemorrhagic type, i.e. insofar as the mechanism of the production of anaemia is concerned.

I should like to make one point regarding the secretion of gastric hydrochloric acid. In iron deficiency of nutritional origin, a high percentage of patients show achlorhydria. In the majority of cases the acid returns after a course of iron treatment, and this achlorhydria is in fact generally reversible. From our follow-up data we are of the opinion that achlorhydria is the effect and not the cause of iron deficiency in the average type of case we see in India.

---

[1] GRANICK, S.: Bull. N. Y. Acad. Med. **25**, 403 (1949).

BEARN: I wonder whether there is any relationship between the iron-deficiency anaemias and the abnormal haemoglobins. Are any particular gene types relatively protected?

CHATTERJEA: In accordance with the suggestion of HALDANE[1], as supported by SIJPESTEIN[2], we attempted to find out whether or not the haemoglobinopathy trait would offer resistance to the development of iron deficiency. Our findings did not provide any evidence to confirm this notion. I should perhaps point out in this connection that the assumption that iron absorption is increased in the thalassaemia trait also derives no support from recent studies on iron absorption (ERLANDSON[3]). Incidentally, it may be worth-while mentioning that our patients suffering from haemoglobin E-thalassaemia did appear to show resistance to induced *P. vivax* infection[4].

FIGUEROA: Dr. HEILMEYER, you had a slide that showed serum iron levels in haemolytic anaemia – with some high, some normal, and some low. I have been impressed by the number of patients with haemolytic anaemia who had a normal serum iron; I was therefore wondering whether you could establish any correlation between the serum iron levels and the type of haemolytic anaemia, the stage of the disease, its duration, and the number of transfusions.

HEILMEYER: We were unable to find any correlation with the type of haemolytic anaemia, the duration of the disease, or the number of transfusions. The height of the serum iron level is determined primarily by the outflow of iron due to enhanced erythropoiesis and by the inflow of iron resulting from the breakdown of erythrocytes. If these two are equally balanced, then the serum iron level will be normal; if erythropoiesis predominates, the serum iron decreases; if the destruction of erythrocytes predominates, it increases. Thus, even in one and the same case, one may observe marked fluctuations in the serum iron at different times.

SCHUBERT: I should just like to make one comment that cytochrome oxidase activity is directly related to iron metabolism, at least in experimental animals, monkeys and rats. But you cannot inhibit the enzyme *in vivo* chronically by means of iron deficiency; such inhibition can only be induced by administering cuprous chelating agents such as cyanide or azide or by means of copper deficiency. In copper-deficient animals, administration of copper, but not of iron, reactivates the cytochrome oxidase. It might be interesting to see whether cytochrome oxidase activity is affected in disturbances of iron metabolism and whether correlations with the clinical picture exist. There is a direct relationship between cytochrome oxidase activity and iron metabolism in that the synthesis of protohaem and haem is diminished, leading to an anaemia. For further details I would refer you to the paper by GALLAGHER[5].

---

[1] HALDANE, J. B. S.: Ric. sc. (It.) Suppl., p. 75 (1949).

[2] SIJPESTEIN, J. A. K.: Enige vormen van erfelijke niet-spherocytaire anaemie bij kinderen. Oppenheim, Groningen, 1955.

[3] ERLANDSON, M. E., et al.: Blood (U.S.A.) **19**, 359 (1962).

[4] CHATTERJEA, J. B., et al.: Bull. Calcutta School Trop. Med. **4**, 105 (1956).

[5] GALLAGHER, C. H., et al.: Proc. Roy. Soc. London **145**, 134, 195 (1956).

Iron overload

The metabolism of iron in haemochromatosis

By

J.-C. Dreyfus and G. Schapira

In the present study, we propose to confine our remarks to idiopathic haemochromatosis, this being the only illness in which the primary and essential disorder is an overload of iron in the organism which cannot be ascribed to any external cause.

Many of the characteristics of idiopathic haemochromatosis have long been known. Having described its biochemical manifestations, we shall concentrate particularly on two of the three fields with which recent research has mainly been concerned, i.e. genetics and pathogenesis, the third aspect being therapeutics, which will be dealt with elsewhere in this Symposium.

I. Biochemical diagnosis and modifications in the metabolism of iron

There are a number of tests by which the diagnosis of idiopathic haemochromatosis can be confirmed, these tests revealing abnormalities in various facets of iron metabolism.

1. Determination of the serum iron concentration (sideraemia) and of the iron-binding capacity of the serum sheds light on disturbances affecting iron transport.

a) *The increase in the serum iron concentration (hypersideraemia)* was the first anomaly to be discovered in patients suffering from idiopathic haemochromatosis and is also the easiest to determine. Hypersideraemia is, in fact, present in the great majority of cases; but, since serum iron levels are liable to range between wide extremes, strict criteria must be adopted when interpreting the results of serum iron determinations. Less than 5 % of normal adult subjects display serum iron levels exceeding 190 μg. % in the case of males, and 180 μg. % in the case of females, although the figures quoted by various authors do vary to some extent.

Table 1 lists the average values obtained from the literature, as compared with the values based on determinations made by ourselves and F. SCHAPIRA and with values obtained by us in cases of haemochromatosis (69 men and 17 women).

Table 1. *Normal serum iron values obtained from the literature and from personal observations, as compared with pathological values from 86 cases of haemochromatosis*

Source of data (values expressed in μg./100 ml.)	Men		Women	
	Average	$+2\sigma$	Average	$+2\sigma$
Normal values selected from the literature	129	193	110	168
Normal values from our own determinations	134	185	123	179
Values obtained by us in 86 cases of haemochromatosis	225	385	213	331

In roughly 80% of cases of haemochromatosis, the serum iron concentrations are pathologically elevated. However, in view of the incidence of normal values in the remaining 20%, absence of hypersideraemia does not exclude the possibility of haemochromatosis.

An increase in serum iron is particularly suggestive of haemochromatosis if anaemia is either absent or merely of a moderate and normochromic type, because hypersideraemia may also be observed in the course of pernicious, haemolytic, Mediterranean, and aplastic anaemia, as well as in patients with acute hepatitis and often in cases of liver cirrhosis.

b) *The iron-binding capacity of the serum.* Iron is transported in the plasma by a protein known as siderophilin or transferrin. In the concentration in which it is normally present in the plasma (0.25–0.30 g./100 ml.), transferrin is capable of binding 300 to 350 μg. iron. Since the level of iron in the serum averages 140 μg., the transferrin is not saturated. The amount of iron which a given serum is capable of binding – in addition to the quantity which it already contains – is referred to as its latent binding capacity; the total amount of iron which it can bind (latent capacity + serum iron) is referred to as its total binding capacity; the coefficient of saturation is the product of $\frac{\text{serum iron}}{\text{total iron-binding capacity}}$. This coefficient normally works out at 0.35–0.40. It is frankly pathological if it exceeds 0.60.

In haemochromatosis, the total iron-binding capacity is somewhat diminished by the decrease in siderophilin; the latent binding capacity is greatly diminished or even reduced to nil; the coefficient of saturation is over 0.8 and sometimes as high as 1.0.

The increase in the coefficient of saturation is the most reliable indicator of haemochromatosis, and only in exceptional cases does this increase fail to occur. It is even observed when the serum iron is normal; in such cases, the relatively low serum iron level is probably due to a marked decrease in the synthesis of transferrin associated with hepatic insufficiency. There are certain other conditions (e.g. hepatitis, haemolysis) in which the coefficient of saturation may rise, but, except in the case of secondary haemosiderosis, it never shows such a high increase as in haemochromatosis.

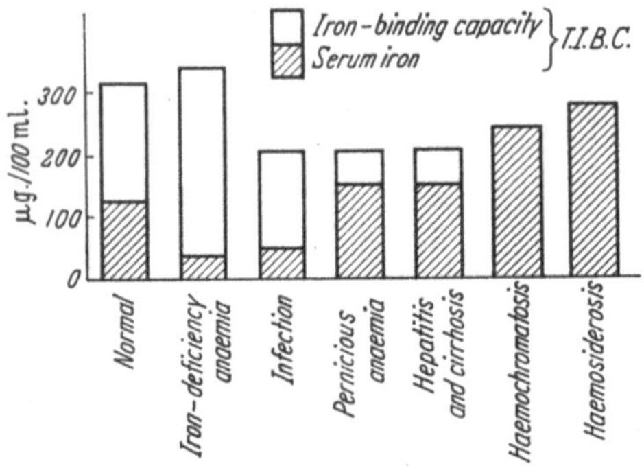

Fig. 1. Serum iron and iron-binding capacity (total iron-binding capacity) in normal subjects and in various pathological conditions

Fig. 1 illustrates the respective serum iron levels and iron-binding capacities encountered in various diseases.

2. Study of the absorption of iron is of major theoretical importance, because it is the rate of iron absorption – and not of its excretion – which regulates the metabolism of iron, and because an overload of iron can result only from an abnormal increase in iron absorption.

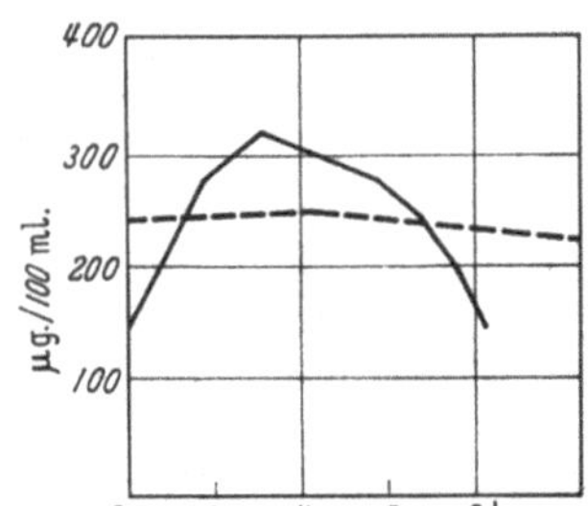

Fig. 2. Normal iron-tolerance curve as compared with the iron-tolerance curve in haemochromatosis. —— control; - - - haemochromatosis

a) *The oral iron-tolerance test* (absorption of a ferrous salt at the rate of 3 or 4 mg./kg.) yields characteristic results, whose significance, however, has long been subject to doubt. In the normal individual, the curve rises and reaches 300 μg. after 4 hours, after which it falls to the initial level within about 10 hours. In patients with haemochromatosis, the curve remains flat and shows no rise at all (Fig. 2).

The first interpretation placed on these curves was that patients suffering from haemochromatosis do not absorb the iron administered, because the intestinal cells are in a refractory state; it was therefore assumed that excessive iron absorption must have occurred at some time prior to the disease. Today, it is generally accepted that the iron is in fact absorbed, but that, since it does not encounter in the plasma any siderophilin capable of retaining it, it passes immediately into the tissues. This interpretation has been borne out by two types of test:

b) *The intravenous iron-tolerance test.* After a prompt rise, the curve in normal subjects gradually drops to initial values, whereas in patients with haemochromatosis the initial values are regained much more rapidly. This rapid decrease is due to the absence of free iron-binding protein in the plasma and possibly also to the fact that the tissues display an avidity for iron for which no explanation has yet been found.

c) *The radioactive iron-absorption test* involves a delicate technique and is difficult to interpret, since, according to various authors, the results vary considerably depending on the dose and on the material employed (ferrous or ferric iron, haemoglobin, dietary iron).

The proportion of the iron absorbed does, in fact, vary within wide limits according to whether the radioactive iron is administered in the form of a tracer dose (a few μg.) either separately or added to a variable amount (1–100 mg.) of ordinary iron. In some cases of haemochromatosis, the test has even yielded negative findings (Chodos et al.; Finch and Finch). In the majority of cases, however, absorption does appear to be increased – as recently confirmed by methods based on the use of a scintillation counter, which enables one to determine the radioactivity in the whole body and thus to make a direct measurement of the quantity absorbed, instead of calculating it by reference to the difference between the dose administered and the amount excreted in the faeces. The situation is complicated, however, by the fact that the results obtained may differ in one and the same patient at various stages of the disease. Finally, studies undertaken with mineral iron yield results which are probably not directly comparable with those obtained in the far less numerous investigations designed to evaluate the absorption of dietary iron.

3. Utilisation of iron. Patients suffering from haemochromatosis usually display no haematopoietic disorders and no anaemia. Hence, the presence of hypochromic anaemia is strongly suggestive of some alternative diagnosis, such as hypochromic hypersideraemic anaemia or sideroachrestic anaemia. Further clues may be obtained from dynamic tests with radioactive iron (ferrokinetics), which reveal characteristic modifications.

a) *Plasma iron* (Table 2). Normally, when a tracer dose of radioactive iron of high specific activity is added to the plasma *in vitro* and then administered intravenously, the radioactive iron disappears according to an exponential law; this reflects the normal flow of plasma iron into the "metabolic pool" of iron. If the values for the iron concentration in the blood and for the plasma volume are known, the rate of renewal of the plasma iron can be calculated.

Table 2. *Rate of renewal of plasma iron (average values)*

	Renewal of plasma iron		Fraction of total plasma iron withdrawn per hour
	in mg./day	in mg./kg./day	
Normal subjects	30	0.46	0.46
Haemochromatosis	50	0.80	0.43
Haemochromatosis treated by venesection	87	1.55	0.89
Cytosiderosis	34	0.46	0.29

Difficulties and errors of interpretation are liable to arise, however, some of which may be related to the conditions of observation. Since the iron-binding capacity of the serum is diminished in patients with haemochromatosis, direct injection of iron salt is out of the question in such cases; on the other hand, incubation of iron salts with the patient's serum *in vitro* may give rise to errors; the amount of iron added must therefore be small (less than 300 μg.) and the injection administered slowly.

The nature of the curves observed in some normal subjects may also result in errors of interpretation. Moreover, in the majority of cases of haemochromatosis, disappearance of the radioactive iron during the first few minutes is extremely rapid and non-exponential, becoming exponential only in the hours that follow.

When interpreting the exponential portion of the curve, it should be borne in mind that the radioactive iron, having first penetrated into the extravascular spaces, does not return to the plasma in any appreciable quantity during this period; the results obtained can therefore be used to calculate the rate of renewal of iron in the plasma.

On the other hand, the fate of the radioactive iron which rapidly disappears during the first few minutes is uncertain. Some of it is undoubtedly accumulated in the liver, and some of it is released into the circulation again, as evidenced by the radioactive iron content of the red-cell mass, which is greater than would be anticipated judging from its initial rate of change in the β_1-globulin of the plasma. The factors responsible for this return of iron into the circulation are still unknown.

The time taken for renewal of the plasma iron is somewhat prolonged, i.e. 160 minutes on the average (extremes: 118–244), as compared with the normal time of 100 minutes (FINCH), a figure which BOTHWELL, too, regards as normal. On the other hand, the quantity renewed each day is increased, i.e. 46 mg., instead of 37 mg., according to FINCH, and 56 mg., instead of 32 mg., according to BOTHWELL; this is equivalent to 0.80 mg./kg./day instead of 0.46 mg./kg./day. The disparity between the renewal time and the quantity renewed is explained by the high concentration of iron in the serum: in the normal subject, the plasma contains a total of about 3.5 mg. iron, as compared with about 6 mg. in patients with haemochromatosis.

The repeated venesections undertaken as a form of treatment in such patients lead to a marked increase in the iron renewal of the plasma.

b) *Red-cell iron* (Table 3). When a tracer dose of radioactive iron is injected intravenously, it is possible to measure its speed of utilisation by reference to the synthesis of haemoglobin and the coefficient of iron utilised during the process of synthesis. If the speed of utilisation is unchanged, the coefficient of utilisation falls from 75 ± 10% to 30–40%: the iron administered seems to be diverted from the synthesis of haemoglobin and stored instead (Fig. 3).

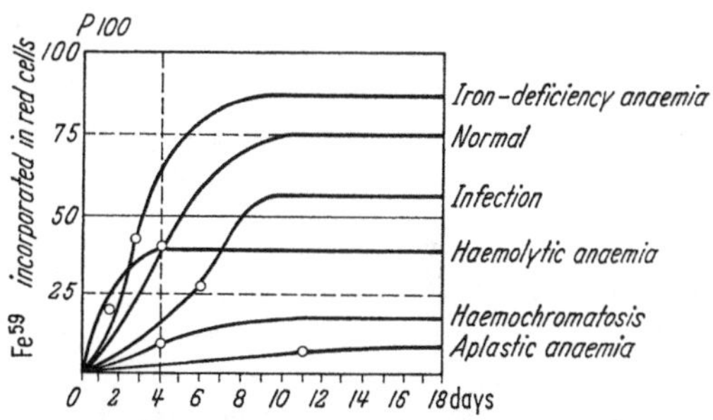

Fig. 3. Utilisation of radioactive iron by the red cells in normal subjects and in various pathological conditions

The utilisation of radioactive iron by the red cells is, in fact, inversely proportional to the

Table 3. *Rate of renewal of red-cell iron (average values)*

	Renewal of red-cell iron		Fraction of red cells renewed each day
	in mg./day	in mg./kg./day	
Normal subjects	24	0.38	0.013
Haemochromatosis	23	0.47	0.017
Haemochromatosis treated by venesection	76	1.36	0.076

amount of iron present in the iron stores, and the total quantity of iron utilised by the red cells remains normal, i.e. 23–29 mg./day.

Knowing the volume of the plasma and the rate of renewal of plasma iron, it is possible to calculate the rate of renewal of haemoglobin iron: since the fraction of red-cell iron renewed each day is normal, the average life-span of the red cells is also normal.

Haematopoiesis being normal, the anomalies affecting the incorporation of radioactive iron in patients with haemochromatosis merely reflect the tendency of the organism to build up excessive stores of this metal.

4. Elimination of iron. The rate of spontaneous iron elimination is very low, both in patients with haemochromatosis as well as in healthy subjects.

a) *Haemosiderin granules.* ROUS advocated investigation of the haemosiderin granules as far back as 1918, but the results yielded by such research proved extremely inconsistent and have no practical value.

b) *Urinary iron.* Though normally amounting to less than 1 mg./day, urinary iron excretion was found by SCHWARZMANN to exceed 1,200 μg. in 6 out of 15 patients studied. This increase in urinary iron excretion, however, is not a consistent finding and would in any case not be sufficient to offset the excessive absorption of iron.

c) *Induced excretion of iron in the urine (induced sideruria).* It was WARTER and WEILL (*46*) who suggested that urinary iron excretion might be enhanced by infusing E.D.T.A. By this means it was found possible in patients with haemosiderosis to increase urinary iron excretion to more than 1 mg./day, as compared with less than 0.60 mg./day in normal subjects and patients suffering from ordinary liver cirrhosis. But this method seemed to us to be of limited practical value, because it is very difficult to determine accurately quantities of iron amounting to less than 1 μg./ml. urine. The principle underlying such treatment, however, is of great interest and might be much more effectively exploited with the more active chelating agents which have meanwhile become available, e.g. D.T.P.A. and desferrioxamine. Following an intramuscular injection of 400 mg. desferrioxamine, normal subjects excrete approximately 1 mg. iron in the 24-hour urine, whereas patients with haemochromatosis excrete at least 15 mg. (see below in the section on treatment).

5. Storage of iron. The essential biochemical disorder responsible for idiopathic haemochromatosis is an excessive deposition of iron in the tissues, demonstration of which furnishes indisputable confirmation of the diagnosis (*32*). Excessive iron storage occurs not only in the liver and spleen, but also in the pancreas and other endocrine organs, with the exception of the sexual glands.

a) *Needle biopsy of the liver* is still the most important bioptic test (Fig. 4), despite the interest which attaches to other forms of biopsy.

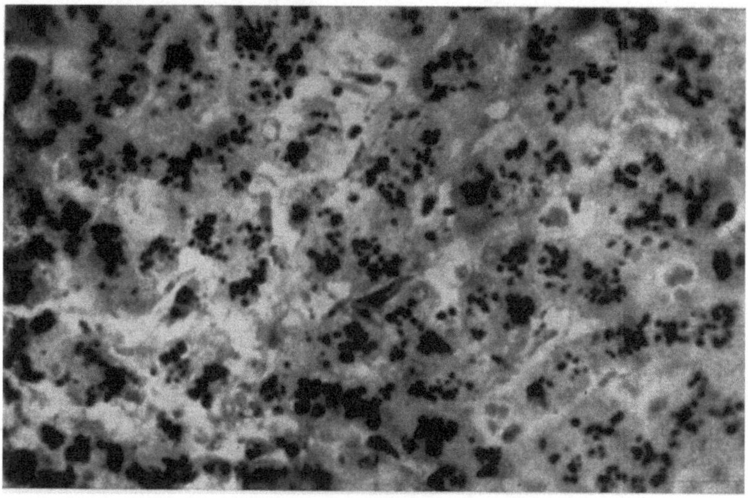

Fig. 4. Liver biopsy section stained for iron

In the initial phase of the disease, haemosiderin granules are found within the hepatic cells, including especially the cellular elements dispersed in the periphery of the lobule. The granules first appear as fine granulations accumulated towards the biliary pole of the cell, but tend later to invade the whole of the cell. When the accumulation has become massive and the structure of the cell altered, the granulations adhere to one another, forming irregular and intensely coloured clumps of pigment. If the cells are finally destroyed, these clumps of pigment are released into the sclerous tissue and may simulate macrophages. This siderosis is coupled with sclerosis, which is at first insular and perilobular, but which ultimately involves the parenchymal tissue and may sometimes be associated with lymphoplasmocyte infiltrations.

Deposition of pigments also affects – though at a later stage – the Kupffer cells. The view generally accepted is that, in idiopathic haemosiderosis, deposition of pigments primarily involves the parenchymal tissues, whereas in transfusion haemosiderosis it is in the Kupffer cells that the pigments are primarily deposited. But exceptions to this rule have been reported (Caroli and Etévé). Two main difficulties are encountered with regard to the histological interpretation of material obtained by liver biopsy (*1*, *25*):

Firstly, in cases examined in the initial stages of the illness, iron deposition associated with a minimal degree of sclerosis poses the problem of defining the limits of the disease. This is often the case with siblings or with the children of parents with a confirmed history of haemochromatosis.

Secondly, in certain forms of liver cirrhosis, there is marked sclerosis with moderate siderosis – which often makes it difficult to distinguish between cirrhosis complicated by siderosis and true haemochromatosis.

Needle biopsy of the liver usually lends itself only to histological interpretation. According to certain authors [Warter; Bueckel et al. (cf. *46*)], however, chemical determinations might also yield information of great interest. It seems reasonable to assume that in haemochromatosis there must be a correlation between chemistry and histology. On the other hand, in cases of liver cirrhosis, there would presumably be no such correlation, because the haemosiderotic pigmentation would be far more intense than justified by the amount of iron present. The haemosiderin is more easily visible through the light microscope than the ferritin, and one possible hypothesis is that the haemosiderin is relatively increased at the expense of the ferritin[1].

b) *Other forms of biopsy,* such as skin biopsy or gastric biopsy, which may also be envisaged, will not be discussed in detail here.

Skin biopsy, the results of which can be regarded as valid only if they are positive, yields findings that are too inconsistent.

Gastric biopsy has been proposed by Althausen. In normal subjects, no iron deposits seem to occur in the gastric mucosa, whereas in patients with haemochromatosis pigmentation is found in the tubular glands and in the interstitial tissue. Gastric secretion, however, remains unaffected. The significance of gastric biopsy has been demonstrated by the studies of Debray, of Cachin, and of Besançon; but the method is not widely employed and has not replaced needle biopsy of the liver.

c) *Sternal puncture.* Advocated in 1948 by Rath and Finch, and investigated in detail by Mouriquand (*32*), sternal puncture yields material showing intense ferric pigmentation, and the results

[1] The lysosomes (containing proteolytic enzymes and phosphatases) are rich in ferritin, as was also found to be the case in a patient with haemochromatosis studied by Novikoff and Essner (*34*).

obtained by MOURIQUAND have recently been confirmed by electron-microscopic studies (*2*). Nevertheless, some authors refuse to ascribe much diagnostic value to this method on the grounds that the results are allegedly unreliable and might also prove positive in other conditions besides haemochromatosis, e.g. infections, haemolytic syndromes, and hypersideraemic hypochromic anaemia.

6. Conclusions. The preceding account shows that haemochromatosis is associated with disorders affecting most of the stages in the metabolism of iron. For the clinician, the two indispensable biological tests are determination of serum iron and calculation of the coefficient of saturation of the serum; these, coupled with his assessment of the clinical picture, should enable him to diagnose haemochromatosis with a high degree of accuracy. However, before regarding the diagnosis as confirmed and instituting treatment accordingly, there is much to be said for performing needle biopsy of the liver, since, in established cases of haemochromatosis, the results of the biopsy will generally leave no doubts as to the correctness of the diagnosis. It is in doubtful cases or in patients in whom the disease is still in its initial stages that further diagnostic tests – such as measurement of urinary iron excretion following administration of iron-chelating agents or chemical determination of the iron content of material obtained by liver biopsy – may well prove of additional value.

II. Treatment

We wish to make only a brief reference to treatment, since this very important subject will be discussed in detail in other papers to be presented here. We would merely recall in this connection that since 1950 the method of repeated venesection has offered us one means by which to remove from the organism much of the excess iron accumulating in patients with haemochromatosis (*8*, *11*, *12*, *18*). This method, which has now become the classic form of treatment, has lately been supplemented by the use of chelating agents: following initial attempts at treatment with B.A.L. (*46*) and E.D.T.A., compounds such as D.T.P.A. and desferrioxamine (*30*, *40*) have now been developed which are capable of removing large quantities of iron or even of preventing the absorption of iron (*49*).

Interestingly enough, it would seem that these two types of treatment, i.e. venesection and the use of chelating agents, are not mutually exclusive; on the contrary, employed simultaneously, they may even help to rid patients of their excess iron at a faster rate. The outlook for patients suffering from haemochromatosis – and particularly for those with transfusion haemosiderosis – thus now appears to be much brighter than only a few years ago.

III. Genetic problems

Since the publication of SHELDON's studies, idiopathic haemochromatosis has been regarded as a congenital disease. In view of the slowness of its evolution, and the fact that the iron accumulates day by day in such minute quantities, it must indeed be assumed that the onset of the accumulation dates back to childhood. As a congenital metabolic disease, it is in all probability also a familial one. Numerous authors have endeavoured to demonstrate its familial character and, subsequently, to discover more about its genetic transmission.

1. General remarks. The problem arising in this connection can be considered on either the clinical or the biological plane. From the clinical aspect, there undoubtedly exist families in which several members directly related to one another, e.g. siblings or cousins, have presented the full clinical picture of haemochromatosis. Such families, however, are rare, and the incidence of haemochromatosis within them is usually only sporadic. For the purposes of statistical study, we are therefore obliged to invoke biological stigmata and to consider, first and foremost, signs and symptoms of iron-overloading. But before entering into details of such studies and the results which they may furnish, we should perhaps first discuss their validity.

Here we are confronted with two opposing points of view. According to one view, except in cases of idiopathic or induced haemochromatosis (transfusional, nutritional cytosiderosis), liver biopsy – particularly if performed in young subjects – will fail to reveal any iron deposition. According to the other view, haemochromatosis may be regarded as one aspect of liver cirrhosis, in the course of which deposition of iron is provoked by the selfsame causes as led to the cirrhosis. Thus, for example, MACDONALD and MALLORY (*28*, *29*), as well as CACHIN, CAROLI, and their colleagues, report that, when autopsies are performed on cirrhotic patients, an association between alcohol-induced cirrhosis and deposits of haemosiderin is to be found in a large number of cases. Moreover, experimental overloading with iron does not in itself lead to typical pigmentary cirrhosis. This problem is difficult to resolve. In some cases (CAROLI and ETÉVÉ), successive needle biopsies carried out in the same cirrhotic patient have revealed the presence and accumulation of iron-containing pigment. Considering the problem from the opposite angle, however, it must be acknowledged that, as pointed out by DARNIS (*11*), haemochromatosis is rare within the general category of cirrhosis. Moreover, it may be argued that, though overloading with iron does not induce haemochromatosis in animals, it might perhaps nevertheless do so in man: the cytosiderosis occurring in the Bantu often bears a very close resemblance to idiopathic haemosiderosis, and the latter is indistinguishable – except by reference to the aetiology – from the terminal haemosiderosis seen in patients who have received multiple blood transfusions.

One may hope to solve the problem by a statistical study of siderosis in livers examined at autopsy or by biopsy. The work most often quoted in this context is that of ZIMMERMANN et al. (*50*), who were able to detect iron histologically in 13% of the patients on whom they performed autopsies; these included cases in which the presence of iron deposits could be ascribed to haemolysis. It may be objected, however, that findings obtained at autopsy are not necessarily identical with the results which one might expect to find *in vivo*; it is interesting to note in this connection that, when SCHEUER, WILLIAMS, and MUIR (*42*) examined the livers of 29 persons who had died following accidents or by suicide, PERLS' test showed a weakly positive reaction in 8 cases, whereas in a series of 200 routine biopsies the proportion was much lower.

In view of such considerations, one must therefore adopt a rather cautious attitude when discussing genetic aspects of haemochromatosis. It may be that certain forms of hypersiderosis described as familial or hereditary are in fact acquired as the result of a deficient diet or some digestive disorder. Be that as it may, we are of the opinion that this is likely to apply only very exceptionally, if at all, to those cases of iron-overloading which occur mainly in young individuals and which are in no way related to cirrhosis; hence, we feel that the findings we are about to report may be accepted as valid.

2. Familial forms. The number of familial forms of haemochromatosis is relatively limited. FINCH and FINCH were able to find only 7 histologically demonstrable cases among a total of 707 patients. In many cases, of course, no histological data are available. In France, cases have been reported by HARVIER et al., LESIEUR, and BOULIN and BAMBERGER; the latter studied a family which appears to offer the most striking example of its type recorded in the whole of the world literature on this subject. Four of the 8 siblings in the family were affected, and anomalies were observed in several of their descendants, many of whom unfortunately refused to submit to tests. One clear fact emerges from these observations: the fully developed picture of the disease is much more often encountered in the siblings of a patient than in previous or subsequent generations. A full clinical picture of haemochromatosis in members of two successive generations has, in fact, only very rarely been observed.

These findings should be interpreted with reservation, particularly in view of the fact that it takes such a long time for the clinical picture of haemochromatosis to become fully developed – a fact which also makes it difficult to study a patient's forebears and which at the same time means that his descendants will probably not yet present any clinical signs of the disease. It was on the basis of such findings, however, that haemochromatosis – at least in its fully established form – was first thought to be transmitted as a recessive autosomal character.

3. Systematic exploration has been conducted on a very limited number of families and, depending on the case, has consisted either in biological investigation or in a study of the pathology. We have been pursuing this research since 1952; meanwhile, other authors have also published the results of similar studies.

DAVISON (*13*), MORGAN (*31*), BOTHWELL et al. (*4*), BRICK (*6*), JOHNSON and FREY (*21*), PIRART (*36*), and CONTE et al. (*9*) have all been able to demonstrate anomalies, usually in siblings and sometimes in a son. JOHNSON and FREY examined 36 members from three generations of the same family; needle biopsy, performed in 7 cases, revealed iron in the liver of one of the sons and one grandson.

An analysis of the literature shows that, of those studies which are concerned not with a systematic exploration of the descendants, but with an examination of the patient's family as a whole, the most exhaustive investigation is that undertaken by WILLIAMS, SCHEUER, and SHERLOCK (*47*). These authors studied 46 relatives of 17 patients, and needle biopsy yielded positive findings in 28 of the 46 cases, as shown in Table 4. Of these 28 subjects, 12 presented abnormal skin pigmentation, though the abnormality was not so marked as in the patients themselves. Hepatomegaly was noted in 3 of the 28. A significant difference was observed between the serum iron levels in the subjects with iron deposits (average 170 μg.) as compared with those showing no iron deposits (average 109 μg.). Convincing though the difference between the averages may be, there were a certain number of exceptions which did not conform to the average pattern. The average serum iron levels in the haemochromatosis patients themselves worked out at 230 μg.

Table 4 shows the presence of histologically detectable iron deposits according to the degree of family relationship; in 6 further cases, electron-microscopic studies revealed an excess of ferritin. It is surprising to see that the sisters are more affected than the brothers, whereas all the sons (except one) and the nephews (except one) show an excess of iron, although only one of the 10 daughters and none of the 3 nieces were affected.

Table 4. *Presence of histologically detectable iron deposits according to the degree of family relationship*

	+	—
Brothers	7	3
Sisters	4	0
Sons	11	1
Daughters	1	9
Nephews	4	1
Nieces	0	3
Grandsons	1	0
Granddaughters	0	1

Despite the importance of such a study, no statistical conclusions can be drawn from it. All that we can say for the moment is that of 46 subjects, 28 (i.e. 61%) showed histologically detectable iron in their livers and that, if we also take into consideration the results obtained by electron microscopy, the percentage rises to 74%.

4. Personal investigations (*14, 15, 40, 41*). Since 1952, we – together with DEBRÉ and subsequently with LAMY et al. – have been investigating the heredity of haemochromatosis. To date, our studies have covered 161 direct descendants (81 females and 80 males). One difficulty encountered is the fact that the patients are frequently sterile. In order to avoid alarming members of the families concerned, the examinations carried out up to the year 1960 consisted only of blood tests: the serum iron was measured, often on repeated occasions, and the coefficient of saturation calculated. The results of the serum iron determinations are presented in Fig. 5, which shows the values for 38 controls (average 140 μg.) and for 40 patients with haemochromatosis (average 250 μg.); the children of the patients have been classified according to age and sex. We have found in these studies that anomalies are much more common in the boys than in the girls, which is consistent with the difference in the incidence of the disease itself in relation to sex. On the other hand, in the boys prior to puberty, the syndrome has usually not yet developed; it will be seen, in fact, that there is no difference between the girls above and below 15 years of age, whereas the values for boys over 15 years of age (average 195 μg.) are significantly higher than for those aged less than 15 (average 135 μg.). The values for boys over 15 fall midway between those for the controls and for the patients.

From these investigations we have concluded that the most acceptable group for study is that of the boys over 15 years of age; the younger boys have not had sufficient time to develop hypersiderosis, while in the girls the latter is to some extent offset after puberty by the menstrual loss of blood.

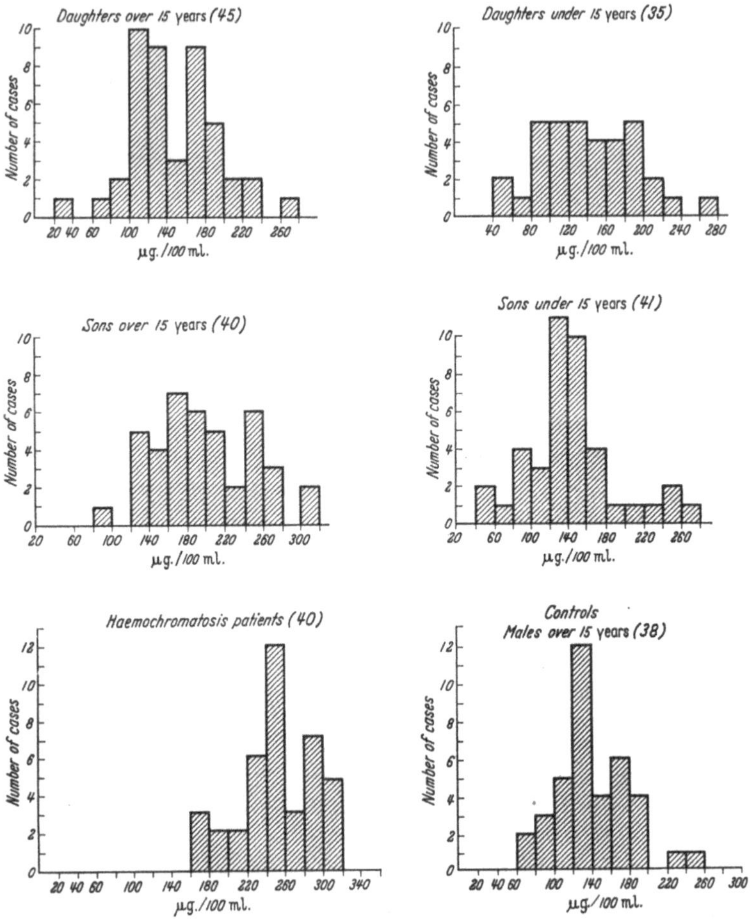

Fig. 5. Serum iron levels in haemochromatosis patients and their children

In the boys over 15 years of age, approximately 50% show elevated serum iron levels and an elevated coefficient of saturation. Moreover, in a group of 30 sons (DEBRÉ et al.), the variance was found to be much greater than in the other groups mentioned above. Since the variance in heterozygotes is often greater than in homozygotes, this is evidence in favour of the heterogeneity of the group of sons.

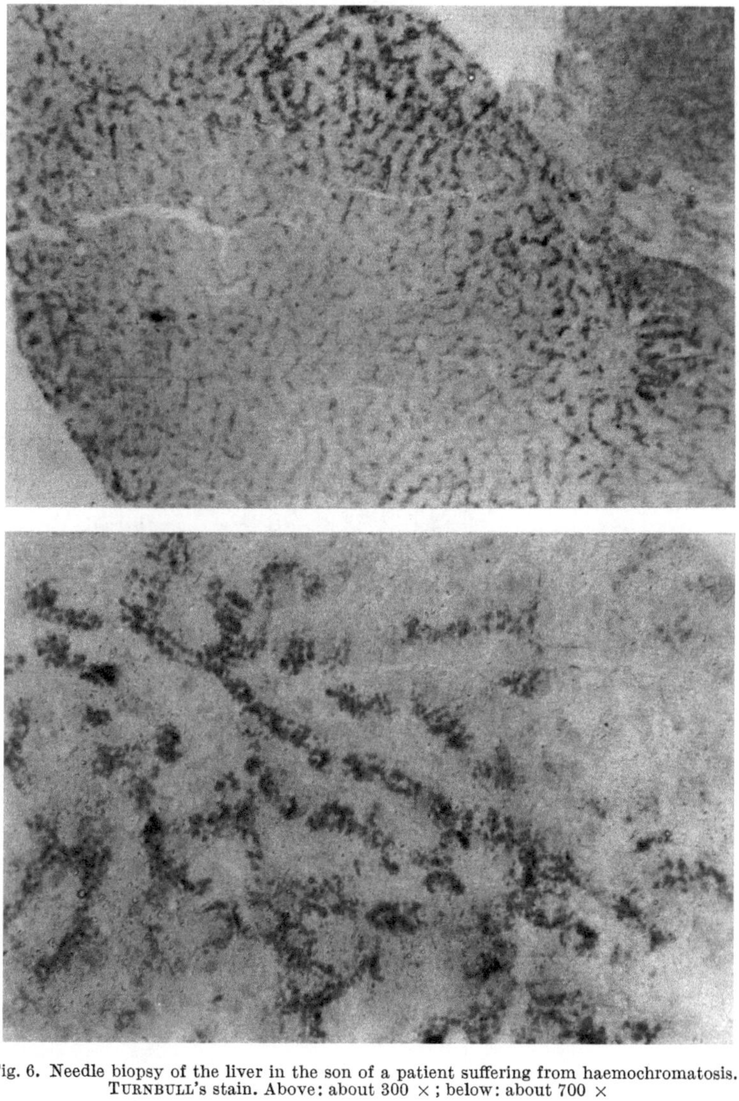

Fig. 6. Needle biopsy of the liver in the son of a patient suffering from haemochromatosis. TURNBULL's stain. Above: about 300 ×; below: about 700 ×

Since 1960, we have undertaken, together with SCHWARZMANN, needle-biopsy studies of the children, although so far only in cases which have presented elevated serum iron levels. To date, biopsy has been performed in 8 of these cases (Fig. 6).

In 7 of the 8 subjects (6 men and 2 women), iron deposits were found in the biopsy material. In 4 cases the amount of iron present was small, in 2 cases moderate, and in one case large enough to constitute haemochromatosis. The only negative case was that of a 19-year-old girl who, following a bout of anaemia, the precise nature of which it was impossible to determine, showed a marked reduction in serum iron (*41*). In 2 of the positive cases, alcoholism was involved, and the slides revealed steatosis without sclerosis.

These histological studies confirmed that excessive iron deposits were present in all the subjects in whom repeated tests had shown hypersideraemia. But they shed no light on the question as to whether the hypersideraemia precedes or follows deposition of iron in the tissues.

Table 5. *Induced sideruria with desferrioxamine in relatives of patients with haemochromatosis and in patients with haemochromatosis or transfusion haemosiderosis*

Patient	Age	Urinary iron excretion (mg./day) in response to desferrioxamine	Serum iron (μg./100 ml.)	Remarks
1. Male control	39	0.655	190	
2. Daughter	19	1.66	100	Previous serum iron 210 μg. Biopsy: iron +
3. ,,	16	0.825	380	
4. Son	24	1.22	290	
5. ,,	37	0.950	185	
6. ,,	42	1.44	150	Venesection for 6 months Previous serum iron 410 μg. Biopsy: iron + +
7. Brother	54	0.206	210	Biopsy: iron +
8. Haemochromatosis	60	14.3	230	
9. ,,	41	13.4	235	
10. ,,	60	6.75	165	Treated by venesection
11. ,,	38	10.4	190	Treated by venesection
12. ,,	50	36		
13. Transfusion haemosiderosis	3	7 to 15	360	
14. Transfusion haemosiderosis	8	5 to 20	295	

In a recent attempt to determine the degree of iron-overloading in the children of patients with haemochromatosis, we have employed desferrioxamine (Desferal). Desferrioxamine (400 mg. or 1,000 mg.) was injected intramuscularly, and the urine was collected over a 24-hour period. Since we did not wish to cause any undue inconvenience to the subjects, we gave them only one injection each. Of the 6 persons thus tested (one sibling and five offspring of haemochromatotic patients), all showed hypersideraemia. According to the literature, the normal rate of urinary iron excretion is accepted as being up to 2 mg./24 hours. This has been compared with values obtained in confirmed cases of haemochromatosis or transfusion haemosiderosis; the results are given in Table 5.

From this table it will be seen that, despite a high serum iron level, none of the subjects tested showed a high urinary iron excretion, whereas this is the case in haemochromatosis (the values recorded by us are somewhat lower than those reported by most other authors, because we administered only one injection). It may therefore be concluded that in these subjects the iron overload must certainly have been slight.

5. Comparison of different studies. All the investigations to which we have referred, including especially those of Williams et al. and ourselves, leave little doubt as to the possibility that haemochromatosis is a disorder of iron metabolism which can be inherited. But do the results obtained enable one to determine with certainty just how the disease is transmitted?

Our own investigations, based on measurement of the serum iron and calculation of the coefficient of saturation, have revealed anomalies in half of the sons over 15 years of age. They point to dominant transmission, if not of the disease, then at least of the disorder affecting iron metabolism.

Williams et al. (*47*) have reported anomalies in roughly 75% of the members of their patients' families. They conclude from this that transmission is of an intermediate type – the patients being homozygotes, and the heterozygotes presenting only an anomaly of iron metabolism. If two heterozygotes marry each other, one out of every four of their children will be completely unaffected, two will display a disorder of iron metabolism, and one will develop the full clinical picture of the disease. Consistent with this concept is the higher incidence of the disease in the patients' siblings than in their children and also the occurrence – admittedly rare – of haemochromatosis in the children of couples having a close consanguinity (Lesieur; Nussbaumer et al.). On the other hand, if this concept were correct, then all the descendants of homozygote patients – or at least those of male sex – should display stigmata of the heterozygous type. This is far from being the case in our series, although one cannot be dogmatic on this point, since half of the sons in the series studied by WILLIAMS et al. showed iron in their biopsy material despite the fact that their serum iron levels were normal. It is therefore impossible at present to decide in favour either of dominant heredity or of intermediate heredity. In all cases, however, the disorder of iron metabolism is evidently of the dominant type.

6. Prophylactic measures. One is justified in resorting to all means, including needle biopsy, in order to demonstrate iron deposition in the offspring of patients with haemochromatosis. In younger individuals the excessive iron seems to cause little harm and one can be virtually certain of preventing any further development of the condition by insisting that the subjects in question enlist as regular blood-donors.

IV. Pathogenic mechanisms

We do not propose to discuss here the role of iron in the pathogenesis of clinical disorders, since this subject has already received much attention. However, the fact that venesection, and especially prolonged treatment with chelating agents, elicits a marked clinical improvement leaves little room for doubt as to the part played by iron in the diseases in question – although, on the other hand, it is impossible to reproduce the full syndrome experimentally by means of iron alone. An attempt to explain the biochemical mechanisms involved has been made by WITZLEBEN and CHAFFEY (*48*); these authors have shown that many enzymes, including particularly the glucose-6-phosphatase in the microsomes, are sensitive to an excess of iron, and they suggest as an hypothesis that such an excess may reduce the number of sulphydryl groups available in the proteins, thereby interfering with the biochemical function of the cells.

The most important problem seems to be that of the excessive accumulation of iron: in the course of haemochromatosis, the organism stores very excessive quantities of iron, i.e. it may accumulate several tens of grammes, as compared with the normal figure of 4–5 g. An excess of 20 g. iron, built up over a period of 40 years, implies an average increase of 1.5 mg. daily. Is this increase due to a disorder affecting the mechanism of absorption, of transport, or of storage, and does the mechanism of utilisation – as seems to be the case – remain intact? Numerous studies have lately been undertaken in an effort to answer these questions, but so far without success. The very slow rate at which the iron deposits accumulate is one of the chief difficulties encountered in this connection[1].

1. Iron absorption. In haemochromatosis, the rate of iron absorption is undoubtedly increased; since, as we have already seen, iron excretion is normally minimal, it must be the spontaneous limitation of iron absorption which prevents the organism from accumulating an excess of this metal. But the mechanism by which the absorption of iron is restricted is still obscure. The only coherent hypothesis to have gained any support is GRANICK's theory that the mucosa becomes "blocked", thereby preventing the absorption of further iron; this concept, however, is rather a vague one and has recently been challenged on the grounds that, despite a prior intake of iron, a subsequent dose of radioactive iron is duly absorbed (*7*). Thus, the regulation of iron absorption and the disorders occurring in this mechanism of regulation are still shrouded in mystery.

A diet very rich in iron (cf. cytosiderosis in the Bantu), or prolonged treatment with iron, has sometimes given rise to haemosiderosis. Similarly, in animals it is possible to produce feed-induced hypersiderosis. Siderosis of this type may be reversible both in animals (*17*, *24*) and in man (*33*).

2. Iron transport. Disorders affecting iron transport may be considered from two aspects: the quantitative and the qualitative.

a) *The regulation of gastro-intestinal absorption* may depend on the degree of saturation of the siderophilin. However, no definite conclusions have emerged from experiments on the absorption of radioactive iron before and after saturation of the siderophilin or after intravenous injection of iron-free siderophilin. Tests conducted on normal subjects do not, in fact, shed any particular light on the question as to whether iron absorption is conditioned by the degree of saturation of the siderophilin. In patients with haemochromatosis, on the other hand, total or subtotal saturation of the siderophilin does not appear in most cases to prevent excessive iron absorption.

b) *The qualitative properties of siderophilin* do not seem to have any bearing on this subject. Neither its affinity for iron, its coloration, its electrophoretic (or immuno-electrophoretic) behaviour, nor – as revealed by more recent studies – its chemical nature appear to undergo any changes [SAADI, unpublished experiments; BOTHWELL et al. (*5*)].

[1] Two observations of haemochromatosis in the newborn have, however, recently been reported (*10*, *27*).

3. Iron utilisation. In patients with haemochromatosis, iron utilisation is evidently normal, as evidenced by the absence of anaemia. Indeed, the passage of iron from the siderophilin to the erythroblasts would actually appear to be facilitated, since research on the utilisation of iron by the reticulocytes has shown that the more saturated it is with iron, the more readily the siderophilin releases this metal (*35*). Admittedly, when radioactive iron is administered, the proportion of the dose utilised for haematopoiesis is less than normal, but this seems to be merely due to the increase in stored iron.

4. Iron elimination cannot be held responsible for haemochromatosis. We have already seen that the rate of iron excretion is very low even under normal circumstances; and in some patients with haemochromatosis, the rate of urinary iron excretion is if anything above normal.

5. Iron storage. It is upon this aspect that most of the research is now being concentrated.

a) *The nature of the constituents* poses one problem from the start. Two pigments have been described: one is probably of lipoid character (haemofuscin) and the other contains iron (haemosiderin). Much work has been done to clarify the nature of haemosiderin and to determine in what way it is related to ferritin. Chemically, ferritin is well defined: it is a protein resulting from the union of iron (up to 23%) with apoferritin, which has a molecular weight of 460,000 and is made up of 20–25 identical subunits (*19*, *39*). From the biochemical aspect, ferritin is a soluble protein, maintained in equilibrium with siderophilin by a mechanism which is still the subject of controversy. In the electron microscope it is visible in the form of micelles of 4–6 elements (*2*, *3a*, *37*). In the light microscope it was at one time alleged to be invisible, but this has now been disclaimed.

In contrast to ferritin, haemosiderin is by no means as well defined (*31*); it contains a larger amount of iron than ferritin, but the character of its protein moiety has not yet been established with any degree of precision (*43*); the fact that it resembles ferritin when examined in the electron microscope (*2*, *37*) suggests that the two proteins are closely akin to each other.

There is at present no unanimously accepted definition for haemosiderin. The only properties about which all agree are that it is an insoluble substance and that it contains histologically detectable iron. Endogenous haemosiderin does not display the same characteristics as the haemosiderin which forms deposits following injection of colloidal iron.

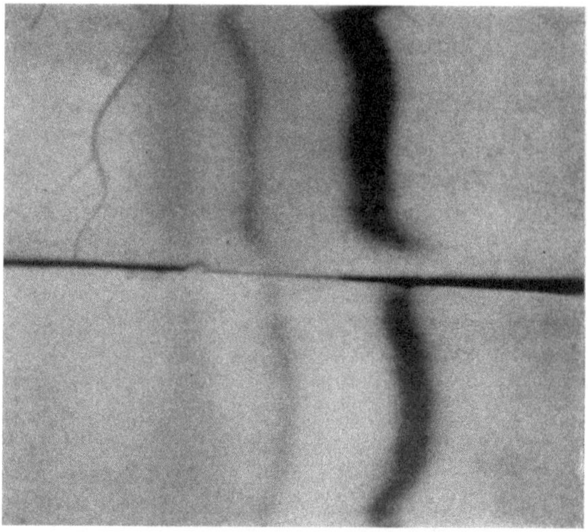

Fig. 7. Electrophoresis pattern obtained using starch gel and Tris-borate buffer. Ferritin from a normal subject (above) shows the same three bands in the same positions as ferritin from a patient with haemochromatosis (below)

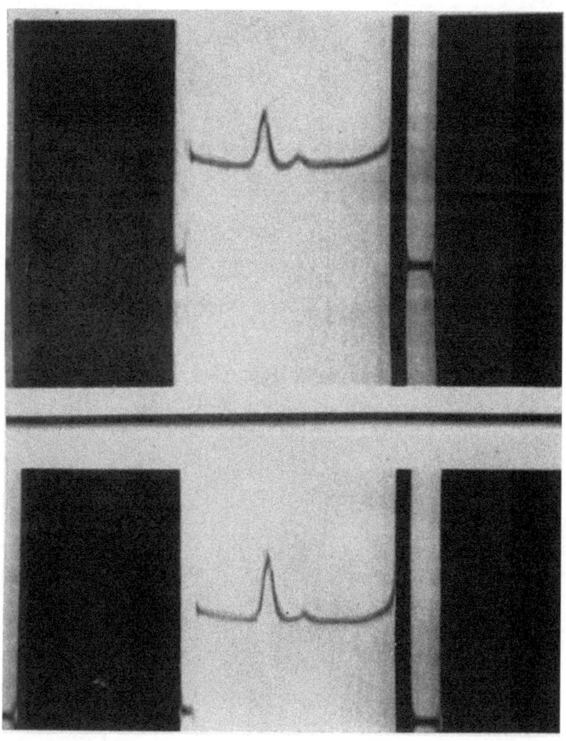

Fig. 8. Ultracentrifugation of apoferritin from a normal subject and from a patient with haemochromatosis under the same conditions. Above: normal liver, 11.9 S; below: haemochromatosis, 11.7 S

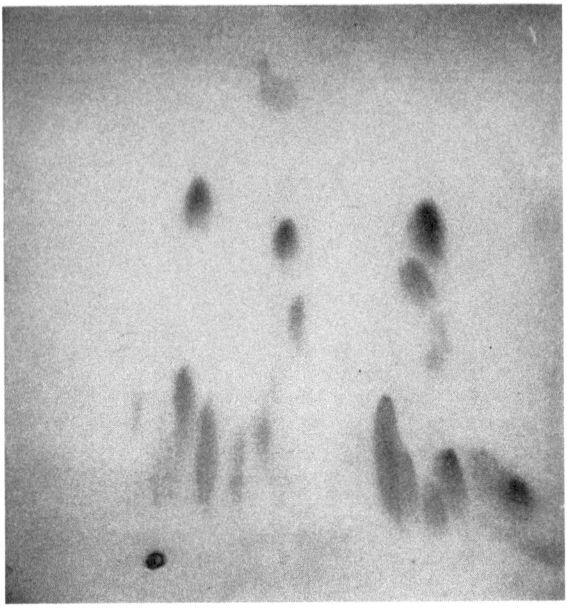

Fig. 9. Electrophoresis chromatogram of a trypsin digest of ferritin from a normal subject (INGRAM's technique)

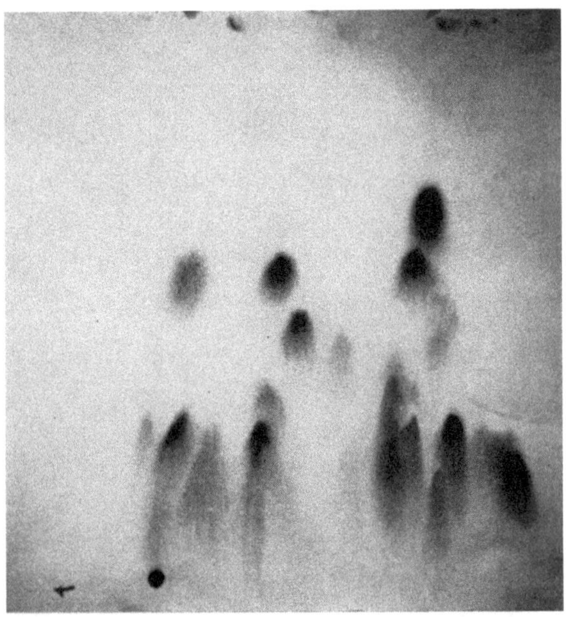

Fig. 10. Electrophoresis chromatogram of a trypsin digest from a patient with haemochromatosis (INGRAM's technique)

b) *Modification of the metabolism of ferritin.* The most likely hypothesis so far suggested is that haemochromatosis is associated with some disorder affecting the regulation of ferritin metabolism. Assuming that haemochromatosis is a genetically determined metabolic disease, there are two possibilities which may be considered in this connection: that the disorder is attributable to a so-called "structural" gene or to a "regulator" gene.

If we suppose that the disorder is of structural origin, i.e. a pathological alteration in the ferritin itself, then haemochromatosis would appear to be a molecular disease analogous to the molecular diseases affecting haemoglobin; so far, however, no chemical modifications have been discovered in the ferritin of patients with haemochromatosis. On the contrary, SAADI has shown in our laboratory (*38*) that neither electrophoresis using starch gel (Fig. 7) or a starch block, nor centrifugation (Fig. 8), nor, in particular, a study of chromatograms of the isolated protein (Figs 9 and 10) obtained by electrophoresis-chromatography of a trypsin digest reveal any differences between ferritin in the normal subject and in the patient with idiopathic haemochromatosis. Nor have we any evidence for supposing that there is a biochemical lesion or an enzymatic deficiency involved at any of the various stages of iron metabolism.

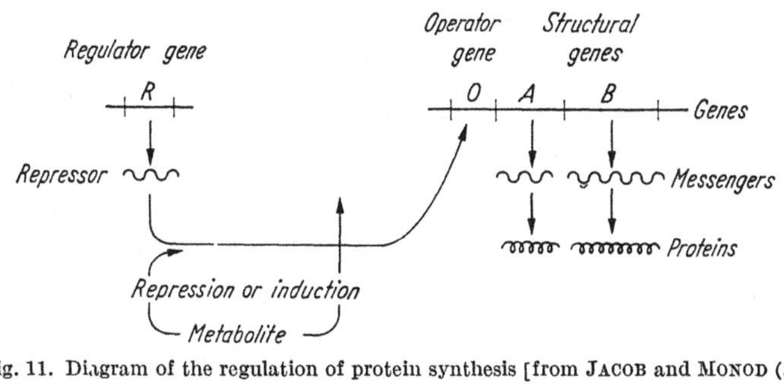

Fig. 11. Diagram of the regulation of protein synthesis [from JACOB and MONOD (*20*)]

It is also tempting to consider this disease in the light of the concepts postulated by JACOB and MONOD (*20*) with regard to the "regulator" gene (Fig. 11).

In line with this hypothesis, it might be assumed that there is some genetically determined fault in the regulation of the biosynthesis of ferritin. If the biosynthesis of ferritin is excessive – owing possibly to the absence of an inhibitor whose activity might in turn perhaps be regulated by the intake of iron – this would lead to an accumulation of ferritin, since the quantity required for haematopoiesis would remain unchanged; the production of haemosiderin might thus result from the catabolism of ferritin.

Though much has now been learned about the biochemical aspects of haemochromatosis, and though considerable progress has lately been made in the treatment of this disease, we still need to know much more about its heredity.

A more thorough understanding of the genetics of the haemochromatosis would already enable us to institute more effective prophylactic measures. Finally, if we can also elucidate the disease at a molecular level, we may even hope to evolve a rational and causal form of treatment.

Summary

Iron metabolism undergoes many changes in idiopathic haemochromatosis, the fundamental feature being the enormous increase in the iron stores.

1. Metabolism displays the following modifications:

a) An increase in serum iron and an even greater increase in the saturation of transferrin.

b) An increase in the absorption of iron; this cannot be seen from the iron-loading curve, which is flat, but only from radioactive iron-absorption studies.

c) A decrease in the utilisation of radioactive iron, pointing to an increase in the iron stores.

d) An increase in iron excretion in response to chelating agents.

e) Histologically detectable iron in sections of liver and other tissues.

Of practical value for purposes of diagnosis are, firstly, measurements of serum iron and transferrin saturation and, secondly, the response to chelating agents. Definite proof can be obtained only by liver biopsy.

2. Therapy:

Treatment consists essentially in eliminating the excess of iron in two ways:

a) Repeated venesection, the purpose of which is to deplete the iron stores to replace iron lost with the blood.

b) Administration of iron-complexing agents, which now hold out promise of good results.

A combination of these two techniques should be attempted, since their effects may be expected to be additive.

As supplementary therapy, oral treatment with chelating agents might to some extent prevent the absorption of iron.

3. Genetics:

Haemochromatosis is a familial disease, but it is very seldom seen in successive generations. A review of the literature is given. We ourselves have examined 160 offspring of patients with haemochromatosis. In 8 of them, liver biopsy was performed, and in 10, urinary iron excretion following administration of desferrioxamine was measured. In half of the male offspring, abnormalities of iron metabolism were detected and were confirmed histologically, but the overload must have been slight in view of the results of the iron-excretion test. The transmission of this abnormality of iron metabolism is either dominant or intermediate, and the offspring are unlikely to present the full clinical picture.

4. Pathogenesis:

It is difficult to elucidate the mechanism by which haemochromatosis occurs, because the process is such a slow one.

a) Iron absorption is increased, and is estimated at 1—3 mg./day, but the mechanism involved is still obscure. Though a diet very rich in iron can give rise to cytosiderosis, this is not the cause of idiopathic haemochromatosis.

b) Transport: Neither changes in the amount or in the saturation of transferrin nor alterations in its chemical constitution appear to play a role in the disease; the chemical constitution of transferrin is apparently unchanged.

c) Iron utilisation is normal.

d) No importance attaches to the excretion of iron, which does not normally have any significant bearing on the regulation of iron metabolism, although it is of potential therapeutic importance.

e) Storage mechanisms are at present receiving much attention. The relationships between ferritin and haemosiderin are still not well defined, owing to the latter's lack of chemical homogeneity. Ferritin seems to be chemically unchanged in haemochromatosis. One attractive hypothesis is to postulate a disorder in the regulation of ferritin biosynthesis, giving rise to an excess of ferritin, part of which would be secondarily transformed into haemosiderin.

Zusammenfassung

Bei der idiopathischen Haemochromatose liegen verschiedene Veränderungen im Eisenstoffwechsel vor, von denen die außerordentlich starke Zunahme der Eisenspeicher im Vordergrund steht.

1. Der Stoffwechsel zeigt folgende Abweichungen:

a) Zunahme des Serumeisens und noch stärkere Sättigung des Transferrins.

b) Vermehrte Resorption, die nach Eisenbelastung nicht deutlich wird, da die Kurve hierbei flach verläuft, sondern nur in Resorptionsversuchen mit radioaktiv markiertem Eisen.

c) Verminderte Ausnutzung von radioaktivem Eisen, die auf eine Ablagerung in den Eisenspeichern hinweist.

d) Vermehrte Eisenausscheidung unter der Einwirkung von Chelatbildnern.

e) Histologisch nachweisbares Eisen in Leberschnitten und anderen Geweben.

Von praktischer Bedeutung für die Diagnose sind zuerst Bestimmungen des Serumeisens und der Sättigung des Transferrins, dann die Reaktion auf die Gabe von Chelatbildnern. Der Beweis ist nur durch eine Leberbiopsie zu erbringen.

2. Behandlung.

Sie besteht im wesentlichen in der Entfernung von überschüssigem Eisen auf zwei Arten:

a) Wiederholte Aderlässe mit dem Ziel, die Eisenspeicher zu entleeren, aus denen das mit dem Blut verlorene Eisen ersetzt wird.

b) Eisenkomplexbildner, die neuerdings erfolgversprechende Resultate ergeben.

Die Kombination der beiden Methoden sollte versucht werden, da die Wirkungen additiv sein dürften.

Als zusätzliche Behandlung perorale Gabe von Chelatbildnern, um die Resorption von Eisen bis zu einem gewissen Grade zu verhindern.

3. Genetik.

Die Haemochromatose ist eine familiäre Erkrankung, die aber nur selten in aufeinanderfolgenden Generationen auftritt. Wir untersuchten 160 Nachkommen von Patienten; bei 8 von ihnen wurde eine Leberbiopsie vorgenommen, bei 10 eine Bestimmung der Eisenausscheidung nach Gabe von Desferrioxamin. Bei der Hälfte der männlichen Nachkommen fanden sich Abweichungen im Eisenstoffwechsel. Sie wurden histologisch bestätigt, aber die Speicherung dürfte im Hinblick auf den Ausfall des Ausscheidungstestes nur geringgradig sein. Die Vererbung der Abweichung im Eisenstoffwechsel ist entweder dominant oder intermediär, und das voll ausgeprägte Bild ist wahrscheinlich nicht bei den direkten Nachkommen zu erwarten.

4. Pathogenese.

Die Aufklärung des Entstehungsmechanismus ist besonders durch den langsamen Verlauf der Erkrankung erschwert.

a) Die Eisenresorption ist vermehrt, sie beträgt 1—3 mg. pro Tag, aber der zugrundeliegende Mechanismus ist unklar. Eine an Eisen sehr reiche Ernährung kann zu Zytosiderose führen, ist jedoch nicht die Ursache der idiopathischen Haemochromatose.

b) Transport: Weder Änderungen der Menge noch der Sättigung von Transferrin spielen bei der Erkrankung eine Rolle; die chemische Konstitution ist nicht verändert.

c) Die Ausnutzung von Eisen ist unverändert.

d) Die Ausscheidung ist nicht verantwortlich, da sie normalerweise keinen entscheidenden Regulator im Eisenstoffwechsel darstellt. Sie ist lediglich von potentieller therapeutischer Bedeutung.

e) Speichermechanismen finden zur Zeit Beachtung. Die Beziehungen zwischen Ferritin und Haemosiderin sind noch nicht genügend geklärt, besonders weil das letztere chemisch nicht homogen ist. Ferritin scheint chemisch bei der Haemochromatose nicht verändert zu sein. Dagegen ist die Hypothese verlockend, eine Störung in der Regulierung der Ferritinbiosynthese anzunehmen, die zu einem Überschuß an Ferritin führt, das seinerseits sekundär in Haemosiderin umgewandelt wird.

Résumé

Le métabolisme du fer subit de nombreux changements dans l'hémochromatose idiopathique, le fait fondamental étant l'énorme accroissement des dépôts de fer.

1. Le métabolisme présente les modifications suivantes:

a) Augmentation du fer sérique et encore plus de la saturation de la sidérophiline.

b) Augmentation de l'absorption: ceci ressort non pas de la courbe de surcharge en fer, qui est plate, mais seulement des études d'absorption de fer radioactif.

c) Diminution de l'utilisation du fer radioactif, indiquant une augmentation des dépôts de fer.

d) Augmentation de l'excrétion du fer sous l'action des agents chélateurs.

e) Fer histologiquement décelable dans les coupes de foie ou d'autres tissus.

Ont une valeur pratique pour le diagnostic: d'abord le dosage du fer sérique et de la saturation du sérum, puis la réponse aux agents chélatants. Seule la ponction-biopsie du foie apporte la preuve.

2. Thérapeutique.

Elle consiste essentiellement à éliminer le fer en excès, de deux façons:

a) Saignées répétées visant à diminuer les dépôts dont le fer remplacera celui soustrait avec le sang.

b) Agents formant des complexes avec les métaux et qui semblent aujord'hui prometteurs.

L'association de ces deux méthodes devrait être essayée, car leurs effets devraient être additifs.

Les chélateurs par voie orale pourraient, en tant que thérapeutique complémentaire, empêcher dans une certaine mesure l'absorption du fer.

3. Génétique.

L'hémochromatose est une maladie familiale, mais elle est très rarement observée dans des générations successives. Nous avons nous-mêmes examiné 160 descendants de malades. Chez 8 d'entre eux une ponction-biopsie a été faite et chez 10 une détermination de l'élimination du fer après desferrioxamine. Chez la moitié des descendants mâles, des anomalies du métabolisme du fer ont pu être décelées. Elles ont été confirmées histologiquement, mais la surcharge devait être légère, étant donné les résultats du test d'excrétion. En conclusion, la transmission de l'anomalie du métabolisme du fer est soit dominante soit intermédiaire, et on ne doit probablement pas s'attendre à un tableau complet chez le descendant.

4. Pathogénie.

Il est difficile de découvrir le mécanisme de production de l'hémochromatose idiopathique en raison de la lenteur du processus.

a) Il existe une augmentation de l'absorption du fer, qui peut être évaluée à 1 à 3 mg. par jour, mais le mécanisme en reste obscur. Un régime très riche en fer peut donner lieu à une cytosidérose; ce n'est pas la cause de l'hémochromatose idiopathique.

b) Transport: ni la quantité de sidérophiline ou sa saturation, ni la constitution chimique de la sidérophiline, apparemment inchangée, ne semblent jouer un rôle dans la maladie.

c) L'utilisation est normale.

d) L'élimination n'est pas en cause, puisqu'elle n'est pas normalement un régulateur notable du métabolisme du fer. Elle a seulement une importance thérapeutique potentielle.

e) Les mécanismes de stockage sont actuellement à l'ordre du jour. Les relations entre ferritine et hémosidérine ne sont pas encore bien définies en raison du manque d'homogénéité chimique de cette dernière. La ferritine semble être chimiquement normale dans l'hémochromatose. Une hypothèse séduisante est celle d'un trouble de la régulation de la biosynthèse de la ferritine, donnant lieu à un excès de ferritine dont une partie serait secondairement transformée en hémosidérine.

Acknowledgements

We wish to thank the Institut National d'Hygiène, the Caisse Nationale de Sécurité Sociale, and the Délégation Générale à la Recherche Scientifique et ses Comités Scientifiques (Fonds de Développement) for their help in connection with this work.

References

For references prior to 1958, readers are requested to consult the study by J.-C. Dreyfus and G. Schapira entitled "Le Fer" (Expansion Scientifique Française, Paris, 1958).

1. André, J.: Rev. internat. hépat. (Fr.) **11**, 113 (1961). — 2. Bessis, M.: Blood (U.S.A.) **19**, 635 (1962). — 3. Bessis, M., and J. Caroli: Gastroenterology (U.S.A.) **37**, 538 (1959). — 3a. Bessis, M., J. Breton, J.-C. Dreyfus, and G. Schapira: Rev. franç. étud. clin. biol. **3**, 981 (1958). — 4. Bothwell, T. H., I. Cohen, O. L. Abrahams, and S. M. Perold: Amer. J. Med. **27**, 730 (1959). — 5. Bothwell, T. H., P. Jacobs, and J. D. Torrance: S. Afr. Med. J. **27**, 35 (1962). — 6. Brick, I. B.: Gastroenterology (U.S.A.) **40**, 210 (1961). — 7. Cantrill, S., and R. J. Walsh: Austral. J. Exper. Biol. **40**, 17 (1962). — 8. Cazal, P., and J. Mirouze: Path. biol. (Sem. hôp. Paris) **34**, 845 (1958). — 9. Conte, M., J. Ristelhueber, J. C. Malvezin, and C. Julien: Bull. Soc. méd. hôp. Paris **74**, 267 (1958). — 10. Cottier, P.: Schweiz. med. Wschr. **87**, 39 (1957). — 11. Darnis, F.: Rev. praticien (Fr.) **8**, 2985 (1958). — 12. Darnis, F.: Path. biol. (Sem. hôp. Paris) **34**, 873 (1958). — 13. Davison, R. H.: Brit. Med. J. **1961**/II, 1262. — 14. Debré, R., J.-C. Dreyfus, J. Frezal, D. Labie, M. Lamy, P. Maroteaux, F. Schapira, and G. Schapira: Ann. Hum. Genet. (G.B.) **23**, 16 (1958). — 15. Dreyfus, J.-C., G. Schapira, V. Schwarzmann, and R. Abbou: Presse méd. (Fr.) **68**, 577 (1960). — 16. Fahey, J. L., C. E. Rath, J. V. Princiotto, I. B. Brick, and M. Rubin: J. Laborat. Clin. Med. (U.S.A.) **57**, 436 (1961). — 17. Gillman, T., M. Hathorn, and P. A. S. Canham: Amer. J. Path. **35**, 349 (1959). — 18. Girard, M.: Rev. praticien (Fr.) **8**, 3041 (1958). — 19. Harrison, P., and T. Hofmann: J. Mol. Biol. (G.B.) **4**, 239 (1962). — 20. Jacob, F., and J. Monod: J. Mol. Biol. (G.B.) **3**, 318 (1961). — 20a. Jandl, J. H., J. K. Inman, R. L. Simmons, and D. W. Allen: J. Clin. Invest. (U.S.A.) **38**, 161 (1959). — 21. Johnson, G. B., and W. G. Frey III: J. Amer. Med. Ass. **179**, 747 (1962). — 22. Justin-Besançon, L., M. Lamotte, S. Lamotte-Barillon, M. Grivaux, R. Deuil, and E. di Prisco: Rev. méd. franç. **41**, 491 (1960). — 23. Kerr, D. N. S., and A. R. Muir: J. Ultrastruct. Res. (U.S.A.) **3**, 313 (1960). — 24. Kinney, T. D., N. Kaufman, and J. V. Klavius: Nature (G.B.) **195**, 604 (1962). — 25. Lamache, A., and M. Bourel: Path. biol. (Sem. hôp. Paris) **34**, 857 (1958). — 26. Lange, J., and B. Endler: Dtsch. Arch. klin. Med. **208**, 53 (1962). — 27. Laurendeau, T.: A. M. A. Arch. Path. **72**, 410 (1961). — 28. MacDonald, C. A., and G. K. Mallory: Arch. Int. Med. (U.S.A.) **105**, 686 (1960). — 29. MacDonald, R. A.: Arch. Int. Med. (U.S.A.) **107**, 606 (1961). — 30. Moeschlin, S.: Schweiz. med. Wschr. **92**, 1295 (1962). — 31. Morgan, E. H.: Australas. Ann. Med. **10**, 114 (1961). — 32. Mouriquand, C.: Path. biol. (Sem. hôp. Paris) **9**, 1557 (1961). — 33. Mukherjee, K. L., and N. Y. Sarkar: Brit. J. Nutrit. **12**, 1 (1958). — 34. Novikoff, A. B., and E. Essner: Amer. J. Med. **29**, 102 (1960). — 35. Paoletti, C., M. Boiron, M. Tubiana, R. Truhaut, and J. Bernard: Sang (Fr.) **29**, 492 (1958). — 36. Pirart, J., and P. Gatez: Sem. hôp. Paris **34**, 1044 (1958). — 37. Richter. G. M.: J. Exper. Med. (USA) **112**, 551 (1960). — 38. Saadi, R.: Rev. franç. étud. clin. biol. **4**, 408 (1962). — 39. Saadi, R., G. Schapira, and J.-C. Dreyfus: Bull. Soc. chim. biol. (Fr.) **43**. 409 (1961). — 40. Schapira, G., J.-C. Dreyfus, V. Schwarzmann, and J. Etévé: Rev.

franç. étud. clin. biol. **5**, 485 (1962). — 41. SCHAPIRA, G., and J.-C. DREYFUS: In: Eisenstoffwechsel. Thieme, Stuttgart, 1959, p. 238. — 42. SCHEUER, P. J., R. WILLIAMS, and A. R. MUIR: J. Path. Bact. (G.B.) **84**, 53 (1962). — 43. SHODEN, A., and P. STURGEON: Acta haemat. (Switz.) **27**, 33 (1962). — 44. THIBAULT, P.: Presse méd. (Fr.) **67**, 731 (1959). — 45. VAN HOEK, R., and M. E. CONRAD: J. Clin. Invest. (U.S.A.) **40**, 1153 (1961). — 46. WARTER, J., and J. P. WEILL: Path. biol. (Sem. hôp. Paris) **34**, 829 (1958). — 47. WILLIAMS, R., P. J. SCHEUER, and S. SHERLOCK: Quart. J. Med. (G.B.) **31**, 249 (1962). — 48. WITZLEBEN, C. L., and N. J. CHAFFEY: J. Exper. Med. (U.S.A.) **115**, 1370 (1962). — 50. ZIMMERMAN, H., R. CHOMET, M. H. KULESH, and C. A. MCWHORTER: Arch. Int. Med. (U.S.A.) **107**, 494 (1961).

Surcharge ferrique dans les cirrhoses (à l'exclusion de l'hémochromatose idiopathique)

par

J. Caroli et J. André

Le plus grand nombre des auteurs, en accord avec Sheldon (*16*), Debré (*8*), Lamy (*13*), etc., admet une forme primitive constitutionnelle d'hémochromatose, par erreur innée du métabolisme du fer. Elle vient d'être exposée par J.-C. Dreyfus (p. 313). Parmi les hémochromatoses secondaires, on a décrit les formes post-transfusionnelles, secondaires aux anémies hypochromes achrestiques avec ou sans hémoglobinopathie. Aujourd'hui vient de naître une nouvelle variété par atransferrinémie (Heilmeyer, *10*). L'hémochromatose nutritionnelle des Bantous est admise depuis les travaux des Gillman. Je crois que, dans le démembrement étio et physiopathologique de l'hémochromatose, on doit faire une place (elle est large en France) à une forme greffée sur une cirrhose, le plus souvent alcoolique, du foie. Autrement dit, il existerait une cirrhose alcoolique de Laënnec secondairement hémochromatosique. Ce point de vue que nous soutenons depuis longtemps (*1*, *4*) est très discuté. Les opinions sont divergentes, car, pour certains auteurs, l'alcool ne serait qu'une cause déclenchante ou aggravante.

Du point de vue de l'hépatologie, nous croyons pouvoir affirmer que les hémochromatoses secondaires des cirrhoses se distinguent des formes constitutionnelles primitives par leurs signes cliniques, leur tableau biologique et surtout par l'évolution des lésions anatomiques.

Les indications thérapeutiques sont à discuter.

La répartition des observations d'hémochromatose recueillies pendant les 5 dernières années dans notre service de l'Hôpital St-Antoine se fait pour 40 cas en 50% d'hémochromatoses constitutionnelles, sans doute héréditaires, et 50% de formes acquises greffées sur une cirrhose alcoolique.

Signes cliniques différentiels entre hémochromatose primitive et hémochromatose secondaire des cirrhoses alcooliques

Ils sont résumés sur le Tableau 1.

On voit que la mélanodermie est constante dans les deux formes. Les femmes sont comparativement plus souvent atteintes

Tableau 1. *Signes cliniques différentiels entre hémochromatose primitive et hémochromatose secondaire des cirrhoses alcooliques*

	Hémochromatose	
	idiopathique	alcoolique
Sexe		
masculin	92,3%	80%
féminin	7,7%	20%
Mélanodermie	100 %	100%
Volume du foie		
hypertrophique	100 %	70%
atrophique		5%
normal		25%
Hypertension portale	0 %	40%
Signes endocriniens	69,2%	50%
Signes cardiaques		
cliniques	30,7%	0%
électriques	46,1%	10%
Diabète	54 %	30%

de cirrhose alcoolique hémochromatosique. Le diabète, les signes endocriniens et surtout les signes cardiaques y sont peut-être moins fréquents. Les deux faits distinctifs fondamentaux concernent: 1) l'hypertension portale qui, dans notre série, est absente aussi bien cliniquement qu'à l'autopsie dans la forme primitive, tandis qu'elle est fréquente dans la forme secondaire. 2) l'hépatomégalie, qui est précoce, extensive, dans l'hémochromatose constitutionnelle. Dans la forme secondaire, au contraire, le foie est ou atrophié ou de volume normal. Quand l'hépatomégalie existe, elle est dans la règle modérée.

Signes biologiques différentiels entre hémochromatose primitive et hémochromatose secondaire des cirrhoses alcooliques

Ils sont résumés sur le Tableau 2.

Les différences, en ce qui concerne le métabolisme du fer (sidérémie moyenne plus basse dans les formes secondaires), sont moins significatives que celles qui affectent les épreuves hépatiques, en particulier l'épuration de la Bromesulfonephthaléine (B.S.P.). La *clearance* du colorant est dans la règle normale en cas d'hémochromatose primitive, tout au moins pendant la plus grande partie de l'évolution. L'épuration de la B.S.P. est précocément et fortement altérée (surtout pour la pente P_1) dans tous les cas de cirrhose de Laënnec devenus hémochromatosiques. Si on utilise l'Indocyanin Green, les mêmes constatations sont plus formelles.

Tableau 2. *Signes biologiques différentiels entre hémochromatose primitive et hémochromatose secondaire des cirrhoses alcooliques*

	Hémochromatose	
	idiopathique	secondaire des alcooliques
Biologie hépatique		
cholestérol total < 1,5 g.	58,3%	66,6%
Floculations + ...	7,7%	40 %
Forte rétention de la B.S.P.	0 %	88,2%
Elévation des gamma-glob.	83,3%	100 %
Métabolisme du fer		
taux moyen du fer sérique	244 gammas	192 gammas
saturation complète de la sidérophiline . .	87,5%	68,7%

Signes différentiels tirés de l'évolution anatomique des lésions

Ces deux formes d'hépatopathies s'opposent à la fois par l'évolution des lésions et le tableau anatomique auquel elles aboutissent.

A. Dans l'hémochromatose primitive constitutionnelle, la sidérose du foie est primitive, la sclérose est secondaire. L'aboutissant n'est pas une vraie cirrhose au sens strict du mot, mais une sidérofibrose hyperplasique diffuse.

Les documents suivants illustrent les étapes anatomiques évolutives de l'hémochromatose constitutionnelle en ce qui concerne les lésions hépatiques.

1ère étape — Elle est représentée par les ponctions-biopsies pratiquées chez des enfants, à transferrine saturée, de sujets hémochromatosiques qui nous ont été confiés par SCHAPIRA et J.-C. DREYFUS (5 observations). Dans chacun de ces cas, la cytosidérose hépatique est déjà abondante, souvent généralisée et massive, et il n'y a pas trace d'hyperplasie fibreuse portale ou trabéculaire.

2ème étape — Elle est représentée par des observations *d'adultes jeunes* atteints d'hémochromatose constitutionnelle. Je mentionne le cas d'un homme de 36 ans, amaigri, traité pour colopathie allergique, se plaignant d'impuissance sexuelle. On découvre un foie très augmenté de volume, mais très induré et tranchant, associé à une mélanodermie cervicale. Tous les tests biologiques d'altération hépatique sont négatifs (B.S.P. 45′ 2,5%; électrophorèse normale, transaminases et aldolases normales; cholestérol 1,75 g.). En *laparoscopie*, 3 signes doivent être soulignés: 1) le foie est lisse, sans nodules; 2) sa couleur rouille est flagrante; 3) au niveau du ligament rond et du péritoine, on ne découvre aucun signe d'hypertension portale. Une *ponction-biopsie* a été pratiquée dans 3 cas: la coloration de Perls à faible et à fort grossissement révèle une cytosidérose hépatique généralisée et massive (Fig. 1). Or sur la coloration de Masson correspondante

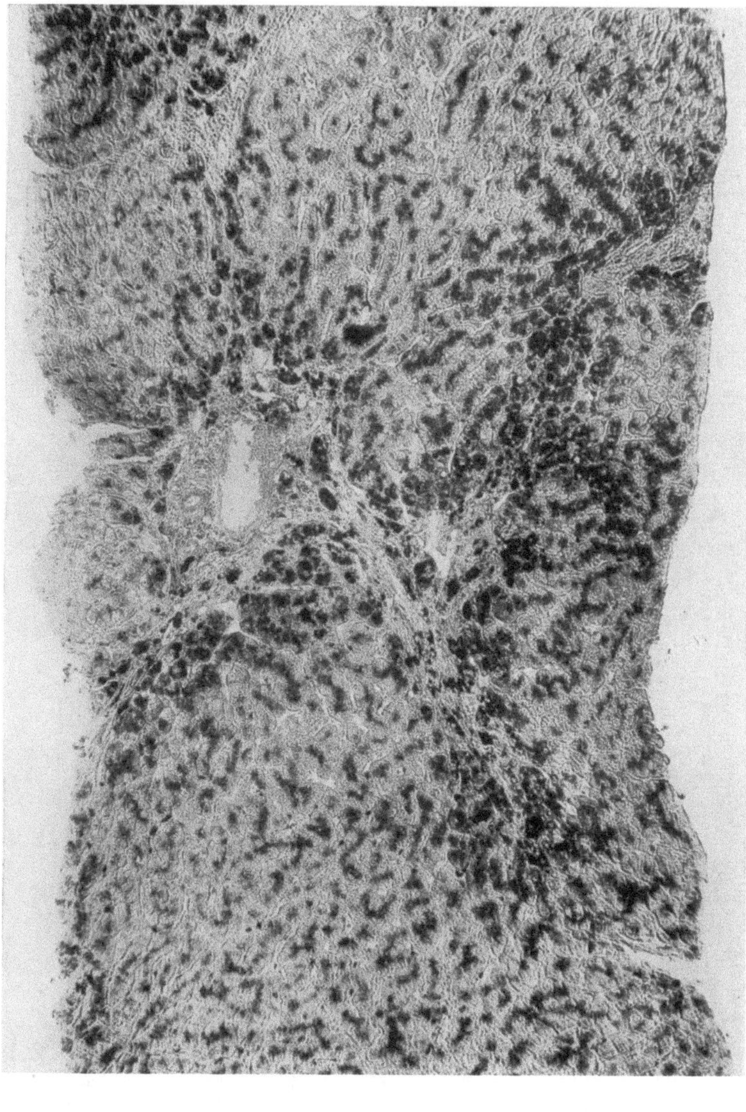

Fig. 1. Ponction-biopsie de foie. Coloration de Perls: hépatosidérose massive et diffuse; 100 ×

(Fig. 2), on peut affirmer que la fibrose est hors de proportion avec la cytosidérose; elle n'est représentée que par quelques septa élargis prolongeant les espaces portes. L'hémochromatose du jeune

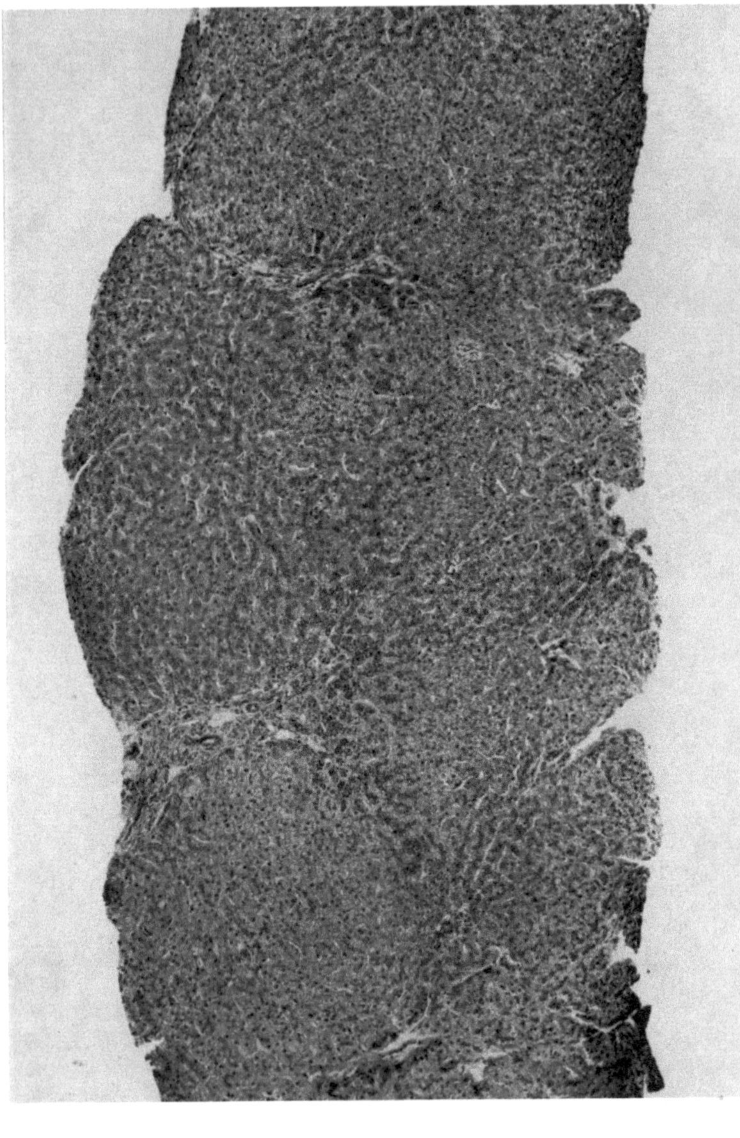

Fig. 2. Ponction-biopsie de foie. Coloration trichromique de MASSON. Sclérose très discrète; 75 ×

adulte n'est que l'agrandissement des lésions de l'enfant avec parfois seulement un début de fibrose. Dans ce cas, les saignées répétées aboutissent à une réduction complète de l'hépatomégalie.

3ème étape – Elle concerne les lésions tardives d'aboutissement. Les prélèvements de ponction-biopsie ne peuvent suffire pour leur étude analytique. On doit se baser sur de larges prélèvements d'autopsie. Etudions les documents obtenus dans 2 cas d'hémochromatose constitutionnelle ayant succombé à un adéno-cancer du foie. Nous n'étudions ici que les zones non transformées.

Les *photographies au contact* montrent que ces foies hémochromatosiques primitifs de taille énorme ne comportent aucun remaniement nodulaire apparent.

Les faits histologiques fondamentaux sont les suivants: 1) les veines hépatiques restent au centre des lobules; 2) ceux-ci sont extraordinairement agrandis par les lésions de fibrose hyperplasique, la surcharge ferrique, les néocanaux etc.; 3) les espaces portes sont écartelés. Les éléments de la triade sont normaux et en aucun cas on n'observe de multiplication des fentes vasculaires et les "angiomes" artério-veineux caractéristiques des cirrhoses portales.

En conclusion, à la phase terminale, l'hémochromatose constitutionnelle réalise une fibrose géante et non une cirrhose vraie. Il n'y a qu'un étirement des structures canalaires et non un remaniement (*Umbau*). Nous avons démontré ce fait avec CHENDEROVITCH (*6*) par la technique de BARCLAY.

B. Dans l'hémochromatose secondaire des cirrhoses, l'évolution des lésions histologiques se fait dans un sens opposé: d'une part, l'hépatopathie est primitive et la surcharge hémochromatosique secondaire, d'autre part, la lésion fondamentale est un remaniement *centrolobulaire.*

1 – Précession de la cirrhose. Un certain nombre d'auteurs, par ponction-biopsie en série le plus souvent, ont pu découvrir que chez les alcooliques en particulier, les signes histochimiques des hémochromatoses se greffent secondairement sur des lésions de cirrhose nodulaire déjà constituées.

Deux biopsies ont été prises à un an d'intervalle. La première montre un remaniement de cirrhose typique sans aucun dépôt ferrique. Il s'agissait alors d'un homme de 55 ans, alcoolique avéré. Foie gros, tests de floculations perturbés, galactosurie positive, B.S.P. 45′ 19%. Le second prélèvement, un an plus tard, montre une surcharge ferrique déjà notable avec hyperplasie et hypersidérose.

L'observation de CASTELMAN (*5*) est encore plus démonstrative. Il s'agissait d'un grand alcoolique atteint de cirrhose hypertrophique confirmée par les examens biologiques, la laparoscopie et la ponction-biopsie hépatique. Quatre ans et demi plus tard, le malade est revu dans un tableau grave: état septicémique, ictère, oedèmes, ascite, mélanodermie et hyperglycémie. A l'autopsie, on constate un foie clouté, surchargé d'hémosidérine, un pancréas fibreux et pigmenté, des ganglions lymphatiques de coloration brunâtre. Revoyant alors la première biopsie pratiquée quatre ans et demi auparavant, les auteurs ont retrouvé une cirrhose portale évidente, mais alors non accompagnée de surcharge sidérosique.

Citons également un cas de CACHERA et DARNIS (*3*).

2 – Les documents analogues deviennent plus nombreux depuis les cas publiés d'hémochromatose secondaire aux shunts porto-caves.

Il s'agit de faits récemment individualisés. La première observation a été publiée en effet par TUTTLE (*18*) en 1959. Depuis cette date, 5 observations détaillées ont été rapportées. Le tableau 3 résume les faits essentiels concernant 5 cas d'hémochromatose après shunt porto-cave jusqu'ici publiés. Deux cas concernent

Tableau 3. *Principaux faits cliniques et anatomiques concernant 5*

	TUTTLE (*18*)	HOFFBAUER (*11*) cas 4
Age Sexe	50 — H	55 — F
Alcoolisme	+	?
Type de cirrhose	Hypertrophique	Biliaire primitive
Intervention		
Motif	Hémorragie	Hémorragie
Type	porto-cave	porto-cave
Hémochromatose		
Date du diagnostic après l'intervention	3 ans	10 mois
Signes cliniques		
— Mélanodermie	+	
— Diabète	+	
Fer sérique	330 gammas	
Cause de la mort	Coma hépatique	Coma hépatique
Autopsie	Cirrhose nodulaire (2.330 g.) Sidérose hépatique et pancréatique Sclérosidérose de myocarde, surrénales, tractus digestif	Cirrhose à gros nodules Sidérose hépatique et pancréatique

des hommes, mais 3 autres des femmes. Dans chacune de ces observations, une biopsie pré- ou per-opératoire avait démontré l'absence de sidérose hépatique. L'hémochromatose s'est développée plus ou moins rapidement après l'intervention, entre 10 mois et 9 ans. Dans tous les cas, à l'autopsie, non seulement la sidérose hépatique était importante, mais la surcharge atteignait pancréas, myocarde, surrénales, tractus digestif et reins.

3 – Les documents suivants concernent 3 de nos 20 observations d'hémochromatose permettant de préciser le tableau anatomo-clinique de ces cirrhoses alcooliques de Laënnec hémochromatosiques. Deux cas sont morts, l'un est encore en vie.

Cas n° 1 – Mme P.

Alcoolisme très important. Début par asthénie, anorexie, amaigrissement. La décompensation se manifeste par ascite et oedème des membres inférieurs. Il y a des troubles psychiques, des varices oesophagiennes et une surinfection avec ulcération cutanée. Les tests biologiques sont de haute gravité, y compris et surtout la fibrinolyse. Les documents anatomiques *in vivo*, surtout la laparophotographie de contact, montrent l'atrophie du lobe droit

observations d'hémochromatose après anastomose porto-cave

TISDALE (*17*) cas 23	TISDALE (*17*) cas 32	SCHAEFER (*15*)
27 — F	53 — F	37 — H
+	—	+
Post-nécrotique	Post-nécrotique	Post-nécrotique
Hémorragie splénorénale	Hémorragie porto-cave	Hémorragie porto-cave
9 ans $^1/_2$	2 ans $^1/_2$	3 ans
—	+ antérieure au shunt	+
—	—	+
Coma hépatique Cirrhose atrophique (1.020 g.) Sidérose hépatique Sclérosidérose pancréatique Sidérose modérée de myocarde, surrénales, tubes rénaux	Coma Cirrhose à petits nodules (1.650 g.) Sidérose de foie et pancréas	Coma hépatique Cirrhose atrophique (800 g.) Sidérose de foie, pancréas, myocarde, estomac, surrénales

entrainant l'érection de la vésicule, la surface hépatique est en damier, mais dans l'intervalle des travées scléreuses, la surcharge rouillée intra-lobulaire est parfaitement représentée sur la photographie, le caractère massif de l'hémochromatose est confirmé par

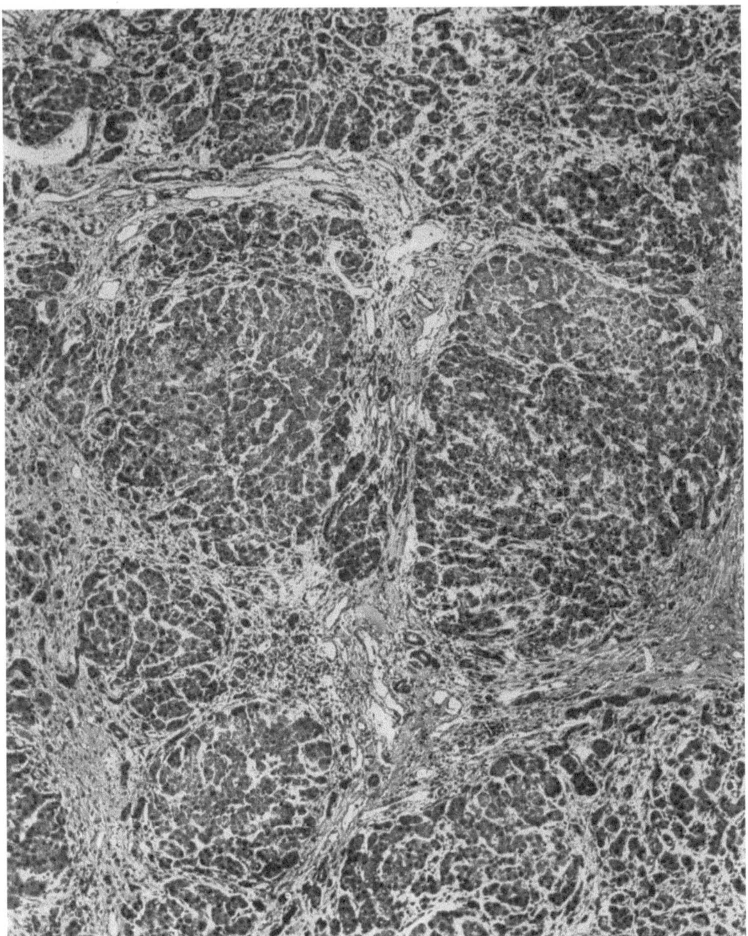

Fig. 3. Coupe de foie. Coloration trichromique de MASSON. Remaniement architectural de la lobulation avec réorganisation de la circulation intra-hépatique; 75 ×

la ponction-biopsie. Malgré les soins, le cas a évolué vers la mort. L'autopsie montre que la particularité des hémochromatoses alcooliques réside essentiellement dans les faits suivants: la structure hépatique est bouleversée (Fig. 3) les veines hépatiques ne sont plus repérables au centre d'un lobule; les espaces portes

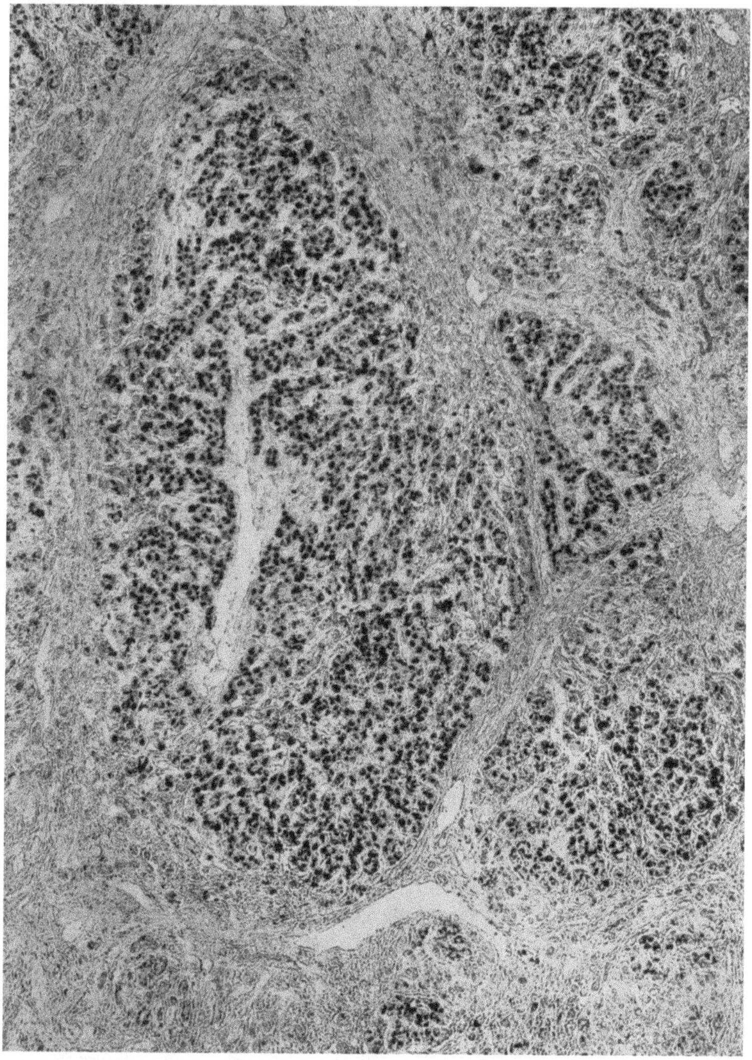

Fig. 4. Coupe de foie. Coloration de PERLS. Surcharge de pigment ferrique correspondant à une hémochromatose secondaire; 85 ×

paraissent rapprochés les uns des autres, unis par des travées fibreuses, au sein desquelles le signe anatomique le plus flagrant est la multiplication et la dilatation des vaisseaux de structure veineuse qui témoignent du remaniement intra-hépatique du système circulatoire et répondent à des signes d'hypertension portale qui, statistiquement, caractérisent l'hémochromatose secondaire des alcooliques, par son association (Fig. 4).

Cas n° 2 — Mme D.

Il s'agit là d'un cas comparable. Cette femme est une grande alcoolique chez qui on note des perturbations de la biologie hépatique considérables, surtout en ce qui concerne la rétention de la B.S.P. Néanmoins, le tableau anatomique n'est pas tout à fait le même, car le foie est augmenté de volume et, comme dans les antécédents on retrouve que la mère et un frère étaient pigmentés, on peut à la rigueur admettre qu'un élément constitutionnel a favorisé l'action de l'alcool. Le diagnostic anatomique *in vivo* confirme le diagnostic d'hémochromatose, mais contrairement à ce qu'on observe dans la forme constitutionnelle, la surface hépatique n'est pas lisse, mais franchement micronodulaire. L'évolution a été mortelle. L'autopsie montre que la surcharge ferrique viscérale est non seulement très importante, mais généralisée.

Comme dans le cas précédent, il s'agit d'une vraie cirrhose et non pas seulement d'une fibrose (Fig. 5). En effet, la veine centrolobulaire est déplacée, la circulation hépatique est remaniée et la fibrose est disloquée par une néoangiomatose veineuse témoignant du remaniement dans la distribution circulatoire du foie, signe indiscutable de cirrhose hépatique vraie.

Cas n° 3 — M. G.

Il s'agit d'un homme de 45 ans. La pigmentation est évidente, les complications sont très graves (ascite infectée), les perturbations biologiques dans les fonctions hépatiques sont considérables. Quant à la biopsie, la fibrose est tellement mutilante et la surcharge ferrique si intense qu'aucune structure lobulaire normale n'est reconnaissable, qu'il s'agisse des coupes colorées au trichrome de MASSON ou de la coloration de VILDER pour la réticuline.

La transferrine était saturée. L'évolution a été émaillée des complications les plus graves qui peuvent survenir au cours des cirrhoses portales: melaena, encéphalopathie porto-cave transitoire avec hyperammoniémie. Néanmoins, l'état s'est actuellement stabilisé, et nous allons pouvoir tenter un traitement par le Desféral.

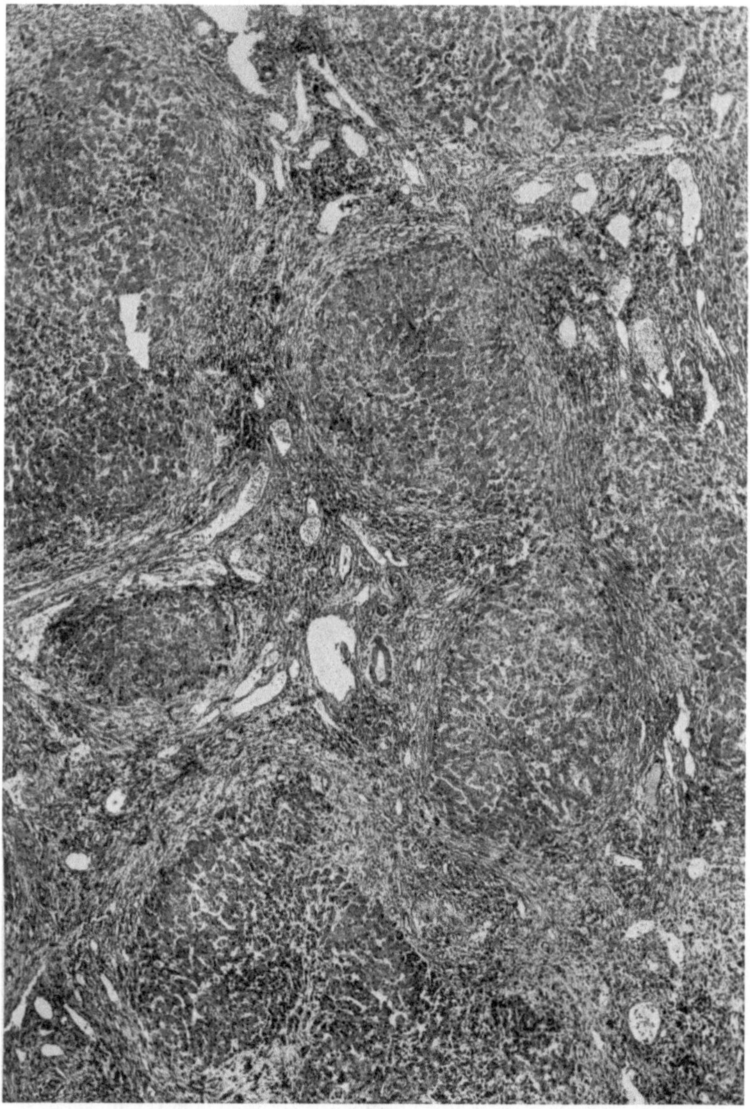

Fig. 5. Coupe de foie. Coloration trichromique de Masson. Remaniement de la distribution circulatoire associée à une fibrose qui disloque les lobules; 42 ×

Nous sommes incapables de fournir l'explication de l'hémochromatose secondaire des cirrhoses, alcooliques ou non. On a évoqué un facteur nutritionnel et le rôle de l'hémolyse. Aucun auteur n'a pu encore fournir une raison valable expliquant l'influence, en apparence favorable, d'un shunt porto-cave chirurgical. Comme pour les Bantous, le rôle d'un apport excessif de fer alimentaire doit surtout, à notre avis, être retenu. Cette hypothèse que nous avions soulevée a été reprise par Aron (*2*) qui a montré que, chez le rat, l'ingestion prolongée de vin déterminait une cytosidérose. Une enquête personnelle nous a révélé que le vin de consommation courante contenait en moyenne 15 mg. de fer par litre: un sujet buvant 2 l. de vin par jour aura un apport de fer 3 fois supérieur aux apports normaux. MacDonald (*14*) considère la teneur en fer du vin comme un facteur étiologique important dans l'hémochromatose, et Zimmerman (*19*) a avancé une opinion comparable. Lamache et Bourel (*12*), pour leur part, ont incriminé le rôle de l'eau de boisson.

Les indications thérapeutiques ne peuvent pas être les mêmes en principe dans les hémochromatoses secondaires et dans les hémochromatoses constitutionnelles. Aucune de nos hémochromatoses alcooliques, en raison de la dysprotidémie dont ces malades étaient atteints dans la règle, n'a été soumise aux saignées répétées. Ce traitement cependant est préconisé par Conte (*7*), qui soustrait les globules rouges et réinjecte le plasma. Le domaine des hémochromatoses secondaires devrait être l'indication élective des chélateurs du fer, si leur action se révèle dans l'avenir suffisante. Le seul cas d'hémochromatose secondaire que nous ayons eu jusqu'ici l'occasion de traiter n'a pas répondu, de façon aussi satisfaisante, à l'action de la desferrioxamine que les 6 cas d'hémochromatose constitutionnelle traités par ce chélateur. Mais la surcharge ferrique, dans cette observation, malgré une saturation complète de la transferrine, était trop faible pour que nous puissions la retenir comme un cas défavorable.

Résumé

A côté de l'hémochromatose congénitale il existe une hémochromatose acquise secondaire à la cirrhose alcoolique. Elle s'en différencie cliniquement par l'existence d'une hypertension portale et l'inconstance de l'hépatomégalie. Elle en diffère également par l'existence d'importantes perturbations de la biologie hépatique, lesquelles sont en règle modérées dans la forme idiopathique. Enfin et surtout l'évolution anatomique est fondamentalement différente dans ces deux variétés d'hémochromatose: dans la variété primitive, la sidérose précède et vraisemblablement détermine le développement de la sclérose, alors que dans la variété secondaire, la cirrhose précède l'apparition de la surcharge sidérosique. Le mécanisme pathogénique de l'hémochromatose secondaire aux cirrhoses alcooliques est encore mal élucidé; le rôle d'un apport alimentaire excessif de fer paraît probable.

Summary

In addition to congenital haemochromatosis there also exists a form of acquired haemochromatosis secondary to alcoholic cirrhosis. The latter differs clinically from the former in that it is associated with portal hypertension and that hepatomegaly is not a consistent finding. It also differs from the idiopathic form of haemochromatosis inasmuch as marked biological disorders occur in the liver, whereas in idiopathic haemochromatosis such disorders are usually only mild. Lastly and above all, the anatomical evolution of the disease is fundamentally different in these two types of haemochromatosis: in the primary form, the siderosis precedes and probably induces the development of sclerosis, whereas in the secondary form it is the cirrhosis which precedes the siderosis. The pathological mechanism leading to haemochromatosis as a sequel to alcoholic cirrhosis is still poorly understood, but it seems likely that an excessive uptake of dietary iron plays a role in this process.

Zusammenfassung

Neben der kongenitalen Haemochromatose gibt es eine erworbene Form, die sekundär als Folge einer alkoholisch bedingten Leberzirrhose auftritt. Sie unterscheidet sich klinisch dadurch, daß ein Pfortaderhochdruck vorliegt, und daß sie nicht immer mit einer Hepatomegalie einhergeht. Während bei der idiopathischen Form die Störungen der Leberfunktion meist nur geringgradig sind, sind sie bei der sekundären Zirrhose erheblich. Schließlich ist vor allem der anatomische Verlauf dieser beiden Arten von Haemochromatose der Leber verschieden: bei der idiopathischen Form geht die Siderose voraus und bestimmt die Entwicklung der Sklerose, während sich bei der sekundären Form die Zirrhose vor dem Erscheinen von Eisendepots manifestiert. Der Mechanismus der sekundären Haemochromatose im Verlauf einer alkoholischen Zirrhose ist nicht geklärt; wahrscheinlich wird sie durch eine übermäßige Aufnahme von Eisen mit der Nahrung begünstigt.

References

1. André, J.: Rev. internat. hépat. (Fr.) **11**, 113 (1961). — 2. Aron, E., C. Paoletti, P. Jobard, et C. Gosse: Arch. mal. app. digest. (Fr.) **50**, 745 (1961). — 3. Cachera, R., et F. Darnis: Rev. internat. hépat. (Fr.) **6**, 163 (1956). — 4. Caroli, J., et J. Étevé: Arch. biol. méd. (Sem. hôp. Paris) **30**, B 19 (1954). — 5. Castelman, B.: N. England J. Med. **235**, 798 (1946). — 6. Chenderovitch, J., et J. Caroli: Rev. internat. hépat. (Fr.) **6**, 907 (1956). — 7. Conte, M., J. Ristelhueber, C. Julien, et A. Leclercq: Sem. hôp. Paris **35**, 465 (1958). — 8. Debré, R.: Arch. biol. méd. (Sem. hôp. Paris) **30**, B 145 (1954). — 9. Gillman, J., et T. Gillman: Gastroenterology (E.-U.) 8, 19 (1947). — 10. Heilmeyer, L., W. Keller, O. Vivell, W. Keiderling, K. Betke, F. Wöhler, et H. E. Schultze: Dtsch. med. Wschr. **86**, 1745 (1961). — 11. Hoffbauer, F. W.: Amer. J. Digest. Dis. **5**, 348 (1960). — 12. Lamache, A., et M. Bourel: Path. biol. (Sem. hôp. Paris) **34**, P.B. 857 (1958). — 13. Lamy, M., et J. Frezal: Bull. Soc. méd. hôp. Paris **74**, 369 (1958). — 14. MacDonald, R. A.: Arch. Int. Med. (E.-U.) **107**, 606 (1961). — 15. Schaefer, J. W., C. J. Amick, Y. Oikawa, et L. Schiff: Gastroenterology (E.-U.) **42**, 181 (1962). — 16. Sheldon, J. H.: Haemochromatosis. Oxford Univ. Press, London, 1935. — 17. Tisdale, W. A.: N. England J. Med. **265**, 928 (1961). — 18. Tuttle, S. G., W. G. Figueroa, et M. I. Grossman: Amer. J. Med. **26**, 655 (1959). — 19. Zimmerman, H. J., B. Chomet, M. H. Kulesh, et C. A. McWhorter: Arch. Int. Med. (E.-U.) **107**, 494 (1961).

Discussion

BRICK: I should like to present a couple of tables featuring some data from two families in which haemochromatosis occurred. Like Dr. DREYFUS, I believe that the most accurate determinant in these genetic studies is liver biopsy. Table 1 illustrates a family in which the propositus is dead. We have an autopsy of him. We also have available a study of the succeeding generation. There were seven siblings in all, three of whom showed clinical haemochromatosis; the others displayed evidence of increased iron stores, including the two female siblings. One of the sons of the propositus, at the age of 25, had increased serum iron. We have recently received a report that he now has diabetes. We have not had an opportunity to do a biopsy on this individual.

All of the siblings shown in Table 1 are above the age of 40. This brings up the question that Dr. DREYFUS raised: should asymptomatic siblings really be treated, should they have a venesection, or should they be given a chelating agent? It is not certain that these patients will go on to haemochromatosis, and, if they are treated, how are we going to be able to know whether they would have developed haemochromatosis? Two of the members of this family died — not from their haemochromatosis, but one from pneumonia and one from a myocardial infarct. This raises the question as to whether such patients, particularly if over the age of 40, should be treated because they are known to be suffering from this genetic disease. I think that, as Dr. DREYFUS has shown, if these asymptomatic siblings are much younger they should possibly be given intermittent treatment. As there is not a complete correlation between liver iron and serum iron, I would suggest that liver biopsy is still the best way to diagnose both the disease and the trait.

Table 2 has a bearing on what Dr. CAROLI has already said. In this family the propositus is a priest who has overt haemochromatosis. When he was first seen 10 years ago, he had very large oesophageal varices, so we had a prophylactic portacaval shunt done. Since then I have been impressed by Dr. SHERLOCK's work to the effect that we shouldn't do prophylactic shunts, and we don't do them any more. This patient's brother, who is 9 years older, came for treatment 7 years later. The first clinical manifestation was massive gastro-intestinal haemorrhage, and extremely large varices were noted. I can't agree if you are saying that portacaval hypertension doesn't present itself in familial or idiopathic haemochromatosis. Incidentally, this last brother has not been shunted, but has been treated for the past 3 years by venesection. He has not had any further haemorrhage, and repeat oesophagoscopy has revealed that the varices are still present, but that they are smaller. Three of our other patients with haemochromatosis have had to be shunted for bleeding from oesophageal varices.

KATZ: I'd just like to emphasise again the problem of the histological criteria for haemochromatosis. I think one of the difficulties is that many different methods for fixation of the tissue are used. PECHET and MACDONALD[1] report a very high incidence of significant amounts of stainable iron in the

[1] PECHET, G. S., and R. A. MACDONALD: N. England J. Med. **267**, 6 (1962).

Table 1. *Data on Family D, showing evidence of familial haemochromatosis in all of 7 siblings*

Name	Sex	Age	Serum Fe/U.I.B.C.*	Glucose tolerance test	Liver biopsy
W. (propositus)	M	50	180/0	110—230—184—143—96	Pigment cirrhosis
J.	M	52	220/0	230—380—460—375—360	Pigment cirrhosis
T.	M	54	125/50	125—208—252—133—79	Haemosiderosis, moderate
H.	M	48	158/100	98—159—200—155—115	Haemosiderosis, severe; fatty infiltration, moderate
R.	M	43	215/0	95—154—206—171—155	Haemosiderosis, marked; fatty infiltration, severe; portal fibrosis, mild
Rs.	F	40	155/50	120—183—200—152—149	Haemosiderosis, mild
M.	F	45	130/50	100—320—340—115—156	Haemosiderosis, mild

* U.I.B.C. = unsaturated iron-binding capacity.

Table 2. *Data on Family H, in whom 2 of the siblings showed large oesophageal varices in addition to familial haemochromatosis*

Name	Sex	Age	Oesophagoscopy	Liver biopsy
1. Propositus	M	50	Large varices (shunted)	Pigment cirrhosis
2. P.	M	59	Large varices	Pigment cirrhosis
3. W.	M	49	Negative	Haemosiderosis, moderate
4. H.	M	48	Negative	Haemosiderosis, moderate
5. C.	F	53	Negative	Haemosiderosis and fibrosis, moderate

liver of patients from a particular hospital in Boston. But they use a buffered formalin to fix the tissues. I think that what is required is a world-wide study, using a single technique for fixation and staining of tissue, before we can know for certain what constitutes an abnormal amount of iron in a biopsy.

There is one other point that I wanted to make regarding the difficulty of distinguishing idiopathic haemochromatosis from the haemosiderosis that is found in cirrhotics. CROSBY [1] very recently reported at a meeting an interesting case of a man with alcoholic cirrhosis whose liver was loaded with iron and who was treated by venesection. He very promptly became anaemic — in contrast, of course, to the usual haemochromatotic in whom the haemoglobin levels remain stable in the face of repeated venesection. I think, therefore, that it's very important to distinguish between local iron stores and total body stores, and I don't think one can do this simply on the basis of the liver biopsy.

BEARN: The evolution of the history of the genetics of haemochromatosis has been most instructive, with the hypothesis shuttling back and forth between a dominant and a recessive mode of inheritance. It is perhaps worth emphasising that these two terms could be eliminated from our vocabulary without too much loss. I should like to raise the question of possible heterogenicity. Is there any evidence of genetic heterogenicity? Do you have any calculations on the gene frequency? In Dr. BRICK's pedigree all the offspring were either affected or carriers. This made me wonder whether one parent was affected and the other a carrier. I also wonder whether you have done any studies in which you were able to compare the age of onset within families and between families.

BOTHWELL: In a disease such as haemochromatosis, where the aetiology is at present completely unknown, we tend to clutch at any straw that presents itself. In this context there is one point which I think may be significant. In family studies we have found that the plasma iron level is often considerably raised in affected relatives at a time when stores are only mildly increased, and examination of the results obtained by others indicates that this association is not uncommon. Now in animal studies — and Dr. MOORE's studies in dogs exemplify this beautifully — there is no rise in the plasma iron level with massive overload, even after several years. This raises the question as to whether there isn't some disordered reticulo-endothelial function in idiopathic haemochromatosis which leads to an alteration in the iron gradient between these cells and the plasma.

With regard to the question raised by Dr. BEARN, our own data suggest that the time of onset of clinical manifestations in a given family is moderately constant if due allowance is made for the additional iron losses in menstruating females.

VERLOOP: Dr. CAROLI pointed out that it is difficult to distinguish *in vivo* between primary haemochromatosis and haemochromatosis secondary to alcoholic siderosis. Now when you give a test dose of desferrioxamine to patients with primary haemochromatosis, there is a large excretion of iron in the urine, whereas patients with alcoholic cirrhosis excrete only a little more than usual. We have had a patient with alcoholic cirrhosis and haemochromatosis, to whom we gave a test dose of 800 mg. desferrioxamine, and he excreted only 1.3 mg. iron. I know that Dr. VANNOTTI has had the same ex-

[1] CROSBY, W. H.: The Control of Iron Metabolism: Lecture given at the Boston City Hospital, Boston (U.S.A.), 16th April, 1963.

perience; this may be of some help to Dr. CAROLI in attempting to differentiate between his haemochromatosis patients.

VANNOTTI: I should like to add that we, too, studied the urinary excretion of iron during desferrioxamine treatment in normal subjects and in patients suffering from cirrhosis. We observed that in cirrhosis the iron excretion in response to this treatment remains very low (less than 2.5 mg. per 24 hours). The mean value for the iron excretion in our 12 cases of cirrhosis was even lower than in normal subjects under treatment with desferrioxamine. The iron excretion also remains low in cases of liver cirrhosis which are characterised by marked siderosis of the liver.

It is difficult to explain these facts, although one could assume that, in cirrhotic patients with siderosis of the liver, the deposited iron becomes fixed in the fibrotic infiltrated tissue of the liver, whence it is probably more difficult to remove it. Observations concerning the lymphatic circulation in the liver, through which appreciable quantities of iron may be released into the systemic circulation, offer perhaps another explanation for this phenomenon. By means of a subcapsular injection into the liver of human albumin labelled with I^{131} MAGNENAT and DELALOYE[1] demonstrated that, in our patient suffering from cirrhosis without ascites, the subcapsular lymphatic circulation was decreased. In this case it seems reasonable to suppose that the lymphatic circulation of desferrioxamine was reduced.

Finally I should like to repeat that our quantitative immunochemical determination of transferrin (VANNOTTI and BLANC[2]) showed a very pronounced decrease in the transferrin level in the blood of patients with haemochromatosis (the average being 87—130 mg.% as compared with a normal level of 200—300 mg.%). We have also observed a diminution in serum transferrin in the presence of infectious hepatitis (average for our cases: 130 mg.%) as well as in liver cirrhosis (average: 175 mg.%).

FRICK: I should like to show how it is possible, by reference to ferrokinetics, to diagnose hereditary haemochromatosis in children before the development of any organic changes[3]. To illustrate what I mean, let me

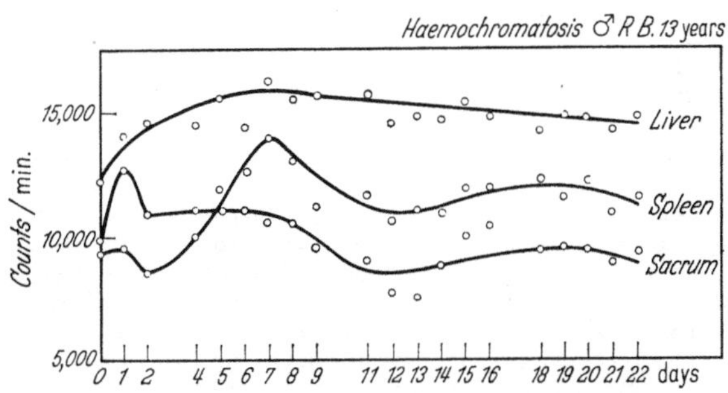

Fig. 1. Surface counts over liver, spleen, and sacrum after injection of Fe^{59} in a case of familial idiopathic haemochromatosis

---

[1] MAGNENAT, P., and B. DELALOYE: Rev. méd.-chir. mal. foie (Fr.), in press (1963).

[2] VANNOTTI, A., and B. BLANC: Schweiz. med. Wschr. **93**, 1189 (1963).

[3] BRUNNER, H. E., P. G. FRICK, and W. H. HITZIG: Schweiz. med. Wschr. **92**, 343 (1962).

describe the case of a 13-year-old child who was taken to the out-patient department by his mother because the father had died of haemochromatosis at the age of 35. The child showed no functional or organic changes indicative of the disease; liver biopsy disclosed no excessive iron deposits, but ferrokinetics revealed the typical findings of haemochromatosis. The half-life of the plasma iron was prolonged to 140 minutes, and the iron turnover was elevated to 33 mg./day; the total iron-binding capacity was slightly decreased to 195 μg.% and showed virtual saturation. The most important findings were the surface counts over the liver: these were much higher throughout the study than the counts over the bone marrow and spleen, indicating excessive hepatic iron storage (Fig. 1). The child was bled, and it was found possible to remove 800 mg. iron over a period of 3 months without making him anaemic, a fact which suggests that his iron storage must have been appreciable.

ALBAHARY: With reference to the sideruria test with desferrioxamine in families with a history of idiopathic haemochromatosis, I have had experience of two cases; one of them was sent to me by Dr. DREYFUS last year. This case, the son of a patient with severe haemochromatosis, did not respond at all to the treatment. I also had another case, the nephew of a patient with haemochromatosis whom I had seen; here, I was able to obtain a urinary iron excretion of up to almost 10 mg. a day. Admittedly, this is not very much, but it's a little more than in the usual cases that you have reported.

TUBIANA: A few years ago, we compared the ferrokinetics in two groups of patients: in idiopathic haemochromatotics and in alcoholic cirrhotics with high levels of blood iron[1]. In the patients with idiopathic haemochromatosis we observed the classic findings: a slow disappearance of plasma iron, a low rate of incorporation into the red cells, and a high uptake by the liver. By contrast, in patients suffering from alcoholic cirrhosis with haemochromatosis, the plasma iron disappearance rate was normal and the turnover of plasma iron accelerated. The rate of incorporation of iron into the red cells was higher than normal, and the uptake by the liver was absolutely normal. The erythropoiesis of iron was thus accelerated in these patients with alcoholic cirrhosis —probably in order to compensate for the shortening of the red-cell life-span, as shown with chromium. Furthermore, this study seems to indicate that the functional iron pool is either normal or certainly not higher than normal in these patients, a finding which would confirm what Dr. KATZ has reported.

MOESCHLIN: We, like Dr. VERLOOP and Dr. VANNOTTI, encountered no enhancement of iron excretion in response to desferrioxamine in patients with secondary haemochromatosis due to alcoholic cirrhosis or to cirrhosis associated with chronic hepatitis — two forms of cirrhosis that are both very common in Switzerland; this lack of response contrasts with the striking increase in urinary iron excretion seen in primary homozygote idiopathic haemochromatosis. I think the reason for the difference is that, in secondary haemochromatosis due to alcoholic cirrhosis, there is much more haemosiderin and less ferritin than in the idiopathic primary form of haemochromatosis.

VENTURA: May I ask Dr. CAROLI a question concerning the biochemical differences between idiopathic haemochromatosis and haemochromatosis secondary to alcoholic cirrhosis? Has he seen any difference between porphyrin metabolism in these two diseases? I ask this question because there exists a primary porphyrin disease — porphyria cutanea tarda — which

[1] ROSSELIN, G., et al.: Path. biol. (Sem. hôp. Paris) 8, 1833 (1960).

develops in alcoholic patients and is characterised by hepatic siderosis with cirrhotic evolution of the hepatic lesions[1,2].

FIGUEROA: We, too, have carried out ferrokinetic studies in patients with primary haemochromatosis and haemochromatosis secondary to alcoholism and have found such studies very useful as a means of investigating the distribution of iron in the body; this is particularly true of cases where the patient refuses a liver biopsy or where this procedure is clinically contra-indicated. There have been two publications[3,4] that have drawn attention to the fact that measuring the serum iron and the saturated iron-binding capacity can no longer be regarded as an adequate means by which to detect relatives of patients with haemochromatosis who are showing early excessive iron storage; the authors of these publications argue that one has to do a liver biopsy in order to detect all such individuals, i.e. because some of the patients with normal ferrous iron levels have shown excessive iron in the liver when subjected to liver biopsy. I should like to know whether Dr. DREYFUS has any information on this point. I believe he stated that he had done biopsies on patients with high serum iron, but I am not clear whether he also biopsied the individuals with normal serum iron.

Among the cases published was one involving the son of a patient with haemochromatosis who had normal serum iron levels and showed "moderate" amounts of iron in the liver, and the patient became severely anaemic after only a brief period of treatment by venesection. If one estimates the amount of iron withdrawn and corrects for the anaemia produced, one reaches the conclusion that this particular individual had no more than 2.5 to 3.0 g. storage iron. Now I would like to ask Dr. DREYFUS whether he can take an individual with haemochromatosis and give some kind of an estimate as to how much iron there is in that particular body and therefore provide the clinician with some guide as to how long it will take to remove it.

J.-C. DREYFUS: I am afraid that many of the problems you have raised I cannot answer. First of all, with regard to the problem of determining the amount of iron accumulated in primary and secondary haemochromatosis, some authors think that in cases where the haemochromatosis is secondary to liver cirrhosis, most of the iron is in the stainable form, so that a chemical determination would show that the total iron is in fact much less in this form than in primary haemochromatosis. However, this assumption is very difficult to check by means of needle biopsies, because the amount of tissue available is too small for both chemical and histological examinations. The 1—2 mg. of tissue which the chemist would be left with is enough for him to determine the iron content accurately, but it may consist either of fibrotic tissue or of blood, and the results would therefore not be reliable.

In reply to Dr. FIGUEROA, I must confess that we have not studied ferrokinetics in the offspring of our haemochromatosis patients. It would certainly be desirable to do so, but we were reluctant to give radioactive iron to apparently healthy subjects, so we confined ourselves to measuring the serum iron and the unsaturated iron-binding capacity, performing a liver biopsy, and determining the rise in urinary iron excretion in response to desferriox-

---

[1] BRUGSCH, J., D. KLAUS, and A. BIENENGRÄBER: Zschr. inn. Med. (G.) **12**, 887 (1957).

[2] VENTURA, S.: Minerva med. (It.) **50**, 2381 (1959).

[3] FREY, W. G., III, J. MILNE, G. B. JOHNSON Jr., and F. G. EBAUGH Jr.: N. England J. Med. **265**, 7 (1961).

[4] BRICK, I. B.: Gastroenterology (U.S.A.) **40**, 210 (1961).

amine. There are two reasons for supposing that the iron deposits in the offspring of these patients are small: the normal elimination of iron in response to desferrioxamine, and the fact that in two of these subjects anaemia was beginning to develop after venesection treatment had been in progress for six months. However, in one of them (a man of 40), venesection had been carried out once a week, as the result of which 5 litres of blood had been removed. So, once again, I would recommend for these children of haemochromatosis patients only a very mild form of treatment (e.g. removal of 300 ml. blood once a month) and I would certainly not advise the use of chelating agents, which would be quite ineffective at such low levels of iron overload.

With reference to Dr. BOTHWELL's remark, I would point out that we have performed liver biopsies only on subjects who had high serum iron levels. All the biopsies yielded positive findings. The only negative case was that of a patient with normal serum iron. So we think that serum iron is a good test — although, of course, not absolutely infallible — and our opinion seems to be borne out by the results of WILLIAMS, SCHEUER, and SHERLOCK[1].

Finally, in reply to Dr. BEARN, I cannot give any definite answer to the question about genetic heterogenicity. We have studied about 50 families, but the results are not statistically significant. One of them shows evidence of possible homozygosity, since both parents of the patient had high serum iron levels. But no other members of the family whom we were able to examine showed any abnormalities.

CAROLI: Dr. BRICK has referred to two brothers with idiopathic haemochromatosis in whom gastro-intestinal haemorrhages occurred owing to rupture of oesophageal varices. We ourselves have never observed portal hypertension in cases of familial haemochromatosis, whereas we have frequently encountered this complication in patients with haemochromatosis secondary to alcoholic cirrhosis. We think that this difference can be explained by the fact that in idiopathic haemochromatosis there is no alteration in the circulation such as one sees in true nodular cirrhosis.

Dr. KATZ in his remarks emphasised the importance of distinguishing between, on the one hand, local cytosiderosis of the mild kind occurring in alcoholics and, on the other hand, genuine haemochromatosis. In this connection, he stressed that one cannot distinguish between the two simply by doing a liver biopsy, because the latter will merely indicate a local storage of iron without reference to any increase in the total body stores. We are fully in agreement with him on this; however, I would point out that autopsy examinations have shown us that, in some patients suffering from alcoholic cirrhosis, one finds a massive and diffuse iron overload involving all the parenchymal tissues of the glands in the same way as in the most authentic cases of idiopathic haemochromatosis.

The desferrioxamine test which Dr. VERLOOP has suggested as a means of distinguishing primary from secondary haemochromatosis will undoubtedly prove of great interest if it can be confirmed that desferrioxamine does in fact produce only a slight increase in urinary iron excretion in patients with alcoholic siderosis. In this regard, our own findings have been in agreement with those of Dr. VERLOOP and Dr. VANNOTTI.

In reply to Dr. VENTURA's question, I am afraid we have not had an opportunity of doing any comparative studies on porphyrin metabolism in our patients suffering from idiopathic haemochromatosis and in those with secondary haemochromatosis, nor have we had any patients with porphyria cutanea tarda.

---

[1] WILLIAMS, R., P. J. SCHEUER, and S. SHERLOCK: Quart. J. Med. (G.B.) **31**, 249 (1962).

Post-transfusional haemosiderosis

By

F. J. CLETON and A. P. R. BLOK

In the last ten years more refined procedures in blood-group immunology and blood banking have enabled us to treat more patients with refractory anaemia over a prolonged period. Multiple transfusions, however, inevitably burden the body with large amounts of iron, and clinical manifestations of iron overload are observed with increasing frequency. While the clinical signs and the histological features of transfusional iron overload may vary considerably from one patient to another, it is apparent that the deposition of excessive amounts of iron in the cells may in some instances be associated with tissue damage and impairment of organ function. The exact pathogenesis of this acquired condition has not yet been clarified, and it is difficult to understand why some individuals appear to be more susceptible than others.

This problem has assumed practical importance now that the withdrawal of excessive storage iron from the body can be brought about by administering synthetic chelating agents.

It is the purpose of this paper to discuss several aspects of the pathogenesis of transfusional iron overload and to present observations on one unusual case.

Present knowledge of the development of post-transfusional haemosiderosis has been acquired by means of accurate histological observation (BOTHWELL, 1953; DUBIN, 1955; CAPPELL et al., 1957; OLIVER, 1959). The iron derived from donor erythrocytes is initially accumulated by cells of the reticulo-endothelial system, mainly in the liver, spleen, lymph nodes, and bone marrow. After a variable interval of time, a redistribution of the iron may take place within the body, part of the storage iron being transferred to the parenchymal cells (FINCH and FINCH, 1955). This form of iron storage, occurring predominantly in the reticulo-endothelial cells and associated with few signs of tissue damage, is commonly referred to as haemosiderosis.

A second pattern of post-transfusional iron overload, marked by the accumulation of greater quantities of iron in the parenchymal cells and associated with significant tissue damage and fibrosis, has been designated secondary or post-transfusional haemochromatosis (Kent and Popper, 1960). In the latter condition, considerable amounts of iron may also be found in the parenchymal cells of the endocrine glands and in the heart. Here, the histological picture is reminiscent of that observed in idiopathic haemochromatosis, but on careful examination certain differences in the distribution of the iron and in the connective-tissue reaction can usually be found. These differences relate to the amount of iron in the reticulo-endothelial cells, to the deposition of iron in the spleen and in the bone marrow, and to the degree of fibrosis. Though it must be admitted that the two patterns of iron storage are at times difficult to differentiate, the establishment of a clear distinction between them has been very helpful in studying the pathogenesis of post-transfusional iron overload.

Variations observed in the degree of the pathological changes occurring in the tissues following multiple transfusions have raised the question whether factors other than iron alone play a role in this acquired disease. An analysis of the reported cases of transfusion haemochromatosis confirms that the majority of the patients were suffering from refractory anaemia associated with a cellular erythroid marrow and usually with defective erythropoiesis (Ellis et al., 1954; Caroli et al., 1957; Bothwell and Finch, 1962). In several instances where chemical determination of tissue iron was performed at autopsy, more iron was found than could be accounted for by the transfused blood, suggesting that part of the iron was accumulated through absorption from the gut (Mackey, 1942; Zeltmacher and Bevans, 1945; Chesner, 1946; Muirhead et al., 1949; Wyatt and Goldenberg, 1949; Womack and Brownlee, 1950; Wyatt et al., 1950; Cottier, 1952). The concept that oral iron contributes to the development of post-transfusional haemochromatosis is supported by the finding of signs of tissue siderosis in patients with this type of refractory anaemia who had not received blood transfusions (Block et al., 1952; Wallerstein and Robbins, 1953; Ellis et al., 1954; Wyatt, 1956; Bowdler and Huehns, 1963). Further corroborative evidence stems from experimental work on iron absorption, indicating that absorption is in some way linked with the activity of the erythroid marrow, being higher when the red-cell marrow is hyperplastic and lower when it is hypoplastic (Dubach et al., 1948; Bothwell, 1953; Bothwell et al., 1958). It could therefore be argued that the condition of secondary haemochromatosis in these patients is primarily caused by oral iron overload. In corroboration of this concept, the histological findings show many similarities with those observed in idiopathic haemochromatosis and in advanced stages of nutritional siderosis in the African Bantu (SHELDON, 1935; FINCH and FINCH, 1955; BOTHWELL and ISAACSON, 1962). Individual differences in erythropoietic activity, iron kinetics, and the duration of the anaemia might well explain the variations in the degree of post-transfusional iron overload and tissue fibrosis. There are many other factors, however, which might also affect the iron overload in these subjects, e.g. the anaemia itself, serum hepatitis, nutritional deficiencies, and oral iron medication, but in practice it is not feasible to assess accurately the individual contribution made by each factor. One possible explanation for the development of a parenchymal iron overload might be the high iron saturation of transferrin. This plasma protein appears to protect the tissues against siderosis (LAURELL, 1952). A good example of this function has recently been described by HEILMEYER et al. (1961) in a report on atransferrinaemia associated with anaemia and severe tissue siderosis.

Subjects with refractory anaemia and a hypoplastic bone marrow provide better material for a study of the effects of post-transfusional iron overload, since it can be expected that in such cases increased iron absorption will not present a complication. Here it is very important to select those cases in which there is adequate evidence for the existence of a hypocellular red-cell marrow throughout the course of the disease. A number of such cases have been reported in which several hundred transfusions were given, resulting in a body iron load far in excess of that found in advanced stages of idiopathic haemochromatosis (MORNINGSTAR, 1955; PLATZER et al., 1955; CAPPELL et al., 1957). Although intense iron deposition is observed in many organs, there are as a rule few signs of tissue damage and only slight to moderate fibrosis. Iron is deposited chiefly in the cells of the reticulo-endothelial system, but variable amounts may also be found in parenchymal cells of the endocrine glands, the skin, and the heart. The findings in the liver are of special interest; here, intense iron loading of parenchymal cells takes place; in contrast to the condition of the liver in idiopathic haemochromatosis, true nodular cirrhosis is an exception and some broadening of the portal tracts is usually all that can be observed (VAN RIJSSEL and STENFERT KROESE, 1951; PENGELLY and JONES, 1956; OLIVER, 1959). The clinical symptoms, on the other hand, may closely mimic those of idiopathic haemochromatosis with the complete triad of enlarged liver, skin pigmentation, and overt diabetes. Although the pathological and clinical signs of extreme post-transfusional iron overload in subjects with aplastic anaemia certainly have several characteristics in common with those of oral iron overload, one has the overall impression that red-cell iron is far better tolerated.

Experiments have been undertaken on a variety of animal species in an attempt to elucidate the role of iron in the production of tissue damage in man, but these efforts have largely failed (BROWN et al., 1957), even when very large amounts of iron were injected – either as blood or in the form of a colloidal preparation – and although the animals were observed for many years. Iron storage in such animals was mainly confined to the liver, with minimal parenchymal deposition and no organ fibrosis.

The liver occupies a central position in iron metabolism and therefore shows the most characteristic alterations in response to a body iron overload. Although it has not been established with certainty that iron has a toxic effect on the cells, results of experimental work indicate that the siderotic liver is more vulnerable to toxic influences (GOLDBERG and SMITH, 1960). Fibrosis and cirrhosis are most frequently observed when the iron is predominantly deposited in the parenchymal cells.

There are two ways in which parenchymal iron deposition may take place:

(1) In conditions associated with an increased rate of iron absorption, plasma iron is presumably directly released from the portal blood into the liver cells.

(2) In severe long-standing post-transfusional haemosiderosis, iron may be transferred from the Kupffer cells to the liver parenchyma.

If we accept the hypothesis that parenchymal iron causes tissue damage, the development of structural alterations in the liver in post-transfusional haemosiderosis is presumably conditioned by the ability of the reticulo-endothelial system to retain iron. Individual variations in the development of liver fibrosis and fibrosis of other organs might accordingly be due to differences in the function of the reticulo-endothelial system (Fig. 1).

We should now like to present our observations on severe post-transfusional haemosiderosis in a pair of identical twins suffering from refractory anaemia with hypoplastic erythropoiesis. The patients in question were two girls who had had a normal growth and were in good health until the age of 15. At that age, anaemia was found when one of the girls was admitted to hospital suffering from severe tonsillitis. Since that time the disease ran an almost identical course in both twins. There was no history of an intake of drugs or of contact with agents which might have caused bone-marrow aplasia. The family history revealed nothing of significance, and no haematological abnormalities were found when the relatives were extensively investigated. Physical examination disclosed no abnormalities except for pallor. Liver, spleen, and lymph nodes could not be palpated. The relevant haematological laboratory data were as follows: — haemoglobin: 7.5 g.%; R.B.C.: 2.48 mill./μl.; W.B.C.: 2,500/μl.; reticulocytes: 1.5–2.3%; and platelets: 55,000–128,000/μl. The red blood cells showed marked anisocytosis, poikilocytosis, and targeting.

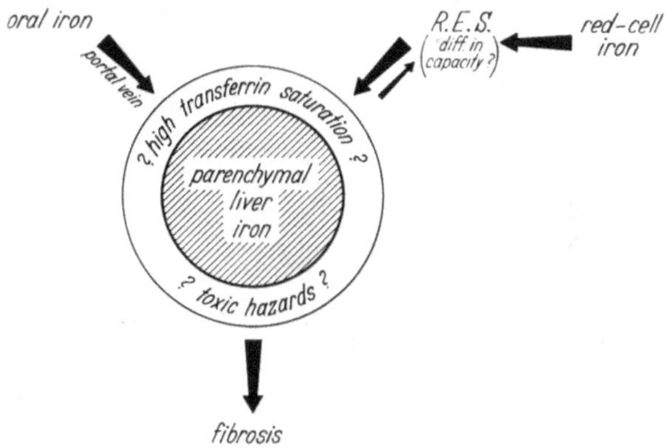

Fig. 1. Schematic representation of the development of post-transfusional liver fibrosis

A surgical bone-marrow biopsy showed the white-cell series and the megakaryocytes to be of normal appearance, but there was hypoplasia of the red-cell series. Serum iron: 195 μg. %. Urobilinogen excretion in the faeces was 150 mg. in 24 hours, and the serum bilirubin varied from 0.5 to 0.9 mg. %. Treatment with vitamin B_{12}, folic acid, and oral iron for several months did not improve the condition of either patient. Because of increasing anaemia the two girls were maintained on blood transfusions, i.e. about one pint per month.

In 1959, at the age of 21 years and after 60 transfusions, diabetes mellitus developed, which proved very difficult to control with 40 units of long-acting insulin daily. The patients had to be admitted to hospital on several occasions because the diabetes had got out of control and because of severe hypoglycaemia. One girl (W.V.) died in November 1961, shortly after entering hospital in a comatose condition. For the sake of brevity, we shall not discuss the autopsy findings at this point, because they were very similar to those found at the autopsy of the twin sister one and a half years later. Suffice it to say that extreme siderosis and fibrosis of the adrenals was found.

The other sister was then referred to us for further clinical evaluation and treatment. When we gave her a physical examination we noted generalised greyish pigmentation of the skin and atrophy of the genital organs. The spleen and liver were not enlarged. The relevant laboratory data were as follows:—haemoglobin: 4.4 g.%; R.B.C.: 1.16 mill./μl.; reticulocytes: 2.3%; haematocrit: 23%; W.B.C.: 2,300/μl.; and platelets: 62,500/μl. The erythrocytes showed anisocytosis with several target cells and polychromasia. Serum iron: 182 μg.% with complete saturation of transferrin. Haemoglobin: A_2 fraction 2.1%. Alkaline-resistant haemoglobin: 2%. Serum bilirubin: 0.85 mg.%. Alkaline phosphatase: 29.8 U. (KING and ARMSTRONG). Total serum protein: 7.7 g.%, with a normal distribution between the albumin and globulin fractions. Erythrokinetic studies: — urobilinogen excretion: 58 mg./24 hours. Mean red-cell survival of a mixture of the patient's own red cells and donor cells (Cr^{51} technique): 50 days. Splenic sequestration index (JANDL, 1956): 183. Plasma iron turnover (BOTHWELL et al., 1957): 0.7 mg./100 ml. whole blood/day. Red-cell incorporation of iron: 8%.

These measurements indicate a decrease in erythropoiesis. Investigation of the function of the endocrine glands revealed that the pituitary and the thyroid gland were functioning normally. Adrenal function was minimal, as evidenced by the fact that less than 1 mg. of 17-ketosteroids and 17-ketogenic steroids was excreted per day and that A.C.T.H. failed to stimulate the excretion of steroids. In view of these findings the patient was given cortisone as substitution therapy. Further treatment consisted of insulin, desferrioxamine, and blood transfusions. Under this regimen the urinary iron excretion varied from 10 to 30 mg./day. The disease subsequently followed a gradual down-hill course, with frequent infections and periods during which the diabetes went out of control. The patient died in May 1963, after having received a total of 98 transfusions.

Since the autopsy findings were quite similar in both instances, we shall describe only those for one of the patients. The heart weighed 190 g. and the cut surface was light brown in colour. The liver weighed 1,940 g., had a smooth surface of rusty brown colour, and showed no nodules when cut. The spleen weighed 160 g., but was otherwise normal. The pancreas weighed 40 g. and was brown. The cut surface of the atrophic adrenals was also brown, the two glands weighing only 3 g. each.

Microscopic examination disclosed marked deposition of iron in the heart, liver, spleen, pancreas, adrenals, and bone marrow. In the liver, iron was found in the parenchymal cells, in the Kupffer cells, and in the portal tracts (Fig. 2). A connective-tissue stain revealed increased portal fibrosis with bile-duct proliferation and minimal fibrosis around the central veins. There was some pseudo-lobulation, but no regenerative nodules were seen. Large quantities of iron in the pancreas were located predominantly in the acinar cells and in smaller quantities in the fibrous tissue. There was a striking degree of fibrosis, and no island tissue could be found in the sections available for examination (Fig. 3). The adrenals showed iron deposition in the parenchymal cells of the cortex and medulla, as well as in the fibrous tissue. The anatomical structure was severely distorted, and here again there was marked fibrosis (Fig. 4). Haemosiderin deposition was also a prominent feature in the muscle cells of the heart, in the macrophages of the spleen and bone marrow, and in the tubular cells of the kidney. The bone marrow was hypocellular.

Chemical estimates were made of the inorganic iron content of the liver, pancreas, spleen, heart, and kidneys. The pancreas had an extremely high concentration of iron, i.e. 3.30 g./100 g. of dried tissue (total iron content: 303 mg.). The concentration in the liver was 1.84 g./100 g. of dried tissue (total iron content: 9.6 g.). The iron content of the other organs was as follows: — heart: 58 mg.; spleen: 554 mg.; and kidneys: 38 mg.

These two patients presented several unusual features: from the clinical aspect, the development of severe diabetes and subsequent adrenal insufficiency; from the morphological aspect, the moderate fibrosis of the liver without true nodular cirrhosis, combined with severe lesions of the pancreas and adrenals.

While the total amount of iron in the body was certainly not much higher than could be accounted for by the blood transfusions, its distribution in the tissues was different from that reported in post-transfusional haemosiderosis (Cappell et al., 1957; Oliver, 1959). In contrast to the general observation that the iron concentration in the liver is higher than in the pancreas, the reverse was true of these patients. The iron concentrations in the liver and pancreas appeared to be roughly related to the degree of tissue damage.

These observations in patients with refractory anaemia and a hypocellular bone marrow offer a good example of the extreme variation observed in reaction to a transfusional iron overload. On the basis of the hypothesis that parenchymal iron deposition is

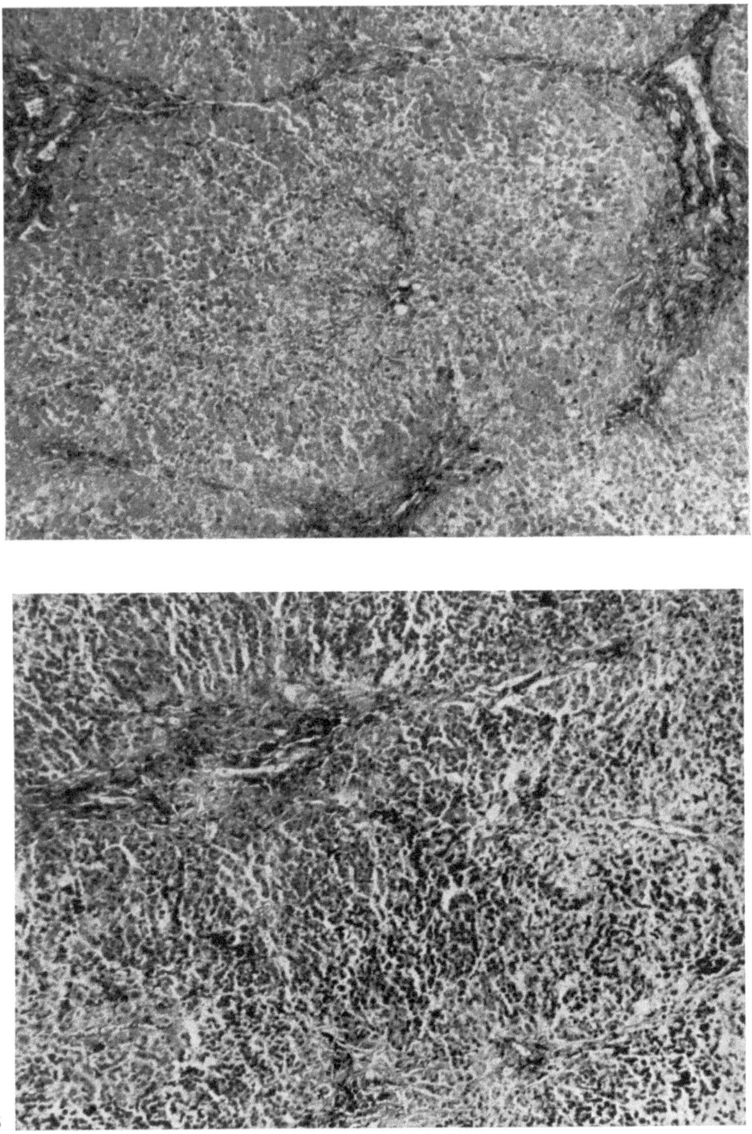

A

B

Fig. 2. Autopsy specimen of the liver. A. Moderate fibrosis of the portal tracts. Azan stain, 65 × ; B. Iron pigment in connective tissue, R.E.S. cells, and parenchymal cells. Prussian blue stain, 65 ×

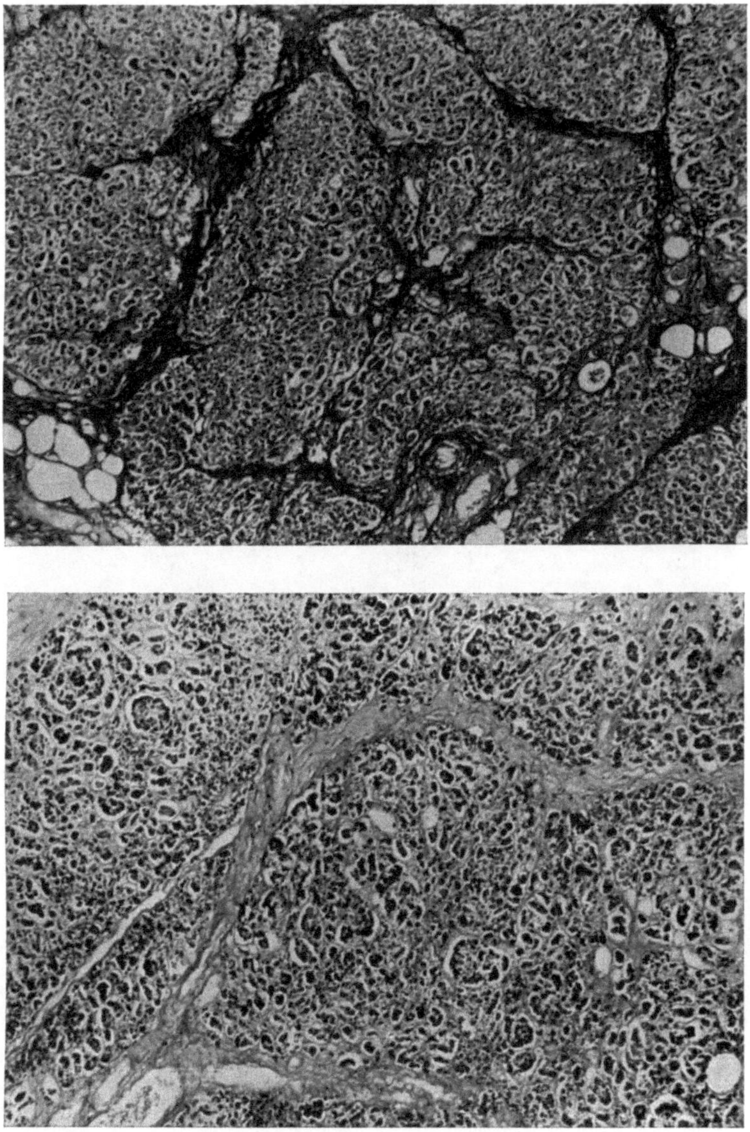

A

B

Fig. 3. Autopsy specimen of the pancreas. A. Marked fibrosis. Azan stain, 65 × ; B. Large amounts of iron pigment in the parenchymal cells. Prussian blue stain, 65 ×

conditioned by the reticulo-endothelial system, it might be supposed that in these patients the disease was not confined to the bone marrow, but that it also affected the function of the reticulo-endothelial cells.

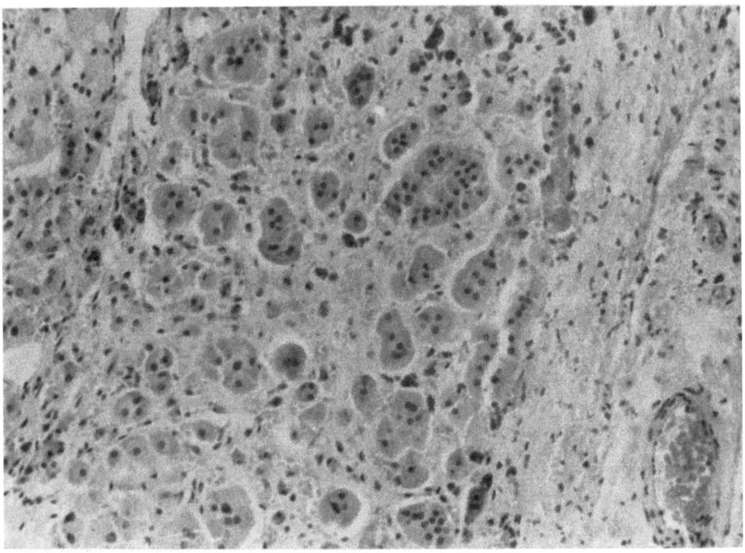

Fig. 4. Autopsy specimen of the adrenals. Severe fibrosis. Iron pigment in the parenchymal cells and connective tissue. Haematoxylin eosin, 140×

Summary

Several aspects of the pathogenesis of post-transfusional haemosiderosis are discussed. Two patterns of iron storage can be distinguished: in the first, it is mainly the reticulo-endothelial cells that are involved, and in the second chiefly the parenchymal cells. Parenchymal storage is often associated with tissue damage and may be caused either by an increase in the absorption of iron through the gut or by a transfer of iron from the reticulo-endothelial cells.

The hypothesis is put forward that it is differences in reticulo-endothelial cell function which account for the wide individual variation of symptoms in patients with post-transfusional haemosiderosis.

Two cases of severe post-transfusional haemosiderosis in a pair of identical twins with refractory anaemia and hypoplastic bone marrow are described.

Zusammenfassung

Verschiedene pathogenetische Aspekte der Haemosiderose nach Transfusionen werden diskutiert. Zwei Arten von Eisenspeicherung können unterschieden werden; bei der einen wird Eisen vorwiegend im retikulo-endothelialen System abgelagert, bei der anderen hauptsächlich in Parenchymzellen. Speicherung im Parenchym geht oft mit Gewebsschädigung einher und kann entweder durch eine vermehrte intestinale Resorption hervorgerufen werden oder durch eine Übertragung von Eisen aus dem retikulo-endothelialen System.

Es wird die Auffassung vertreten, daß Verschiedenheiten in der Funktion des R.E.S. verantwortlich für die großen individuellen Schwankungen der Symptome bei Patienten mit Transfusions-Haemosiderose sind.

Zwei Fälle von schwerer Transfusions-Haemosiderose bei eineiigen Zwillingen mit refraktärer Anaemie und hypoplastischem Knochenmark werden beschrieben.

Résumé

Plusieurs aspects de la question de la pathogénie des hémosidéroses post-transfusionnelles sont discutés. On peut distinguer deux tableaux de surcharge en fer: dans le premier c'est plutôt le système réticulo-endothélial qui est impliqué, et dans le second ce sont plutôt les cellules parenchymateuses. Le stockage du fer dans les parenchymes est souvent associé à des lésions tissulaires et peut être dû soit à une augmentation de l'absorption intestinale du fer, soit à un transfert de ce métal hors des cellules du système réticulo-endothélial.

On avance l'hypothèse que ce sont des différences dans la fonction des cellules réticulo-endothéliales qui répondent des larges variations individuelles dans les symptômes observés chez des malades présentant une hémosidérose post-transfusionnelle.

Deux cas d'hémosidérose post-transfusionnelle grave chez deux jumeaux univitellins présentant une anémie réfractaire avec hypoplasie médullaire sont décrits.

Acknowledgement

We are indebted to Dr. J. J. M. Cooymans and Dr. A. E. Harmsen of the St. Ignatius Ziekenhuis, Breda, for referring the patients to us and for allowing us to examine the tissues.

References

Block, M., W. Bethard, and L. Jacobson: J. Laborat. Clin. Med. (U.S.A.) **40**, 781 (1952). — Bothwell, T. H.: S. Afr. J. Clin. Sc. **4**, 53 (1953). — Bothwell, T. H., and C. A. Finch: Iron Metabolism, Little, Brown & Co., Boston, 1962. — Bothwell, T. H., and C. Isaacson: Brit. Med. J. **1962**/I, 522. — Bothwell, T. H., G. Pirzio-Biroli, and C. A. Finch: J. Laborat. Clin. Med. (U.S.A.) **51**, 24 (1958). — Bothwell, T. H., A. V. Hurtado, D. M. Donohue, and C. A. Finch: Blood (U.S.A.) **12**, 409 (1957).— Bowdler, A. J., and E. R. Huehns: Brit. J. Haemat. **9**, 13 (1963). — Brown, E. B., R. Dubach, E. D. Smith, C. Reynafarje, and C. V. Moore: J. Laborat. Clin. Med. (U.S.A.) **50**, 862 (1957). — Cappell, D. E., H. E. Hutchison, and M. Jowett: J. Path. Bact. (G.B.) **74**, 245 (1957). — Caroli, J., J. Bernard, M. Bessis, A. Combrisson, R. Malassenet, and J. Breton: Presse méd. (Fr.) **2**, 1991 (1957). — Chesner, C.: J. Laborat. Clin. Med. (U.S.A.) **31**, 1029 (1946). — Cottier, H.: Schweiz. med. Wschr. **82**, 873 (1952). — Dubach, R., S. T. Callender, and C. V. Moore: Blood

(U.S.A.) **3**, 526 (1948). — DUBIN, I. N.: Amer. J. Clin. Path. **25**, 514 (1955). — ELLIS, J. T., I. SCHULMAN, and C. H. SMITH: Amer. J. Path. **30**, 287 (1954). — FINCH, S. C., and C. A. FINCH: Medicine (U.S.A.) **34**, 381 (1955). — GOLDBERG, L., and J. P. SMITH: Amer. J. Path. **36**, 125 (1960). — HEILMEYER, L., W. KELLER, O. VIVELL, W. KEIDERLING, K. BETKE, F. WÖHLER, and H. E. SCHULTZE: Dtsch. med. Wschr. **86**, 1745 (1961). — JANDL, J. H., M. S. GREENBERG, R. H. YONEMOTO, and W. B. CASTLE: J. Clin. Invest. (U.S.A.) **35**, 842 (1956). — KENT, G., and H. POPPER: Arch. Path. (U.S.A.) **70**, 623 (1960). — LAURELL, C. B.: Pharmacol. Rev. (U.S.A.) **4**, 371 (1952). — MACKEY, R.: Med. J. Australia **1**, 172 (1942). — MORNINGSTAR, W. A.: Arch. Path. (U.S.A.) **59**, 355 (1955). — MUIRHEAD, E. E., G. CRASS, F. JONES, and J. M. HILL: Arch. Int. Med. (U.S.A.) **83**, 477 (1949). — OLIVER, R. A.: J. Path. Bact. (G.B.) **77**, 171 (1959). — PENGELLY, C. D. R., and P. JONES: Lancet (G.B.) **1956**/II, 445. — PLATZER, R. F., L. E. YOUNG, and C. L. YUILE: Acta haemat. (Switz.) **14**, 185 (1955). — SHELDON, J. H.: Haemochromatosis. Oxford University Press, London, 1935. — VAN RIJSSEL, T. G., and W. F. STENFERT KROESE: Ned. tschr. geneesk. **95**, 3843 (1951). — WALLERSTEIN, R. O., and S. L. ROBBINS: Amer. J. Med. **14**, 256 (1953). — WOMACK, C. R., and R. C. BROWNLEE: Amer. Pract. Digest. Treatm. **1**, 731 (1950). — WYATT, J. P.: Arch. Path. (U.S.A.) **61**, 56 (1956). — WYATT, J .P., and W. GOLDENBERG: Arch. Int. Med. (U.S.A.) **83**, 67 (1949). — WYATT, J. P., H. K. MIGHTON, and V. MORAGUES: Amer. J. Path. **26**, 833 (1950). — ZELTMACHER, K., and M. BEVANS: Arch. Int. Med. (U.S.A.) **75**, 395 (1945).

Discussion

Sherlock: Did any of your patients have steatorrhoea?

Cleton: We wondered about that, but these patients did not cooperate very well. We just did a normal exploration of the faeces and we couldn't find any steatorrhoea.

Najean: I should be interested to hear what experience Dr. Dreyfus, Dr. Cleton, and Dr. Verloop have had with regard to ferrokinetics in haemochromatosis. It seemed to me from Dr. Pollycove's methods of calculation that the movement of iron from the plasma pool to the storage pool was no greater in idiopathic haemochromatosis than in hypersideraemia caused by aplasia; this contrasts with the findings in hypochromic hypersideraemic anaemia (thalassaemia, achrestic anaemia, or Dacie's anaemia), in which this movement was 2 or 3 times greater. The quantities were 0.15 to 0.25 mg./kg./day in the first group of cases and 0.3 to 0.5 mg./kg./day in the second group. If this observation is correct, this would probably account for the difference in the rate at which haemochromatosis develops in the two groups of cases.

J.-C. Dreyfus: I'm afraid I have no answer to that. I think we should refer to Dr. Pollycove.

Cleton: In sideroachrestic anaemias with iron loading of the tissues, there is usually a marked elevation of the plasma iron turnover. We have not performed calculations of plasma versus storage pool exchange.

Pollycove: It is true that patients with idiopathic endogenous haemochromatosis usually have a smaller exchange between plasma and storage than is demonstrable in cases of refractory anaemia with erythroid hyperplasia and iron overload. Of interest in this connection is the considerable number of patients in whom haemochromatosis is associated with intramedullary haemolysis and in whom there is not an erythroid hypoplasia, but hyperplasia. Ironkinetic body-surface measurements may be misinterpreted inasmuch as, though hepatic radioactivity may not initially show an abnormal increase, there may yet exist a marked increase in plasma-storage iron exchange. Because there may also be a marked increase in plasma-erythropoietic exchange, such as a tenfold increase, a tenfold increase in plasma-storage exchange would not be detected by external measurements, since the fractional partition of plasma iron movement would be normal, ten times as much going each way. Quantitative analysis of plasma radio-iron measurements, however, clearly demonstrates the marked increase in plasma-storage iron exchange. It seems that in these cases of refractory anaemia with erythroid hyperplasia and intramedullary haemolysis there is frequently an associated haemochromatosis which sometimes develops rapidly to a fatal conclusion. All too common is the fatal secondary haemochromatosis occurring in patients with thalassaemia major, which may be classified functionally as congenital refractory anaemia with erythroid hyperplasia. We have studied a boy who had received only 6 litres of blood and no parenteral iron but who, at the age of 19, died of haemochromatosis secondary to such an anaemia. An increased absorption of iron seems to be the explanation for this massive accumulation of iron.

The increase in iron absorption associated with increased erythropoiesis is understandable in terms of the elegant studies of HALLBERG and SOLVELL as reported in their recent monograph on iron absorption[1]. Their data clearly demonstrate that increased saturation of transferrin is associated with decreased absorption of iron from the intestinal lumen into the circulating plasma. Normally, when iron is absorbed from the diet, there occurs an increased saturation of transferrin which may then diminish further absorption. In patients with increased erythropoiesis, however, the rapid removal of iron from the plasma, which is balanced by the enormous influx from destroyed blood cells, is so great that the amount absorbed from the gastro-intestinal lumen does not produce a significant elevation of the transferrin saturation. As a result, iron absorption continues at a relatively high level without the normal feed-back control. This seems to be a reasonable explanation for the increased iron absorption seen in conditions with enhanced erythropoiesis. Iron absorption is particularly increased in those patients with intramedullary haemolysis in whom a marked increase in erythropoiesis and a coexistent marked anaemia both increase iron absorption.

CLETON: Are you certain that, in the case of completely saturated transferrin, iron cannot be absorbed and transferred to the liver in another chemical form?

POLLYCOVE: Oh no! I don't want to get involved in this controversy, although I agree that there is considerable evidence obtained in rodents and dogs to support your statement. I am merely saying that — on the basis of the data presented by HALLBERG and SOLVELL — as transferrin saturation was increased in humans, minute-to-minute absorption of iron from the intestinal lumen into the plasma was decreased, and that this feed-back control is probably not significantly operative in patients with marked intramedullary haemolysis and increased erythropoiesis. This seems to be a plausible explanation for the increased iron absorption observed in patients with enhanced erythropoiesis. This is not to say that the absorption of iron ceases when transferrin is entirely saturated.

BRICK: We, too, have observed a case somewhat similar to that of the Italian woman of 45 to whom you referred. We have now had under observation for 10 years a patient with thalassaemia major who has received 100 transfusions over a 20-year period. In 1957 she developed rather severe diabetes of sudden onset. She has hepatomegaly, but her liver function has been fairly normal, which is rather characteristic in this type of case. We have done 6 liver biopsies over a period of 10 years, and we have been able to observe the gradual development of slight fibrosis; the last biopsy a year ago yielded material fairly similar to that from the biopsy which you presented. It's interesting that you have raised the question of adrenal insufficiency, because in our patient we have been plagued at times with episodes of hypotension in the hospital that we haven't been able to explain.

FIGUEROA: I was not quite clear about what you said with reference to the role which the absorption of iron from the gut plays in the aggravation of transfusion haemosiderosis. Dr. POLLYCOVE mentioned that an increase occurs in the absorption of iron in the individual with hypoplastic anaemia. I wonder in how many patients you have studied iron absorption. We investigated three patients in whom we administered Fe^{59} orally (using 10 μc.

[1] HALLBERG, L., and L. SOLVELL: Acta med. Scand. **168**, Suppl. 358 (1960).

and 25 mg. elemental iron) and then measured the red-cell uptake, examined the stools, and carried out whole-body studies. We were unable to detect any excessive absorption of iron in these three patients. We have also studied several individuals with secondary transfusion haemosiderosis. Here again we failed to detect any excessive iron absorption. The absorption of iron was either normal or slightly reduced; and I was just wondering how many of the patients you studied have shown this excessive iron absorption with hyperplastic marrow and refractory anaemia.

CLETON: We have also found normal absorption on two occasions, using a 5 mg. dose of ferrous sulphate. However, I would not rely too much on the absorption test when inorganic iron is used, and when no information is obtained as to what happens to food iron. There is the additional problem of the dose used. It may well be that an increased absorption can only be demonstrated when very small amounts of iron are employed, as shown by the results of CROSBY's group[1]. Dr. CALLENDER also mentioned this point when she reported normal absorption of haemoglobin iron in thalassaemia three years ago.

CALLENDER: Yes, that's true.

POLLYCOVE: We have demonstrated increased iron absorption in approximately 8 patients with enhanced erythropoiesis. For this purpose we used a whole-body counter with 4 mg. doses of ingested elemental iron.

---

[1] VAN HOEK, R., M. E. CONRAD, and W. H. CROSBY: J. Clin. Invest. (U.S.A.) **40**, 1153 (1961).

Iron overload in the Bantu

By

T. H. Bothwell

Over 30 years have passed since it was first noted that the majority of adult Bantu in South Africa have varying degrees of tissue siderosis (Strachan, 1929). These findings have been confirmed in a number of subsequent studies (Gillman and Gillman, 1951; Bothwell and Finch, 1962), and there is evidence to indicate that iron overload is not only common in South Africa but also occurs in the Bantu of Rhodesia, Bechuanaland, Nyasaland, Moçambique (Higginson et al., 1953), and Ghana (Edington, 1959). In these various areas it is almost exclusively confined to the

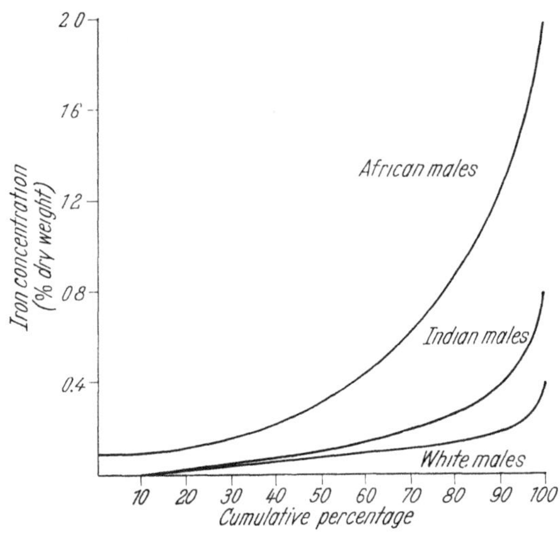

Fig. 1. The cumulative percentage incidence of various iron concentrations in the livers of 240 Bantu males (mean age 34 years), 40 Indian males (mean age 48 years), and 60 withe males (mean age 40 years). All subjects died acute traumatic deaths

Bantu; it is not found in white subjects and is rare in Indians (Fig. 1). Although the incidence and severity of the siderosis is variable, the usual pattern is a remarkably constant one with most of the excess iron confined to the liver and reticulo-endothelial system (Higginson et al., 1953).

The condition first becomes manifest in late adolescence and reaches its greatest degree between the ages of 40 and 60 years (WAINWRIGHT, 1957; BOTHWELL and ISAACSON, 1962). It occurs in both sexes, but the most severe involvement is usually found in males. The extent of the problem in the Johannesburg area was recently defined by estimating the chemical concentrations of iron in the livers of several hundred Bantu adults dying in hospital

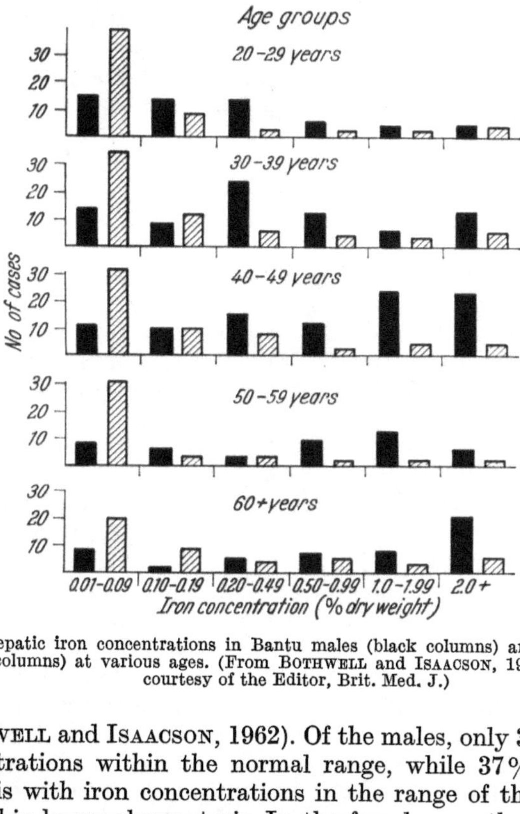

Fig. 2. Hepatic iron concentrations in Bantu males (black columns) and females (cross-hatched columns) at various ages. (From BOTHWELL and ISAACSON, 1962. Reprinted by courtesy of the Editor, Brit. Med. J.)

(BOTHWELL and ISAACSON, 1962). Of the males, only 30% had iron concentrations within the normal range, while 37% had severe siderosis with iron concentrations in the range of those found in idiopathic haemochromatosis. In the females, on the other hand, results were far less striking: 75% had hepatic iron concentrations within or just above the normal range, while only 12% showed severe involvement (Fig. 2).

Although it is accepted that the iron overload must be the result of increased absorption from the gut, there has been controversy in the past as to why this should occur. Originally it was postulated that there was an alteration in the behaviour of the bowel mucosa induced by chronic malnutrition (Gillman and Gillman, 1951). More recently, however, it has been shown that the Bantu diet contains large amounts of iron (Walker and Arvidsson, 1953), and there is evidence to indicate that this is a more likely cause of the tissue siderosis. Most of the iron is derived from the utensils used in cooking and in the preparation of fermented alcoholic beverages (Walker and Arvidsson, 1953). Although it is difficult to estimate the actual quantities of iron being ingested, analyses of various alcoholic drinks have shown a mean iron concentration of about 4.0 mg./100 ml. (range: 0.5 to 15). Calculations from these figures suggest that the average Bantu male consumes between 50 and 100 mg. iron daily in beer alone (Bothwell et al., 1963). The high daily iron intake of the Bantu has also been shown by measuring the iron concentrations present in faeces. When this has been done, the values have been found to be several times greater than in a comparable white population. In one study, a mean figure of 144 mg./100 g. was found in faeces collected from males on Monday mornings as compared with a figure of 34 mg./100 g. on Thursday mornings. These variations almost certainly reflect the week-end drinking habits of urban Bantu. Over 80% of the iron present in drinks is in the ionisable form, and isotopic studies have demonstrated that it is absorbed to the same degree as simple ferric salts, and about one-third as well as ferrous salts (Bothwell et al., 1963) (Fig. 3). It is of interest that most Bantu have been found to have lesser percentage absorptions than white subjects. This can be ascribed to the fact that the majority have varying degrees of iron overload, as it has been shown that even a moderate increase in iron stores depresses absorption (Pirzio-Biroli and Finch, 1960). It is, however, apparent that Bantu ingesting 100 mg. daily in alcoholic beverages absorb enough from this source (approximately 2–3 mg. daily) to account for the degrees of siderosis found in middle age. The fact that isotopic

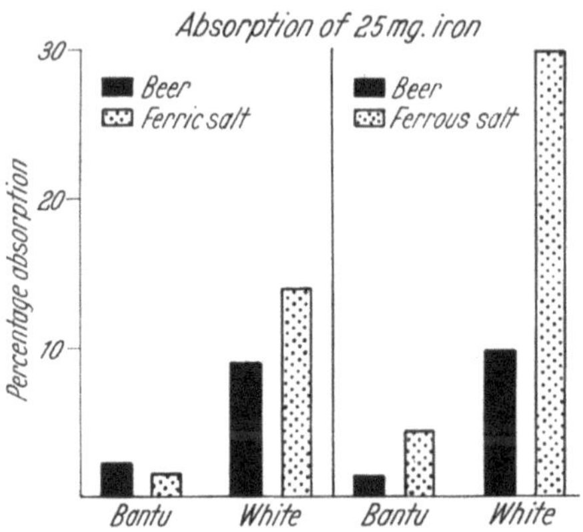

Fig. 3. A comparison in Bantu and white subjects of the absorption of iron in Bantu beer with a similar dose of iron given as ferric chloride or ferrous ascorbate. (Data from Bothwell et al., 1963)

studies have not revealed any evidence of abnormally *high* absorption rates can be taken as good evidence that the siderosis so commonly found in the Bantu is not the result of any intrinsic mucosal defect.

In the earliest phases of iron overload, the iron can be detected as haemosiderin granules in the parenchymal cells of the liver, particularly in the periportal areas (BOTHWELL and BRADLOW,

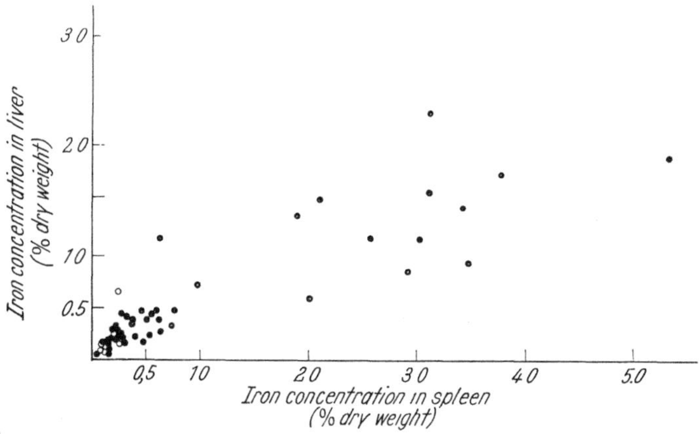

Fig. 4. A comparison of the iron concentrations in the livers and spleens of Bantu adults. The closed circles represent males and the open circles females. (From BOTHWELL and BRADLOW, 1960. Reprinted by courtesy of the Editor, Arch. Path.)

1960). As the condition progresses, the iron granules become dispersed throughout the hepatic lobules, and iron is also visible in the Kupffer cells. When the iron concentration reaches levels between 5 and 10 times normal, increasing amounts of haemosiderin are present in parenchymal and Kupffer cells, and at this stage the portal tracts also show involvement. With concentrations over 20 times normal, heavy deposits are usually present in all three sites. Although it is evident that Bantu siderosis initially manifests itself in the liver as parenchymal deposits, it is interesting to note that the splenic concentration rises at the same time as the liver concentration, and that with increasing levels of iron the splenic concentrations are often greater than those in the liver (Fig. 4). Deposits in the reticulum cells of the bone marrow are also a feature, and the results of a recent *in vivo* study using an isotopic dilution technique indicate that as much as 10 g. may be stored in this site (GALE et al., 1963). Epithelial involvement of significant degree is uncommon in Bantu siderosis, and the iron is usually confined to the liver and reticulo-endothelial system, even when marked overload is present (HIGGINSON et al., 1953; ISAACSON et al., 1961). The pattern in the majority of subjects is, therefore, different from that in idiopathic haemochromatosis but is very similar to the distribution described in animals placed on deficient diets with heavy iron supplements (KINNEY, et al., 1949).

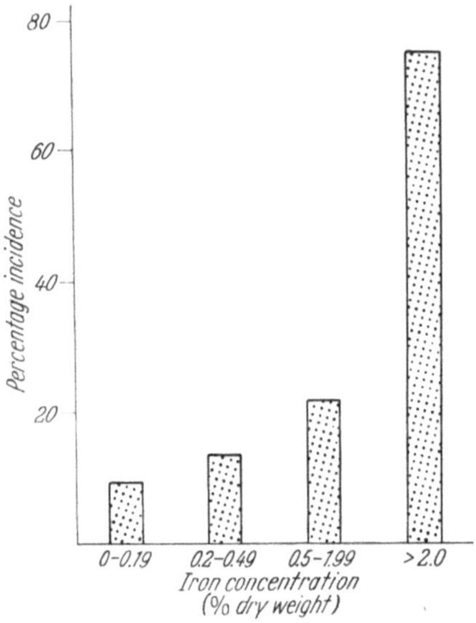

Fig. 5. The combined incidence of moderately severe portal fibrosis and portal cirrhosis in Bantu subjects with different concentrations of iron in the liver. (Data from BOTHWELL and BRADLOW, 1960; and BOTHWELL and ISAACSON, 1962)

In assessing the possible relationship between iron overload in the Bantu and tissue damage, most attention has been paid to the liver, since a major portion of the excess iron is located in this site. The results of several studies have shown a close relationship between the degree of overload and the presence of portal fibrosis or cirrhosis (HIGGINSON et al., 1957; GILLMAN et al., 1958). For example, moderately severe portal fibrosis or frank cirrhosis has been found in the great majority of livers in which the concentration of iron was more than 20 times normal (BOTHWELL and BRADLOW, 1960; BOTHWELL and ISAACSON, 1962) (Fig. 5). As a corollary to this it has been noted that subjects exhibiting portal cirrhosis at autopsy almost invariably have heavy siderosis (ISAACSON et al., 1961) (Fig. 6). This is in marked contrast to the findings in post-necrotic cirrhosis, where it has not been possible to demonstrate any relationship with iron overload (ISAACSON et al., 1961).

These various observations all suggest that there is a close relationship between the presence of heavy hepatic deposits of iron and the development of a fibrous reaction in the liver. This is, however, not the only point of interest that has emerged from these studies. Another feature of note in cases of portal cirrhosis has been the finding of significant epithelial deposits in a number of organs (BRADLOW et al., 1961; ISAACSON et al., 1961). This is especially so in the pancreas, thyroid, adrenals, pituitary, and myocardium. The microscopic findings in such cases are, therefore, similar to those in idiopathic haemochromatosis, and chemical analyses of various organs have demonstrated iron concentrations in the same

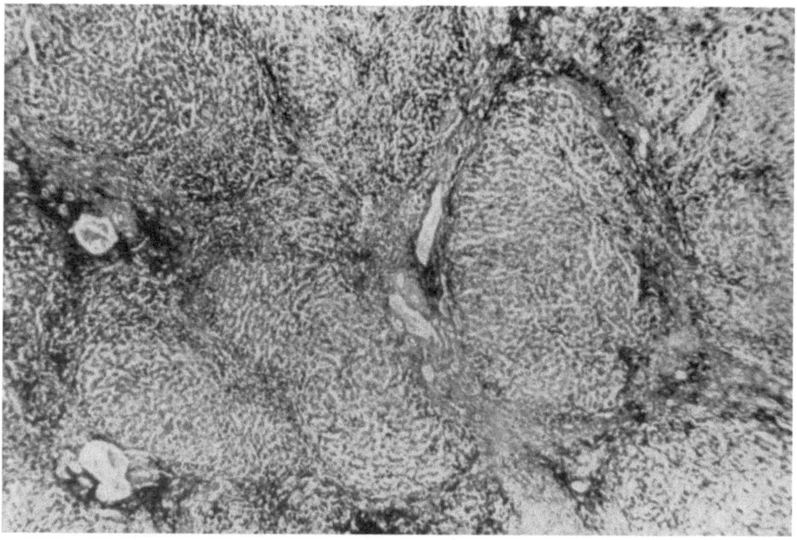

Fig. 6. A section of the liver from a Bantu adult with fully developed haemochromatosis. PERLS' stain. Original magnification 30 × (From ISAACSON et al., 1961. Reprinted by courtesy of the Editor, J. Laborat. Clin. Med.)

range as are found in this classic iron-storage disease (Fig. 7). Why the development of cirrhosis should be associated with an

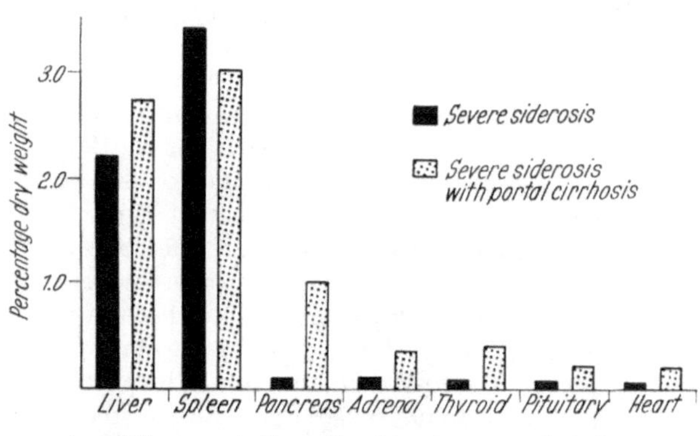

Fig. 7. A comparison of the concentrations of iron in various organs in 20 Bantu subjects with severe siderosis and 20 Bantu subjects with severe siderosis plus portal cirrhosis. (Data from ISAACSON et al., 1961)

iron distribution so different from that found in the majority of Bantu is not clear. It may, however, be related to the percentage saturation of circulating transferrin. In Bantu with siderosis but no cirrhosis, the plasma iron level is higher than normal, but there is, in addition, an increased amount of circulating transferrin with the result that the percentage saturation is normal or only moderately raised (Hathorn et al., 1960). On the other hand, when cirrhosis is present, transferrin levels tend to be lower, and the percentage saturation is very high (Seftel et al., 1961). It has been shown experimentally that iron is taken up more readily by tissues under such circumstances (Jandl et al., 1959), and it is therefore possible that this mechanism may be of importance in the transfer of iron to epithelial cells in cirrhotic subjects.

Whatever the explanation for these findings, there is no doubt that a small proportion of adult Bantu exhibit pathological findings indistinguishable from those in idiopathic haemochromatosis. The similarity between the two conditions is further underlined by the clinical manifestations (Seftel et al., 1960). Analyses of clinical records have shown that more than 20% of Bantu with pathological evidence of haemochromatosis at autopsy were diabetic prior to death (Isaacson et al., 1961), while a recent survey of living diabetics has revealed that approximately 7% were suffering from fully developed haemochromatosis (Seftel et al., 1961). The clinical picture in such subjects is a fairly characteristic one. The condition is commoner in males (male to female ratio 2 : 1), and the majority of subjects are between the ages of 40 and 60 years. All give a history of excessive consumption of alcoholic beverages. They are almost invariably underweight, a firm hepatomegaly is always present, and insulin is needed for control of the diabetes. These features serve to distinguish the condition from the common form of late-onset diabetes found in the Bantu, since this usually occurs in middle-aged, obese females and can often be controlled by diet or by oral hypoglycaemic agents (Seftel et al., 1961). The prognosis in Bantu subjects with haemochromatosis is poor, and death usually results from liver failure and/or portal hypertension.

Although these various findings support the concept that long-term oral iron overload in the Bantu can cause severe damage to body tissues, it is important to stress that there are still certain puzzling discrepancies. While it is clear that the majority of subjects with marked hepatic siderosis develop portal fibrosis or cirrhosis, an appreciable percentage do not do so. For example, in one study 30% of subjects over the age of 50 years with hepatic iron concentrations above 2.0% dry weight showed no significant portal fibrosis (Both-

WELL and ISAACSON, 1962). A finding such as this raises the possibility that iron is only a low-grade fibrogenic agent and that other potentiating factors are often present. It is perhaps noteworthy that the major source of iron in the Bantu is an alcoholic drink which is adulterated in a number of ways. There is, therefore, the added insult of alcohol on the liver together with the possible harmful effects of the unidentified adulterants and the associated malnutrition. A concept such as this would fit in with the experimental observation that the siderotic liver is particularly vulnerable to toxic, metabolic, and nutritional hazards (GOLBERG and SMITH, 1960).

The preceding discussion has been primarily concerned with the pattern of iron overload in Bantu adults and with the possible effects exerted locally on tissues by the iron deposits when they have been present in high concentrations for long periods. While most attention has been directed to this aspect, there are certain interesting associations between iron overload in the Bantu and other diseases. These include porphyria cutanea tarda, scurvy, and vertebral collapse. Although the incidence of porphyria cutanea tarda is higher in subjects with siderosis (LAMONT and HATHORN, 1960), there is no evidence that its occurrence is directly related to the iron deposits *per se*, and it seems more reasonable to suppose that the major link is the high intake of adulterated alcoholic drinks. The relationship with scurvy is a more direct one. Severe siderosis is almost invariably present in scorbutic Bantu (BOTHWELL et al., 1963), and the results of one recent study suggest that it is extremely difficult to saturate such subjects with ascorbic acid even after adequate therapy (SCHULZ and SWANEPOEL, 1962). These observations have led to the intriguing suggestion that persons living on a borderline diet may be precipitated into clinical scurvy as a result of irreversible oxidation of available ascorbic acid by the excessive deposits of ferric iron (SCHULZ and SWANEPOEL, 1962). The last association is perhaps the most interesting one. It has been recognised for several years that collapse of lumbar vertebrae secondary to gross demineralisation of bone occurs commonly in middle-aged Bantu males (GRUSIN and SAMUEL, 1957) (Fig. 8). Current studies indicate that all such subjects have severe siderosis and give a history of excessive consumption of brewed alcoholic beverages (SEFTEL and BOTHWELL, 1963). Although the cause of the vertebral collapse has not yet been fully elucidated, it is noteworthy that the calcium content of the drinks is low, while the iron content is high. There is some experimental evidence to show that iron and calcium compete for active transport in the duodenum (Manis and Schachter, 1962), and it therefore seems possible that the presence of excessive iron in a diet which contains suboptimal amounts of calcium may be of critical importance in promoting a negative calcium balance. Whatever the significance of the association between iron overload and vertebral deformities,

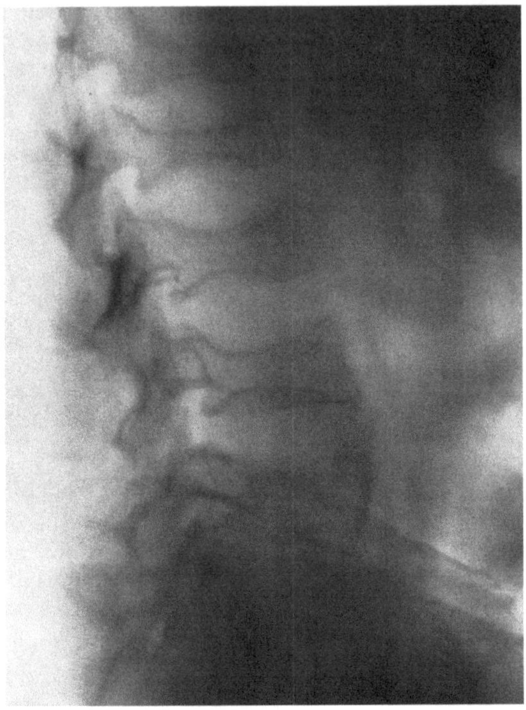

Fig. 8. An X-ray plate of the lumbar spine of a Bantu male with severe sidercsis, showing a marked diminution in bone density and vertebral collapse

it is of interest to note that the present observations are not new. A syndrome with similar features was described almost a century ago in Manchurian subjects (Kaschin, as cited by Hiyeda, 1939). These people seem to derive the excess iron from well-water and at autopsy exhibit pathological findings similar to those in the Bantu (Hiyeda, 1939).

Current evidence, derived from a number of different studies over the years, indicates that a small proportion of Bantu adults suffer both directly and indirectly from the effects of long-term oral iron overload. At the same time it must be appreciated that the majority exhibit only mild to moderate degrees of siderosis, and there is no evidence that these deposits exert deleterious effects. In fact, under special circumstances they may well be beneficial. This is especially so in pregnancy. The mean haemoglobin level at term in untreated Bantu females has been found to be 13 g./100 ml. (GERRITSEN and WALKER, 1954; EDELSTEIN et al., 1963), which must be quite unique for a population subsisting on a diet that is in many ways suboptimal.

Summary

The Bantu of Southern Africa consume a diet with a high iron content, and the majority of adults at autopsy show varying degrees of tissue siderosis. Isotopic studies suggest that the iron overload is directly related to the high intake, and there is no evidence to indicate any abnormality in gut behaviour.

In most Bantu the iron deposits are confined to the liver and reticulo-endothelial system. The distribution is, therefore, different from that found in idiopathic haemochromatosis. In the liver there is a fairly close correlation between the degree of siderosis and the presence of significant portal fibrosis or portal cirrhosis. This is especially so when the iron concentration is above 2.0% dry weight. When portal cirrhosis is present, the distribution of iron is different from that normally found, since epithelial deposits in a number of organs are invariably present. In this small group of cases, the histological findings and chemical concentrations of iron in organs such as the liver, pancreas, adrenals, thyroid, pituitary, and heart are very similar to those found in idiopathic haemochromatosis. In addition, clinical manifestations are also similar, and insulin-dependent diabetes is often present.

Although the findings in severe Bantu siderosis support the concept that long-term oral iron overload is noxious to tissues, there are enough exceptions to suggest that added factors, such as alcoholism and malnutrition, may be important aggravating factors.

Zusammenfassung

Die Nahrung der südafrikanischen Bantus ist sehr reich an Eisen, und die Mehrzahl der zur Sektion gelangenden Erwachsenen zeigt verschiedene Grade von Gewebssiderose. Untersuchungen mit radioaktivem Eisen sprechen dafür, daß die Überladung des Organismus mit Eisen in Beziehung zur hohen Einnahme steht und nicht auf einer abnormen enteralen Resorption beruht.

In den meisten Fällen beschränken sich die Eisendepots auf die Leber und auf das retikulo-endotheliale System. Die Verteilung unterscheidet sich somit von der bei der idiopathischen Haemochromatose gefundenen. In der Leber besteht eine recht enge Korrelation zwischen dem Grad der Siderose und dem Vorliegen einer deutlichen portalen Fibrose oder Zirrhose. Dies ist besonders der Fall, wenn der Eisengehalt der Nahrung über 2% ihres Trockengewichtes liegt. Ist eine portale Zirrhose vorhanden, so unterscheidet sich die Verteilung von Eisen von der normalerweise gefundenen dadurch, daß regelmäßig Ablagerungen in den Epithelien verschiedener Organe auftreten. Bei dieser kleinen Gruppe von Patienten sind die histologischen und biochemischen Befunde in verschiedenen Organen — Leber, Pankreas, Neben-nieren, Schilddrüse, Hypophyse und Herz — sehr ähnlich wie bei der idiopathischen Haemochromatose. Auch die klinischen Erscheinungen sind vergleichbar, und oft ist ein Insulin-empfindlicher Diabetes vorhanden.

Obgleich die Beobachtungen bei den Bantus mit schwerer Siderose dafür sprechen, daß die langdauernde Zufuhr großer Mengen von Eisen in der Nahrung die Gewebe schädigt, gibt es genügend Ausnahmen, die darauf hinweisen, daß zusätzliche schädigende Faktoren wie Alkoholismus oder Mangelernährung ebenfalls von Bedeutung sind.

Résumé

Le régime des Bantous d'Afrique du Sud a une haute teneur en fer, et la majorité des adultes présente à l'autopsie une sidérose plus ou moins marquée des tissus. Des études radio-isotopiques suggèrent que la surcharge en fer est en relation directe avec l'apport élevé, et il n'y a aucune raison d'invoquer une anomalie dans le comportement de l'intestin.

Chez la plupart des Bantous les dépôts de fer sont localisés au foie et au système réticulo-endothélial. Leur distribution est donc différente de celle trouvée dans l'hémochromatose idiopathique. Dans le foie, il existe une relation assez étroite entre le degré de la sidérose et la présence d'une fibrose, ou d'une cirrhose portale importante. C'est en particulier le cas quand la concentration du fer dépasse 2,0% du poids sec. Quand il existe une cirrhose portale, la distribution du fer est différente de celle trouvée normalement, puisque des dépôts épithéliaux sont invariablement retrouvés dans un certain nombre d'organes. Dans ce petit groupe de cas, les constatations histologiques et les concentrations chimiques du fer dans des organes tels que le foie, le pancréas, les glandes surrénales, la thyroïde, l'hypophyse et le coeur sont très semblables à celles trouvées dans l'hémochromatose idiopathique. De plus, les manifestations cliniques sont également semblables, et un diabète insulino-sensible est souvent présent.

Bien que ces constatations dans la sidérose grave du Bantou soient en faveur de la conception selon laquelle la surcharge perorale de fer au long cours est nocive pour les tissus, il existe des exceptions, assez nombreuses pour que l'on soit amené à penser que des facteurs surajoutés, comme l'alcoolisme et la malnutrition, peuvent jouer un rôle aggravant important.

Acknowledgement

This work was supported by grants from the National Institutes of Health, U.S.A. (AM-04912-02) and from the Council for Scientific and Industrial Research, South Africa.

References

BOTHWELL, T. H., and B. A. BRADLOW: Arch. Path. (U.S.A.) **70**, 279 (1960). — BOTHWELL, T. H., and C. A. FINCH: Iron metabolism. Little, Brown & Co., Boston, 1962. — BOTHWELL, T. H., and C. ISAACSON: Brit. Med. J. **1962**/I, 522. — BOTHWELL, T. H., H. SEFTEL, P. JACOBS, J. D. TORRANCE, and N. BAUMSLAG: Amer. J. Clin. Nutr. (in press, 1963a). — BOTHWELL, T. H., B. A. BRADLOW, P. JACOBS, K. J. KEELEY, S. KRAMER, H. SEFTEL, and S. ZAIL: Brit. J. Haemat. (in press, 1963b). — BRADLOW, B. A., J. DUNN, and J. HIGGINSON: Amer. J. Path. **39**, 221 (1961). — EDELSTEIN, T., J. METZ, and T. H. BOTHWELL: Unpublished data (1963). — EDINGTON, G. M.:

Centr. Afr. J. Med. **5**, 186 (1959). — GALE, E., J. TORRANCE, and T. H. BOTHWELL: J. Clin. Invest. (U.S.A.) (in press, 1963). — GERRITSEN, T., and A. R. P. WALKER: J. Clin. Invest. (U.S.A.) **33**, 23 (1954). — GILLMAN, J., and T. GILLMAN: Perspectives in Human Malnutrition. Grune & Stratton, New York, 1951. — GILLMAN, T., M. HATHORN, and N. M. LAMONT: S. Afr. J. Med. Sc. **23**, 187 (1958). — GOLBERG, L., and J. P. SMITH: Amer. J. Path. **36**, 125 (1960). — GRUSIN, H., and E. SAMUEL: Amer. J. Clin. Nutrit. **5**, 644 (1957). — HATHORN, M., T. GILLMAN, P. A. S. CANHAM, and N. M. LAMONT: Clin. Sc. (G.B.) **19**, 35 (1960). — HIGGINSON, J., T. GERRITSEN, and A. R. P. WALKER: Amer. J. Path. **29**, 779 (1953). — HIGGINSON, J., B. G. GROBBELAAR, and A. R. P. WALKER: Amer. J. Path. **33**, 29 (1957). — HIYEDA, K.: Jap. J. Med. Sc.**4**, 91 (1939). — ISAACSON, C., H. SEFTEL, K. J. KEELEY, and T. H. BOTHWELL: J. Laborat. Clin. Med. (U.S.A.) **58**, 845 (1961). — JANDL, J. H., J. K. INMAN, R. L. SIMMONS, and D. W. ALLEN: J. Clin. Invest. (U.S.A.) **38**, 161 (1959). — KINNEY, T. D., D. M. HEGSTED, and C. A. FINCH: J. Exper. Med. (U.S.A.) **90**, 137 (1949). — LAMONT, N. M., and M. HATHORN: S. Afr. Med. J. **34**, 279 (1960). — MANIS, J. G., and D. SCHACHTER: Amer. J. Physiol. **203**, 73 (1962). — PIRZIO-BIROLI, G., and C. A. FINCH: J. Laborat. Clin. Med. (U.S.A.) **55**, 216 (1960). — SCHULZ, E. J., and H. SWANEPOEL: S. Afr. Med. J. **36**, 367 (1962). — SEFTEL, H., and T. H. BOTHWELL: Unpublished data (1963). — SEFTEL, H., C. ISAACSON, and T. H. BOTHWELL: S. Afr. J. Med. Sc. **25**, 89 (1960). — SEFTEL, H., C. ISAACSON, K. J. KEELEY, and T. H. BOTHWELL: J. Laborat. Clin. Med. (U.S.A.) **58**, 837 (1961). — STRACHAN, A. S.: M. D. Thesis, Glasgow, 1929. — WAINWRIGHT, J.: S. Afr. J. Laborat. Clin. Med. **3**, 1 (1957). — WALKER, A. R. P., and U. B. ARVIDSSON: Transact. Roy. Soc. Trop. Med. (G.B.) **47**, 536 (1953).

Discussion

Mouriquand: Dr. Bothwell, you have mentioned that there was a close relationship between liver iron and bone-marrow iron in your cases. Are you referring to the parenchymal iron or to the Kupffer-cell iron in the liver? May I also ask if you have studied the sideroblasts in the bone marrow of these cases and, if so, how they compared with the reticular-cell iron in the marrow of patients with idiopathic haemochromatosis? I was especially interested in your reference to the occurrence of scurvy in your cases. Did you notice any peculiar distribution of iron in the bone marrow of these scorbutic patients, i.e. accumulation of iron in the reticular cells together with a marked lowering of the sideroblast count, as is the case in scorbutic guinea-pigs?

Bothwell: With regard to the comparisons we made between iron concentrations in the bone marrow and liver, our results represent total non-haem iron concentrations in the two organs. As for the percentage of sideroblasts in the marrows of siderotic and scorbutic subjects, although we have made no special study in siderosis, it is my impression that the percentage of sideroblasts is increased in those subjects with saturated transferrin levels. In untreated scurvy the plasma iron level is low, and sideroblasts are usually absent from the marrow. On the other hand, reticular cells in the bone marrow contain large amounts of haemosiderin. In response to therapy there is a prompt and dramatic rise in the plasma iron level which is probably the result of increased release from the reticulo-endothelial system.

Albahary: I should like to know the frequency of secondary cancer encountered by Dr. Bothwell in Bantu patients with alimentary siderosis of the liver.

Saadi: Dr. Bothwell did not mention what happened to the heart and to the skin in his patients with nutritional siderosis.

Bothwell: Although primary carcinoma of the liver is common in the Bantu, it occurs in subjects with post-necrotic cirrhosis and is uncommon in Bantu haemochromatosis. I have not seen any patient exhibiting clinical evidence of myocardial involvement. This, however, is not surprising, since the heart is one of the last organs to accumulate iron, and the rapidly progressive liver failure tends to cause death before the myocardial deposits have reached significant proportions.

Pollycove: Dr. Bothwell, you mentioned the very interesting association of two patterns of iron distribution, between the liver and other organs and epithelial tissues, with two groups of subjects differentiated by the absence or presence of hepatic cirrhosis, the latter group having a distribution of iron closely resembling that observed in patients with endogenous haemochromatosis. You also mentioned that the cirrhotic individuals have an increased plasma iron concentration and marked saturation of plasma transferrin, since the concentration of transferrin is not increased; the non-cirrhotic group, however, shows an increased concentration of transferrin with adequate latent iron-binding capacity of the plasma. Now the question is: do you think that the following sequence of events occurs? All subjects develop varying degrees of haemosiderosis; then, as a result of various injurious factors — perhaps excessive alcohol in a certain percentage — some individuals develop hepatic cirrhosis. Owing to the cirrhosis, transferrin production is impaired, with consequent inadequate latent iron-binding capacity. As a result there occurs a different distribution of the iron with marked deposition in other organs and tissues, mimicking the iron distribution observed in patients with endogenous haemochromatosis.

BOTHWELL: The relationship between the percentage saturation of circulating transferrin and the development of epithelial deposits is an interesting point. We believe that this is the most plausible explanation for the differences in iron distribution between non-cirrhotic and cirrhotic subjects. It should, however, be emphasised that this is merely an hypothesis and we only have indirect evidence to support it.

BRICK: Dr. BOTHWELL, for what length of time have you been able to follow the patients who had mild to moderate siderosis without any clinical evidence of liver failure? This, I think, brings up once again the important point as to whether or not we ought really to treat asymptomatic siblings. I fancy this issue has already been raised before, and your data may perhaps help towards answering the question.

BOTHWELL: I am sorry to have to disappoint Dr. BRICK on this question of following up subjects with mild to moderate siderosis. Although I agree that it would be most important to know the answer to this, I regret to have to say that we have not done any studies along these lines.

Hereditary hypochromic hypersideraemic anaemia

By

M. C. Verloop, W. Ploem, and J. Leunis

Cooley in 1945 and Rundles and Falls in 1946 described a form of hereditary hypochromic hypersideraemic anaemia which proved to be sex-linked and occurs only in males. In 1957, Heilmeyer suggested the name *anaemia hypochromica sideroachrestica hereditaria* for this condition, in which there is a disturbance in haemoglobin synthesis associated with accumulation of iron in the bone marrow and in other iron depots.

In the bone marrow, large quantities of iron are found in the reticulo-endothelial system, i.e. in the marrow fragments, in the erythroblasts, and in the erythrocytes. Iron staining reveals not only that the number of sideroblasts is larger than normal but that the iron granules in the sideroblasts are often strikingly coarse and arranged in a ring immediately round the nucleus – giving rise to so-called ringed sideroblasts (Bowman).

Electron-microscopic studies (Bessis; Sorenson) have shown that these coarse iron granules are located in the mitochondria.

We should first like to present some data on 6 patients suffering from primary hypochromic hypersideraemic anaemia (Table 1). Our follow-up studies on these patients covered periods of 4 to 7 years, during which time the clinical features showed no significant changes. Two of the patients (No. 3 and No. 5 in Table 1) had a history of anaemia dating back more than 25 years (Verloop, Bierenga, and Diezeraad-Njoo).

"Ringed sideroblasts", as encountered in this hereditary condition, occur only sporadically, if at all, in normal subjects and in other forms of hypochromic hypersideraemic anaemia. It is important to know this, because there are patients with hypochromic hypersideraemic anaemia who, both clinically and haematologically, show a striking similarity to those suffering from so-called primary hereditary hypochromic sideroachrestic anaemia.

Firstly, one must distinguish the latter from patients with *thalassaemia minor.* In the past few years we have examined patients from 4 families – all of Dutch descent as far as could be established – who were suffering from hypochromic hypersider-

Table 1. *Some data on 6 patients belonging to 5 families with "primary" hereditary hypochromic hypersideraemic anaemia*

Patients	Sex and age	Hb. g./100 ml.	Erythrocytes mill./cu. mm.	M.C.H.C.[1] %	M.C.V.[2] μ 3
Normal range:				32—36	76—96
1. Vi.. . .	M. 6	7.3	5.2	27	59
2. Sm. . .	M. 47	9.5	5.1	27	67
3. Ja.. . .	M. 50	8.4	4.9	23	73
4. de Jo. .	M. 39	10.6	5.3	27	75
Fam. { 5. Ve. . .	M. 54	7.5	5.0	24	52
Fam. { 6. Ve. . .	M. 57	11.4	5.3	29	74

	Serum iron		Bone marrow			
	Fasting μg./100 ml.	Saturation %	Ratio Red: White	R.E.S. iron	Sideroblasts	Ringed sideroblasts %
Normal range:	80—180	25—60	1:(2.5—5)	±	±	0
1.	310	100	1 :2	++	++	30
2.	305	100	1 :1	++	++	51
3.	365	100	3 :2	+++	+++	52
4.	236	95	1 :1	+++	+++	48
Fam. { 5.	262	80	1½:1	+++	++	38
Fam. { 6.	141	36	1 :1	+++	++	20

1 M.C.H.C. = mean corpuscular haemoglobin concentration.
2 M.C.V. = mean corpuscular volume.

aemic anaemia and showed an increased haemoglobin A_2 and/or haemoglobin F concentration (cf. Table 2). Ringed sideroblasts are lacking in this condition or occur only sporadically.

Secondly, there may be difficulties with regard to differential diagnosis between haemoglobin-H disease. We studied 3 families which included several patients with hypochromic hypersideraemic anaemia; in haemolysates from these patients, haemoglobin H was demonstrable in concentrations amounting sometimes to less than 1%, and in some cases only after recourse to special electrophoretic techniques (Table 3). Fortunately, the typical inclusion bodies seen in vitally or semi-vitally stained blood samples usually indicate the diagnosis, although these inclusion bodies are sometimes found only after prolonged search (Hedenberg et al.; Malanos et al.).

Thirdly, we encountered a family with hypochromic iron-saturated anaemia without ringed sideroblasts in the bone-marrow smears (Table 4); in haemolysates from these patients we found no anomalies, no haemoglobin H, no increase in haemoglobin A_2 or F, and no abnormal inclusion bodies in the blood samples. Are

Table 2. *Some data on 5 patients belonging to 4 families with thalassaemia minor (β-thalassaemia)*

Patients	Sex and age	Hb. g./100 ml.	Erythrocytes mill./cu. mm.	M.C.H.C.[1] %	M.C.V.[2] $\mu 3$	Reticulocytes ‰	Serum iron: Fasting μg./100 ml.	Serum iron: Saturation %
Normal range:				32—36	76—96	2—20	80—180	25—60
Fam. { 1. v. E.	F. 18	10.1	4.3	29	60	39	138	37
Fam. { 2. v. d. V.	M. 34	10.6	5.4	30	63	39	167	51
3. Ko.	M. 19	10.9	4.8	29	83	21	142	33
4. Vi.	F. 61	9.8	4.5	27	80	30	136	44
5. Si.	F. 5	9.8	4.3	26	84	10	151	36

	Bone marrow: Ratio Red:White	Bone marrow: R.E.S. iron	Bone marrow: Sideroblasts	Bone marrow: Ringed sideroblasts %	Haemoglobin: Alkaline resistance %	Haemoglobin: A_1 %	Haemoglobin: A_2 %	Haemoglobin: H %
Normal range:	1:(2.5—5)	±	±	0	max. 3	max. 98	max. 3	0
Fam. { 1.	1:2	++	+	0	0.9	94.3	*4.8*	0
Fam. { 2.	1:1	++	+	0	2.2	93.1	*4.7*	0
3.	2:1	+	+	0	1.4	93.9	*4.7*	0
4.	1:1	++	+	0	*9.3*	98.5	*5.7*	0
5.					*3.8*	91.3	*4.9*	0

[1] M.C.H.C. = mean corpuscular haemoglobin concentration.
[2] M.C.V. = mean corpuscular volume.

these to be regarded as cases of thalassaemia (i. e. of alpha-thalassaemia), or should such patients, despite the absence of ringed sideroblasts, be included in the group suffering from primary hereditary hypochromic anaemia? We do not know the answer to this question, but for the time being we still prefer to distinguish them from our patients with primary hereditary hypochromic hypersideraemic anaemia.

Iron staining of bone-marrow smears is thus of great importance for purposes of differential diagnosis. For a good evaluation of the sideroblasts, we favour a combination of staining techniques as described by Douglas and Dacie and by Kaplan et al. We fix the specimens in formaldehyde vapour and stain them at 56°C.

In taking a closer look at some of the results obtained in our study of the first group of patients showing many ringed sideroblasts in the bone marrow (Table 5), we shall confine our attention chiefly to data reflecting the disturbance in iron metabolism. We shall not discuss the anomalies in the pre-stages of haem found by

Table 3. *Some data on 5 patients belonging to 3 families with haemoglobin-H disease (α-thalassaemia)*

Patients	Sex and age	Hb. g./100 ml.	Erythrocytes mill./cu. mm.	M.C.H.C.[1] %	M.C.V.[2] $\mu 3$	Reticulocytes ‰	Serum iron: Fasting μg./100 ml.	Serum iron: Saturation %
Normal range:				32—36	76—96	2—20	80—180	25—60
1. M.	M. 29	10.3	5.0	28	66	38	127	46
Fam. 2. Ch. H.	M. 10	8.9	4.1	28	78	25	78	23
Fam. 3. L. H.	M. 3	9.8	4.7	30	71	17	157	33
Fam. 4. F. H.	M. 40	13.3	4.3	29	94	8	112	34
5. Ne.	M. 45	10.5	5.9	26	67	44	98	37

	Bone marrow: Ratio Red: White	Bone marrow: R.E.S. iron	Bone marrow: Sideroblasts	Bone marrow: Ringed sideroblasts %	Haemoglobin: Alkaline resistance %	Haemoglobin: A_1 %	Haemoglobin: A_2 %	Haemoglobin: H %	Inclusion bodies %
Normal range:	1:(2.5—5)	±	±	0	max. 3	max. 98	max. 3	0	0
1.	2:1	+++	+	1	0.6	97.9	*1.5*	<1	21
Fam. 2.	1:1	+	+	0	1.3	97.3	*1.4*	1—2	15
Fam. 3.					1.0	97.5	*1.5*	<1	16.5
Fam. 4.					1.5	96.1	2.4	0	0.5
5.	2:1	++	+	0	0.9	98.4	*0.7*	<1	73

[1] M.C.H.C. = mean corpuscular haemoglobin concentration.
[2] M.C.V. = mean corpuscular volume.

Heilmeyer and his co-workers in the erythrocytes of patients with hereditary hypochromic hypersideraemic anaemia. These anomalies would seem to be correlated with one or several of the mechanisms by which haem synthesis is blocked, and may lead – among other things – to a pathological increase in the coproporphyrins. This disturbance in haem synthesis, whatever its cause may be, often leads in the course of the years to massive haemosiderosis and sometimes haemochromatosis.

We should first like to present various data on two of our patients in whom 10 μc. Fe^{59} was injected intravenously as ferri-citrate (Bothwell and Finch).

The first patient, Ve. (No. 5 in Table 1), in whom liver biopsy revealed extensive haemosiderosis, had a firm, enlarged liver and spleen. The plasma iron clearance $t^1/_2$ was 24 minutes (normal: over 60 minutes). The plasma iron turnover (mg./day/100 ml. whole blood) was 5.8 mg. (normal: under 1 mg.). The curve for the percentage of radioactive iron in the plasma during the hours and days

Table 4. *Some data on 3 patients belonging to a family with hereditary hypochromic hypersideraemic anaemia without "ringed sideroblasts" (α-thalassaemia?)*

Patients	Sex and age	Hb. g./100 ml.	Erythrocytes mill./cu. mm.	M.C.H.C.[1] %	M.C.V.[2] μ3	Reticulocytes ‰	Serum iron Fasting μg./100 ml.	Serum iron Saturation %
Normal range:				32—36	76—96	2—20	80—180	25—60
Fam. 1. K.	M. 7	10.9	5.3	30	72	30	186	56
Fam. 2. K.	M. 30	13.4	5.2	32	80	46	138	43
Fam. 3. K.	F. 25	11.6	4.5	33	78	44	202	59

	Bone marrow Ratio Red:White	Bone marrow R.E.S. iron	Bone marrow Sideroblasts	Bone marrow Ringed sideroblasts %	Haemoglobin Alkaline resistance %	Haemoglobin A_1 %	Haemoglobin A_2 %	Haemoglobin H %	Inclusion bodies %
Normal range:	1:(2.5—5)	±	±	0	max. 3	max. 98	max. 3	0	0
Fam. 1.	1:1	++	+	0	1.3	96.2	2.5	0	absent
Fam. 2.	1:1	++	+	0	1.8	95.8	2.4	0	absent
Fam. 3.	1:1	++	+	0	0.8	97.5	1.7	0	absent

[1] M.C.H.C. = mean corpuscular haemoglobin concentration.
[2] M.C.V. = mean corpuscular volume.

Table 5. *Comparison of some data on the patients listed in Tables 1 to 4*

	Ringed sideroblasts present	Hb.A_2 increased	Hb.F increased	Hb.H present	Inclusion bodies present
Primary hereditary hypochromic hypersideraemic anaemia	yes	no	no	no	no
Thalassaemia minor (β-thalassaemia)	no	yes	yes	no	no
Haemoglobin-H disease	no	no	no	yes	yes
Hereditary hypochromic hypersideraemic anaemia (α-thalassaemia?)	no	no	no	no	no

following the injection initially showed a steep descent, but soon swung back to the horizontal, to remain almost horizontal on the second and third days (Fig. 1). Unfortunately, we failed to measure the plasma radioactive iron concentration over a sufficiently long period for us to be able to predict its further course with any degree of certainty. The slope of the curve, and the plasma radioactive iron concentration of 0.28% on the third day, however, would seem to indicate a significant interchange between the plasma iron and one or several unstable iron pools. No calculations were made to determine the size of these iron compartments (POLLYCOVE). One reason for the fact that the plasma radioactive iron concentration remained slightly above normal might be random pathological haemolysis (POLLYCOVE and MORTIMER), because in patient Ve. the life-span of the circulating erythrocytes was shortened (Cr^{51} $t^1/_2$: 15 days).

In this patient, the maximum red-cell utilisation of radioactive iron after 25 days amounted to 19% of the Fe^{59} injected, which is considerably below normal (Fig. 2). A remarkable feature was the protracted gradual increase in the percentage of utilisation. This is probably correlated with re-utilisation of radioactive iron, re-offered to the bone marrow after premature abnormal haemolysis, and with re-cycling of iron removed by the spleen from the iron-loaded siderocytes. Surface scanning (Fig. 2) revealed a rapid increase in radioactivity over the bone marrow (although less than normal!), followed by an initially rapid and then more gradual decrease. The blood activity (heart) ran roughly parallel with the curves for plasma iron clearance and red-cell utilisation. Over the liver the radioactivity measured was above normal from the onset; this indicates that a portion of the radioactive iron injected is directly taken up by the liver and remains there. The radioactivity over the spleen diminished during the first few hours, roughly in parallel with the blood (heart) activity, but during the following days there was a marked abnormal increase in Fe^{59} activity over the spleen.

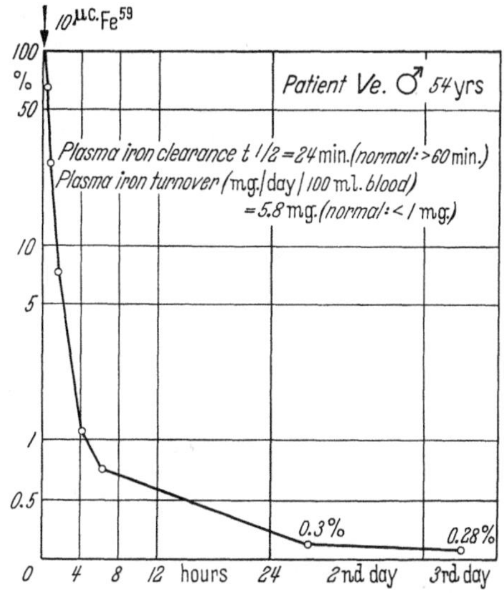

Fig. 1. Plasma Fe^{59} clearance with a $t^1/_2$ of 24 min. in patient Ve. (No. 5 in Table 1). After the second day the curve remains almost horizontal, which seems to indicate a significant interchange between the plasma iron and one or more unstable iron pools

It seems most probable that this marked increase occurred because siderocytes loaded with Fe^{59} entered the circulation and released their iron load in the spleen. As CROSBY has demonstrated, the spleen is capable of retaining the iron granules of the siderocytes. The bone marrow of patients with primary hereditary hypersideraemic anaemia often contains a large number of siderocytes with coarse iron granules (patient Ve.: 13%). Another possible explanation for the marked increase in radioactivity over the spleen may have been the above-mentioned random pathological haemolysis.

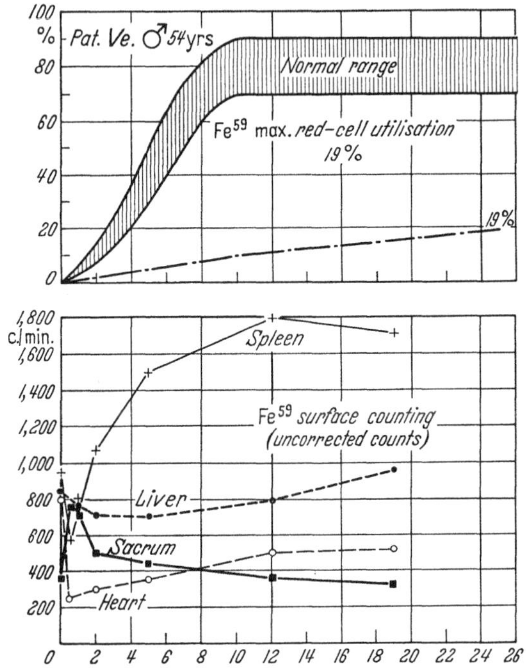

Fig. 2. Red-cell utilisation of intravenously injected Fe^{59} in patient Ve. (No. 5 in Table 1), which is considerably below normal. The results of the surface counts reveal that the radioactivity over the liver is above normal and that there is a marked increase in radioactivity over the spleen in the weeks following the Fe^{59} injection. This last feature may be mainly due to the fact that the spleen retains the coarse iron granules present in the siderocytes

In the second patient, Ja. (No. 3 in Table 1), liver biopsy showed unmistakable haemochromatosis, and he also had a firm enlarged liver and spleen. He, too, showed an accelerated plasma iron clearance $t^1/_2$ of 32 minutes, with a plasma iron turnover of 4.5 mg./day/100 ml. whole blood (Fig. 3). The radioactive iron concentration in the plasma on the second day was still 0.7%, i.e. slightly higher than in the first patient. This is not surprising, because this patient's iron stores (and therefore probably also his unstable iron pools) were probably larger than those of the first

Fig. 3. Plasma Fe^{59} clearance with a $t^{1}/_{2}$ of 32 min. in patient Ja. (No. 3 in Table 1). On the second day the radioactive iron concentration in the plasma was still 0.76%, which indicates a significant interchange between the plasma iron and one or more unstable iron pools

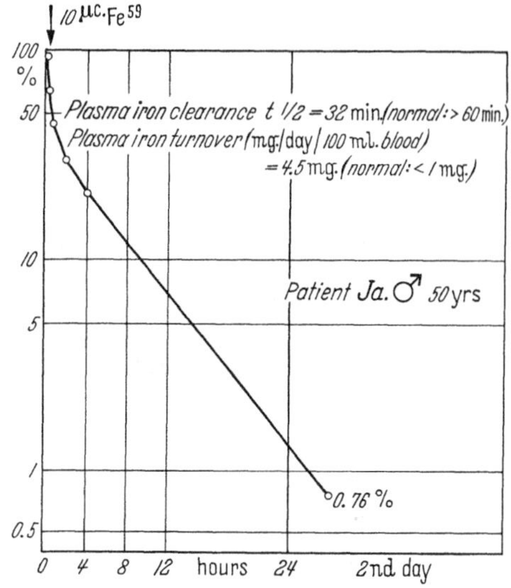

patient, since he showed clear evidence of haemochromatosis. The maximum red-cell iron utilisation was only 16% (Fig. 4). The results of surface measurements were largely the same as in patient Ve. (Fig. 4).

Patient Ve. received oral iron medication only for a period of a few months. He was given five intravenous iron injections of 100 mg. and never received a blood transfusion. Oral iron medication of patient Ja. covered a period of a few years and must have exceeded 50 g. In addition he was given two blood transfusions of 400 ml. each.

The haemosiderosis and haemochromatosis in these two patients cannot therefore be explained by reference to parenterally administered

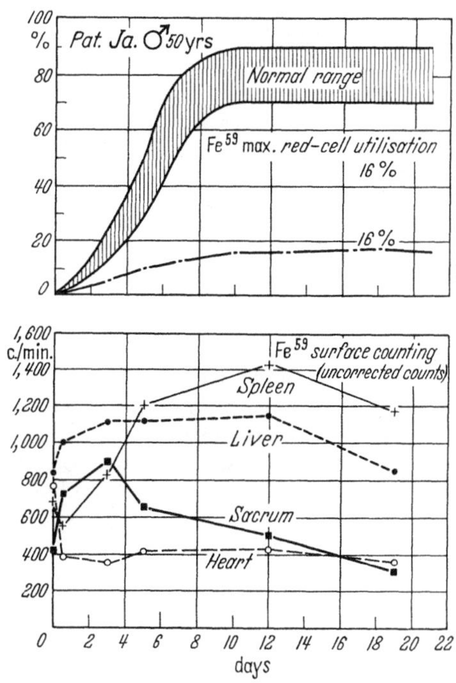

Fig. 4. As in patient Ve. (Fig. 2), the red-cell utilisation of intravenously injected Fe^{59} in patient Ja. (No. 3 in Table 1) is considerably below normal. Fe^{59} surface counts reveal a greatly increased radioactivity over the liver and spleen. For further details, see text

iron. The patients must for years have been absorbing increased amounts of iron in the gastro-intestinal tract. While more than the normal quantity must have been absorbed from the iron administered orally, it has to be assumed that extra iron was also taken up from the food.

The fact that iron absorption may be pathological in such patients has been established by various investigators, including ERLANDSON et al., who reported that the absorption of medicinal iron is sometimes greatly increased in patients with chronic anaemia and a hyperplastic red-cell system.

Thus, patients who are suffering from chronic anaemia which is not due to iron deficiency, and who have a hyperplastic erythropoietic system, can apparently absorb much more iron than normal in the course of the years. It is in this way that generalised haemosiderosis may occur. At the same time, however, there are probably additional factors involved in the pathogenesis of haemochromatosis which we shall not discuss here.

We measured iron absorption by the method of NAJEAN and ARDAILLOU, which makes it possible to calculate the quantity of radioactive iron absorbed by reference to the proportion of Ba^{131} and Fe^{59} prior to ingestion and the proportion of the two radioactive isotopes in the faeces. The range of absorption of radioactive iron established in five test subjects was 13–30%. In patient Ve., practically no iron was absorbed when 5 μc. Fe^{59} was administered in a dose of 625 mg. ferrous sulphate, whereas in patient Ja., with haemochromatosis, we found a mean absorption of 54%!

What is the explanation for this great difference in absorption? In both patients, the iron depots were overfilled with iron. It has been established (BOTHWELL and FINCH) that, in patients of this kind, iron absorption diminishes when iron accumulates in the organism, and this may be the reason why patient Ve. absorbed almost no radioactive iron. Patient Ja., however, had been subjected to repeated venesection over a period of several years, and PIRZIO-BIROLI et al. have pointed out that this procedure may stimulate iron absorption.

Both patients were known to have been anaemic for at least 25 years; thus, for decades there had probably been an increase in absorption which, in the long run, gave rise to generalised haemosiderosis.

Finally, we should like to refer briefly to the problem of treatment. In hereditary hypochromic hypersideraemic anaemia, we are confronted with an anomaly of haemoglobin synthesis, for which there is at the moment no causal therapy. Treatment must be aimed at combating the anaemia, when it assumes a serious form, and at controlling or preventing haemochromatosis.

In a number of patients, *the anaemia requires no treatment*, because the haemoglobin concentration is 10 g./100 ml. or higher. Blood transfusions are sometimes needed, however, if the anaemia is more serious. It is often found that the anaemia shows a favourable response to the administration of substances of which the bone marrow has apparently become deficient. This deficiency is probably relative and is perhaps related to the hyperplasia of the erythropoietic system. Agents described as having a beneficial effect include vitamin B_6 (Verloop and Rademaker), vitamin C (Vuylsteke et al.), folic acid, and certain liver extracts such as Valentine's liver extract.

In our patients we have so far observed only partial remissions of the anaemia. When medication which has improved the anaemia is discontinued, the haemoglobin concentration is seen to diminish again to pre-treatment levels. Persistent therapy is therefore required. Intercurrent infections can exert an unfavourable influence on the anaemia and may even cause a latent folic acid deficiency to become manifest.

How can secondary haemochromatosis best be controlled or prevented? In the case of our patient Ja., we have eliminated in the course of $3^1/_2$ years a total of more than 30 g. iron by means of weekly venesections of 0.5 litre. The haemoglobin concentration has continued to fluctuate between 9.5 and 11 g./100 ml., and no complications have occurred during this period (Verloop and Rademaker). The greatly enlarged liver and spleen diminished in size, and there was an improvement in liver function tests and in the glucose tolerance test. The patient also felt better. A second liver biopsy revealed, however, that, although the quantity of stainable iron had diminished, there was still a marked degree of haemosiderosis. When we measured the absorption of a dose of Fe^{59} we found that this patient still absorbed considerable quantities of iron — possibly, i.e. under the influence of repeated venesections, even more iron than before (Pirzio-Biroli et al.).

At present we are employing desferrioxamine to treat this patient, as well as patient Ve. whom we have already discussed. Both patients have learned to give themselves two daily injections of 500 mg. desferrioxamine methane sulphonate intramuscularly; their average urinary excretion is now 10–20 mg. iron per 24 hours, which is equivalent to a maximum weekly urinary excretion of 70–140 mg. iron. By means of weekly venesections of 0.5 litre, we had been removing from our patient with haemochromatosis about 150 mg. iron per week over a period of several years, and this treatment was well tolerated. We therefore consider that it may be desirable in the future to revert to repeated venesections in these cases should chelating agents fail to ensure a greater weekly excretion of iron; alternatively, we may perhaps combine both forms of treatment.

It has been established – as we have also seen in one of our patients – that, when the iron stores are reduced by treatment in cases of haemosiderosis or haemochromatosis, there may be a marked increase in intestinal iron absorption (PIRZIO-BIROLI et al.). It would be useful if a means could be discovered of controlling this increased intestinal iron absorption. It is alleged that at the moment oral desferrioxamine medication cannot prevent the absorption of iron from the food (BANNERMAN et al.). It is to be hoped that this problem, too, will eventually be solved.

Summary

The staining of iron in bone-marrow smears is a valuable aid to the diagnosis of primary hereditary hypochromic hypersideraemic anaemia. "Ringed sideroblasts" are invariably encountered in this condition. An exhaustive study of the haemolysate and an investigation into the presence of abnormal inclusion bodies in the red cells is required to exclude the presence of beta-thalassaemia or alpha-thalassaemia.

Much remains to be discovered about the pathophysiology of haemoglobin synthesis and iron metabolism in these patients. Further study may well reveal that patients included collectively under the heading of primary hereditary hypochromic hypersideraemic anaemia will have to be further classified under various subheadings.

It is frequently possible to ensure partial remission of anaemia in such cases with the aid of certain anti-anaemic agents. In addition, attention must be paid to the treatment or prevention of secondary haemochromatosis. Desferrioxamine undoubtedly constitutes an important acquisition in this respect. However, in the two patients described in the present paper, who have been treated with desferrioxamine, the amount of iron eliminated did not exceed the amount of iron removed by weekly venesection.

Zusammenfassung

Die Färbung von Eisen in Knochenmarkausstrichen ist ein geeignetes Hilfsmittel für die Diagnose der primären hereditären hypochromen hypersideraemischen Anaemie. „Ringförmige Sideroblasten" werden dabei regelmäßig gefunden. Um eine β- oder α-Thalassaemie auszuschließen, ist es notwendig, sowohl das Haemolysat eingehend zu untersuchen als auch nach abnormen Einschlußkörperchen in den Erythrozyten zu fahnden.

Zahlreiche Fragen über die Pathophysiologie der Haemoglobinsynthese und des Eisenstoffwechsels sind bei diesen Patienten noch ungeklärt. Möglicherweise werden weitere Untersuchungen ergeben, daß die jetzt unter der Diagnose der primären hereditären hypochromen hypersideraemischen Anaemie zusammengefaßten Zustände in einzelne Untergruppen zerfallen.

Mit Hilfe einer antianaemischen Behandlung ist es möglich, partielle Remissionen der Anaemie bei diesen Patienten zu erzielen. Zusätzlich ist es notwendig, der Behandlung oder Verhütung einer sekundären Haemochromatose Beachtung zu schenken. Desferrioxamin stellt zweifellos einen wichtigen Fortschritt in dieser Richtung dar. Allerdings war bei zwei Patienten, über die in dieser Arbeit genauer berichtet wird, die Menge von Eisen, die unter Behandlung mit Desferrioxamin ausgeschieden wurde, nicht größer als diejenige, die durch wöchentliche Aderlässe entfernt wurde.

Résumé

La coloration du fer dans les étalements de moelle est une aide appréciable au diagnostic d'anémie primaire héréditaire hypochrome avec hypersidérémie. Des «sidéroblastes annulaires» se rencontrent de façon constante dans cet état pathologique. Une étude complète de l'hémolysat et une recherche de la présence de corps d'inclusion anormaux dans les globules rouges sont nécessaires pour exclure l'existence d'une β- ou d'une α-thalassémie.

Il reste encore beaucoup à apprendre sur la physiopathologie de la synthèse de l'hémoglobine et sur le métabolisme du fer chez ces malades. Il est bien possible que des études ultérieures montrent que ce groupe de l'anémie primaire héréditaire hypochrome avec hypersidérémie, dans lequel sont actuellement classés tous ces malades, devrait en fait être démembré en différents sous-groupes.

Il est fréquemment possible d'obtenir une rémission partielle de l'anémie dans de tels cas à l'aide de certains facteurs anti-anémiques. De plus, le traitement ou la prévention de l'hémochromatose secondaire ne doit pas être négligé. La desferrioxamine constitue sans aucun doute une acquisition importante à ce point de vue. Cependant, chez les deux malades décrits dans cette présente communication, et qui ont été traités par la desferrioxamine, la quantité de fer éliminée n'excède pas celle soustraite par la saignée hebdomadaire.

References

Bannerman, R. M., S. Callender, and D. L. Williams: Brit. Med. J. **1962**/II, 1573. — Bessis, M.: Nouv. rev. fr. hémat. **2**, 153 (1962). — Bothwell, T. H., and C. A. Finch: Iron Metabolism. Little, Brown & Co., Boston, 1962. — Bowman, W. D.: Blood (U.S.A.) **18**, 662 (1961). — Cooley, T. B.: Amer. J. Med. Sc. **209**, 561 (1945). — Crosby, W. H.: J. Clin. Invest. (U.S.A.) **38**, 997 (1959). — Douglas, A. S., and J. V. Dacie: J. Clin. Path. (G.B.) **6**, 307 (1953). — Erlandson, M. E., B. Walden, G. Stern, N. W. Hilgartner, J. Wehman, and C. H. Smith: Blood (U.S.A.) **19**, 359 (1962). — Hedenberg, F., U. Müller-Ebenhard, S. Sjölin, and L. Wranne: Acta paediatr. (Sweden) **47**, 652 (1958). — Heilmeyer, L.: Schweiz. med. Wschr. **92**, 1285 (1962). — Heilmeyer, L., J. Emmerich, M. H. Hennemann, H. Schubothe, W. Keiderling, M. H. Lee, R. Bilger, and W. Bernauer: Schweiz. med. Wschr. **87**, 1237 (1957). — Kaplan, E., W. W. Zuelzer, and C. Mouriquand: Blood (U.S.A.) **9**, 203 (1954). — Malanos, B., P. Fessas, and G. Stamatoyannopoulos: Brit. J. Haemat. **8**, 5 (1962). — Najean, Y., and N. Ardaillou: Nouv. rev. fr. hémat. **3**, 82 (1963). — Pirzio-Biroli, G., T. H. Bothwell, and C. A. Finch: J. Laborat. Clin. Med. (U.S.A.) **51**, 37 (1958). — Pollycove, M.: J. Clin. Invest. (U.S.A.) **40**, 1071 (1961). — Pollycove, M., and R. Mortimer: J. Clin. Invest. (U.S.A.) **40**, 753 (1961). — Rundles, R. W., and H. F. Falls: Amer. J. Med. Sc. **211**, 641 (1946). — Sorenson, G. D.: Amer. J. Path. **40**, 297 (1962). — Verloop, M. D., M. Bierenga, and A. Diezeraad-Njoo: Acta haemat. (Switz.) **27**, 129 (1962). — Verloop, M. C., and W. Rademaker: Brit. J. Haemat. **6**, 1 (1960). — Vuylsteke, J., M. C. Verloop, and A. C. Drogendijk: Acta med. Scand. **169**, 1 (1961).

Discussion

HEILMEYER: "Hereditary hypochromic hypersideraemic anaemia" strikes me as being not a very suitable term to apply to congenital sideroachrestic anaemia, because thalassaemia is also a form of hereditary hypochromic hypersideraemic anaemia which can be clearly distinguished from congenital sideroachrestic anaemia. In contrast to thalassaemia, congenital sideroachrestic anaemia — as can be demonstrated both by electron microscopy and by light microscopy — is associated with a different form of iron deposition in the erythroblasts and a different pattern of haem precursors in the erythrocytes (i.e. an increase in coproporphyrin but no increase in protoporphyrin). In addition, the values for haemoglobin F and haemoglobin A_2 are invariably normal. In patients with thalassaemia one of the most distinctive features is the increase in protoporphyrin. We have encountered only one case of congenital sideroachrestic anaemia in which the behaviour of the haem precursors was different from what I have just indicated; in this case, there was a decrease in all the haem precursors in the erythrocytes, a finding which suggests a disorder affecting the first step in haem synthesis. In this patient, a stable derivative of α-amino-β-keto-adipic acid was in fact found in the urine. The metabolic disturbance in this case is at present under further chemical study.

With regard to the treatment of sideroachrestic anaemia, I feel that this disease constitutes a very good indication for desferrioxamine, particularly because the iron overload represents a far greater danger to the patient than does the anaemia. It was for this reason that CROSBY[1] suggested such patients should be treated by venesection; but it seems rather paradoxical to treat anaemia by venesection. Desferrioxamine is therefore preferable. There have been cases in which, in response to elimination of excess iron, the sideroachrestic disorder improved, i.e. the erythrocytes and haemoglobin showed an increase.

VERLOOP: I made no reference to porphyrin metabolism in connection with haem synthesis, because I preferred to discuss our own results and to deal with the question of iron metabolism. I'm afraid I do not quite agree with your statement that these patients with anaemia have to be treated with desferrioxamine. I hope I have succeeded in demonstrating that such patients — or at least some of those suffering from anaemia and hypersiderosis — can be treated by venesection for years without sustaining any ill effects. The patients we have treated in this way are doing well; their haemoglobin values sometimes rise during the course of treatment by venesection, and they are able to carry on at work.

GAJDOS: I should like to add just a few words to the remarks made by Dr. HEILMEYER. In a case of hypochromic hypersideraemic achrestic anaemia, on which MALLARMÉ, BESSIS, and myself have already reported[2], we also found an increased level of coproporphyrin and a decreased level of proto-

[1] CROSBY, W. H., and T. W. SHEEHY: Brit. J. Haemat. **6**, 56 (1960).

[2] MALLARMÉ, J., M. BESSIS, A. GAJDOS, M. GAJDOS-TÖRÖK, P. BOIVIN, and F. NICOLLO: Sang (Fr.) **31**, 757 (1960).

porphyrin in the red blood cells. But our *in vitro* experiments with the blood of this patient do not confirm Dr. HEILMEYER's hypothesis, which ascribes the accumulation of coproporphyrin to a defective synthesis of protoporphyrin. After incubating the patient's blood with glycine for 4 hours, we observed a very significant degree of protoporphyrin synthesis, despite the fact that reticulocytosis was quite normal. This is an interesting finding, because normal human red cells do not synthesise protoporphyrin in these conditions. On the other hand, we have also incubated our patient's blood with δ-aminolaevulinic acid, labelled with C^{14}. The haemin isolated after incubation has shown a highly significant radioactivity. I think these experiments clearly demonstrate that protoporphyrin synthesis by the red blood cells of patients with achrestic anaemia is not diminished; on the contrary, it is actually increased.

CAROLI: I should like at this point to tell you about an additional case involving one of our patients suffering from achrestic hypersideraemic anaemia complicated by haemochromatosis. A preliminary report on this case was already published in 1957[1]. The patient, a man aged 39 years, showed very pronounced enlargement of the liver. Peritoneoscopy and liver biopsy revealed massive haemochromatosis. From the biological aspect the condition of the liver was largely normal, whereas haematological examination indicated hypochromic anaemia with hypersideraemia and a decrease in the life-span of the erythrocytes. Studies of iron metabolism showed not only elevated serum iron levels and complete transferrin saturation, but also an increase in the non-haemoglobin iron content of the erythrocytes and a considerable acceleration of the plasma iron turnover, as well as a very low rate of incorporation of Fe^{59} into the red cells. BESSIS[2] found in the electron microscope that the liver cells where packed with ferritin and haemosiderin and that in the bone marrow there were also very large numbers of granules containing iron; in the cytoplasm of the erythroblasts the electron microscope revealed appreciable quantities of iron in the form either of ferritin molecules or of iron-bearing micelles in the mitochondria.

In this case, pyridoxine was partially effective in reversing the anaemia, but did not prevent the patient's condition from progressively deteriorating; he developed ascites, diabetes, and finally pericarditis. At autopsy, haemochromatosis of a most severe and generalised type was found, with massive siderosis of the liver, spleen, pancreas, anterior pituitary, thyroid, adrenal cortex, gastro-intestinal tract, heart, and choroid plexus.

BEUTLER: I was very interested in Dr. VERLOOP's introductory comments, which indicated that the cases reported by RUNDLES and FALLS[3] almost 20 years ago probably belong to this group of disorders. I would appreciate some further clarification of the mode of genetic transmission of this disease. In the family reported by RUNDLES and FALLS, although a question mark was placed after the term "sex-linked" in their title, it seems that the evidence of the sex-linkage is fairly good. There was evidence that the mothers of involved males had some degree of abnormality. They had a few hypochromic cells, or in some instances splenomegaly was present, even in the absence of abnormal cells in the circulation. Of the cases that Dr. VERLOOP has presented today, all 6 were males, and while this certainly is in good accord with the hypothesis of sex-linkage, it cannot be considered as evidence.

[1] CAROLI, J., J. BERNARD, et al.: Presse méd. (Fr.) **65**, 1991 (1957).
[2] BESSIS, M.: Personal communication.
[3] RUNDLES, R. W., and H. F. FALLS: Amer. J. Med. Sc. **211**, 641 (1946).

The transmission could also be sex-limited. If these patients are of the same variety as those described by RUNDLES and FALLS, one would expect abnormalities in their mothers; and one would also expect that male relatives of the mothers would be affected by the same disease. I wondered whether extensive predigrees were available in the cases described by Dr. VERLOOP and also in those that have been reported by other groups, and whether this is indeed a homogenous group of sex-linked anaemia.

VERLOOP: Our 6 patients belonged to 5 families, and in 3 of these 5 families we were unable to find any abnormalities. In the remaining 2 families, however, there were several brothers with the disease. The 6-year-old boy had been suffering from anaemia for a long time, so we think that this was an hereditary form too, although in his family we couldn't find any abnormalities. But I think that the genetics have not yet been sufficiently thoroughly investigated in these families; this is something we hope to do in the future.

UNDRITZ: In many cases, bone-marrow puncture, which is a safe method, ought to be given preference over liver biopsy as a means of detecting haemochromatosis, because liver biopsy is not completely without danger and is contra-indicated in some conditions. The advantages of bone-marrow biopsy are also clearly apparent from the instructive results obtained by Dr. VERLOOP.

Let me illustrate this by the case of a 40-year-old man with "occult leukaemia" (observed together with Dr. P. MULLER, Bassecourt, and Dr. M. AUROI, Delémont). Examination of the bone marrow revealed neutrophil blasts and promyelocytes amounting to about 20% of the leucocytes, in addition to many highly polyploid erythroblasts as seen in erythraemia. No immature elements were found in the blood; there was merely severe anaemia and leucopenia with pseudopelgerisation of the neutrophils, which is so common in leukaemia. This clinical picture, which has probably not previously been diagnosed, was treated with two courses of Endoxan therapy. The first course of treatment elicited an excellent response, inasmuch as the neutrophil blasts and the polyploid erythroblasts in the bone marrow disappeared, as did also the reactive pelgerisation of the neutrophils. The anaemia regressed completely. The response to the second course of Endoxan therapy was not so impressive; the anaemia failed to improve and the pelgerisation persisted. The patient had to be given regular blood transfusions because of aplasia of the erythropoietic system. In this case, as in so many cases of leukaemia treated with cytostatics, monocytosis of over 50% occurred in the blood and bone marrow, the monocytes of the bone marrow collecting together in the form of granulomas and containing a great deal of iron (sideromonocytes). In view of the risk of haemochromatosis, the patient was given Desferal for 4 months in addition to the blood transfusions, in order to remove the pathological iron deposits. In response to this treatment he excreted in the urine up to 25 mg. iron daily (total 630 mg.). Re-examination of the bone marrow showed that less iron was being stored by the monocytes, which had not declined in number. At first, the patient showed a marked improvement in general condition, but this improvement did not last long owing to the gradual but inevitable progression of the incurable underlying disease; the haemoglobin levels improved only in response to blood transfusions. As a result of the myelosis, the patient died after $2^1/_2$ years, the cause of death being cardiac insufficiency. We had the definite impression that the effect of the transfusions was in no way impaired by Desferal, since despite their diametrically opposed effects the two types of treatment possess entirely different sites of attack: the transfusions replace the erythrocytes in a physiological manner, while Desferal merely removes pathological deposits of useless iron. In this case, bone-marrow puncture offered a perfectly adequate means of checking the iron stores; liver biopsy would in any event have been contraindicated because of the thrombopenia and the occasional tendency towards haemorrhage in this patient.

VERLOOP: I agree that in this type of case you may perhaps be right in using desferrioxamine. If you have to give the patient blood transfusions, this means that you are introducing even more iron into the body; by treating him at the same time with desferrioxamine you may be able to keep him in balance.

POLLYCOVE: I have just one comment to make on the data on iron kinetics which Dr. VERLOOP has presented. They seem quite characteristic of intramedullary haemolysis: the rapid and early marrow uptake of the plasma radio-iron, the delayed and incomplete release of radio-iron from the bone marrow, and the markedly subnormal and prolonged appearance of radio-iron in the circulating red cells. This abnormal pattern is observed in thalassaemia major, pernicious anaemia, and other conditions in which there is considerable intramedullary haemolysis. The data on iron kinetics lend support to the remarks of Dr. GAJDOS in that, although there is defective erythropoiesis with abnormal intermediary metabolism of haem, the over-all synthesis of haem and haemoglobin is actually increased in hereditary hypochromic hypersideraemic anaemia. Erythropoiesis, though increased, is quite defective, so that the red cells formed frequently die in the bone marrow, with release into the circulation of relatively few reticulocytes compared to the erythroid hyperplasia of the marrow.

VERLOOP: I have not done these calculations in our Fe^{59} studies.

STURGEON: I should like to comment briefly on the relation of this condition to thalassaemia. In the few cases that I have seen, it is true that the general qualitative changes of hypochromia and hypersideraemia resemble those observed in thalassaemia; but generally we have been able to distinguish the two conditions quite readily by reference to the hereditary pattern. I think, if one pays attention to the genetic manifestations in the patient and his relatives, that the various forms of thalassaemia can be distinguished quite easily. I should also like to suggest that the four cases which Dr. VERLOOP presented were in fact the α-thalassaemia trait and not thalassaemia haemoglobin-H disease. With refined methods of starch-block electrophoresis of haemoglobin it is possible to find a small amount of haemoglobin H in the traits without the presence of the H gene. I must have misunderstood you about the other four cases; I believe they were ordinary β-thalassaemia rather than hypersideraemic hypochromic anaemia.

VERLOOP: We found only a very small band of haemoglobin H in the three families mentioned (Table 3, p. 379), and only with a pH of 7.3 on a thin layer of starch gel. At a pH of 8.4 or 6.4. we couldn't find anything abnormal at all. So evidently one has to use special techniques. I quite agree with you that this abnormality can better be termed α-thalassaemia trait, although in my opinion α-thalassaemia is still a hypothetical disease.

Introduction to the General Discussion

By

SHEILA SHERLOCK

It is generally accepted that primary haemochromatosis is a genetically determined disease and that the best method of diagnosing affected siblings is by needle liver biopsy. We have found that serum iron values might be normal, although liver biopsy showed significant iron deposition (WILLIAMS et al., 1962)

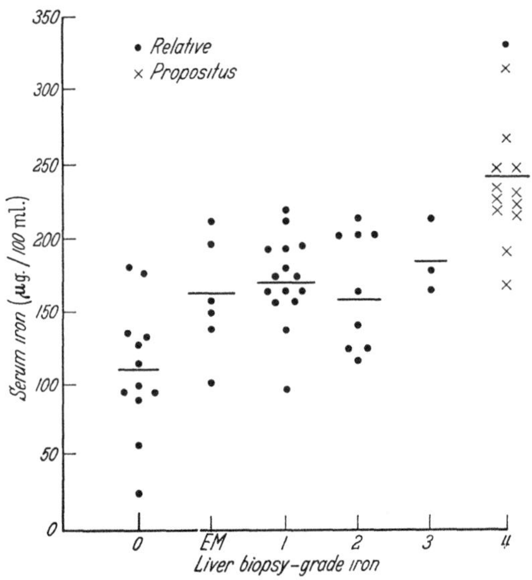

Fig. 1. Relation between the serum iron level and the hepatic biopsy section graded for free iron (EM = electron microscopy only). (WILLIAMS et al., 1962)

(Fig. 1). Dr. BOTHWELL has commented on the reverse situation, namely high serum iron values with no excess iron in the liver on biopsy. This is difficult to explain unless the duration of the elevated serum iron value is also of importance. Further work is needed on this problem.

Liver biopsy is a quite justifiable procedure in relatives of patients suffering from haemochromatosis, since, if iron is found in the liver, useful treatment can be offered to them. The main clinical and biopsy data are given in Fig. 2. We found that 28 of 46 relatives of 16 propositi with the disease showed increased

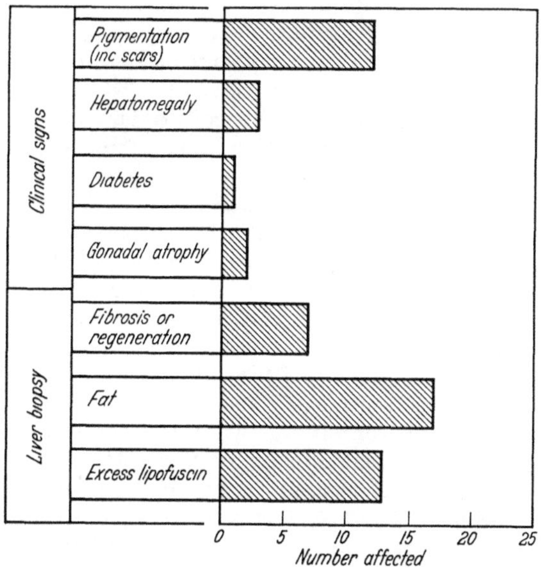

Fig. 2. Main clinical and biopsy findings in the 28 relatives with increased free iron in hepatic biopsy sections on light microscopy. (WILLIAMS et al., 1962)

amounts of iron in the liver on biopsy (Table 1). Six of these required electron microscopy to show the increased amounts of iron. This raises the question as to what is to be regarded as a significant positive for iron excess in the liver. A number of these relatives had really very little excess iron in the liver. In such

Table 1. *Liver biopsy iron in 46 relatives of 16 propositi with idiopathic haemochromatosis* (WILLIAMS et al., 1962)

Grade	0	1	2	3	4
No. of biopsies . .	18	15	9	3	1

cases one is faced with the problem of deciding whether there is more liver iron than one would expect to find in a *normal* person. Certainly some specimens of liver taken at autopsy and some biopsies from a "normal" hospital population showed traces of iron.

These specimens, however, do not come from really normal people, and of course it would not be reasonable to do liver biopsies, say, on everyone in this room. The interpretation of our results, i.e. the percentage regarded as positive, determines what is believed to be the mode of inheritance. At the moment the general impression is that this is of intermediate type.

Iron absorption studies on siblings would be of interest. Using the double isotope technique, we have studied the oral iron absorption of 12 relatives of sufferers from primary haemochromatosis. Preliminary findings are very variable. Some show increased, some normal absorption. Of more interest may be our results in 4 affected relatives *after* venesection treatment. The study was made more than one year after the last venesection, when they were not anaemic and had a normal serum iron level. All 4 showed a greatly increased iron absorption. This work needs extension. Our findings fit in with the observation of Dr. VERLOOP that one of his patients with haemochromatosis showed a greatly increased iron absorption after removal of iron by multiple venesection. The results obtained may depend very much on the state of the disease and on the extent of iron storage when the observation is made.

In our relatives of genetic haemochromatotics the iron deposition in the liver was less than in the propositi in whom the disease was fully developed. Two relatives were venesected until a second liver biopsy showed no iron, but the amount of iron removed was only 5.2 and 4.1 g., respectively. Two other younger siblings were also venesected, and the amount of iron removed was only 2.4 and 2.3 g.; yet serum iron and haemoglobin values were falling (Table 2).

Table 2. *Amount of iron removed during venesection therapy of 4 affected relatives* (WILLIAMS et al., 1962)

Family and case number	Age (years)	Biopsy grade	Initial serum iron (μg./100 ml.)	Iron removed (g.)
D.15	60	3	205	4.1
D.16	56	3	168	5.2
H.34	44	2	125	2.4
H.35	40	2	191	2.3

These quantities are much less than the 25 g. or so of iron stored in the usual patient with haemochromatosis. Moreover it is very rare for the florid disease to appear in more than one generation; in the few such instances recorded, the details given are not sufficient for one to be certain that the disease is in fact florid.

Now, turning from the genetic aspect, we come to the relation between nutrition and haemosiderosis. I was a little sorry that Dr. MacDonald of Boston was not here. He really believes that most instances of haemochromatosis are nutritional, especially in alcoholics. The rest of us seem to be agreeing too much. Undoubtedly, alcoholism is in some way related to iron excess in the liver. In our group of 16 primary haemochromatotics (all with affected relatives), 5 were alcoholics and 2 more had a history of severe malnutrition. Now that is a high incidence in Britain, where alcoholism and malnutrition are unusual. This suggests that if you have the gene, or genes, of haemochromatosis it is unwise to take excessive amounts of alcohol or to become malnourished.

We now come to the difference between primary (genetic) haemochromatosis and the iron deposition in the cirrhotic liver of the alcoholic. Dr. Caroli dealt with this magnificently. I am, in general, in agreement with him. The essential difference between the two types is in the sequence. In the alcoholic, cirrhosis comes first, and then comes the iron. In the primary haemochromatotic, the iron comes first, and then comes the cirrhosis. This was brought out very well in Dr. Caroli's paper. Like a good historian, he was making it all very simple; for, as Dr. Brick emphasised, patients with primary haemochromatosis do have portal hypertension, but that wouldn't make any sort of story!

The relation of iron deposits in the liver to the portal systemic collateral circulation is also very much in the news. Dr. Figueroa, who is here, with Dr. Grossman and Dr. Tuttle, described the first case. The patient, an alcoholic cirrhotic, had a portacaval shunt and received some blood transfusions, and three and a half years later developed iron deposits in the liver. In the table there are 10 cases recorded (Table 3), 2 of which are my own. I learnt this morning that Dr. Caroli and Dr. Léger of Paris had also seen a case, making 12 in all, which is really very few. All of us who are interested in the liver have been searching for these cases over the last four years and yet we can only muster 12. This just seems to be a rather rare complication of portacaval anastomosis. It does not occur only in alcoholics, but in all varieties of cirrhosis, including Wilson's disease and primary biliary cirrhosis. Not only may this complicate surgically made shunts, but also if a patient with cirrhosis develops a really large natural shunt, iron may be found in the liver. For instance, I have seen 2 cases: one with a very large umbilical vein, and one with a large spontaneous splenorenal, natural shunt; neither had had any transfusions (Table 4). Three to eight years after the first biopsy they had developed considerable amounts

Table 3. *Iron deposition in the liver after portacaval anastomosis*

Author	Sex and age	Type of cirrhosis	Shunt	Transfusion	Duration after shunt (years)
TUTTLE et al., 1959	M.50	Alcoholic	P.C.A.[1]	5.4 l.	3 1/2
HOFFBAUER, 1960	F.55	Primary biliary	P.C.A.	11×	1
SCHAEFER et al., 1961	M.37	Alcoholic	P.C.A.	0	3
	F.62	Post-necrotic	P.C.A.	1	3 1/2
	M.54	Alcoholic	Sp. R.[2]	0	3
	F.36	Post-necrotic	Sp. R.	++	6
TISDALE, 1961	F.27	Post-necrotic	Sp. R.	8.5 l.	9 1/2
	F.53	Post-necrotic	P.C.A.	10 l.	2
SHERLOCK, 1963	F.17	Wilson's	P.C.A.	12.5 l.	2 1/2
	F.61	Post-necrotic	P.C.A.	4 l.	4

[1] P.C.A. = portacaval.
[2] Sp. R. = splenorenal.

of iron in the liver. Now, is this unique, or is it part of the general picture of cirrhosis? I am inclined to think that it is probably part of the general picture of cirrhosis, and that it is not very

Table 4. *Iron deposition with a large "natural" portal systemic shunt*

Name	Sex and age	Shunt	Type of cirrhosis	Transfusion	Time (years)
J. B. . . .	M. 39	Umbilical	Post-necrotic	0	3
D. A. . . .	F. 37	Splenorenal	Post-necrotic	0	8

closely related to the portal-systemic shunt. Some results we have obtained recently using the double-labelling isotope absorption technique are summarised in Table 5. In our normal subjects oral iron absorption runs from some 5 to 15%. Here are 5 well-compensated cirrhotics, 4 of whom have considerably increased iron absorption.

Table 5. *Iron absorption in cirrhosis* (WILLIAMS et al., 1964)

Case	Hb. (g./100 ml.)	M.C.H.C.[1] (%)	Serum iron (μg./100 ml.)	Absorption (%)	Liver biopsy iron
D. D. . .	12.8	31	174	50	0
J. M.[2] . .	12.5	31	132	42	+++
M. M. . .	15.6	31	110	38	0
J. D.. . .	11.6	29	49	28	0
T. B.. . .	10.6	28	97	4	0

[1] M.C.H.C. = mean corpuscular haemoglobin concentration.
[2] Alcoholic.

Owing to the presence of anaemia interpretation of the results becomes very difficult. Note also that of these 4 who absorb a lot of iron the alcoholic is the only one who shows excessive iron in the liver biopsy. This again points to the importance of alcoholism in the development of liver iron in cirrhosis. Shown in Table 6 are some

Table 6. *Iron absorption in cirrhosis; large collateral circulation* (WILLIAMS et al., 1964)

Case	Shunt	Hb. (g./100 ml.)	M.C. H.C. (%)	Serum iron (μg./100 ml.)	Absorption (%)	Liver biopsy iron
M. B. . .	Failed P.C.A.	8.6	27	20	60	0
D. K. . .	Failed P.C.A.	7.0	29	65	57	0
B. L. . .	Failed P.C.A.	13.2	27	52	14	0
W. K. .	Umbilical	11.2	28	205	89	0
D. A. . .	Natural splenorenal	10.4	31	140	65	++
S. M. . .	Umbilical	13.2	30	89	11	0

patients with large collateral circulations of one sort or another, failed portacaval shunts, etc.; these also by and large seem to absorb a lot of iron; again some of them are quite obviously anaemic. I think our feeling at the moment is that the development of iron deposits in the liver of patients after a shunt may be an exaggeration of what normally occurs in the cirrhotic liver. The patient who is prevented from losing blood because he has a good collateral circulation, either surgical or natural, is able to deposit iron in the liver.

Fig. 3 could be made far more complicated. Its purpose is merely to emphasise that the interpretation of results for iron in the liver of patients with liver disease may involve many factors. Firstly, we have the genetic ones, and then the emphasis on alcoholism. The iron content of wine has been commented upon by Dr. MOORE. Dr. BOTHWELL has noted the high iron content of Kaffir beers. The alcoholic, by and large, is ingesting much iron. The alcoholic is also suffering from protein malnutrition with increased iron absorption. The protein malnutrition is related to pancreatitis, and this apparently increases iron absorption. The alcoholic also develops cirrhosis. So, when you consider the alcoholic, you immediately have four causes for siderosis: the iron content in the alcohol, the protein malnutrition causing pancreatitis, the protein malnutrition causing increased iron absorption, and the cirrhosis *per se* which may also increase iron absorption. Thus, once cirrhosis has developed in the alcoholic patient, it is associated – as in other forms of liver disease — with a diminished survival of red cells and a haemolytic element. In addition, splenic hyperfunction may be

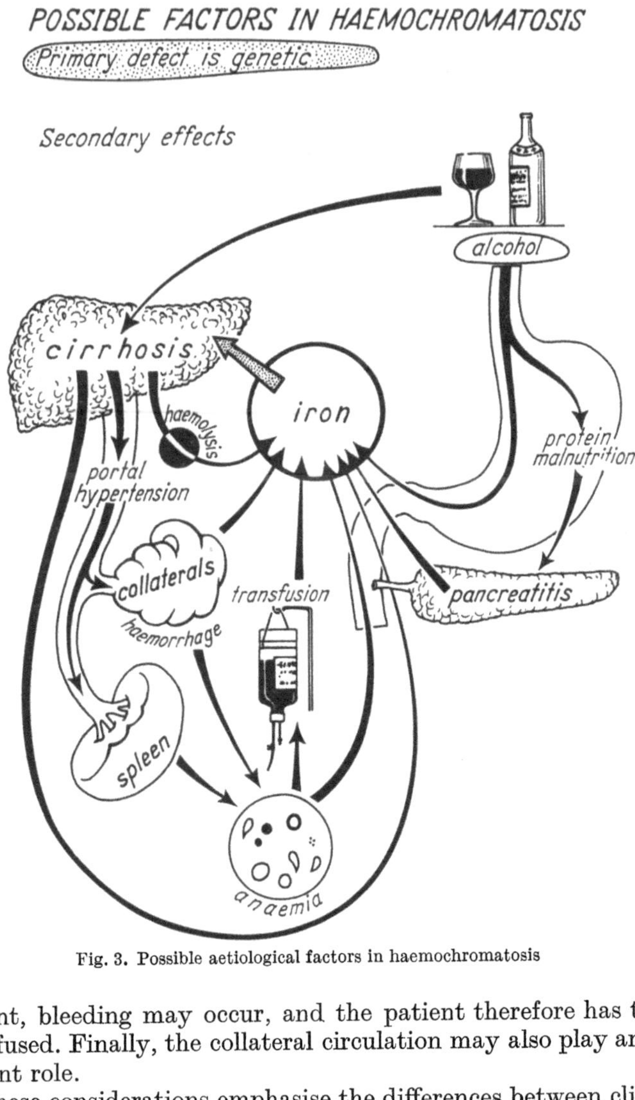

Fig. 3. Possible aetiological factors in haemochromatosis

present, bleeding may occur, and the patient therefore has to be transfused. Finally, the collateral circulation may also play an important role.

These considerations emphasise the differences between clinical observation and work with experimental animals. In the rat, conditions can be strictly controlled, whereas in the human situation things are more complex.

Acknowledgement

The original unpublished observations in this paper were made in collaboration with R. WILLIAMS, C. S. PITCHER, and H. S. WILLIAMS.

References

HOFFBAUER, F. W.: Amer. J. Digest. Dis. **5**, 348 (1960). — MACDONALD, R. A.: Amer. J. Path. **36**, 499 (1960). — MACDONALD, R. A.: Arch. Int. Med. (U.S.A.) **107**, 606 (1961). — MACDONALD, R. A., and G. K. MALLORY: Arch. Int. Med. (U.S.A.) **105**, 686 (1960). — SCHAEFER, J., Y. OIKAWA, and L. SCHIFF: Gastroenterology (U.S.A.) **40**, 692 (1961). — SCHEUER, P. J., R. WILLIAMS, and A. R. MUIR: J. Path. Bact. (G.B.) **84**, 53 (1962). — TISDALE, W. A.: N. England J. Med. **265**, 928 (1961). — TUTTLE, S. G., W. G. FIGUEROA, and M. I. GROSSMAN: Amer. J. Med. **26**, 655 (1959). — WILLIAMS, R., P. J. SCHEUER, and S. SHERLOCK: Quart. J. Med. (G.B.) **31**, 249 (1962). — WILLIAMS, R., H. S. WILLIAMS, C. S. PITCHER, and S. SHERLOCK: In preparation (1964).

General Discussion

Schapira: I should like to ask Dr. Sherlock a question. When, together with J.-C. Dreyfus, we studied the sons of patients with haemochromatosis, we investigated primarily the serum iron content and iron-binding capacity. We observed only 50% of abnormalities, but we knew exactly what the limits of confidence were, because only 5% of normal subjects are liable to display such abnormalities. Since we did not wish to inflict liver biopsy in all the cases, we carried out liver-biopsy studies only in those subjects who had shown an abnormal serum iron content or iron-binding capacity, and in every instance the biopsies yielded pathological findings. On the other hand, when you studied all your cases, although the serum iron was sometimes normal, you invariably found changes, i.e. abnormalities, in the liver-biopsy material. In all our cases we knew that only a 5% error could have occurred. What percentage of error can be expected in the case of your subjects?

Sherlock: I can't answer that question, because it depends on what you are going to accept as the normal amount of iron in a liver biopsy. We graded these liver biopsies according to the amount of iron. This was done by a very capable pathologist, working independently of the clinician, and we took as our standard of reference biopsies from a General Hospital population. We have also used autopsy material, which seems to have more iron. What is needed are biopsies from completely normal people. Even in a suicide there are changes in the liver tissues after death — changes which affect the fixing and the staining of the iron; and one also has to ask the question: why did the person commit suicide in the first place?

Schapira: I feel that this whole problem is a very important one, because the entire future of these people is at stake. If you are right, that is to say, if there are more than 50% abnormal, then you can be quite sure that these people do not need treatment. On the other hand, if less than 50% are abnormal, then perhaps you have to undertake some form of preventive treatment, e.g. repeated venesection. This is the important issue which I suggest we have to solve.

Sherlock: We have venesected those who, by our classification, had grade 2 iron or above. After all, little harm comes from venesection, and you may be saving the patient some further problem. But my personal feeling is that, if the subjects in question are not alcoholics and do not become alcoholics, then they will probably not develop the overt disease. This is a purely clinical impression, and I should be interested to hear what Dr. Brick thinks about this.

Brick: That's the point which I think is terribly important, because it rather looks as if we are coming into an era when we shall have very effective drugs at our disposal. I'm not convinced that we have enough evidence at the present time in the asymptomatic siblings to start them on therapy. I don't think any of us have any information actually obtained from following up over a long period some of these patients who have 2 or 3 + iron in their marrow and liver, but who display perfectly normal liver functions and no other abnormalities. We don't really know that they are going to develop haemochromatosis. I think Dr. BOTHWELL's information is important in this connection, because if we knew how long these asymptomatic Bantu remain siderotic but otherwise normal, then maybe there is no harm done if a little iron is present. In the families we have studied, the two patients that died did not die of haemochromatosis, but of a myocardial infarction in one case and pneumonia in the other. I think this is an important question and one that we ought to try and solve. I certainly don't know the answer, but I have the feeling we shouldn't be suggesting that all of the asymptomatic cases be treated. Are we really accomplishing anything in this way? This is a question I can't answer, and I wonder if there is someone here who can.

POLLYCOVE: With regard to the problem of how to pick the individuals who probably will develop haemochromatosis, we have now studied three families with endogenous haemochromatosis, in which two or more generations have been involved. Dr. SHERLOCK previously said that not a single well-documented instance of florid haemochromatosis in two generations of a single family had been reported. It is obviously very difficult for one investigator to follow this disorder through two generations because of the long time required for the florid complications of endogenous haemochromatosis to develop. The oldest generations of the three families we studied all had individuals with the full-blown clinical picture of endogenous haemochromatosis, sometimes with strikingly advanced involvement of two or three siblings. In one family, three brothers were involved, two dying of the disorder, while the third was severely ill with diabetes mellitus and advanced cirrhosis. The 21-year-old son of one of the dead brothers showed a normal plasma iron concentration of 140 μg./100 ml. and a marked increase in iron absorption measured with a whole-body counter, while iron-kinetic studies in this case revealed an abnormally increased exchange of iron between plasma and storage. Liver biopsy disclosed a marked increase in haemosiderin but no fibrosis. In this young man it seemed very reasonable to go ahead with venesection, and he was started on an intensive programme of prophylactic venesection therapy. We have studied two other families in which 7 children have demonstrated a markedly abnormal increase in iron absorption with normal plasma iron concentrations. In these three families we have observed the manifestation of endogenous haemochromatosis as a metabolic abnormality in at least two or three generations.

We have also encountered two cases of haemochromatosis associated with portacaval shunt; in one of them, a liver biopsy, performed during the shunt operation, showed that the haemosiderin in the liver was only slightly increased. Four years later, when the patient died, a massive deposition of iron was found in the liver. Thus, in this relatively short time, a remarkable increase in iron deposition had occurred. It seems unlikely that iron absorption did not increase following the shunt and that a decrease in the loss of iron due to cessation of bleeding could have resulted in such massive retention of iron.

BEARN: I don't think we should be too surprised if the disease is occasionally seen in two generations, even if it is inherited in an autosomal recessive fashion — although three generations is a bit much. The gene for haemochromatosis is not very rare, since everybody here has seen such cases, and every now and then an affected individual will marry a carrier. This will happen more frequently if marriage occurs between cousins. From such a marriage 50%

of the offspring will be affected and 50% will be carriers. This is in contrast to the more usual marriage between heterozygotes, in which case there will be three categories of offspring: affected children, carriers, and normal subjects. If one could measure the appropriate parameter, and unfortunately we don't know what this is, one would get a trimodal distribution curve, and one could perhaps work out a useful discriminant.

VENTURA: Among the different forms of sideroachrestic anaemia there are first the primary ones which Dr. VERLOOP has discussed in detail and in which — as Dr. HEILMEYER has also shown — a primary derangement of porphyrin metabolism occurs in the erythroblasts which inhibits iron utilisation for haemoglobin synthesis. There are also the secondary forms in which a particular position is occupied by the anaemia that almost unvariably develops in patients affected by a primary alteration of porphyrin metabolism in the erythroblasts (so-called "erythropoietic porphyria"). In this disease, the bone marrow is strongly fluorescent in Wood's light and the fluorescence is electively localised in the nuclei of the erythroblasts. Such a radical alteration in the porphyrin metabolism of the erythroblasts gives rise to typical achrestic anaemia. The *light microscope*[1,2] reveals alterations in the nuclei of the erythroblasts (irregular segmentation) and in their cytoplasm (numerous basophilic granules and iron granules with a perinuclear distribution). The *electron microscope*, as the research I have done in collaboration with Dr. ORLANDI and Dr. CARUSO has recently shown, affords a better understanding of these alterations. The nuclear profile (Fig. 1) is very irregular and sinuous and the nucleoplasm homogeneous. The cytoplasm shows an elective accumulation of iron between the cristae of the mitochondria. The mitochondria undergo pronounced modifications which are not usually seen in primary sideroachrestic anaemia[3]: the cristae and the iron accumulations disappear, giving rise to vacuoles of varying shape and volume which may be occupied by a granular substance or may appear amorphous. Such alterations in the erythroblasts occurring in achrestic anaemia secondary to erythroblastic porphyria may shed further light on the morphological and biochemical alterations associated with primary achrestic anaemia.

FIGUEROA: I would agree with Dr. SHERLOCK that the occurrence of excessive iron storage in patients following portacaval shunt is very rare. I have only seen two other cases, and I know that Dr. FINCH has observed one further case. TUTTLE[4] placed a notice in the journal Gastroenterology in an attempt to locate additional cases, but he was able to obtain only 2 or 3 more. In an article by TISDALE[5] eight further cases are documented.

With reference to the mechanism, we still do not know exactly what happens. We have also wondered about the role that bleeding and subsequent correction by the shunt may play. Another question is whether the shunt may aggravate nutritional problems.

In connection with the study of iron absorption in cirrhotics, especially when they are slightly anaemic, I think that, like Dr. SHERLOCK, one has to be very cautious in interpreting these results. The cirrhotics are notoriously

[1] VENTURA, S., P. CARUSO, and G. ARESU: Haematologica (It.) **44**, 993 (1959).
[2] LARIZZA, P.: Panminerva med. (It.) **4**, 315 (1962).
[3] LARIZZA, P.: Haematologica (It.) **47** (suppl.) 249 (1962).
[4] TUTTLE, S. G.: Gastroenterology (U.S.A.) **39**, 123 (1960).
[5] TISDALE, W. A.: N. England J. Med. **265**, 928 (1961).

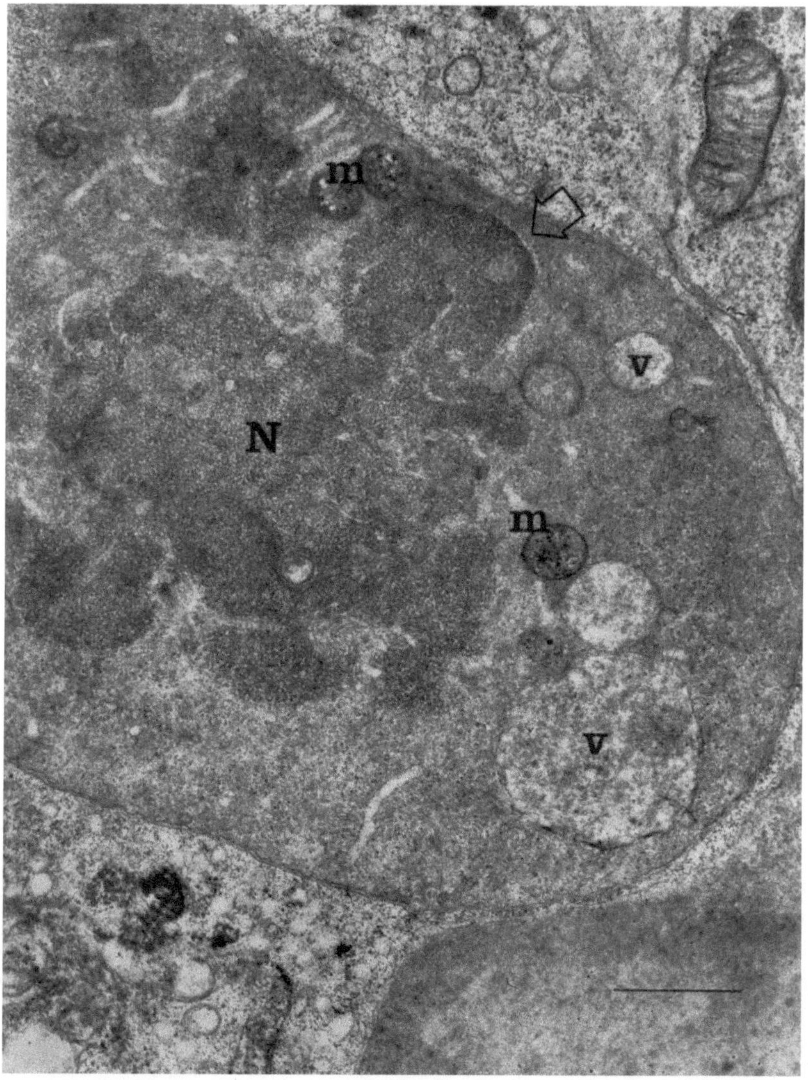

Fig. 1. Erythroblast from a case of erythropoietic porphyria. The nucleus (N) is irregularly segmented. The nuclear membrane is evident only along a limited portion of the nuclear profile (arrow). Iron aggregates are present in the mitochondria (m). Light vacuoles (v), containing an amorphous substance, are also visible in the cytoplasm. Electron micrograph: 15,000 ×

prone to suffer from gastro-intestinal bleeding and to develop iron deficiency; when one studies them, one therefore has to make sure that they are not iron deficient. I wonder if Dr. SHERLOCK has any findings indicating that iron doesn't go to the red cells. I believe that, if Fe^{59} goes to the red cells, it may be just iron-deficiency anaemia. For instance, one can demonstrate that Fe^{59} is going to the liver by means of external body counting; and by doing a whole-body count one can show that the iron is in the liver or is going to other parts of the body.

I should also like to ask Dr. BOTHWELL about the collapse of the vertebrae in Bantu haemosiderosis, as this is difficult to manage, especially in patients of the ages he has mentioned, i.e. between 40 and 60 years. I was wondering whether he had done any studies using large amounts of calcium by mouth with two aims in mind; one possibly to prevent the absorption of iron, and the other to see if calcium can be used clinically to prevent collapse of further vertebrae.

HEILMEYER: Might I just say a word about the case Dr. VENTURA has described? This is quite an exceptional case such as has never been observed before. In congenital erythropoietic porphyria (GÜNTHER), one normally finds no sideroachrestic disorder; the sideroblasts in the bone marrow show no increase, nor do they display any pathological changes (no ringed forms). I think that in Dr. VENTURA's case there must be a combination of several genic defects affecting haemoglobin synthesis. We should be pleased to try and help to clarify this case, and perhaps Dr. VENTURA would care to send us a blood sample.

VENTURA: Regarding this suggestion of Dr. HEILMEYER, I think we should bear in mind that the iron granules of the sideroblasts in the cases I have referred to (two brothers) were smaller and less numerous than those we have usually seen in the sideroblasts of patients with primary sidero-achrestic anaemia.

HALLBERG: I should like to ask Dr. DREYFUS to clarify his statement that there was no increase in iron excretion with desferrioxamine in the siblings of haemochromatotics. We have found, for instance, that when we give a certain amount of desferrioxamine per kg. body-weight intravenously, there is a fairly narrow normal range of iron excretion in men and women. Have you also made such a study? What do you consider as normal, and how do you perform the test?

J.-C. DREYFUS: We have not so far made an extensive study of the normal range. We have accepted as normal a value of 1 to 2 mg. in the urine after desferrioxamine. In any case, in healthy subjects we have never seen an excretion of more than 2 mg. — in contrast to the very high values obtained in confirmed haemochromatosis. But I must point out that most studies by others were made on siblings of patients with haemochromatosis, whereas we — except for one sibling — have confined ourselves to the children of such patients, who were generally younger (16 to 43 years) and always symptomless.

BRICK: In my paper (p. 572) I refer to the effect of D.T.P.A. in some asymptomatic siblings with a minor output of iron in the urine.

POLLYCOVE: Perhaps I can offer a comment to clarify the seeming paradox of venesection therapy in anaemia. I think that the removal of injurious excessive deposits of iron from anaemic individuals becomes paradoxical only if the anaemia is the result of decreased erythropoiesis. If the anaemia is due to a partially compensated haemolytic process, so that erythropoiesis is increased manyfold, then venesection therapy is no longer paradoxical. Since the additional removal of red cells from the circulation by weekly venesection constitutes here only a small fraction of the total number produced and destroyed each week, the resultant decrease in the equilibrium level of red-cell parameters in the blood will be rather small. If it is desirable to remove large amounts of iron, this still seems the best way to do it. However, if erythropoiesis is not significantly increased, then of course venesection therapy is not practicable, as Dr. HEILMEYER has mentioned.

Therapeutics

Oral treatment of iron deficiency

By

E. Undritz

Iron is essential for life, and from birth onwards it is absorbed from the digestive tract. In iron-deficiency states, the most natural form of administration – i.e. by the oral route – is generally employed, since treatment consists essentially in the natural substitution of a vital component of nutrition.

For oral treatment, bivalent organic compounds, which retain their valency for a determinable time (e.g. ferrous gluconate), are preferable to trivalent ones, which are far less effective, or to inorganic compounds, which are much more toxic (e.g. ferrous sulphate). I should like here to discuss a number of findings, resulting from experimental and clinical oral iron therapy, which confirm and complement the observations reported by other authors.

The results I wish to report are based both on clinical studies as well as on more than 20 years of experimental work in this field. Practically all the animal experiments, most of which were undertaken on rats, were performed twice, and some were repeated several times. All the results are reproducible.

First, I should like to touch on the constantly recurring question as to whether the results of animal experiments are applicable to man. My answer – at least as regards iron and copper metabolism, which are inseparably linked with each other in relation to haemoglobin formation – is that such results undoubtedly are applicable to man. We are dealing here with a primitive, fundamental mechanism, common to both the human and the animal organism. Hence, provided of course that species differences are known and taken into consideration, the evidence obtained from animal experiments may well be relevant to the situation in man (*67–71*).

In this connection, I would remind you, for instance, how widely diffused throughout the animal kingdom are the iron-containing respiratory pigments (chromoproteins), which include the haemoglobins and which are encountered not only in all vertebrates, but even in certain worms; similarly, studies in natural history have shown that haemoglobin and red-cell production can be traced back an enormous distance in time – nearly 400 million years, for example, in the case of the coelacanth (*67–71*).

The purely passive action of iron

Our experiments were carried out on rats kept on an iron-deficient diet (pure cow's milk or a combination of cow's milk and

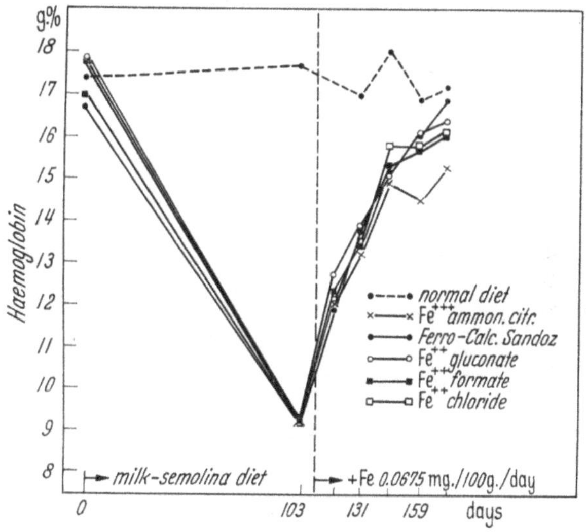

Fig. 1a. Experimental anaemia in rats. Therapeutic experiment. Haemoglobin values in response to a milk-and-semolina diet and to oral treatment with various iron preparations

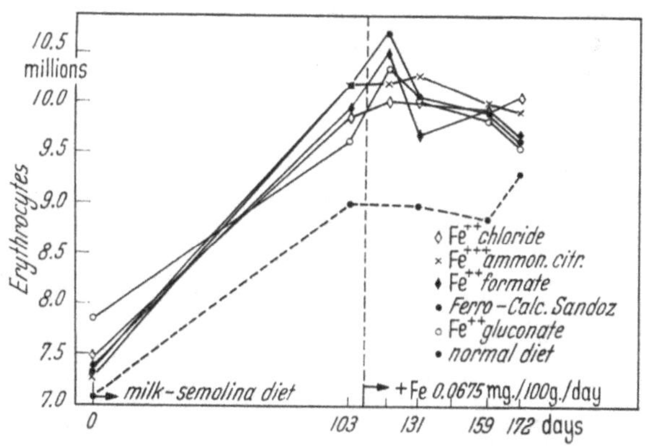

Fig. 1b. The erythrocyte values of these relatively young animals are low at the beginning, rising afterwards. During the period on a preparatory diet, they rise more markedly than in the animals on a normal diet. This typical pattern, which has been confirmed in all experiments, proves that the milk-and-semolina diet causes an absolute erythrocytosis, which is brought back to normal by means of iron therapy

semolina) and took two forms: a) *therapeutic* (Figs 1 a–c and 2, treatment not initiated until anaemia had developed); b) *prophylactic* (Figs

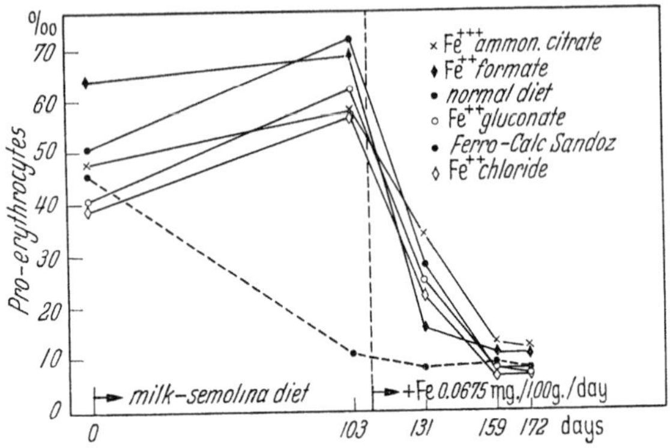

Fig. 1c. The pro-erythrocyte values are high at the beginning, as is to be expected in such young animals. In controls on a normal diet they soon fall, but remain high in the animals on the milk-and-semolina diet. This pro-erythrocytosis is subsequently responsible for the erythrocytosis shown in Fig. 1b. On initiation of iron therapy the pro-erythrocyte values rapidly drop to normal. Compensatory production of erythrocytes is no longer necessary, as the newly formed erythrocytes possess a full complement of haemoglobin

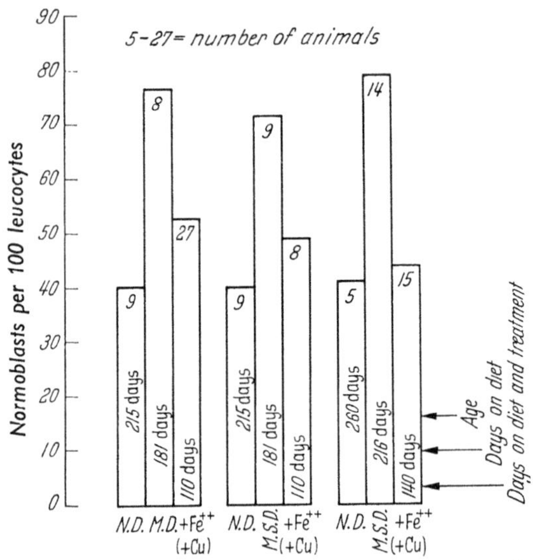

Fig. 2. Experimental anaemia in rats. Bone-marrow normoblasts. Therapeutic experiments. Normoblasts (mean values) per 100 white cells. Findings in animals sacrificed at the ages of 215 and 260 days. Response of the normoblasts to a normal diet (N.D.), to a milk diet (M.D.), and to a milk-and-semolina diet (M.S.D.) with and without oral administration of iron (Fe^{++}) and copper (Cu). In the untreated animals the values are high, whereas treated animals show the normal, comparatively low, values

3a—c and 4, treatment commenced at the same time as the rats were placed on an iron-deficient diet). These experiments confirmed the following. It is not iron that stimulates erythropoiesis, but *lack*

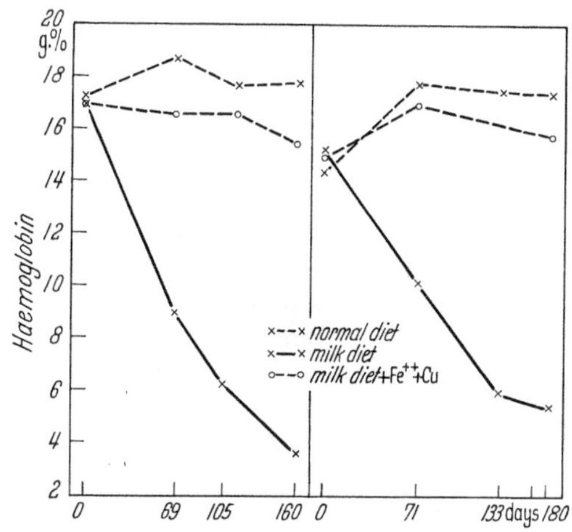

Fig. 3a. Experimental anaemia in rats. Two prophylactic experiments. Haemoglobin values in animals on a pure milk diet, with and without Fe++ and Cu, and on a normal diet

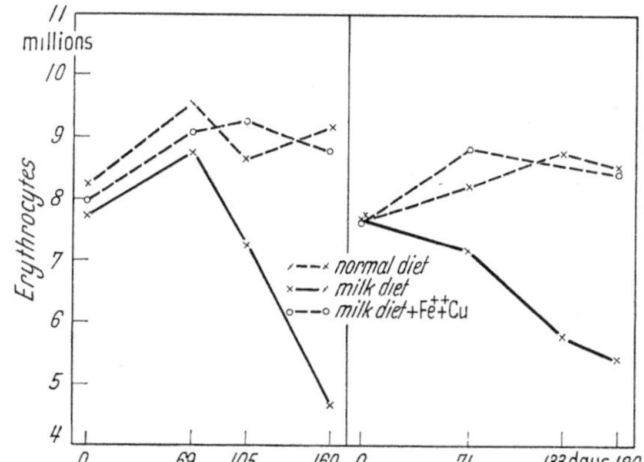

Fig. 3b. Erythrocyte values in rats on a pure milk diet, with and without Fe++ and Cu, and on a normal diet

of iron (*48*, *63*), which — while the haemoglobin level is falling (Figs 1a and 3a) — leads to relative or absolute erythrocytosis (Figs 1b and 3b) and pro-erythrocytosis (so-called reticulocytosis) (Figs 1c and 3c) in the blood and to an increase in the number of

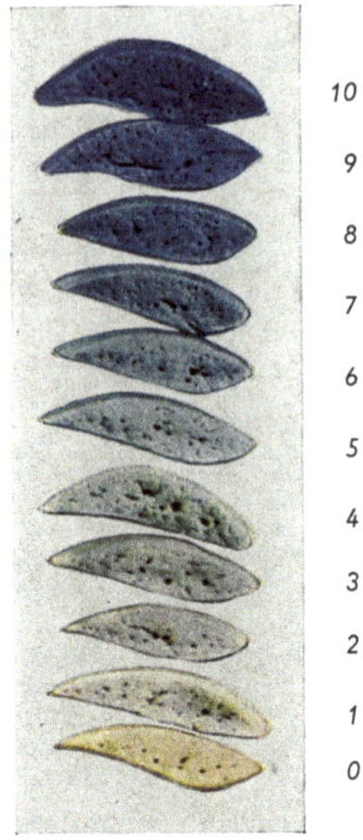

Fig. 5. Colour scale for determining the amount of iron by means of the macroscopic Prussian blue reaction. The liver sections, given here in their original size, are from different animals and show various grades of colour intensity

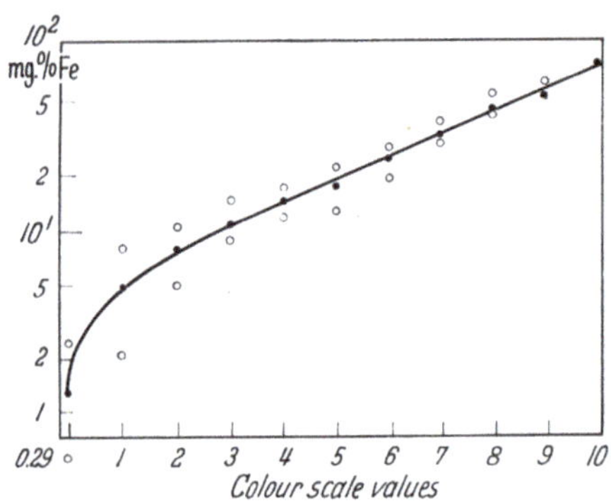

Fig. 6. The mean iron values for the specimens shown in Fig. 5 were determined by a chemical analytical method, using 5—10 livers from each group with the same colour intensity; they give a straight line when entered on a semilogarithmic scale. The colour grade 0 corresponds to a mean value of 1.28, and grade 10 to a mean value of 98.62 mg. % iron in the fresh tissue

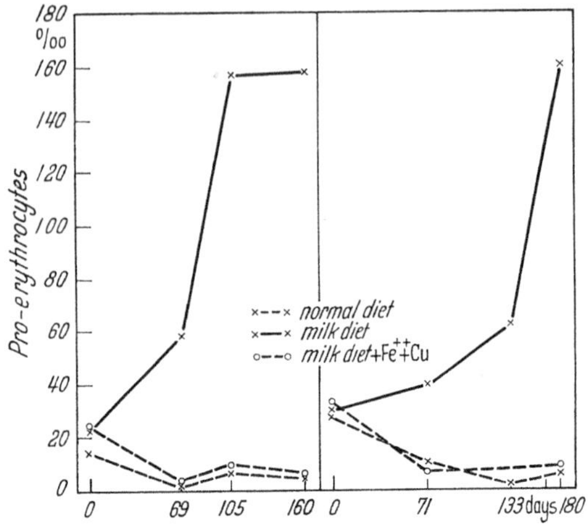

Fig. 3c. Pro-erythrocyte (reticulocyte) values in rats on a milk diet, with and without Fe^{++} and Cu, and on a normal diet

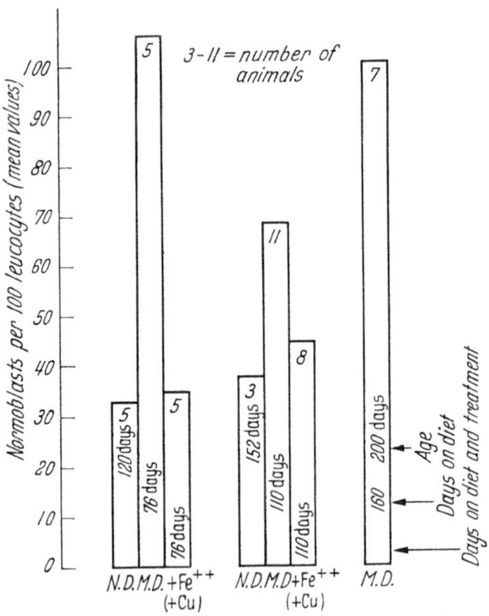

Fig. 4. Experimental anaemia in rats. Two prophylactic experiments. Bone-marrow normoblasts. Findings in animals sacrificed at the ages of 120, 152, and 200 days. Response of the normoblasts to a normal diet (N.D.) and to a milk diet (M.D.), with and without simultaneous oral administration of iron (Fe^{++}) and copper (Cu). In the untreated animals the values are high, whereas treated animals show the normal, comparatively low, values

normoblasts in the bone marrow (Figs 2 and 4). These changes are considerably greater on a pure milk diet (see prophylactic experiment, Figs 3 a – c and 4) than on a milk-semolina diet (see therapeutic experiment, Figs 1 a – c and 2). The haemoglobin falls to a lower level (compare Figs 1 a and 3 a) and the pro-erythrocyte count shows a greater increase (compare Figs 1 c and 3 c); the same applies to the bone-marrow normoblasts (compare Figs 2 and 4). Owing to the profound drop in the haemoglobin level, the ensuing erythrocytosis is relative, rather than absolute (compare Figs 1 b and 3 b). When iron is administered in therapeutic experiments, these changes are reversed in direct proportion to the rise in the haemoglobin level. In the prophylactic experiment, the findings for the treated rats remain normal, while the untreated controls show the expected changes indicative of severe anaemia.

Convincing visual evidence of the stimulant effect of iron deficiency on erythropoiesis is afforded by the histological findings in rat spleen. The spleen of the normal rat displays some – but only slight – erythropoietic activity; in the pulp there are small scanty myelogenic foci containing normoblasts. On the other hand, if the rats are rendered anaemic, the normoblast nests undergo intense proliferation, which subsides again when iron is administered in sufficient quantities.

The action of copper

It had previously been assumed that the rise in the haemoglobin level was stimulated by the iron administered. This, however, proved to be a misconception (*48*, *63*). The iron serves purely as a passive material; all the available evidence indicates that the copper acts as a catalyst in the formation of haemoglobin (*5* – *24*, *27*, *29*, *32* – *35*, *38* – *42*, *48*, *50*, *52*, *53*, *55*, *56*, *58*, *61*, *73*).

In evaluating the effect of copper on iron metabolism in animals we obtained useful results by *demonstrating the presence of iron* in the internal organs with the aid of the *macroscopic Prussian blue reaction* (*4*, *46*, *47*, *62*, *66*). The liver is the most suitable organ in which to demonstrate the presence of iron. The colour scale correlates well with the logarithm of the iron content of the liver as determined chemically (Figs 5 and 6).

If young rats are rendered anaemic by a pure milk diet, their haemoglobin falls to minimal levels (Fig. 7, left), but iron can still be demonstrated in their livers (Fig. 8). If such animals are then given iron only, their haemoglobin rises to 50 – 60% of normal but no higher, while at the same time iron accumulates in the depots, particularly in the liver. If copper alone is given, the

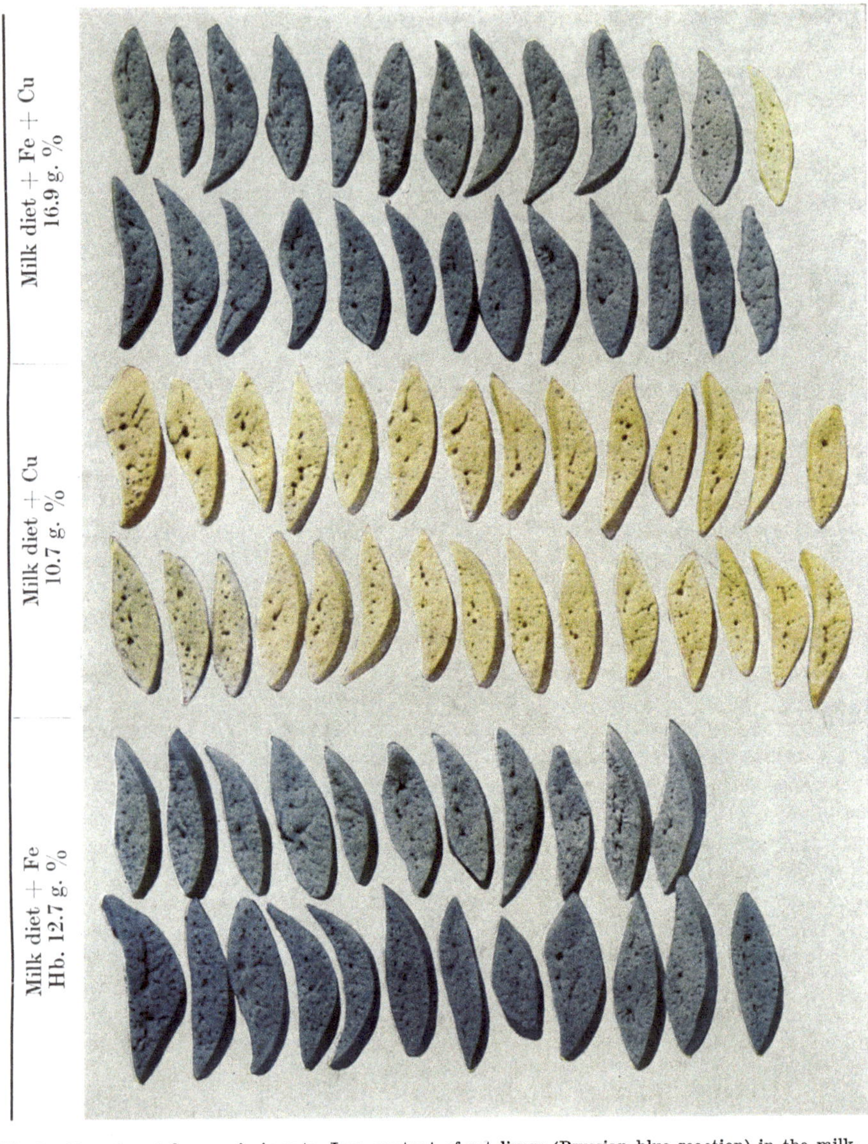

Fig. 8. Experimental anaemia in rats. Iron content of rat livers (Prussian blue reaction) in the milk-diet groups treated orally with iron or copper alone, or with iron and copper combined. *Left*: Milk diet plus iron only. The haemoglobin content (12.7 g. %) is considerably below normal (17—19 g. %), the liver containing a large quantity of iron. *Centre*: Milk diet plus copper only. The haemoglobin values are still considerably below normal. The livers contain no iron whatsoever in the majority of the animals; only three animals show the lowest grade of colour intensity (grade 1). The iron is utilised for haemoglobin synthesis. *Right*: Milk diet plus iron and copper. The haemoglobin values are almost normal and the iron content of the livers is also normal (with one exception)

haemoglobin rises to the same level as after iron alone, but the liver becomes depleted of iron. *Apparently copper mobilises the entire iron reserve for haemoglobin formation.* Only when both iron and copper are given together over a sufficiently long period do the haemoglobin values and the iron depots in the liver revert to

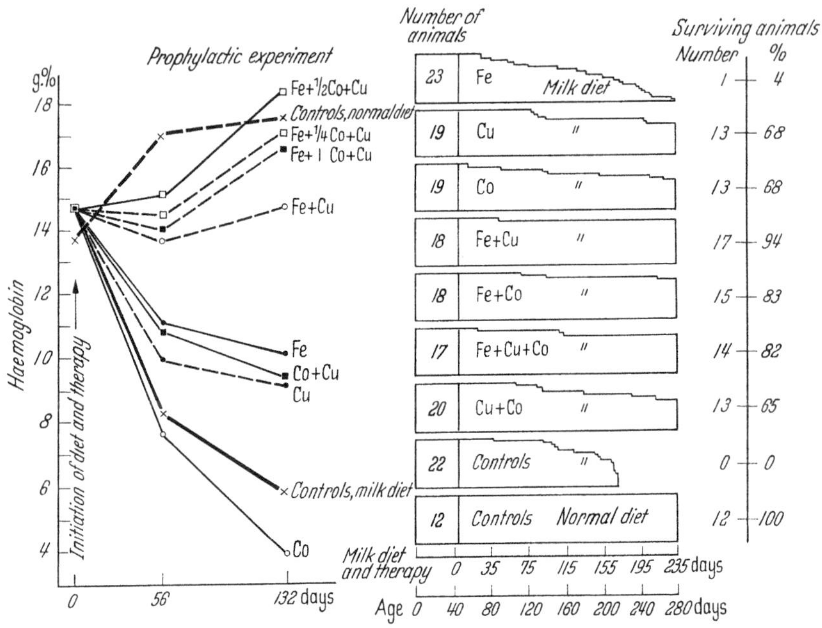

Fig. 7. Left: Haemoglobin curves of rats (♂) on a pure milk diet; oral treatment with 67.5 μg. Fe, 6.75 μg. Cu, and 25 or 50 or 100 μg. Co (= 1/4 or 1/2 or 1 Co)/100 g./day

Right: Mortality trend of rats (♀) on a pure milk diet. Dosage: 67.5 μg. Fe; 6.75 μg. Cu; 100 μg. Co/100 g./day. The Fe and Cu were given orally and the Co subcutaneously

With the milk-diet controls there is a marked fall in the haemoglobin level (left) and the animals all die within approx. 150 days (right). When iron or copper alone are administered the haemoglobin falls to nearly half the normal value; the animals treated with iron alone die, though more slowly than the untreated controls; with copper alone the haemoglobin values fall as low as in the untreated animals, but these animals survive (right). Cobalt alone has no effect on haemoglobin, but the animals do not die, cf. copper-treated group. Iron and copper combined produce a satisfactory effect; the optimal effect, however, is achieved by the addition of cobalt, the smallest dose of which (25 μg. Co) will suffice. The few deaths occurring in the groups with Cu, Co, Fe + Cu, Fe + Co, Fe + Cu + Co, and Cu + Co are incidental, being due chiefly to complications arising from prolonged tube-feeding

normal. The remarkable fact is that rats given iron alone all eventually die, just like the untreated animals on a milk diet, although they take a little longer to succumb than the latter (Fig. 7, right). The rats treated with copper alone survive, despite total depletion of their iron reserves. This shows that *depot iron has no "protective" action, whereas copper has an as yet unexplained "vitalising" effect which, though not exerted by iron, is also displayed by cobalt (51, 52, 53, 64, 65, 67).*

The effect of copper is well demonstrated in the following experiments (Fig. 9). When a diet of milk and semolina (right) in administered, instead of pure milk (left), the fall in haemoglobin

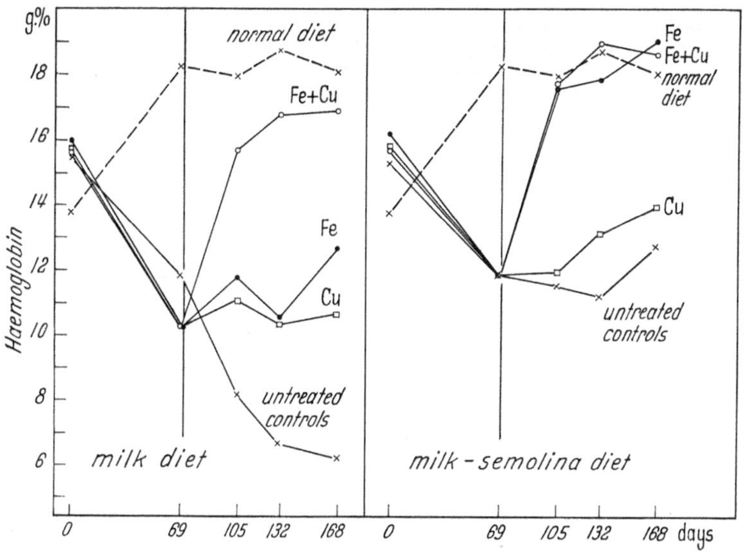

Fig. 9. Experimental anaemia in rats. Therapeutic experiment. Effect of iron and copper therapy on the haemoglobin of rats rendered anaemic by a milk diet (left) or a milk-and-semolina diet (right). Mean values for groups of up to 30 animals. Dosage: 67.5 μg. Fe and 6.75 μg. Cu/100 g. body-weight/day. Animals on a pure milk diet show a very marked fall in haemoglobin. When iron or copper is given alone, the effect is inadequate, but when the two are administered jointly the effect is almost optimal. In the animals on a milk-and-semolina diet, the haemoglobin level is just as high as in those treated with copper alone, since the copper content of the semolina is sufficient to produce a maximum effect. For the same reason, iron alone produces an optimum rise in haemoglobin, additional copper having no further effect

in untreated animals is not significantly greater than in animals on a pure milk diet receiving copper only. Both iron and iron plus copper raise the haemoglobin levels to the same extent. The haemoglobin in the milk-and-semolina rats treated with iron alone does not remain low in the way that it does in the pure-milk rats treated with iron alone. What is more, the milk-and-semolina animals treated with iron alone survive just as well as if they had been treated with iron plus copper. The explanation for this is the fact that semolina always contains copper. Incidentally, cereals such

Diet:	Normal	Milk diet	Milk-and-semolina diet	
Condition:	Normal	Manifest anaemia	Masked iron deficiency	Optimal iron therapy
Hb. g. % (mean values):	18.3	5.1	17.5	17.8

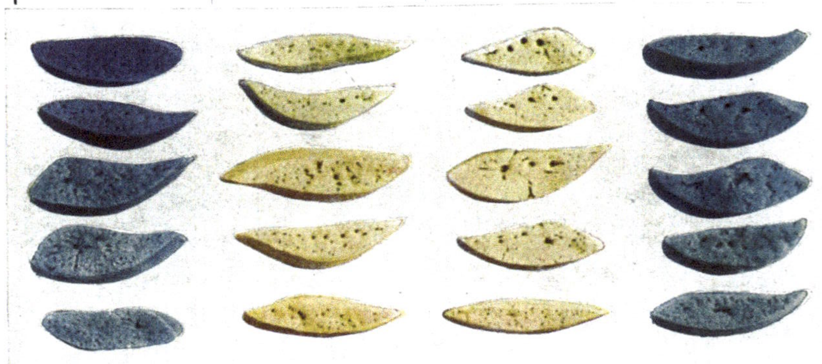

Fig. 10. Masked iron deficiency. Comparison of the haemoglobin values and iron content of rat livers (Prussian blue reaction). Left to right: *1st column*: Normal diet. Normal haemoglobin values and liver iron content. *2nd column*: Milk diet without treatment. Low haemoglobin level and almost complete absence of iron in the liver. *3rd column*: Milk-and-semolina diet with inadequate iron treatment. Normal haemoglobin values but absence of iron in the liver, i.e. "masked iron deficiency" or "iron deficiency with normal haemoglobin values". *4th column*: Milk-and-semolina diet with adequate iron treatment. Both haemoglobin and liver iron content are normal.

Springer Verlag, Berlin - Gottingen - Heidelberg

as wholemeal, oats, etc. are known to be remarkably rich in this metal.

Copper deficiency, as reflected in subnormal serum copper levels, is rare in humans (*59*) and is most likely to be encountered in children fed for long periods on an exclusively milk diet.

The action of cobalt, already mentioned above, calls for a brief explanation in this connection. This element has a "vitalising" effect similar to that of copper, inasmuch as the animals survive (Fig. 7, right) although the severe anaemia is not alleviated (Fig. 7, left). Cobalt exercises its erythropoietic effect only provided adequate iron is available. When iron and copper are employed together for the treatment of anaemia, their therapeutic effect can be slightly enhanced by adding cobalt as well. Unlike iron and copper, however, cobalt is not one of the normally essential heavy metals. The action of cobalt ions is, in fact, a pharmacological, rather than a physiological one – apart, of course, from the physiological action exerted by the cobalt-containing vitamin B_{12}.

The main indications for cobalt therapy are certain anaemias which fail to respond to treatment with iron and vitamin B_{12} owing to an impairment of iron utilisation. Such forms of anaemia are due to infection, including especially tuberculosis, and to renal diseases, malignant neoplasms, and leukaemia. Like iron, cobalt is most conveniently administered by the oral route. Similarly, it is preferable to administer it in the form of organic salts, e.g. cobalt glutamate; the latter is much less toxic and better tolerated than, say, cobalt chloride, which is at present in wide use. A daily dose of 15–30 mg. cobalt generally suffices to restore the formation of haemoglobin to normal.

Women of child-bearing age, as well as children, usually suffer from an iron deficit; thus, when treating the above types of anaemia in these categories of patient, it is necessary to administer iron along with cobalt, since cobalt itself is ineffective in the absence of iron (*50–53*, including the comments of SIMUNIĆ, *64*, *65*, *67*).

Masked iron deficiency

This is a condition in which the haemoglobin level is normal, in spite of the fact that the iron stores are depleted. All the signs and symptoms of frank anaemia may be observed, except for haemoglobin deficiency. This clinical state was first recognised by BECQUEREL and RODIER in 1844 (*1*) and was also described in 1909 by SAHLI (*54*), who referred to it as "masked chlorosis"; subsequently, however, it appears to have been forgotten. During the years

1938 to 1940, WALDENSTRÖM (*74*, *75*), HALLÉN (*26*), and WALDENSTRÖM and KJELLBERG (*76*) reported various monosymptomatic manifestations of iron deficiency, i.e. signs of epithelial atrophy, e.g. koilonychia, atrophy of the tongue, Plummer-Vinson syndrome, etc., associated with normal haemoglobin values. After ROTHLIN and UNDRITZ (*47*) had demonstrated that the syndrome of masked iron deficiency could be readily produced in animals (Fig. 10), JASINSKI (*31*), ROTH (*45*), and other authors resumed its clinical

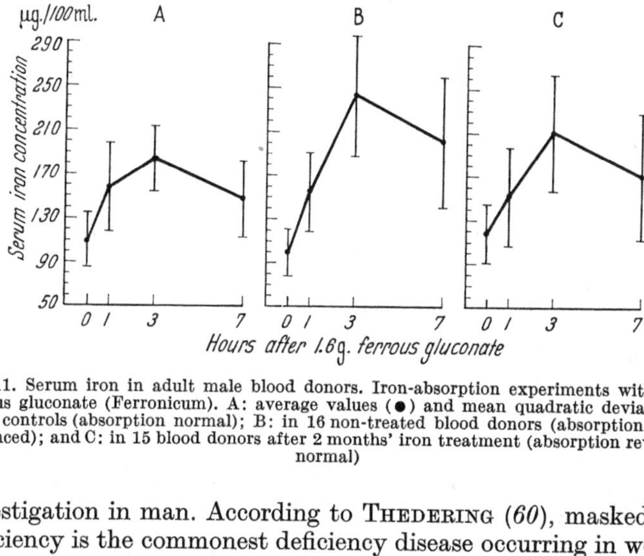

Fig. 11. Serum iron in adult male blood donors. Iron-absorption experiments with 1.6 g. ferrous gluconate (Ferronicum). A: average values (●) and mean quadratic deviation (I) in 11 controls (absorption normal); B: in 16 non-treated blood donors (absorption greatly enhanced); and C: in 15 blood donors after 2 months' iron treatment (absorption reverts to normal)

investigation in man. According to THEDERING (*60*), masked iron deficiency is the commonest deficiency disease occurring in women of child-bearing age in Central Europe.

BERDE, HOLLÄNDER, UNDRITZ, and ZEHNDER (*2*) plotted iron-absorption curves for healthy male *blood donors* (Fig. 11). Their findings confirmed those of other observers that iron deficiency may co-exist with normal haemoglobin values, and the fact that it may occur even in male blood donors is now generally recognised. These authors have found masked iron deficiency in men donating more than one litre of blood per year.

Cytochrome C, iron depots, and haemoglobin

Until recently it has been widely held that in iron deficiency it is the iron reserves which are drawn upon first and then the haemoglobin, and that even in very severe anaemia the important iron-containing enzymes, such as cytochrome C, remain intact.

This view is not borne out by my own finding that, in iron-saturated rats suffering from an isolated copper deficiency, the haemoglobin is low and the depots full of iron, as already mentioned above.

The theory of the inviolability of cytochrome was based on a single experiment in a single animal carried out by HAHN and WHIPPLE (*25*) in 1936. These workers found that the iron content of the perfused liver of an exsanguinated dog after ashing was the same as the enzymatic iron content calculated theoretically. But since 1 g. of completely exsanguinated liver contains in the form of enzymatic iron an amount equivalent to only 1/6,000th of the quantity of iron present in 1 ml. of blood, and since it is not in fact possible to remove all traces of blood from an organ, there are good grounds for supposing that the iron demonstrated in this dog's liver might after all have originated from haemoglobin. The problem was recently taken up again by BEUTLER (*3*), who carried out minute spectrophotometric studies of the cytochrome C and other enzymes contained in the liver and other organs of anaemic and non-anaemic animals. His work has clearly shown that, even in masked iron deficiency, i.e. in the presence of perfectly normal haemoglobin values, the cytochrome content is substantially lowered.

The haemoglobin iron does not interfere with the results obtained by the method used by BEUTLER.

The signs and symptoms of masked iron deficiency in man, a condition in which – as we have already seen – the haemoglobin is normal, are to some extent the same as those of manifest anaemia, in which the haemoglobin is deficient. Clearly, therefore, these signs and symptoms cannot be due to lack of haemoglobin. They consist of fatigue, weakness, headache, tinnitus, vertigo, dyspnoea, palpitation, dysphagia (probably due to oesophageal rhagades – cf. Plummer-Vinson syndrome), koilonychia, perlèche, and atrophy of the tongue. The serum iron is not necessarily lowered. BEUTLER's work and certain clinical observations suggest that these manifestations of anaemia, including especially the mucosal atrophy and diminished secretion in the digestive tract, may be due to depletion of tissue-iron enzymes, such as cytochrome C.

Anaemia in young animals and children

For the investigation of anaemia in small mammals, the rat was selected (*49*). When young rats are fed an iron-deficient diet of cow's milk and semolina, their haemoglobin falls by half, while their weight, as the result of growth, increases threefold. Only after a steady weight has been achieved do the haemoglobin levels slowly recover. In animals left with the mother, from whom they obtain nourishment of normal iron content, the haemoglobin remains normal (Fig. 12).

Anaemia in large mammals was investigated in the young elephant, the work being carried out in collaboration with LANG (*36*). Generally speaking, the elephant, a giant herbivore, is viable only in its natural biotope, since it is dependent upon the high iron

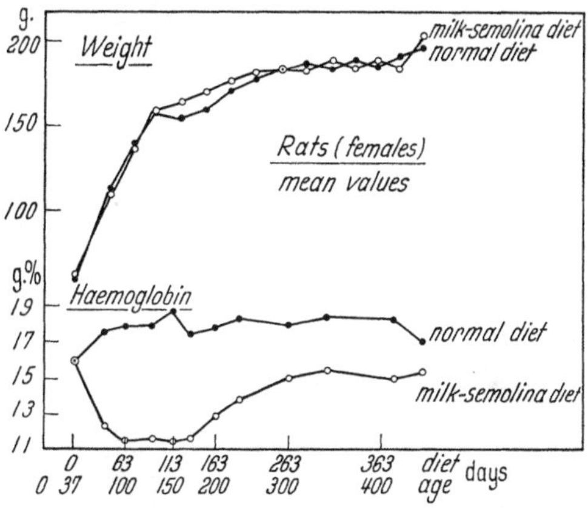

Fig. 12. Mean weight and haemoglobin curves in rats on a normal diet and on a diet of milk and semolina. In the rats on the milk-and-semolina diet, which corresponds to the milk-and-cereal diet which infants throughout the world customarily receive, the haemoglobin level is lowest just after the animals have tripled their weight, as the iron reserves are diminished by growth and the iron contained in the diet is not sufficient. On the other hand, the haemoglobin values remain normal in response to the normal mixed diet

content of red earth and red water. Even in Africa itself, 60% of the young perish if kept in captivity, death being apparently due to anaemia. If, however, elephants in captivity are given iron in the high dosage appropriate to their weight, the anaemia disappears and the animals survive (Fig. 13). This is another example of the relationship between the development of anaemia and the *combined effect of an iron-deficient diet and the "dilution" of body iron resulting from growth.*

Basically the *same situation is found in man.* That in human beings there is a relationship between haemoglobin values and age emerges clearly from the international statistics compiled by LEICHTENSTERN (*37*) in Germany in 1878 and from the excellent statistical study published by WILLIAMSON (*78*) in the U.S.A. in 1919. In more recent years, additional statistics have appeared in many other countries, e.g. Great Britain (*43*), U.S.A. (*44*), Finland

(*57*), Australia (*77*), Canada (*28*), etc. These studies, even the most recent of them, consistently show the same picture: high "supernormal" haemoglobin values in the newborn, a 50% fall during the first 6 months of life, persistence of low values until the 3rd year, and a slow recovery which is not complete until growth ceases at

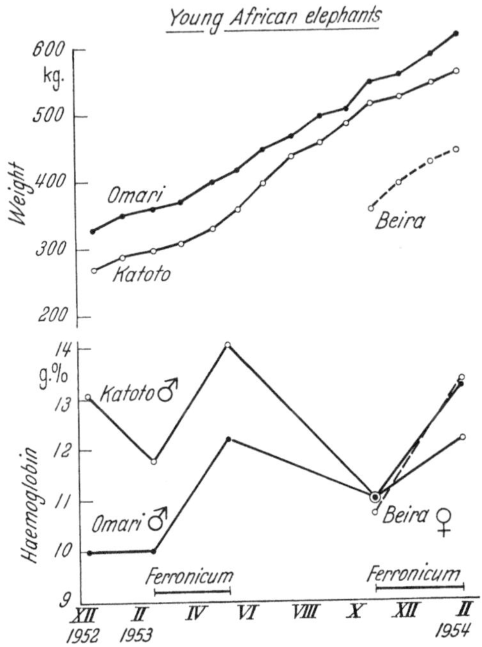

Fig. 13. Weight and haemoglobin curves of 3 young African elephants (2 males and 1 female). The haemoglobin falls when the animals receive no iron, and rises as soon as iron is given. During the period of observation the weight of the 2 males doubled and the female also showed a marked weight gain. Here, too, the reason for the anaemia is to be sought in the disproportion between the increase in weight and the iron content of the food

about the 20th year. *The milk and cereal diet customarily given to infants and young children all over the world contains too little iron* (as in the case of our diet-fed rats and of elephants in captivity) to prevent a "dilution" of body iron by growth and a resultant fall in haemoglobin. The fall in haemoglobin coincides with the period of most intensive growth, since a normal infant trebles its body-weight in the first year of life. The weight of a premature infant may even increase sevenfold during this period – in which case the anaemia will be even more severe.

Together with Heimendinger (*30*) we have shown that this fall in haemoglobin is by no means the normal and physiological phenomenon that it has hitherto been assumed to be; 3 months' oral administration of iron will bring the haemoglobin value in all children, including infants, up to the same level as in adult women (Fig. 14). The incidence of infections and colds decreases significantly as the iron balance improves; nocturnal enuresis also ceases; at the same time the children become livelier and more active.

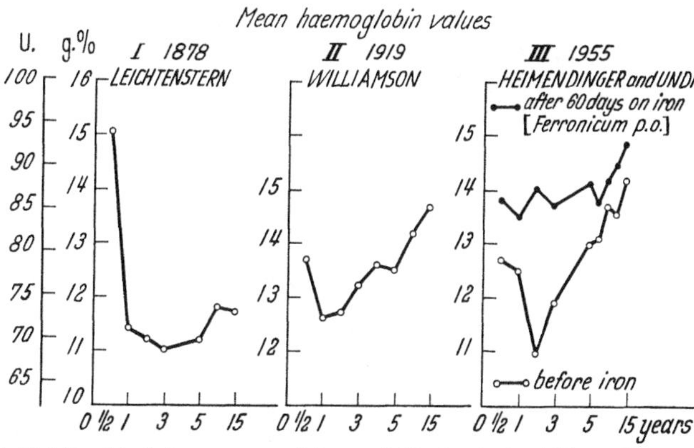

Fig. 14. Relationship between age and haemoglobin levels in children. The curves from LEICHTENSTERN and WILLIAMSON give the mean haemoglobin values in boys and girls not receiving iron treatment. The curves in III show the mean values found by us in 107 children who received iron for approx. 2 months. The values are expressed in units (SAHLI) and in g. %. The curve obtained before treatment has exactly the same pattern as the curves on the left. After iron treatment, the haemoglobin values show a rise in all age groups, corresponding to the normal adult female values. These curves demonstrate that the lower haemoglobin values throughout the entire period of childhood are due to iron deficiency, and that iron therapy is necessary if a diet more rich in iron does not have the desired effect. Iron is indicated in all cases of marked haemoglobin deficiency

Sex variations

VAHLQUIST (*72*) and others have shown that the haemoglobin level is normally higher in men than in women, even in healthy women in a state of iron saturation. No such sex difference has been observed in children. It is not until the onset of puberty that the haemoglobin level in females begins to drop appreciably below that of males. The work I have done on animals (*66*) has confirmed the finding of other investigators that the difference between the sexes is due not to inhibition of haemoglobin formation by oestrogens in the female, but to its stimulation by androgens in the male. The haemoglobin values in women and children are unaffected by the sex-hormonal factors present; it is the large amount of testosterone in the adult male which is responsible for the higher haemoglobin level in men.

The Lepehne reaction

In conclusion, I should like to draw your attention to the Lepehne reaction, an excellent method of demonstrating the haemoglobin content of erythroblasts (*62*, *68*). In the earliest stages of development of the erythroblasts, the pro-erythroblasts – i.e. the promegaloblasts and pronormoblasts – have not yet acquired any haemoglobin. Hence, they do not give the brownish-yellow reaction indicative of haemoglobin. A positive reaction appears in the following stages, i.e. in the basophil erythroblasts (basophil megaloblasts and normoblasts), and increases progressively as the cells mature, so that the mature erythrocyte – in other words, the megalocyte or normocyte – has the highest haemoglobin content (Fig. 31 in *62*).

Summary

Since oral iron therapy corresponds more closely to the physiological intake of iron in the food, the oral route is to be preferred to parenteral administration whenever possible.

In an attempt to discover more about haemoglobin and erythrocyte formation and the processes of iron metabolism underlying them, investigations were undertaken on laboratory animals (rats and rabbits), on wild animals in captivity (elephants), and on human subjects. The findings obtained in mammals are also relevant to man, since the functions involved are basic to all vertebrates and are even extensively encountered among invertebrate animals. Secondary differences between one species and another must, however, be taken into consideration.

Like other authors, we were able to demonstrate that iron plays only a passive role in haemoglobin synthesis and that it does not stimulate erythropoiesis. Iron deficiency, on the other hand, has a very pronounced stimulant effect, as evidenced by absolute or relative erythrocytosis associated with an increase in the normoblasts in the bone marrow and pro-erythrocytosis (reticulocytosis). If iron is administered in iron-deficiency anaemias of this kind, these phenomena recede as the haemoglobin values revert to normal.

Copper is of supreme importance for erythropoiesis. It acts indirectly. Copper deficiency leads to states of anaemia which can readily be produced in animals but which very rarely occur in man, since cereals alone contain sufficient quantities of copper. Young rats fed on a pure diet of cow's milk eventually die. Administration of iron alone merely delays their death, whereas the administration of copper alone keeps them alive, despite the fact that the iron depots are exhausted and the haemoglobin values excessively low.

A "vitalising" action similar to that of copper is also exerted by cobalt, although the latter has a pharmacological rather than a physiological effect. The dose of cobalt required for this purpose is greater than that occurring naturally in food. Cobalt is capable of regulating erythropoiesis in anaemias that are resistant to treatment with iron and vitamin B_{12}, i.e. in infectious diseases, including especially tuberculosis, as well as in renal diseases, malignant tumours, etc. This pharmacological action of cobalt is not identical with that of vitamin B_{12}, which, though it contains cobalt, is effective only in the form of the complete molecule.

The clinical picture of masked iron deficiency presents all the signs and symptoms of anaemia except that the haemoglobin values are normal. The symptomatology is probably due to a deficiency of iron-containing enzymes, which, as demonstrated by BEUTLER, are the first to be affected in cases of iron deficiency. This condition constitutes the initial stage of all chronic manifest iron-deficiency anaemias, and recurs once more when the latter are responding successfully to treatment. Consequently, iron therapy should be continued beyond the point at which the haemoglobin values revert to normal.

Low haemoglobin values are normally encountered in infants and children in all countries, including those of Europe, and are due to iron deficiency. The diet which the child receives — consisting initially mainly of milk and cereals—is not sufficiently rich in iron to meet the iron requirement associated with the rapid growth of infancy. Oral iron administration restores the haemoglobin values to normal in infants and young children. The normal haemoglobin values in older children of both sexes correspond to those of non-anaemic women. They are lower than for men, in whom testosterone appears to be responsible for a higher haemoglobin level.

The Lepehne reaction offers a virtually specific means by which to follow up haemoglobin synthesis in the erythroblasts.

Zusammenfassung

Die perorale Eisentherapie entspricht der physiologischen Eisenaufnahme mit der Nahrung und ist daher, wenn immer möglich, einer parenteralen Applikation vorzuziehen.

Zur weiteren Abklärung der Haemoglobin- und Erythrozytenbildung und des ihr zugrunde liegenden Eisenstoffwechsels wurden Untersuchungen an verschiedenen Laboratoriumstieren (Ratte und Kaninchen), an Tieren in Gefangenschaft (Elefant) und beim Menschen durchgeführt. Die bei Säugetieren erhobenen Befunde lassen sich auf den Menschen übertragen, da es sich bei diesen Funktionen um Grundmechanismen handelt, die bei allen Wirbeltieren und auch bei Evertebraten vorkommen. Sekundäre Artunterschiede sind zu beachten.

Ebenso wie andere Autoren konnten wir nachweisen, daß dem Eisen bei der Haemoglobinbildung eine passive Rolle zukommt. Die Erythropoese wird durch Eisen nicht angeregt. Dagegen ruft Mangel an Eisen einen hochgradigen Reizzustand hervor: absolute oder relative Erythrozytose mit Vermehrung der Normoblasten im Knochenmark, Proerythrozytose (Retikulozytose). Wird Eisen bei derartigen Eisenmangelanaemien verabfolgt, so verschwindet der Reizzustand mit fortschreitender Normalisierung des Haemoglobins.

Kupfer ist für die Erythropoese absolut notwendig. Es wirkt indirekt. Bei Kupfermangel kommt es zu Anaemien, die beim Tier leicht hervorzurufen sind, beim Menschen aber nur sehr selten vorkommen, da schon in den Zerealien genügend Kupfer vorhanden ist. Wenn junge Ratten eine reine Kuhmilchnahrung erhalten, so gehen sie mit der Zeit zugrunde. Eisengabe allein verzögert lediglich den Tod, während die Tiere bei Gabe von Kupfer trotz erschöpfter Eisendepots und ungenügender Haemoglobinwerte am Leben bleiben.

Eine ähnliche „vitalisierende" Wirkung wie dem Kupfer kommt auch dem Kobalt zu, das nicht physiologisch, sondern pharmakodynamisch wirkt. Dafür sind Kobaltdosen erforderlich, die natürlicherweise nicht in der

Nahrung vorkommen. Kobalt normalisiert die Erythropoese bei Eisen- und Vitamin B_{12}-resistenten Anaemien: bei Infekten, insbesondere Tuberkulose, Nephropathien, malignen Tumoren u. a. Dieser pharmakodynamische Kobalteffekt ist nicht identisch mit der Wirkung von kobalthaltigem Vitamin B_{12}, das nur als ganzes Molekül wirksam ist.

Der larvierte Eisenmangel geht mit subjektiven und objektiven Anaemiesymptomen einher, jedoch sind die Haemoglobinwerte normal. Die Symptome beruhen wahrscheinlich auf dem Ausfall eisenhaltiger Fermente, die, wie Beutler nachweisen konnte, bei Eisenmangel zuerst in Mitleidenschaft gezogen werden. Dieser Zustand stellt das Vorstadium aller chronischen manifesten Eisenmangelanaemien dar, bei deren erfolgreicher Therapie er wieder auftritt. Die sich daraus ergebende Konsequenz ist, daß eine Eisenbehandlung länger als bis zur Normalisierung der Haemoglobinwerte durchzuführen ist.

Tiefe Haemoglobinwerte bei Säuglingen und Kindern finden sich üblicherweise in allen Ländern, auch in Europa, und sind durch Eisenmangel bedingt. Die eisenarme Nahrung — zunächst meistens nur Milch und Zerealien — genügt nicht, um den durch das starke Wachstum bedingten Eisenbedarf im Säuglingsalter zu decken. Perorale Gabe von Eisen normalisiert bei Säuglingen und Kleinkindern die Haemoglobinwerte. Knaben und Mädchen haben die gleichen normalen Haemoglobinwerte wie erwachsene Frauen ohne Eisenmangel. Diese Werte liegen tiefer als beim Mann, bei dem das Testosteron für die höheren Haemoglobinwerte verantwortlich ist.

Die Haemoglobinbildung in den Erythroblasten läßt sich gut mit der praktisch spezifischen Lepehnereaktion verfolgen.

Résumé

La thérapeutique martiale par voie buccale réalise les conditions de l'apport physiologique de fer par l'alimentation. On la préférera donc, chaque fois que cela sera possible, à la voie parentérale.

Nos recherches sur la synthèse de l'hémoglobine et la formation des érythrocytes, ainsi que sur le métabolisme du fer qui en constitue la base, comprennent des essais sur divers animaux de laboratoire (en particulier rats, lapins), sur des animaux en captivité (en particulier éléphants), et sur l'homme au cours de mesures thérapeutiques. Les résultats obtenus sur les mammifères sont applicables à l'homme, étant donné qu'il s'agit de processus constituant des mécanismes fondamentaux, communs à tous les vertébrés et à de nombreux invertébrés. Les différences secondaires caractéristiques des espèces sont à prendre en considération.

Confirmant les résultats d'autres auteurs, nous avons pu prouver que le fer joue un rôle passif dans la synthèse de l'hémoglobine. Il ne stimule point l'érythropoïèse. C'est au contraire la carence en fer qui produit la plus grande stimulation: érythrocytose absolue ou relative, proérythrocytose (réticulocytose), augmentation des normoblastes dans la moelle osseuse. Si l'on administre du fer dans un cas d'anémie ferriprive, cette stimulation disparaît à mesure que se normalise le taux d'hémoglobine.

Le cuivre est un métal indispensable à l'érythropoïèse. Il agit de manière indirecte. La carence en cuivre entraîne une anémie, facile à reproduire chez l'animal mais qui est rare chez l'homme, étant donné qu'une alimentation à base de céréales suffit déjà à couvrir les besoins en cuivre. De jeunes rats nourris exclusivement au lait de vache finissent par périr. Ils périssent également, mais plus tardivement, s'ils ne reçoivent que du fer. Par contre, ils restent en vie s'ils ne reçoivent que du cuivre, et ceci malgré l'épuisement des réserves de fer et l'insuffisance des taux d'hémoglobine.

L'ion cobalt exerce, lui aussi, un effet «vitalisant», mais il s'agit d'un effet pharmacodynamique et non physiologique, qui ne se produit qu'à des doses bien plus élevées que celles apportées par les aliments naturels. Le cobalt exerce des fonctions régulatrices de l'érythropoïèse dans des anémies résistant au fer et à la vitamine B_{12}: au cours d'infections, surtout tuberculose, de néphropathies, de tumeurs malignes, etc. Par ailleurs, l'effet pharmacodynamique du cobalt n'est pas identique à celui de la vitamine B_{12}, qui en contient mais n'est active qu'en tant que molécule entière.

La sidéropénie larvée comprend des symptômes subjectifs et objectifs d'anémie, bien que les taux d'hémoglobine soient normaux. Ces symptômes sont probablement dûs à l'absence de ferments ferreux qui, comme a pu le montrer BEUTLER, sont les premiers à souffrir de la carence en fer. La sidéropénie larvée constitue l'état préliminaire de toute anémie ferriprive manifeste chronique, et elle réapparaît au cours du traitement, si celui-ci est efficace. La conséquence pratique est la nécessité de poursuivre le traitement après que le taux d'hémoglobine soit revenu à la normale.

Dans tous les pays, y compris l'Europe, on constate couramment chez les nourrissons et les enfants des taux d'hémoglobine bas, qui ne sont pas physiologiques, mais bien l'expression d'une sidéropénie. L'alimentation pauvre en fer que constituent le lait et les céréales ne suffit pas à couvrir chez le nourrisson les besoins en fer, augmentés par la croissance. Un traitement martial *per os* permet de normaliser le taux d'hémoglobine chez le petit enfant et le nourrisson.

Les taux normaux d'hémoglobine chez la petite fille et le petit garçon sont les mêmes que ceux de la femme adulte ne présentant pas de sidéropénie. Ils sont par contre plus faibles que les taux normaux d'hémoglobine de l'homme, qui, par sa testostérone, atteint des valeurs plus élevées.

La synthèse de l'hémoglobine dans les érythroblastes est facile à étudier au moyen de la réaction de Lepehne qui peut être considérée comme spécifique.

References

1. BECQUEREL, A., and A. RODIER: Gaz. méd. Paris **12**, 751 (1844). — 2. BERDE, B., L. HOLLÄNDER, E. UNDRITZ, and K. ZEHNDER: Schweiz. med. Wschr. **85**, 936 (1955). — 3. BEUTLER, E.: Amer. J. Med. Sc. **234**, 517 (1957). — 4. BIDDER, H. v., and E. UNDRITZ: Helvet. physiol. pharmacol. acta **6**, 765 (1948). — 5. BRENNER, W.: Mschr. Kinderhk. (G.) **102**, 128 (1954). — 6. BRENNER, W.: Der Kupferstoffwechsel. Biologische Daten für den Kinderarzt. 2nd Ed., Vol. 1. Springer, Berlin, 1954, p. 322. — 7. CARTWRIGHT, G. E., C. J. GUBLER, and M. M. WINTROBE: J. Clin. Invest. (U.S.A.) **33**, 685 (1954). — 8. CARTWRIGHT, G. E., B. TATTING, D. KURTH, and M. M. WINTROBE: Blood (U.S.A.) **7**, 992 (1952). — 9. CHASE, M. S., C. J. GUBLER, G. E. CARTWRIGHT, and M. M. WINTROBE: J. Biol. Chem. (U.S.A.) **199**, 757 (1952). — 10. CHASE, M. S., C. J. GUBLER, G. E. CARTWRIGHT, and M. M. WINTROBE: Proc. Soc. Exper. Biol. Med. (U.S.A.) **80**, 749 (1952). — 11. DARBY, W.: J. Amer. Med. Ass. **142**, 1288 (1950). — 12. ELVEHJEM, C. A.: Physiol. Rev. (U.S.A.) **15**, 471 (1935). — 13. ELVEHJEM, C. A., and E. B. HART: J. Biol. Chem. (U.S.A.) **84**, 131 (1929). — 14. ELVEHJEM, C. A., and E. B. HART: J. Biol. Chem. (U.S.A.) **95**, 363 (1932). — 15. ELVEHJEM, C. A., and A. R. KEMMERER: J. Biol. Chem. (U.S.A.) **93**, 189 (1931). — 16. ELVEHJEM, C. A., and N. J. SHERMAN: J. Biol. Chem. (U.S.A.) **98**, 309 (1932).—

17. ELVEHJEM, C. A., A. SIEMERS, and D. R. MENDENHALL: Amer. J. Dis. Child. **50**, 28 (1935). — 18. ELVEHJEM, C. A., H. STEENBOCK, and E. B. HART: J. Biol. Chem. (U.S.A.) **83**, 21 (1929). — 19. FUKUSHIMA, K., N. SENDA, and T. VENOYAMA: Med. J. Osaka Univ. **2**, 157 (1951). — 20. GISINGER, E.: Wien. Zschr. inn. Med. **36**, 168 (1955). — 21. GUBLER, C. J.: J. Amer. Med. Ass. **161**, 530 (1956). — 22. GUBLER, C. J., M. E. LAHEY, M. S. CHASE, and G. E. CARTWRIGHT: Blood (U.S.A.) **7**, 1075 (1952). — 23. GUBLER, C. J., M. E. LAHEY, G. E. CARTWRIGHT, and M. M. WINTROBE: Amer. J. Physiol. **171**, 652 (1952). — 24. GUBLER, C. J., D. S. TAYLOR, E. J. EICHWALD, and G. E. CARTWRIGHT: Proc. Soc. Exper. Biol. Med. (U.S.A.) **86**, 223 (1954). — 25. HAHN, P. F., and G. H. WHIPPLE: Amer. J. Med. Sc. **191**, 24 (1936). — 26. HALLÉN, L.: Acta med. Scand., Suppl. **90**, 398 (1938). — 27. HART, E. B., H. STEENBOCK, J. WADDELL, and C. A. ELVEHJEM: J. Biol. Chem. (U.S.A.) **77**, 797 (1928). — 28. HAWKINS, W. W., E. SPECK, and V. G. LEONARD: Blood (U.S.A.) **9**, 999 (1954). — 29. HEILMEYER, L., W. KEIDERLING, and G. STÜWE: Kupfer und Eisen als körpereigene Wirkstoffe. Fischer, Jena, 1941. — 30. HEIMENDINGER, H., and E. UNDRITZ: Schweiz. med. Wschr. **85**, 919 (1955). — 31. JASINSKI, B.: Schweiz. med. Wschr. **79**, 1255 (1949). — 32. LAHEY, M. E., C. J. GUBLER, M. S. CHASE, G. E. CARTWRIGHT, and M. M. WINTROBE: Amer. J. Physiol. **167**, 804 (1951). — 33. LAHEY, M. E., C. J. GUBLER, M. S. CHASE, G. E. CARTWRIGHT, and M. M. WINTROBE: Blood (U.S.A.) **7**, 1053 (1952). — 34. LAHEY, M. E., C. J. GUBLER, G. E. CARTWRIGHT, and M. M. WINTROBE: J. Clin. Invest. (U.S.A.) **32**, 322 (1953). — 35. LAHEY, M. E., C. J. GUBLER, G. E. CARTWRIGHT, and M. M. WINTROBE: J. Clin. Invest. (U.S.A.) **32**, 329 (1953). — 36. LANG, E., and E. UNDRITZ: Schweiz. med. Wschr. **84**, 1120 (1954). — 37. LEICHTENSTERN, O.: Untersuchungen über den Hämoglobulingehalt des Blutes in gesunden und kranken Zuständen. Vogel, Leipzig, 1878, p. 99. — 38. MAASS, A. R., L. MICHAUD, H. SPECTOR, C. A. ELVEHJEM, and E. B. HART: Amer. J. Physiol. **141**, 322 (1944). — 39. MACELROY, W. D., and B. GLASS: Copper Metabolism. Symposium, Baltimore, 1950. — 40. MACHARGUE, J. S., D. J. HEALY, and E. S. HILL: J. Biol. Chem. (U.S.A.) **78**, 637 (1928). — 41. MACKAY, H.: Arch. Dis. Childh. (G. B.) **8**, 221 and 251 (1933). — 42. MARKOWITZ, H., C. J. GUBLER, J. P. MAHONEY, G. E. CARTWRIGHT, and M. M. WINTROBE: J. Clin. Invest. (U.S.A.) **34**, 1498 (1955). — 43. Haemoglobin Levels in Great Britain in 1941. Medical Research Council, Special Report Series, No. 252, 1945. — 44. MILAN, D., and H. MUENCH: J. Laborat. Clin. Med. (U.S.A.) **31**, 878 (1946) — 45. ROTH, O.: Schweiz. med. Wschr. **80**, 1065 (1950). — 46. ROTHLIN, E., and E. UNDRITZ: Helvet. med. acta **13**, 460 (1946). — 47. ROTHLIN, E., and E. UNDRITZ: Schweiz. med. Wschr. **77**, 58 (1947). — 48. ROTHLIN, E., and E. UNDRITZ: Bibl. paediatr. (Switz.) **58**, 636 (1954). — 49. ROTHLIN, E., and E. UNDRITZ: Analecta Sandoz **1954**, 27. — 50. ROTHLIN, E., E. UNDRITZ, and K. ZEHNDER: 5th Congress of the European Society of Haematology, Freiburg i. B., 1955, p. 161. — 51. ROTHLIN, E., E. UNDRITZ, and K. ZEHNDER: 6th Congress of the International Society of Haematology, Boston, 1956, p. 704. — 52. ROTHLIN, E., E. UNDRITZ, and K. ZEHNDER: Rev. path. comp. (Fr.) **56**, 1540 (1956). — 53. ROTHLIN, E., E. UNDRITZ, and K. ZEHNDER: Schweiz. med. Wschr. **86**, 1428 (1956). — 54. SAHLI, H.: Lehrbuch der klinischen Untersuchungsmethoden. 5th Ed. Deuticke, Leipzig and Vienna, 1909, p. 933. — 55. SCHULTZE, M. O.: J. Biol. Chem. (U.S.A.) **138**, 219 (1941). — 56. SCHULTZE, M. O., C. A. ELVEHJEM, and E. B. HART: J. Biol. Chem. (U.S.A.) **115**, 453 (1936). — 57. SETÄLÄ, A.: Ann. med. int.

Fenniae **38**, Suppl. 4 (1949). — 58. SMITH, E., and M. MEDLICOTT: Amer. J. Physiol. **141**, 354 (1944). — 59. STURGEON, P., and C. BRUBAKER: A. M. A. J. Dis. Child. **92**, 254 (1956). — 60. THEDERING, F.: Med. Klin. (G.) **50**, 1463 (1953). — 61. UNDERHILL, A., J. M. ORTEN, E. R. MUGRAGE, and R. C. LEWIS: J. Biol. Chem. (U.S.A.) **99**, 469 (1932/33). — 62. UNDRITZ, E.: Sandoz Atlas of Haematol. (**1952**). — 63. UNDRITZ, E.: Triangle, Sandoz, **2**, 33 (1955). — 64. UNDRITZ, E.: J. Amer. Med. Ass. **163**, 376 (1957). — 65. UNDRITZ, E.: Recipe (Belg.) **16**, 291 (1957). — 66. UNDRITZ, E.: Proceedings of the 7th Congress of the International Society of Haematology, Rome, 1958. Vol. 2, Communications. — 67. UNDRITZ, E.: Wien. klin. Wschr. **73**, 545 (1961). — 68. UNDRITZ, E.: Palette, Sandoz, No. 11, 10 (1962). — 69. UNDRITZ, E.: Rev. franç. hémat. **2**, 918 (1962). — 70. UNDRITZ, E.: The Physician's Panorama, Sandoz, Febr. (1963). — 71. UNDRITZ, E.: Folia haemat. (G.), N. F. 8, 258 (1963). — 72. VAHLQUIST, B.: Blood (U.S.A.) **5**, 874 (1950). — 73. VAN WYK, J. J., J. H. BAXTER, J. H. AKEROYD, and A. G. MOTULSKY: Bull. Johns Hopkins Hosp. (U.S.A.) **93**, 41 (1953). — 74. WALDENSTRÖM, J.: Acta med. Scand., Suppl. **90**, 380 (1938). — 75. WALDENSTRÖM, J.: Nord. med. tskr. **6**, 940 (1940). — 76. WALDENSTRÖM, J., and S. R. KJELLBERG: Acta radiol. (Sweden) **20**, 615 (1939). — 77. WALSH, R. J., B. J. ARNOLD, H. O. LANCASTER, M. A. COOTE, and H. COTTER: Spec. Report Series No. 5, Nat. Health and Med. Res. Council, Canberra, 1953. — 78. WILLIAMSON, C. S.: Arch. Int. Med. (U.S.A.) **18**, 505 (1919).

Parenteral treatment of iron deficiency

By

W. G. Figueroa

The great majority of patients suffering from iron deficiency can be treated successfully with oral iron. This leaves only a very small number of patients that absolutely require parenteral iron therapy, and this form of treatment should be used only after the diagnosis of iron-deficiency anemia has been established.

There is no question that this small group of patients derives benefit from this type of therapy and that in many instances it minimizes the transfusion needs of the patient and facilitates his clinical management. The extensive use made of parenteral iron preparations by the medical profession in the past few years suggests that there must in fact be a large number of patients in whom this more expensive treatment is being employed unnecessarily, particularly since safer intramuscular iron preparations have appeared on the market.

When a real need for parenteral iron therapy arises, the physician must be adequately acquainted with certain basic facts regarding this form of treatment.

The present review will include a discussion of four pertinent topics relative to parenteral therapy: 1) indications for this type of iron therapy; 2) iron preparations frequently used; 3) anticipated response to parenteral iron therapy; 4) toxic reactions encountered.

Wide use of the medical literature will be made in order to deal with certain of these points.

Historical background

There are many excellent reviews (*2, 9, 12, 24, 50*) describing the early attempts made to give iron parenterally by some of the first investigators. These pioneer studies may be summarized by saying that the preparations originally used were, with rare exceptions, toxic or painful or did not contain sufficient iron to be therapeutically very effective. This limited their clinical usefulness. It was not until Nissim (*43*) introduced intravenous saccharated iron-oxide for clinical use in 1947, followed shortly afterwards by AGNER's introduction of intravenous iron-dextrin (*1*), that the clinician had available for the first time iron preparations which were effective and safer to use than the earlier preparations. Saccharated iron-oxide had the drawback of lack of stability in the plasma, painful local reactions when injected out of the vein, and a moderate incidence of toxic side effects depending on the amount injected. For these reasons its use has diminished markedly, especially with the introduction of iron-dextran in 1954 (*6, 22*). Very recently another intramuscular iron preparation (*3*) has been introduced, but it is too early to evaluate its role in our therapeutic armamentarium.

Indications for parenteral iron therapy

While one can argue that there is no scientifically valid reason for not using parenteral treatment in any given patient with iron-deficiency anemia, the unpredictability of toxic reactions – infrequent and mild to moderate though they may be – dictates judicious use of this form of therapy.

The other argument is that most people with iron-deficiency anemia will respond to oral iron therapy, that there are therefore very few legitimate indications for parenteral iron therapy, and that it is undesirable to inject an expensive and potentially toxic agent. This has been our approach and practice for several years. Among some of the valid indications that have been listed for this mode of treatment are the following:

1) Failure to absorb adequate amounts of oral iron.

2) Where the patient is unable to tolerate adequate amounts of oral iron or, alternatively, is unwilling or cannot be relied upon to take the treatment.

3) To replenish iron stores in severe predictable and frequent recurrent blood loss not amenable to medical or surgical correction.

4) Uncomplicated well-documented iron-deficiency anemia that has been unresponsive to prolonged adequate iron therapy.

Patients belonging to this first category are very rare, but do occur. Using the Fe^{59} oral technique during the past 9 years in over 200 patients, only 2 patients of this type have been found (*21*). Although patients with subtotal gastrectomy show a reduction in Fe^{59} absorption, nearly all will respond to oral iron. The largest contingent of cases in this category is made up of patients with idiopathic steatorrhea (*5, 33*) and those who have undergone extensive surgical removal of small bowel.

In the second group are found some patients with gastro-intestinal disorders, especially inflammatory diseases such as ulcerative colitis, regional enteritis or severe diverticulitis, nausea and vomiting from various causes (especially pregnancy), and several other disorders whose symptoms may be aggravated by oral iron salt. Many of these patients, including those with peptic ulcer, are able to tolerate small doses of iron without difficulty. In this same group are a large number of patients who are either unreliable or unwilling to take iron in sufficient quantities to correct a severe or moderately severe iron-deficiency anemia. This situation is particularly common in the last trimester of pregnancy. Whether the slight to moderate increase in hemoglobin response achieved with large doses of parenteral iron is justification for administering parenteral in preference to oral medication, especially in severe anemia in late pregnancy, is still a debatable point. There are several investigators who believe that such therapy is justified (*31*).

In the third group are included patients losing blood in large amounts, usually from the gastro-intestinal tract, as a result of disorders such as hereditary telangiectasia or from some other undiscoverable cause. These individuals may bleed so frequently and severely that one is unable to keep up with the loss by the oral route alone.

The last category includes individuals whose iron-deficiency anemia is well documented and in whom other complications have been eliminated, but who fail to respond to oral iron therapy for one reason or another. Probably the main reason for patients falling into this group is that they are unreliable in taking their medication or may have an unsuspected absorption defect or unsuspected intermittent bleeding in excess of their iron intake.

Preparations available

While there are many parenteral iron preparations on the market, our discussion will be limited to four of these, as our clinical experience has been confined to these four and as there is already a large volume of medical literature on the clinical use of the first three preparations.

The preparations that have been found satisfactory for parenteral use are listed in Table 1 and are: 1) saccharated iron-oxide; 2) Dextriferron; 3) iron-dextran; 4) iron-sorbitol-citric acid with dextrin; 5) iron-polyisomaltose.

Table 1. *Parenteral iron preparations*

	Daily dosage in mg.
Intravenous	
Saccharated iron-oxide (Ferrivenin) (Proferrin)	100—200
Iron-dextrin complex (Dextriferron) (Astrafer)	100
Intramuscular	
Iron-dextran complex[1] (Imferon)	100—500
Iron-sorbitol-citric-acid complex (Jectofer)	100
Iron-polyisomaltose (Ferrum Hausmann Intramuscular)	100

[1] May also be used intravenously in a dosage of 100—250 mg.

Preparations for intravenous use

Saccharated iron-oxide, although still used, has now been largely replaced by other less toxic iron preparations. Administered intravenously in a dosage of 100–200 mg., saccharated iron-oxide is rapidly cleared from the plasma over a period of 3–6 hours (Fig. 1),

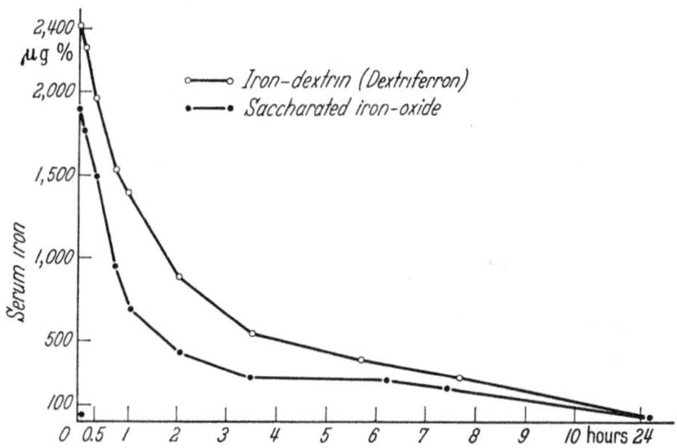

Fig. 1. Serum iron clearance following intravenous injection of 100 mg. each of Dextriferron and saccharated iron-oxide in a patient with moderately severe iron-deficiency anemia. Interval of 5 days between the two injections

and is taken up by the reticulo-endothelial system and later by the parenchymal liver cells. Saturation of transferrin depends on the amount injected. Urinary excretion is negligible (*55*).

Dextriferron (iron-dextrin) (Astrafer) is a colloidal solution of ferric hydroxide in complex with partially hydrolyzed dextrin, which is a carbohydrate of lower molecular weight. It contains 20 mg. iron per ml. in isotonic solution, is stable in saline and plasma, and has a pH of 7.3. This preparation was introduced by Agner

(*1*) in 1948 and has been used by ANDERSSON (*2*), HAGEDORN (*39*), and FIELDING (*18*). The preparation is handled by the body in a similar fashion to saccharated iron-oxide and disappears from the plasma at about the same rate as the latter (Fig. 1). There is practically no urinary iron excretion following its use. Its effect on hemoglobin production is comparable to that of saccharated iron-oxide (Table 2).

Preparations for intramuscular use

Iron-dextran or Imferon is a complex of ferric hydroxide and dextran containing 50 mg. iron per ml. When the complex is absorbed following intramuscular injection, it first enters the lymph system, passing through the regional lymph nodes and subsequently into the bloodstream (*25*). Various studies (*23, 27*) using Fe^{59} have indicated that as much as 20–40% of the injected dose may still be present at the site of injection 40–50 days later. Lower values have been found by STEVENS (*56*) in his studies in moderately severe iron-anemic patients. Within 2–3 hours the serum iron begins to rise and usually reaches 0.7–1.5 mg.% depending on the amount injected. Incorporation of the liberated Fe^{59} into the red cells is still progressing 50–60 days later. This preparation has had extensive clinical use in the past few years and is probably the most frequently employed parenteral iron preparation. The manufacturers (*35*) recommend it solely for intramuscular use, but it has been given intravenously by various clinicians (*17*), with a higher incidence of moderately severe toxic reactions, several years ago (*13*).

Jectofer is a solution of iron-sorbitol-citric-acid complex with dextrin as a stabilizer. It contains 50 mg. Fe/ml., has a pH of 7.5, and is stable in serum. Following intramuscular injection it is promptly absorbed by both blood and lymphatic vessels, raising the serum iron concentration to a maximum of 300–500 μg. at 2–3.5 hours (*3, 38a*). It rapidly binds with transferrin to saturate it in $^1/_2$–3 hours (Fig. 2). Using Fe^{59}, it is estimated that 70% of the dose is absorbed in 3 hours, with only small amounts remaining after 10 hours (*44, 57*). Utilization of iron for hemoglobin production is rapid and very similar to that of transferrin-bound iron (*4, 44*). Approximately 30% of the dose is excreted in the urine in 24 hours. ANDERSSON (*3*) concludes that the hemoglobin regeneration rate following the use of Jectofer compares with that following iron-dextran. FIELDING (*19*) has reported that Jectofer does not produce sarcoma in experimental animals.

Iron-polyisomaltose or Ferrum Hausmann Intramuscular (*8, 40*) is a solution related to iron-dextran. It is a complex of ferric hydroxide and polyisomaltose, the latter occurring in the hydrolytic splitting of dextran. The iron concentration amounts to 5%. We have not had any experience with this preparation.

Selection of parenteral preparations and calculations of dosage. The intramuscular route for parenteral iron has certain practical advantages with regard to ease of administration. The incidence of toxic reactions to iron-dextran is estimated to be low, probably in the neighborhood of 0.5–0.8%. The large amount of iron-dextran remaining at the site of injection has to be taken into consideration, since this iron is not available for red-cell production and may exert a local inflammatory effect which constitutes a possible hazard to the patient. From this point of view, a preparation which is rapidly absorbed offers certain advantages, provided the test of time indicates that it has the same degree of safety as iron-dextran. The intravenous route would bypass the above difficulty, but has been found to involve the risk of severe toxic reactions. Perhaps, as some investigators believe (*18*), the use of Dextriferron or some other preparation will reduce this risk. There are even some authors who advise against any intramuscular injection of iron in principle (*54*).

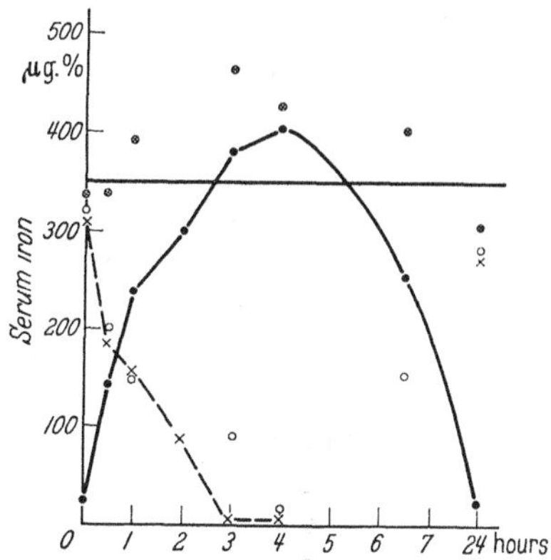

Fig. 2. Hourly serum iron (●——●) and unsaturated iron-binding capacity determination in a patient with moderately severe iron-deficiency anemia following the intramuscular injection (gluteal) of 100 mg. Jectofer. The degree of saturation was determined by two methods — the resin chemical method (values represented by plain circles) and the optical density method (values represented by crosses). Saturation of transferrin was complete at 3 to 4 hours using both methods. The horizontal line at 350 µg. %, showing the total iron-binding capacity, represents the sum of the serum iron value plus the optical density unsaturated iron-binding capacity at zero (0) hour. The total iron-binding capacity (values represented by circles containing a cross) was determined after zero hour by the sum of the serum iron value plus the unsaturated iron-binding capacity as determined by the resin chemical method

Calculation of the amount of iron needed. There are many methods of calculating the dosage of iron needed for hemoglobin regeneration. Some prefer the formula which assumes that 25 mg. iron is needed to raise the hemoglobin 1% on the Haldane scale. The method proposed by Brown and Moore (*12*) is simple and easy to remember: normal hemoglobin minus patient's initial hemoglobin $\times 0.255 =$ grams of iron needed. This method allows for 50% replacement of tissue stores.

Table 2. *Hemoglobin regeneration following parenteral iron therapy*[6]

A. Intravenous therapy

Author	Iron prep.	Mg. elemental Fe/day	Total dose in g. range	No. of subjects	Initial Hb. range (av.)	Initial Hct. range (av.)	Daily increase Hb. g./100 ml. range	Daily increase Hb. g./100 ml. av.	No. of days	Av.	Comments
HORRIGAN (*34*)	Sacc. iron-oxide	100—600	1.2 —2.6	9	4.8 — 6.9[1]	15—34	0.15 —0.34	0.215	11—33	24	8 non-pregnant females 1 male
BROWN (*11*)	Sacc. iron-oxide	100[2]	0.7 —2.0	10	5.8 —9.8		0.106—0.262	0.177	10—29	22	8 non-pregnant females 2 males
CAMERON (*14*)	Sacc. iron-oxide	100—200	1.5 —2.5	3	7.1 — 8.4	28—34	0.23—0.25	0.24	24—32	29	
SLACK (*55*)	Sacc. iron-oxide	200[4]	920	60	50%[5]			0.184 0.215[7]	21—35		57 non-pregnant females 3 males
ANDERSSON (*2*)	Astrafer	100	0.4 —2.24	10	< 8		Not stated	0.21	Not stated		
ANDERSSON (*2*)	Astrafer	100	0.4 —2.24	30	> 8		Not stated	0.13	Not stated		
LUCAS and HAGEDORN (*39*)	Astrafer	100—200[3]	0.75—1.35	6	6.8 —10.3 (7.3)	27—36 (31)	0.021—0.173	0.094	13—36	21	Pregnant
LUCAS and HAGEDORN (*39*)	Astrafer	100—200[3]	1.2 —1.4	5	5.8 —7.8 (6.6)	27—32 (28)	0.094—0.355	0.268	8—48	26	Non-pregnant Hb. < 8 g.%
LUCAS and HAGEDORN (*39*)	Astrafer	100—200[3]	0.57—1.25	6	8.2 —10.4 (8.9)	32—36 (34)	0.055—0.284	0.154	12—42	23	Non-pregnant Hb. > 8 g.%
FIELDING (*18*)	Astrafer	100	0.6 —1.2	9	5.98— 7.88 (7.15)		0.067—0.18	0.138	21—42	29	Non-pregnant Hb. < 8 g.%
FIELDING (*18*)	Astrafer	100	0.55—1.2	4	8.46— 9.63 (9.26)		0.076—0.116	0.094	21—44	28	Non-pregnant Hb. > 8 g.%
FIELDING (*18*)	Astrafer	100	0.95—1.24	3	7.15— 7.88 (7.49)		0.090—0.150	0.112	32—42	35	Pregnant Hb. < 8 g.%
FIELDING (*18*)	Astrafer	100	0.64—1.04	15	8.17—10.0 (9.07)		0.01 —0.14	0.096	13—38	27	Pregnant Hb. > 8 g.%

Table 2. *Hemoglobin regeneration following parenteral iron therapy*[6] (continued)

B. Intramuscular therapy

Author	Iron prep.	Mg. elemental Fe/day	Total dose in g. range	No. of subjects	Initial Hb. range (av.)	Initial Hct. range (av.)	Daily increase Hb. g./100 ml. range	Daily increase Hb. g./100 ml. av.	No. of days	Av.	Comments
GRUNBERG and BLAIR (*28*)	Imferon	250	1.95—3.2	5	4.6— 7.5 (6.42)		0.171—0.390	0.249	10—28	21	4 Non-pregnant females
KARLEFORS (*36*)	Imferon	250	1.0 —2.0	3	6.2— 8.3 (7)		0.23 —0.265	0.242	10—20	16	
KOSZEWSKI and WALSH (*38*)	Imferon	100—250	1.0 —2.0	17	5.4—10.2 (7.8)	26—36	0.071—0.257	0.132	14		
PRITCHARD (*45*)	Imferon	250—500	1.5	6	3.2— 7.2 (5.4)	12—28 (19.5)	—0.34[10]	0.26	10—33	19	Gynecological cases
HAGEDORN (*32*)	Imferon	200	0.75—2.0	10	4.6— 9.7 (7.4)	37	0.02 —0.31	0.12	19		3 males 7 non-pregnant females
ANDERSSON (*3*)	Jectofer	100	1.0	7	5.4— 7.8		0.077—0.142	0.108	35		
ANDERSSON (*3*)	Imferon	100	1.0	7	5.0— 8.0		0.091—0.145	0.111	35		
ANDERSSON (*3*)	Jectofer	100	1.0	23	8.1—12			0.065	35		
ANDERSSON (*3*)	Imferon	100	1.0	16	8.1—12			0.071	35		
SCOTT (*52*)	Imferon	100—250	Not given[9]	200[8]	8.5			0.095	21		Pregnant
SCOTT (*52*)	Imferon	100—250	Not given[9]	44	< 8			0.142	21		Pregnant
MULLA (*42*)	Imferon	100—500	1.25—1.60	14	7.4— 9.3 (8.64)	24—29 (24.93)	0.141—0.275	0.209	14—28	21	

1 One case had 10 g. Hb./100 ml.
2 A few received 200 mg.
3 Single dose did not exceed 100 mg.
4 25, 50, 100 mg. first 3 days, occasionally 200 mg. b.i.d.
5 100% value in grams not given.
6 Final Hb. minus initial Hb. ÷ days of therapy.
7 Value obtained in last 42 cases treated.
8 Figure includes the 44 cases listed below.
9 Amount given calculated 0.3 × weight in lbs. × Hb. deficit in % Haldane.
10 Lower figure not given.

Anticipated hemoglobin response

When parenteral iron is given to non-pregnant adults with iron-deficiency anemia the hemoglobin rises from 0.1 to 0.35 g. per 100 ml. per day during the period of maximum hemoglobin production. Table 2, which is not intended to be complete in any sense, lists some of these results. Coleman et al. (*15*), using saccharated iron-oxide, found a value of 0.25 g. hemoglobin per 100 ml. per day when the initial hemoglobin was below 7 g. In one investigation using blood-volume studies, Bass (*7*) reported that in over 20% of his 70 patients he obtained values of 0.35 to 0.4 g. hemoglobin per 100 ml. per day or over. The higher values for hemoglobin regeneration of between 0.2 and 0.35 g. hemoglobin per 100 ml. per day appear to be obtained when larger doses of iron, i.e. between 200 and 500 mg., are administered. The hemoglobin response in children appears to be somewhat greater (*15*).

When he treated pregnant patients with saccharated iron intravenously and with Imferon intramuscularly and compared the results, Scott (*51, 52*) found that they were about equal as regards their effect on the rate of hemoglobin production. Scott (*26*) noticed that, in pregnant women receiving intravenous saccharated iron-oxide, hemoglobin production was more rapid than in those taking oral iron. Cope (*16*), after studying a group of ante-partum, post-partum, and medical cases in receipt of oral ferrous succinate, saccharated iron-oxide, and Imferon, concluded that intramuscular iron was as effective as intravenous iron except that it did not exert such a rapid effect in the medical cases. The response to oral iron was a little slower in the ante-partum group as compared with the response to intramuscular Imferon (average daily hemoglobin increase: 0.9−1.2%).

Pritchard (*45*), treating two small groups of hospitalized gynecological bleeding problems, one with oral iron, the other with a large dose of Imferon (200−500 mg.), concluded that the oral therapy was about 80% as efficient as parenteral therapy. A comparison between these two groups is shown in Table 3.

In children suffering from iron deficiency in an out-patient clinic, Yu (*58*) found hemoglobin-regeneration rates, following the use of Imferon intramuscularly, of 2.1, 2.2, and 1.0 g. hemoglobin per 100 ml. during the first, second, and third weeks, whereas comparable oral iron therapy yielded values of 0.9 g. hemoglobin per 100 ml. during each of the first three weeks.

It appears that comparable hemoglobin-regeneration rates can be obtained with parenteral and oral iron therapy, but that with large amounts of parenteral iron (250−500 mg.) a slight to moderate

Table 3. *Comparison of hemoglobin regeneration following oral and intramuscular iron therapy in a group of patients with uterine bleeding*

	Iron preparation	
	Imferon (i.m.)	Fe gluconate (oral)
Mg. elemental Fe		
Day	250—500	230
Total	>1,500	
No. of cases	6	6
Hb. g./100 ml.		
Initial	5.4 (av.)	5.1 (av.)
Final	10.4	10.0
No. of days	19	24
Daily increase Hb. g./100 ml.	0.26	0.20

From PRITCHARD, J. A.: J. Amer. Med. Ass. **175**, 478 (1961).

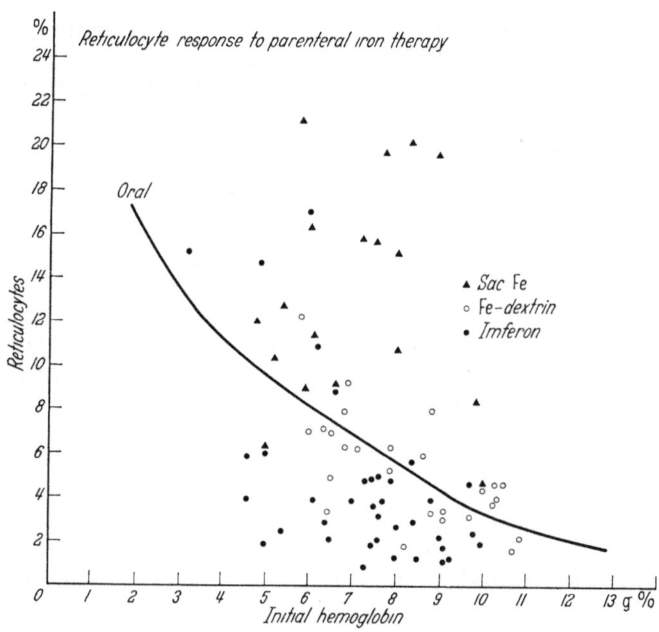

Fig. 3. Comparison of maximum reticulocyte response in adults receiving various parentera iron preparations and in patients receiving oral iron therapy. The data on oral iron therapy are from MINOT (*41*) and those on parenteral iron therapy from various authors (*7, 11, 28, 32, 34, 36, 38, 39*)

increase in hemoglobin regeneration is seen over and above that obtained with oral therapy. Although there is no agreement on this point, the usual figure quoted for hemoglobin regeneration following oral therapy is 0.1–0.25 g. hemoglobin per 100 ml. per day. RESNIKOFF (*46*) has reported one case in which a rate of 0.536 g. hemoglobin per 100 ml. per day was recorded following administration of 324 mg. elemental iron per day in the form of ferrous gluconate.

A comparison of maximum reticulocyte responses in adults receiving various parenteral iron preparations and MINOT's (*41*) data on the response to oral iron is given in Fig. 3. This indicates that reticulocytosis is maximal with saccharated iron-oxide and exceeds that obtained with either oral or intramuscular therapy. Imferon appears in many instances to yield values below those recorded with oral iron.

Toxicity of iron preparations

The toxicity of the various parenteral iron preparations has been one of the principal difficulties associated with their use. It has not been possible to attribute this toxicity to any single cause. The suggestion that the toxicity is due to the release of ionic iron, with subsequent saturation of transferrin, does not appear to offer a full explanation. Since complete saturation can be demonstrated with both saccharated iron-oxide and iron-sorbitol without evidence of toxicity (*3, 30*), FIELDING (*20*) states: "It is unlikely that a single factor is responsible for all or even most of the observed toxic reactions. Instability of the complex in plasma with possible precipitation *in vivo* is a likely cause in the case of the saccharated oxide but improbable with the dextran, dextrin, or sorbitol complexes. The rate of reticulo-endothelial uptake from the circulation, the rate of release of dissociated iron from reticulo-endothelial cells, dissociation of the complex in the circulation, the intrinsic ionic iron content of the complex, and anaphylactic phenomena have all been postulated. It is clear that each complex needs to be considered separately in detail."

The toxicity manifestations of saccharated iron-oxide have been fully documented by NISSIM (*43*) and BROWN (*12*), and the reader is referred to their excellent papers. Toxicity manifestations of Imferon have been estimated at around 0.5% by SCOTT (*51*), who cautions against its use in patients with asthma or skin rashes. In 1960 the product was temporarily withdrawn from the market following the reports by RICHMOND (*47, 48*) and HADDOW and

HORNING (*29*) of the induction of sarcomas in rats and mice at the site of injection after repeated massive doses of the drug. Comparable tissue changes in man are confined to a single report of a possible sarcoma which developed in the deltoid muscle at a site of probable injection 3 years previously (*49*). It is now believed that the danger of producing malignancy in man is very remote, and Imferon accordingly reappeared on the market in the U.S.A. in 1962. Its chief toxic manifestations are listed in Table 4.

Table 4. *Side effects after injection of Imferon*

A. *Local:*	Pain at the site of injection Skin discoloration Tender inguinal lymphadenopathy Abdominal pain in the lower quadrant.
B. *Systemic:*	Fever, chills, headache, nausea, vomiting Bronchospasm with dyspnea Arthralgia, backache, constricting chest pain Urticaria with or without eosinophilia, rash Generalized lymphadenopathy Leukemoid reactions Flushing of the face, hypotension and dizziness.

Dextriferron toxicity has been reported to be mild and infrequent. Leakage of the preparation from the vein results in minor inflammation which usually subsides in 24–48 hours with no tendency to thrombophlebitis. Flushing, nausea, headaches, and abdominal pain may occur. Delayed side effects include a feeling of stiffness in the extremities or face, chills, and fever. Recently two severe reactions were documented in two patients receiving this preparation while on oral iron therapy (*10*).

The initial studies with iron-sorbitol-citric-acid complex indicated only mild toxicity consisting mainly of local pain at the site of injection and interference with the sense of taste starting about one hour after injection and lasting for several hours. Although initially no general reactions were observed, SCOTT (*53*) has reported three episodes involving a general reaction in the form of headaches and vomiting in two cases and dizziness and disorientation in a third; all three patients were receiving simultaneous oral iron therapy. SCOTT suggests that the association of oral iron with the above complex is the determining factor and utters a warning against the possible hazards of such a combination. KINLOCH (*37*) has observed four similar reactions in patients who were not receiving oral iron at the same time. At present it is probably best not to give iron-sorbitol in association with oral iron.

Summary

Since the great majority of patients with iron-deficiency anemia will respond successfully to oral iron, parenteral iron therapy has a limited scope of usefulness. Parenteral treatment with iron should be reserved for the rare patient in whom, for various reasons, oral iron is either ineffective or poorly tolerated. Some of the indications for this form of therapy are listed, together with several useful parenteral iron preparations.

There is no question that, when the rare need arises for their use, parenteral iron preparations are effective in increasing hemoglobin regeneration from 0.1 to 0.35 g. hemoglobin per 100 ml. per day during the first 2—3 weeks. Comparison of hemoglobin-regeneration rates following oral and parenteral iron therapy indicates that there is a slightly more rapid rate in response to injectable iron, especially when administered in amounts of 250—500 mg. per day. Several studies have revealed no appreciable difference in hemoglobin regeneration between the two forms of therapy, particularly when the amount of iron injected was 100 mg. per day. Because of the mild to severe toxic reactions which may develop with all the parenteral iron preparations at present available, the indications for their use should be evaluated carefully.

Zusammenfassung

Da die Mehrzahl der Patienten mit Eisenmangelanaemie auf orale Gabe von Eisen anspricht, kommt der parenteralen Eisentherapie nur eine begrenzte Bedeutung zu. Sie beschränkt sich auf wenige Patienten, bei denen aus verschiedenen Gründen oral zugeführtes Eisen entweder ungenügend wirkt oder schlecht vertragen wird. Einzelne Indikationen für diese Form der Eisenbehandlung werden angegeben, ebenso eine Reihe geeigneter Präparate für die parenterale Therapie.

In den seltenen Fällen, bei denen Eisenpräparate parenteral angewendet werden müssen, sind sie zweifellos wirksam und steigern die Haemoglobinregeneration von 0,1 auf 0,35 g. Haemoglobin pro 100 ml. pro Tag während der ersten 2—3 Wochen. Ein Vergleich der Haemoglobinregeneration nach oraler und parenteraler Zufuhr von Eisen ergibt einen etwas rascheren Anstieg nach Injektion von täglichen Dosen von 250—500 mg. Die Regeneration von Haemoglobin ist jedoch bei den beiden Arten der Behandlung gleich, wenn 100 mg. Eisen täglich injiziert werden. Im Hinblick auf die mitunter schweren toxischen Reaktionen, die nach Gabe aller heute verfügbaren parenteral applizierbaren Eisenpräparate auftreten können, ist ihre Anwendung sorgfältig abzuwägen.

Résumé

Puisque la grande majorité des malades présentant une anémie ferriprive réagit bien à l'administration orale de fer, la thérapeutique par voie parentérale ne présente donc qu'un intérêt limité. Cette voie ne devrait être réservée qu'aux rares malades chez qui, pour diverses raisons, le fer par voie orale est inefficace ou mal toléré. Quelques indications de cette forme d'administration sont énumérées ainsi que plusieurs utiles préparations parentérales de fer.

Il ne fait aucun doute que, dans les rares cas où elles sont indiquées, les préparations de fer parentérales sont efficaces et remontent les taux d'hémoglobine de 0,1 g. à 0,35 g. par 100 ml. de sang et par jour au cours des 2 ou 3 premières semaines. Des comparaisons entre les taux de restitution de l'hémoglobine après administration orale et après administration parentérale de fer montrent que la réponse est légèrement plus rapide avec le fer injectable, en particulier quand il est administré à des doses de 250 à 500 mg. par jour. Plusieurs études n'ont montré aucune différence appréciable dans la restitution de l'hémoglobine entre les deux formes de traitement, en particulier quand la dose injectée de fer était de 100 mg. par jour. En raison des réactions toxiques, moyennes à graves, que peuvent déclencher toutes les préparations parentérales de fer actuellement disponibles, la justesse de leurs indications doit être soigneusement établie.

References

1. Agner, K. J., N. S. E. Andersson, and N. G. Nordenson: Acta haemat. (Switz.) **1**, 193 (1948). — 2. Andersson, N. S. E.: Acta med. Scand. Suppl., **241**, 5 (1950). — 3. Andersson, N. S. E.: Brit. Med. J. **1961**/II, 275. — 4. Andersson, N. S. E.: Brit. Med. J. **1962**/II, 1260. — 5. Badenoch, J., and S. T. Callender: Blood (U.S.A.) **9**, 123 (1954). — 6. Baird, I. M., and D. A. Podmore: Lancet (G.B.) **2**, 942 (1954). — 7. Bass, R. K., E. R. Halden, and E. E. Muirhead: Texas State J. Med. **55**, 22 (1959). — 8. Bersin, T., and H. Schwarz: Justus Liebigs Ann. Chem. (G.) **623**, 138 (1959). — 9. Beutler, E., V. F. Fairbanks, and J. L. Fahey: Clinical Disorders of Iron Metabolism. Grune & Stratton, New York, 1963, p. 181. — 10. Blazar, A. S., and M. G. del Riego: Obstetr. Gynec. (U.S.A.) **20**, 156 (1962). — 11. Brown, E. B., C. V. Moore, C. Reynafarje, and D. E. Smith: J. Amer. Med. Ass. **144**, 1084 (1950). — 12. Brown, E. B., and C. V. Moore: Progr. Hemat. (U.S.A.) **1**, 22 (1956). — 13. Callender, S., and M. D. Smith: Brit. Med. J. **1954**/II, 1486. — 14. Cameron, D. G., E. H. Bensley, P. Wood, and V. Grayston: Canad. Med. Ass. J. **64**, 27 (1951). — 15. Coleman, D. H., A. R. Stevens, and C. A. Finch: Blood (U.S.A.) **10**, 567 (1955). — 16. Cope, E., R. O. Gillhespy, and R. W. Richardson: Brit. Med. J. **1956**/II, 638. — 17. Dillon, E. D.: Brit. Med. J. **1960**/I, 960. — 18. Fielding, J.: Brit. Med. J. **1961**/II, 279. — 19. Fielding, J.: Brit. Med. J. **1962**/I, 1800. — 20. Fielding. J., and G. M. Smith: J. Clin. Path. (G.B.) **16**, 12 (1963). — 21. Figueroa, W. G.: Personal observation. — 22. Fletcher, F., and E. London: Brit. Med. J. **1954**/I, 984. — 23. Garby, L., and S. Sjolin: Acta med. Scand. **157**, 319 (1957). — 24. Goetsch, A. T., C. V. Moore, and V. Minnich: Blood (U.S.A.) **1**, 129 (1946). — 25. Golberg, L.: In: Iron in Clinical Medicine, Chapter on "Pharmacology and Parenteral Iron Preparations". University of California Press, Berkeley and Los Angeles, 1958, p. 74. — 26. Govan, A. D. T., and J. M. Scott: Lancet (G.B.) **1949**/I, 14. — 27. Grimes, A. J., and M. S. R. Hutt: Brit. Med. J. **1957**/II, 1074. — 28. Grunberg, A., and J. L. Blair: A.M.A. Arch. Int. Med. **96**, 731 (1955). — 29. Haddow, A., and E. S. Horning: J. Nat. Cancer Inst. (U.S.A.) **24**, 109 (1960). — 30. Hagberg, B.: Acta Soc. med. Upsal. **58**, 56 (1953). — 31. Hagedorn, A. B.: Proc. Staff Meet. Mayo Clin. (U.S.A.) **27**, 277 (1952). — 32. Hagedorn, A.: J. Amer. Med. Ass. **164**, 1642 (1957). — 33. Hawkins, C. F., A. L. P. Peeney, and W. T. Cooke: Lancet (G.B.) **1950**/II, 387. — 34. Horrigan, D. L., J. F. Mueller, and R. W. Vilter: J. Laborat. Clin. Med. (U.S.A.) **36**, 422 (1950). — 35. Imferon® Brochure: Milwaukee Lakeside Laboratories (U.S.A.). Revised November, 1961. — 36. Karlefors, T., and A. Norden: Acta med. Scand. Suppl., **342**, 1 (1958). — 37. Kinloch, J. D.: Brit. Med. J. **1962**/II, 605. — 38. Koszewski, B. J., and J. R. Walsh: Amer. J. Med. Sc. **235**, 523

(1958). — 38a. LINDVALL, S., and N. S. E. ANDERSSON: Brit. J. Pharmacol. **17**, 358 (1961). — 39. LUCAS, J. E., and A. B. HAGEDORN: Blood (U.S.A.) **7**, 358 (1952). — 40. MEREU, T., and O. TONZ: Dtsch. med. Wschr. **86**, 1259 (1961). — 41. MINOT, G. R., and C. W. HEATH: Amer. J. Med. Sc. **183**, 110 (1932). — 42. MULLA, N.: Obstetr. Gynec. (U.S.A.) **12**, 325 (1958). — 43. NISSIM, J. A.: Brit. Med. J. **1954**/I, 352. — 44. PRINGLE, A., A. GOLDBERG, E. MACDONALD, and S. JOHNSTON: Lancet (G.B.) **1962**/II, p. 749. — 45. PRITCHARD, J. A.: J. Amer. Med. Ass. **175**, 478 (1961). — 46. RESNIKOFF, P., and W. F. GOEBEL: J. Clin. Invest. (U.S.A.) **16**, 547 (1937). — 47. RICHMOND, H. G.: Scott. Med. J. **2**, 169 (1957). — 48. RICHMOND, H. G.: Brit. Med. J. **1959**/I, 947. — 49. ROBINSON, C. E. G., D. N. BELL, and J. H. STURDY: Brit. Med. J. **1961**/I, 744. — 50. SCHULTEN, H., and W. PRIBILLA: In: Eisenstoffwechsel, Chapter on "Eisentherapie". Georg Thieme, Stuttgart (1959), p. 253. — 51. SCOTT, J. M., and A. D. T. GOVAN: Brit. Med. J. **1954**/II, 1257. — 52. SCOTT, J. M.: Brit. Med. J. **1956**/II, 635. — 53. SCOTT, J. M.: Brit. Med. J. **1962**/II, 480. — 54. SIMON, K. H.: Med. Mschr. (G.) **16**, 511 (1962). — 55. SLACK, H. G. B., and J. F. WILKINSON: Lancet (G.B.) **1949**/I, 163. — 56. STEVENS, Jr., A. R.: In: Iron in Clinical Medicine, Chapter on "The Treatment of Iron-Deficiency Anemia". University of California Press, Berkeley and Los Angeles, 1958, p. 144. — 57. WETHERLEY-MEIN, G., J. G. BUCHANAN, U. H. GLASS, and L. C. PEARCE: Brit. Med. J. **1962**/I, 1796. — 58. YU, W. L. Y., K. MANONMANI, and R. J. WATSON: J. Pediatr. (U.S.A.) **54**, 50 (1959).

Discussion

SCHAPIRA: I should like to ask Dr. UNDRITZ two questions. Firstly, I agree that the lack of iron induces haemoglobinopoiesis. But the diet you used is deficient in cobalt. Can we take it that in human iron deficiency one should also use copper? Secondly, could you tell us some more about the elephants?

UNDRITZ: I would say that cobalt is primarily indicated in those forms of anaemia which respond neither to iron alone nor to vitamin B_{12}. This includes anaemia associated with infectious diseases, such as tuberculosis in particular, and with renal disorders, cancer, leukaemia, myxoedema, etc. In many of these conditions, the mechanism responsible for the fact that under the influence of cobalt the iron, which would otherwise be insufficient by itself, is utilised for haemoglobin production, seems to be the same, because the response to cobalt is the same. The cobalt ion has an indirect effect; in contrast to vitamin B_{12}, which contains cobalt, and to iron and copper, the action of cobalt is not that of an element essential to the organism, i.e. it is not a physiological but a pharmacological action. For an adult, 15—30 mg. cobalt per day is sufficient to restore haemoglobin production to normal; this is a quantity which is not found in any natural form of food and which is 375,000 to 750,000 times greater than the daily dose of vitamin-B_{12} cobalt needed to prevent a relapse in a patient with pernicious anaemia (for this purpose, a daily dose of 1 μg. vitamin B_{12} is adequate, and as vitamin B_{12} contains 4% cobalt, this corresponds to 0.04 μg. cobalt daily). Thus, the pharmacological activity of cobalt has nothing to do with the action of vitamin B_{12} as such.

Since, in the diseases to which I have just referred, cobalt can exert its pharmacological effect only if sufficient iron is also available, it is advisable to administer the cobalt in combination with iron, especially in the case of women or children, who often suffer from iron deficiency or even from frank iron-deficiency anaemia. I personally administer copper as well (a daily dose of 2—5 mg. is sufficient), so as to make sure that this element, which physiologically stimulates haemoglobin production, is not lacking — although, in fact, copper deficiency hardly ever occurs in man. In anaemia associated with infectious diseases, the concentration of copper in the serum is actually enhanced, though most of it is bound to ceruloplasmin. Our knowledge of copper metabolism is at present so limited, however, and the types of anaemia in question tend to be so refractory, that I consider one is justified in administering small doses of copper in addition, particularly since we have at our disposal organic hydro-insoluble copper compounds, e.g. copper leucinate, which, although fully effective, are of very low toxicity. This does not impose any additional strain on the gastro-intestinal tract — a point which one must always consider when prescribing salts of heavy metals.

In uncomplicated cases of iron-deficiency anaemia, which respond well to iron alone, neither cobalt nor, for that matter, vitamin B_{12} is generally indicated. On the other hand, in very severe forms of anaemia in which immunopathological factors are perhaps involved as well, or where a prompt effect is required, e.g. prior to an operation, use of cobalt is to be recommended.

KUNDRATITZ[1] and WEIPPL[2] advocate a combination of cobalt, iron, and copper for the treatment of anaemia in premature infants.

With regard to anaemia in young elephants, I am afraid I have nothing more to add to the findings reported in my paper.

NAJEAN: May I ask Dr. UNDRITZ how he accounts for the very rapid effect of oral iron on the reticulocyte level in hyposideraemic anaemia? What do you think may possibly be the direct effect of iron on normoblast multiplication?

And could Dr. FIGUEROA tell me how many local sarcomas are actually known to have developed in human beings after injection of Imferon? Have there been any other cases besides the one published by ROBINSON[3]?

UNDRITZ: The effect of iron deficiency in stimulating erythropoiesis is a non-specific reaction by which an attempt is made to compensate for the lack of haemoglobin. The heart rate is also accelerated, and in severe anaemia the heart may become markedly enlarged. This enlargement of the heart, like the stimulation of erythropoiesis, subsides once the anaemia has been reversed, a fact which we have been able to demonstrate particularly well in experiments on rats. The iron simply fulfils the role of a passive, albeit necessary, component in the synthesis of haemoglobin.

FIGUEROA: In reply to the question Dr. NAJEAN has asked me, I know only of the case reported by ROBINSON, in which a sarcoma developed in the deltoid area; as you know, the slides were sent to several pathologists, and I think the verdict was about 5 to 1 in favour of its being a sarcoma. Whether this has anything to do with the injection of Imferon, I don't know. The patient is well after 3 years. Dr. CLETON tells me that he believes he has seen another case in a 40-year-old woman with a sarcoma at the site of injection; perhaps he would like to tell us more about this case later on in the discussion.

MOESCHLIN: It was mentioned yesterday that the stimulating action of cobalt is due to intracellular hypoxaemia produced by an enzyme-blocking effect of this metal. If this is the case, I think the "therapeutic use" of cobalt should be avoided.

UNDRITZ: Regarding the toxicity of cobalt, I would remind you that according to some authors the effect of cobalt is described as "histotoxic anoxia", while WEISSBECKER[4] has used the term "aredoxia". The same applies to cobalt as to so many other highly active drugs: they exert a desirable effect when given in relatively small doses, whereas they are toxic when administered in higher doses. Our own investigations have shown that in the case of cobalt, too, one can distinguish between these two dose-dependent patterns of effect. If given to healthy subjects in a sufficiently high dosage, cobalt leads to "polyglobulia", i.e. to an increase in the erythrocytes and in the haemoglobin, this effect being due to the anoxaemia or "aredoxia" which it induces. But one-half of the dose of cobalt which is just enough to produce polyglobulia in rats is sufficient to restore haemoglobin production to normal in anaemic conditions that are resistant to iron

[1] KUNDRATITZ, K.: Wien. klin. Wschr. **68**, 972 (1956).

[2] WEIPPL, G.: Wien. klin. Wschr. **70**, 859 (1958).

[3] ROBINSON, C. E. G., D. N. BELL, and I. H. STURDY: Brit. Med. J. **1960**/II, 648.

[4] WEISSBECKER, L.: Kobalt als Spurenelement etc. Wissenschaftl. Verlagsges., Stuttgart, 1950.

and to vitamin B_{12}; as far as I know, this is not possible with any other drug. Thus, though one may conceivably regard this dose-dependent, incipient polyglobulia as a toxic effect — despite the fact that it resembles the anoxaemia occurring in rarefied air at great altitudes and, like the latter, is also reversible — I do not see how the normalisation of pathologically reduced haemoglobin production in forms of anaemia refractory to iron therapy, a response which is obtained with a smaller dose of cobalt, can possibly be described as a toxic effect; on the contrary, it is surely a very desirable pharmacological effect. Of course, as the dose needed to elicit a pharmacological effect is not far short of the "toxic" dose, one must avoid using poorly tolerated inorganic cobalt salts that are in any case more toxic, e.g. cobalt sulphate; instead, one should employ an organic preparation which is just as effective but less toxic, i.e. a preparation such as cobalt glutamate, which is only half as toxic as the sulphate or chloride and is therefore much better tolerated.

WITTS: I must disagree with Dr. UNDRITZ on his view that iron does not stimulate erythropoiesis. Stimulation was clearly demonstrated by FOWLER and BARER[1], both in normal subjects and in patients with anaemia. The rise in the blood haemoglobin on treatment with iron reaches a peak at the end of 10 to 12 weeks, and following this there is a gradual reduction to the normal haemoglobin level for the subject, regardless of whether or not the treatment with iron is continued. WIDDOWSON[2] showed in 1939 that the same kind of thing happens in women in pregnancy, who can maintain a normal haemoglobin if iron is given, whereas immediately the iron is stopped the haemoglobin falls to the levels characteristic of pregnancy, although presumably the store of iron has increased. It must be admitted that STURGEON[3] has questioned the statistical significance of FOWLER and BARER's results.

With regard to the injection of iron, I would emphasise the value of this in steatorrhoea. We have at least one patient with steatorrhoea who apparently absorbs no iron whatsoever when it is given by mouth. The question of pigmentation after intramuscular injection of iron is an important one. We have had one threat of an action for damages, and I know of another case where an action was settled out of court for a substantial sum of money. The patient must therefore be warned of the risk of pigmentation and given the alternative of intravenous injections.

UNDRITZ: The investigations cited by Dr. WITTS, from which the authors concluded that iron does not act solely as a form of replacement therapy but that it has an additional stimulating effect, were carried out with trivalent iron ammonium citrate or reduced metallic iron. The dosage was 1 g. daily. We can say today with certainty that the absorption figure of 37 mg. Fe per day accepted by the authors is far too high. Moreover, their assumption that the higher the serum iron, the greater the amount of iron used for haemoglobin formation, does not necessarily correspond to the facts — as, for example, in hepatitis, hereditary haemoglobinopathies, etc. This consequently invalidates their conclusions regarding the stimulating action of iron. Almost all the "healthy" subjects in the group studied by FOWLER and BARER were anaemic, since haemoglobin values of 8.68 to 11.78 and 8.68 to 10.94, and an average value of 11.53 g.% are well below the norm and in fact

[1] FOWLER, W. M., and A. P. BARER: Amer. J. Med. Sc. **201**, 642 (1941).
[2] WIDDOWSON, E. M.: Lancet (G.B.) **1939**/II, 640.
[3] STURGEON, P.: In: Iron in Clinical Medicine. Ed. by R. O. WALLERSTEIN and S. R. METTIER. University of California Press, 1958, p. 183.

constitute anaemia. In healthy, iron-saturated subjects one does not encounter such low "individual normal values" as those for which the authors believe they have to make allowances. There is only one of their groups which may perhaps have included no subjects suffering from anaemia, i.e. the group with haemoglobin values ranging from 13.33 to 15.74 g. %; unfortunately no details are given about the sex distribution, so that here, too, it is impossible to draw any reliable conclusions.

If individuals receiving a normal diet suffer from anaemia, there must be either a disorder of absorption — due to achylia, for instance — or a regular blood loss, as caused, for example, by an excessively copious menstrual flow. If trivalent iron is given to subjects in whom absorption is disturbed, only a very small amount of iron is absorbed, and its effect is merely temporary. This is due to the absence of hydrochloric acid and of other factors promoting absorption. If patients suffering from chronic loss of iron merely receive supplementary iron, without any attempt being made to discover the cause of the anaemia, the effect of the iron administration is also liable to prove of short duration. Moreover, the preparations administered may quite possibly have deleterious effects on the mucosa of the gastro-intestinal tract. In the dosage mentioned they are liable, like all heavy-metal compounds, to cause gastric and intestinal catarrh. This inevitably leads to a fall in the haemoglobin levels in the course of further iron administration, as described by the investigators. The lack of continued haemoglobin formation in pregnant women can also be explained on the same grounds; another reason is that the affinity of the placenta for iron, when pregnancy is well advanced, is greater than that of the mother's depots and blood-formation centres, with the result that the bulk of the iron absorbed is deposited in the placenta. Stable bivalent iron preparations, especially organic ones, are absorbed even by patients suffering from achylia, and the amount required is 10 to 100 times less than the corresponding quantity of trivalent or metallic iron, particularly in the case of anaemias due to disorders of absorption. What is more, administration of bivalent iron exerts a lasting effect, provided the cause of the anaemia is eliminated. Gastro-intestinal disorders which inhibit further absorption do not as a rule occur. In animal experiments in which adequate oral iron is administered, the type of paradoxical effect reported by FOWLER and BARER never occurs.

I have in addition analysed the cases described in quite a number of such papers — starting with the hypothesis advanced by VON NOORDEN[1] at the end of the last century — and I still see no reason, even on clinical grounds, to depart from the view postulated by SCHMIEDEBERG[2] at the beginning of this century that iron merely serves as material for erythropoiesis and has no stimulant effect on the latter *per se*. One point which must be taken into account is that the situation in man, particularly as regards the absorption of iron from the food ingested, is more complicated than in a straightforward animal experiment. Similarly, pregnancy in humans is also a very complex process: it is my view that the non-physiological signs and symptoms encountered here — e.g. nausea, vomiting, accelerated E.S.R., leucocytosis, regenerative shift to the left of the neutrophils, and sometimes refractory anaemia occurring in the advanced stage in pregnant patients who have received no treatment — are evidence of immunopathological reactions. For this reason, I make it a practice to administer bivalent iron to all expectant mothers from the moment when pregnancy is diagnosed until a few

[1] VON NOORDEN, C.: Berliner klin.-therap. Wschr. **32**, 181 and 214 (1895).
[2] SCHMIEDEBERG, O.: Grundriß der Pharmakologie. Vogel, Leipzig, 1902.

weeks after delivery; in women thus treated I have never observed such pronounced decreases in the haemoglobin values as in patients who have not come for treatment until late in the course of their pregnancy and in whom the haemoglobin sometimes fails to rise in response to therapy.

POLLYCOVE: I should like to make two comments. The first concerns and agrees with Dr. UNDRITZ's statement with regard to the lack of stimulation of erythropoiesis by iron. The primary erythropoietic stimulus in an iron-deficiency anaemia occurs as a result of the anaemia and is not a consequence of the iron administered therapeutically. With a view to understanding the therapeutic action of iron by integrating the results of iron-kinetic studies with the sideroblast measurements of BAINTON and FINCH[1], let us retrace the pathogenesis of iron-deficiency anaemia. As bleeding continues, storage iron is obtained for erythropoiesis by means of a small decrease in the plasma iron concentration. This decrease is not sufficient to affect significantly the rate of iron transfer to immature red cells and the excess labile iron in the red cells. Consequently, erythropoiesis remains normal or increased. The subsequent decrease in serum iron in response to continued blood loss facilitates the transfer of iron from the stores to maintain the plasma iron concentration at a useful level for erythropoiesis. This goes on until finally the stores are exhausted. When the stores are exhausted, the plasma iron concentration decreases to the very low levels characteristic of iron-deficiency anaemia. When transferrin saturation falls below a certain level — this may very well be the 15% saturation level mentioned by Dr. FINCH — then the plasma iron pool is so small that the immature red cells are unable to obtain enough iron per cell from transferrin to maintain normal haemoglobin synthesis. From this point on, then, I think that the immature red cells become progressively more defective and that the intramedullary haemolysis becomes progressively more severe in association with increasing anaemia and increasing erythroid hyperplasia. Iron therapy produces an increase in the plasma iron concentration with adequate plasma-erythropoiesis iron transfer per cell, thereby terminating the intramedullary haemolysis. As a result, the numerous immature red cells now mature normally into reticulocytes, which are released into the circulation with consequent reticulocytosis. The stimulation and the erythroid hyperplasia are both present before iron therapy is instituted, but the cells are defective because the amount of iron per cell is inadequate; this is similar to what occurs — though to a much more severe degree — in pernicious anaemia. The former type of anaemia is the result of a lack of iron, whereas pernicious anaemia is due to a deficiency of vitamin B_{12}. Therapeutic administration of the requisite factor, either iron or vitamin B_{12}, ends the intramedullary haemolysis and results in the release of reticulocytes into the circulation.

The second point I should like to make refers to Dr. FIGUEROA's remarks on the use of Imferon. Following its intramuscular administration we have been impressed by the noxious side effects of skin discoloration and, more especially — even if we bypass the difficult problem of the possible subsequent development of sarcoma — the very annoying and persistent pain, the lymphadenitis, and the fever which occur in a high percentage of our patients. When first administering Imferon intravenously, as WALLERSTEIN[2] had previously done, we proceeded very cautiously, because of early reports in the literature on alarming reactions. Gradually, however, we became more

[1] BAINTON, D. L., and C. A. FINCH: Amer. J. Med. in press (1964).

[2] WALLERSTEIN, R. O.: Clin. Res. (U.S.A.) 8, 105 (1960). — MARCHASIN, S., and R. O. WALLERSTEIN: Blood (U.S.A.) in press (1964).

confident and injected the drug more rapidly; but in a new patient we still take at least three minutes to give 5 ml. (250 mg. iron) intravenously. We have not found even mild reactions, except in extremely rare instances; in fact, in several hundred intravenous injections administered to over 40 patients, I can recall only one reaction, consisting of mild flushing. Subsequently, in this one individual who had slight flushing, we avoided this reaction simply by slowing the injection rate to 5 minutes per 5 ml. Intravenous administration of Imferon appears to be quite safe, and it by-passes the problems of the local and systemic side reactions — discoloration and questionable induction of sarcoma — that are associated with intramuscular administration.

UNDRITZ: I was very interested in the observations and remarks made by Dr. POLLYCOVE, which I can only confirm. In my experience, however, what he has said only holds true provided there is a normal supply of copper; this applies particularly to the utilisation of depot iron for haemoglobin production before the haemoglobin values decrease. If there is a deficiency of copper, the depot iron is withheld, and any iron that is administered also finds its way into the depots, only a small portion being utilised for haemoglobin synthesis. This becomes very obvious from the experiments on rats, in which it is possible to induce a state of copper deficiency by feeding the animals a diet of pure cow's milk. On the other hand, observations to date indicate that in man copper deficiency is extremely rare, so that the sequence of iron utilisation which Dr. POLLYCOVE has outlined, and which we, too, have always accepted as being correct, can be regarded as constituting the rule.

VERLOOP: I should like to ask Dr. FIGUEROA a question about toxic reactions produced by Imferon. Sometimes we have had the impression that a severe haemolytic reaction can occur after Imferon therapy. After we gave 2 g. to a patient with iron deficiency, her haemoglobin decreased sharply, and we thought that this was due to abnormal haemolysis. In another patient with iron-deficiency anaemia we were surprised to find that she had a relapse when given Imferon. We had treated her with Imferon for 4 weeks, after which we interrupted the treatment and then resumed it again. She relapsed quickly, so we thought that perhaps this, too, was a case of abnormal haemolysis probably caused by Imferon. Have you had any experience of haemolytic reactions during or after parenteral iron administration?

FIGUEROA: There is no question that some of these preparations do produce haemolysis *in vitro;* as a matter of fact, this is one of the procedures that investigators such as FIELDING[1] use when determining the amount of ionised iron that is present. Not all the preparations tested have a tendency to produce haemolysis of the red blood cells *in vivo*. One study, for example, has shown that Jectofer has no haemolytic effect in high concentrations, but that, on the contrary, it can even prevent some of the haemolysis produced by other preparations — probably by chelating the excess ionised iron.

GROSS: I should like to ask Dr. FIGUEROA two questions. Firstly: is anything known about the excretion of the iron-carbohydrate complexes, and particularly whether they are eliminated as such through the kidneys? Secondly: are these anaphylactoid reactions due to the iron or are they due to the dextran or to the carbohydrate moiety? Is there any indication that, when these complexes are administered repeatedly, the anaphylactoid

[1] FIELDING, J., and G. M. SMITH: J. Clin. Path. (G.B.) **16**, 12 (1963).

reactions become less pronounced? It could be that they may provoke histamine liberation or the liberation of histamine-like substances, with the result that, when these complexes are given repeatedly, the anaphylactoid reaction may be reduced.

FIGUEROA: My recollection is that with saccharated iron a large amount of the sucrose is excreted in the urine during the first 24—36 hours, whereas only a small fraction of the iron is excreted, i.e. probably less than 0.2% of the dose. As for the iron-citric-acid-sorbitol complex, I understand that, owing to its low molecular weight of under 5,000, the whole complex is excreted in the urine in amounts equivalent to approximately 30% of the administered dose in 24 hours. The urine during the first few hours following administration of the dose is fairly dark.

With regard to anaphylactoid reactions, these are probably due to the dextran moiety, as some patients will develop reactions to the dextran alone. But, in one or two instances, patients who developed reactions to Imferon did not develop a reaction to dextran, so it may be a combination of both.

SALERA: As to whether or not iron provides a stimulus for erythropoiesis, I think that first of all one has to define what one means by stimulation. By studying the peripheral blood we can, in fact, only determine the consequences resulting from stimulation or inhibition of erythropoiesis. But if we analyse the elementary phenomena occurring in the bone marrow, we have to distinguish between at least three fundamental processes, namely differentiation, maturation, and proliferation. I do not believe that the iron is capable of influencing differentiation, i.e. that it can affect the processes by which the stem cell develops into an erythropoietic cell; this process is influenced by erythropoietin. On the other hand, iron does constitute an indispensable constructive material for the formation of haemoglobin. To this extent, then, we may regard iron as exerting a stimulant action on the maturation of the erythropoietic cells. When iron is administered to an organism suffering from iron deficiency, maturation of the erythroblasts is accelerated, because the iron thus supplied is a material which enables haemoglobin formation to occur. I think this is the idea that Dr. UNDRITZ is propounding.

This brings me to the question of proliferation. Fifteen years ago I did some work together with Dr. ASTALDI[1] in the laboratory of the Medical Clinic at the University of Pavia. In the course of this work we carried out some experiments on the proliferation and maturation of erythropoietic cells cultivated *in vitro*. We found that the erythroblasts of patients suffering from iron-deficiency anaemia matured more slowly than normal when they were cultivated in the same patient's plasma, and that this defect could be corrected by cultivating the erythroblasts in the plasma of a healthy subject. However, it was not possible to demonstrate that culturing the erythroblasts in normal plasma stimulated their proliferation. I do not therefore believe that the presence of iron can constitute a stimulus to the proliferation of erythroblasts.

UNDRITZ: I think Dr. SALERA's bone-marrow studies are very informative and that, from the morphological aspect, they shed further light on the concept of erythropoiesis stimulation. His findings form a welcome supplement to the broad outline of facts known to date; in particular they also tally well with our own observations that in iron-deficiency anaemia the increase in haemoglobin in response to iron therapy is not a sign that erythropoiesis is being stimulated, as postulated according to the classic concept, but that this

[1] ASTALDI, G., C. MAURI, and U. SALERA: Rev. hémat. (Fr.) **5**, 634 (1950).

increase tends, if anything, to occur at a time when erythropoiesis is already diminishing, as the signs of stimulation are all the more intensive the greater the iron deficiency and the more severe the anaemia. On the other hand, the classic signs of stimulation can still be accepted as valid; these include erythrocytosis, which is either relative or (as in chlorosis) absolute, pro-erythrocytosis, often wrongly referred to as "reticulocytosis", and normoblastosis of the bone marrow and, in laboratory animals, of the spleen as well.

And now I should just like, if I may, to revert to the question of parenteral iron therapy. It has been rightly emphasised that parenteral iron therapy should only be undertaken in exceptional cases when iron is absolutely necessary and cannot be administered by mouth.

Together with BETTINA FRAENKEL[1] I carried out tests on the production of localised sarcomas in the rat by long-term intramuscular injection of organic iron preparations. The results of these tests confirm Dr. FIGUEROA's view, particularly with regard to the dangers of intramuscular injection.

The normal life-span of our albino rats ranges from $1^1/_2$ to $3^1/_2$ years, 50% of the animals barely attaining an age of 2 years.

708 rats were given weekly injections of iron preparations into the flexor muscle of the left limb. 122 rats served as controls. The experiment was continued throughout the life-span of the animals, in some cases for more than three years. The following iron-carbohydrate preparations were studied: inulin, sinistrin, starch, two dextrans, and 10 dextrins of our own manufacture; two proprietary preparations, a dextran and a polyisomaltose, were also included. We have not yet been able to test iron sorbitol for its sarcoma-inducing effect, because this preparation was only recently introduced and the experiment takes at least three years. The occurrence of an iron-induced sarcoma at the injection site in response to an unphysiologically high dosage of this preparation, however, has been reported.

All the compounds induced local sarcomas at the site of injection, these being the only sarcomas that were taken into account. The maximum single dose in man is 250 mg. iron. According to the literature, a pregnant woman with a haemoglobin level of 30% (= 5 g.%) and a body-weight of 60 kg. requires a total of 3,650 mg. iron = 6.1 mg./100 g. body-weight, if we calculate for the weight of the rats. A premature baby weighing 2 kg. needs a total of 250 mg. iron = 12.5 mg./100 g.

The iron compounds were administered at three dosage levels:

A) An excessively high dosage of 20 mg. Fe/animal = approx. 7 mg. Fe/100 g./week (Fig. 1). 212 rats received this dose up to 78 times. The first sarcoma occurred within 3 months, i.e. after 13 injections amounting to a total of 87 mg. Fe/100 g. had been administered. The last animal developed a sarcoma after 78 injections (totalling 520 mg./100 g. administered over a period of 534 days); the sarcoma in this animal developed 260 days after the treatment had been stopped — i.e. 794 days, or 2 years and 2 months, after the beginning of treatment. It died 2 months later, after 857 days (2 years and 4 months). The sarcoma rate is as high as 80% in animals which are young when selected for the experiment.

B) A dose corresponding to the single therapeutic dose in man, i.e. 0.35 mg. *Fe/100* g.*/week* (Fig. 2). The total dose/100 g. body-weight exceeded that which would be administered to a patient, since as many as up to 148 injections were given. The group comprised 252 rats. The first sarcoma occurred after 614 days (1 year and 8 months), i.e. following 87 injections totalling

[1] UNDRITZ, E., and B. FRAENKEL: Proceedings of the 9th Congress of the European Society of Haematology, Lisbon, 1963.

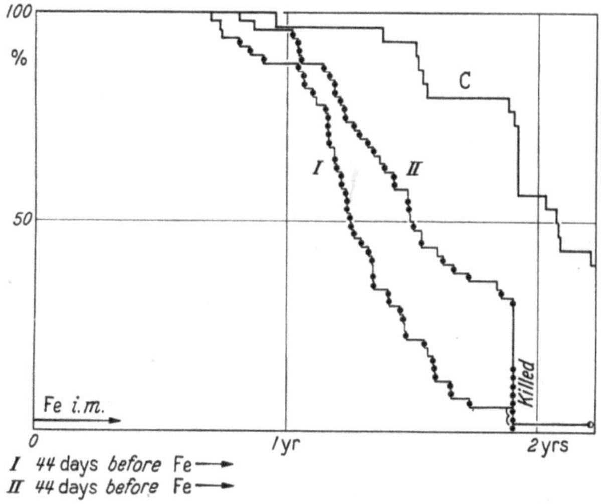

Fig. 1. Mortality rate of rats treated intramuscularly with 7 mg. iron/100 g./week in the form either of a commercial preparation of iron-dextran (I) or of iron-dextrin (II). Tumour rate in group I (50 animals): 80%; in group II (50 animals): 68%. C = controls (30 animals)

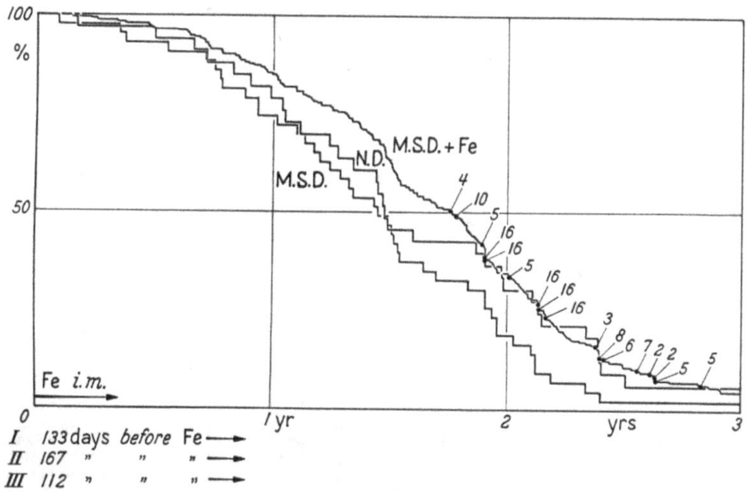

Fig. 2. Mortality rate of rats treated with a therapeutic dose of iron (0.35 mg./100 g./week i.m.) and receiving various diets. N.D. = normal diet (33 animals); M.S.D. = milk-semolina diet (43 animals); M.S.D. + Fe = milk-semolina diet plus various iron-carbohydrate preparations (252 animals); I, II, III: experiment started at three different dates.
The reference figures adjacent to the curve for M.S.D. + Fe indicate the iron preparations which the animals were receiving when a tumour appeared at the corresponding date (1: Fe-inulin; 2: Fe-sinistrin; 3 and 4: Fe-dextrans; 5 and 6: commercial preparations of Fe-dextran; 7: Fe-starch; 8—16: Fe-dextrin)
Percentage of tumours occurring in the total group: 7.1% (17 out of 240); percentage of tumours occurring in the animals still alive at the time of appearance of the first tumour: 14.9% (17 out of 114)

30 mg. Fe/100 g. By this time 50% of the rats had died. Of the 242 dead animals, 18 had developed localised sarcomas, a sarcoma rate which works out at 7.5%. The last sarcoma occurred on the 1,081st day, i.e. after 3 years. This animal received 122 injections, totalling 42.7 mg./100 g., over a period of 858 days (2 years and 4 months). The sarcoma developed 223 days (7 months) after the last injection. The experiments have not yet been concluded in 10 animals.

C) A subtherapeutic single dose of 0.07 mg. Fe/100 g./week administered up to 141 times in 164 rats (Fig. 3). In this group only 2 sarcomas were observed, since most of the animals died. The first sarcoma occurred after 949 days (2 years and 7 months), i.e. 91 days after the end of the treatment. This animal had received 122 injections, totalling 8.5 mg. Fe/100 g., i.e. *a total dose corresponding to that given in man* (see above). The second animal to develop a sarcoma had likewise received a total dose of 8.96 mg./100 g., which is also equivalent to the total dose in man. Seven animals were then still surviving; hence the sarcoma rate *from the first occurrence* was 28.6%, or 1.2% of all 164 rats. Experiments on a series of 80 animals have not yet been concluded.

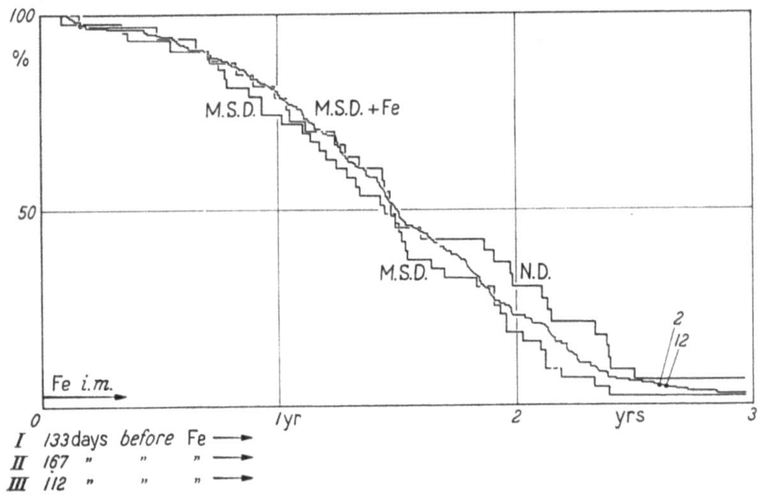

Fig. 3. Mortality rate of rats treated with a subtherapeutic dose of iron (0.07 mg./100 g./week i.m.) and receiving various diets. N.D. = normal diet (33 animals); M.S.D. = milk-semolina diet (43 animals); M.S.D. + Fe = milk-semolina diet plus various iron-carbohydrate preparations (244 animals, in 80 of which the experiments have not yet been concluded); I, II, III: experiment started at three different dates.

Reference figures for the preparations as in Fig. 2

Percentage of tumours occurring in the total group: 1.2% (2 out of 164); percentage of tumours occurring in the animals still alive at the time of appearance of the first tumour: 28.6% (2 out of 7)

The rats in group A were on a normal diet. Those in groups B and C received a milk-semolina diet, poor in iron so as to render the experimental conditions more closely similar to those in human iron-deficiency anaemia.

Our tests show that, when conducting animal experiments designed to demonstrate the sarcomagenic effect of intramuscular injections of iron, it is not sufficient to prolong the tests for one year only, as most investigators have done in the past. Since the smaller the dosage, the longer the time that elapses before the sarcomas appear, sarcomas do not develop for 2—3 years in rats subjected to repeated treatment with therapeutic and subtherapeutic doses.

Our experimental procedure differs from the usual methods adopted for the treatment of human beings inasmuch as the latter receive only a small number of injections. On the other hand, injections of 200 mg. Fe, for example, each impose a far greater strain per unit of muscle in the human being than in the rat, although the muscle areas are far larger. In our tests, however, the animals received far more injections than human beings — with rare exceptions — have ever received, even though the total dose employed for the tests at subtherapeutic levels does correspond, in relation to body-weight, to the total dose received by human beings. The number of stimuli resulting from the repeated injections in rats is far higher, and the injections were always given at approximately the same site.

We agree with HADDOW[1] when he says: "From the nature of the case we cannot have a useful answer to this question under something of the order of 15—20 years. The statistics of the hazard (if indeed it exists in man) are quite unknown. We cannot therefore say it is negligible." With respect to their delayed appearance, iron-induced tumours may behave similarly to thorium-induced tumours, if the results of iron injections in animal experiments can be applied to man. The sarcomagenic effect is also dependent on the preparation used. For example, our results confirm the observations reported by other authors that the tumours occur later with iron-dextrin than with iron-dextran. Perhaps one day an iron compound will be found which does not exert any sarcomagenic effect following intramuscular injection and is in fact well tolerated locally.

Local iron-induced tumours in the rat metastasise, but only at a later stage. If local tumours should occur in human beings as a result of intramuscular iron injections — of which millions must have been administered by now — our experience in rats suggests that immediate surgical removal of the region affected is likely to prevent metastasisation and to stop the development of fatal sarcomas.

---

[1] HADDOW, A.: Brit. Med. J. **1960**/II, 664.

Physiopathologic mechanisms of iron excretion

By

C. A. Finch

Almost 30 years ago, McCance and Widdowson (*18*) marshaled evidence that the excretion of iron was a limited process. Further data have accumulated since then to indicate that maintenance of the iron balance is more dependent on the absorption than on the elimination of iron from the body through normal channels. As a result, iron has become known as a one-way substance which remains in the body once absorbed. Such a "no loss" concept has proved eminently satisfactory to the clinician, for it properly focuses attention on bleeding as the usual explanation for iron-deficiency anemia.

Admitting that iron excretion is restricted, our first purpose today is to attempt to define as rigorously as possible the losses which do occur. In the male, such losses are found in the feces, urine, or shed integument. In respect to *fecal iron* both chemical and isotopic data are of interest. Ordinarily, chemical balance techniques permit measurement of the balance between oral intake and fecal output only, without disclosing the amount of iron exchange within the intestinal tract. The close relationship, however, between the amount fed and recovered over a large range of iron intake in itself suggests that the intake by this route is limited (Fig. 1). Further, by reducing the intake to low levels, it is possible to estimate the loss. Ingalls and Johnston (*14*) fed diets of 1, 2, and 3 mg./day and attempted to estimate excretion from a regression line extended

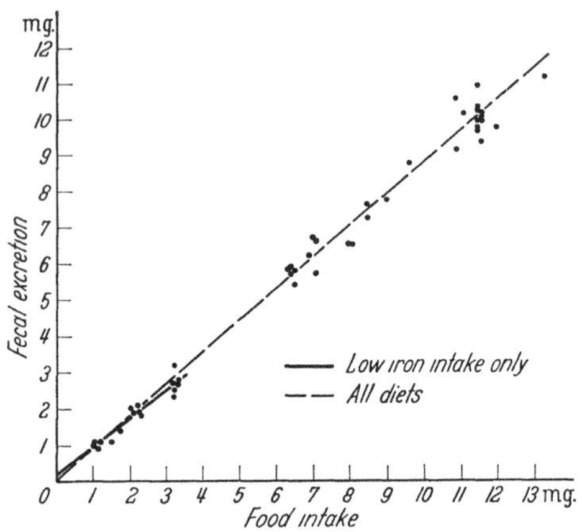

Fig. 1. Chemical iron-balance studies [from Ingalls and Johnston (*14*)]

to zero iron intake. While their 8-day balance periods may have been too short, their value of 0.2 mg./day for the 8 women studied is impressively low. DUBACH, MOORE, and CALLENDER (*6*) injected radio-iron and estimated iron excretion from the amount of isotope in the feces. Their estimate in the 3 men studied was about 0.4 mg./day. In the conversion of isotope in the feces to the amount of iron lost, it was assumed that measurement over 140 days would permit mixing and that the 5.6 mg. of iron ascorbate injected intravenously would be handled physiologically. In this calculation I have chosen their estimate of red-cell mass, as determined by the Evans blue dye, uncorrected for mean body hematocrit to represent the miscible iron pool, since it corresponds reasonably closely to that defined by the isotope dilution technique (*9*). Both types of information would place loss from the intestinal tract at less than 0.5 mg. iron/day.

There is reasonable agreement that *urinary losses* are insignificant, being about 0.05 mg./day in the normal subject (*3*, *11*, *21*).

Integumental loss of iron is at present a matter of some debate. While hair and nail losses amount to no more than 1 to 5 μg./day (*6*, *16*), a number of chemical analyses suggest that sweat losses may amount to several mg./day (*5*). The fact that such iron resides largely in the cellular sediment of the sweat alters not at all the implications of such losses in respect to the iron balance. However, are such chemical measurements physiologically valid? One could suggest that dermal loss may be as easily derived from external contamination as from actual iron excretion. Isotope studies should be useful in differentiating the source of sweat iron, and DUBACH et al. (*6*) have attempted this. Radioactive iron was found in the sweat in small amounts, and their calculations suggest that this could represent no more than 1 mg./day with continuous sweating.

While it is recognized that information concerning fecal and especially dermal losses is inadequate, the difficulties in measuring all the iron excreted and exfoliated from the body are evident. It is likely that the composite loss of iron will be more accurately determined by following *total-body radio-iron turnover*. It would be convenient to measure this by employing a total-body counter, but, unfortunately, the short half-life of Fe^{59} limits the duration of follow-up and does not permit uniform labeling of body iron. Results of 0.1 to 0.2%/day, published by PRICE and associates (*22*) with this isotope, seem unrealistically high when compared with other information. A preliminary report by SAITO et al. (*25*) summarizes a more extensive study employing this technique on 6 normal male subjects over a period of 200 to 300 days.

The average loss was 0.04% of the radio-iron daily. This should be equivalent to about 1.2 mg./day if one assumes complete mixing of injected radio-iron with total-body iron. One must be concerned about the degree of isotope mixing in these studies as well as in those by DUBACH and associates (*6*).

A more likely way of obtaining accurate measurements of total-body iron turnover is through the use of Fe^{55}, with blood sampling over prolonged periods of time (*9*, *24*). Data were obtained in 3 small groups of subjects over a period of 5 years. After a period of 12 to 18 months, blood radioactivity appeared to decline as a simple exponential function, which in the male amounted to 8% annually, in the non-menstruating female to 10%, and in the menstruating female to 20%. On the basis of certain assumptions concerning the miscible iron pool, these percentages are equivalent to a loss in the male and in the non-menstruating female of 0.6 mg./day and in the menstruating woman to a loss of twice this value. These data are not above criticism. The initial studies were technically of questionable quality and carried out on inmates of a mental institution. Since many of these individuals were inactive, it would seem possible that the usual sweat losses might not be adequately represented. Because of this, further studies are in progress on 14 male subjects who are active workers in the temperate zone. The rate of loss of radioactivity from the circulation appears to be similar to that of the original group of men (Fig. 2). We would believe that this reasonably establishes total iron losses in man in the temperate zone at about 0.6 mg./day.

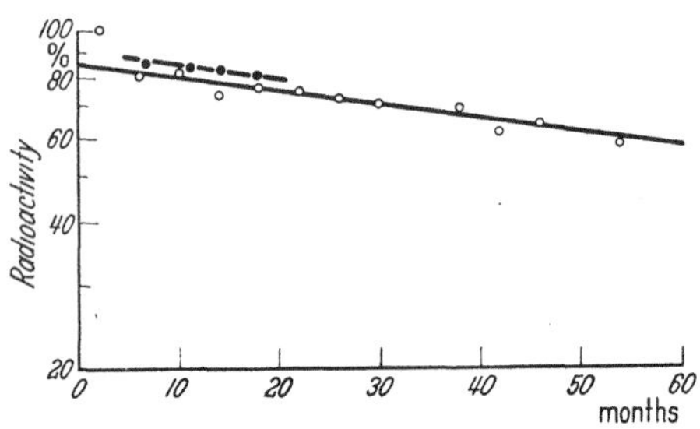

Fig. 2. Body turnover of radio-iron in man. The open circles are from a previous report (*9*); the solid dots are from current studies. Both show a decline in radioactivity of about 8% per year

The woman has other losses superimposed on those already discussed for the male. A tabulation of pregnancy requirements includes an outlay of perhaps 280 mg. for the fetus and 150 mg. for the placenta and blood loss at delivery. Thus, the requirement of pregnancy, plus basal losses, represents an average of about 1.8 mg./day (*2*), although this increases progressively from 0.6 to 4.0 mg./day through pregnancy. Lactation involves about 0.5 mg./day (*8*), but this loss may often be offset by the presence of amenorrhea.

Menstrual bleeding is a much more variable avenue of blood loss. Average values based on direct analysis of menses have been estimated at 0.8 mg. iron/day (*20*), which is not too different from the 0.6 mg. difference between menstruating and non-menstruating women as calculated from the red-cell radio-iron turnover (*9*). However, there is a variation in menstrual iron loss from person to person, and in some women the loss is considerable. For example, FRENCHMAN and JOHNSTON (*10*) found 14% of the women they studied to have a menstrual iron loss of 1.2 mg./day or more, and RANKIN et al. (*23*) found an average daily iron loss of 2.3 mg. in 20 women with the complaint of menorrhagia. Thus, average menstruation doubles the male iron loss, pregnancy triples it, and menorrhagia entails an even greater loss.

Let us now examine the extent to which excretion may regulate the iron balance. Earlier studies gave no indication of an ability to actively excrete iron. For example, McCANCE and WIDDOWSON (*19*) found no evidence of excessive iron excretion in a woman with hemolytic anemia receiving the equivalent of 80 mg. iron/day by transfusion. Her daily oral iron intake was 5.6 mg., and her output in the feces 4.9 and in the urine 0.3, representing a positive balance of 0.4 mg./day. Others have obtained similar results after the injection of parenteral iron (*17*). However, the chemical balance technique may not be sufficiently sensitive for our purpose. Isotope experiments in animals (*4*) suggested that iron losses are modified according to the body iron content of the animal (Fig. 3). The conversion of isotope data to iron losses in this study was predicated on the basis of uniform mixing of radio-iron with total-body iron. While this probably occurred with iron depletion, it is unlikely with iron overload. The greater conservation of iron in iron deficiency is supported by clinical data. DUBACH et al. (*6*) have reported a marked reduction in the fecal excretion of iron in 3 patients with iron-deficiency anemia (Fig. 4), and HUSSAIN and PATWARDHAN (*13*) have shown a reduced iron content of desquamated skin in iron-

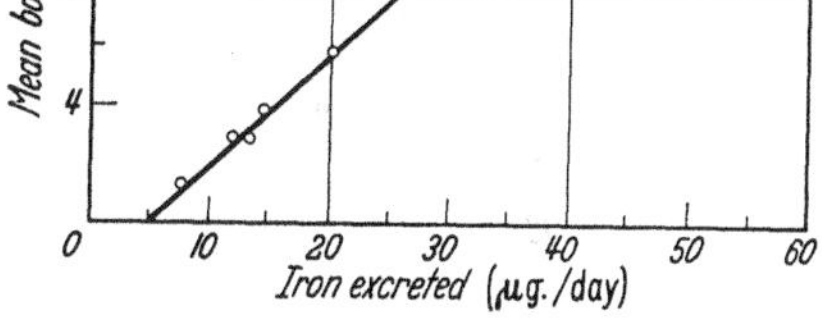

Fig. 3. Relation of total-body iron to iron loss as determined from body iron turnover of radio-iron and body iron content in mice [from CHAPPELLE et al. (*4*)]

deficiency anemia. There seems to be little question that iron loss will be modified according to body iron content, but at the present time it is difficult to place this on an absolute scale, particularly in respect to the maximum amount of iron which may be lost.

Another way to examine the ease with which an altered iron balance regains normalcy is shown in the following experiment (Table 1) (*1*). Two individuals were bled in order to deplete the body iron stores, and two other individuals were injected with parenteral iron to enlarge the stores. In the subsequent 2 years, the absorption of iron was measured on several occasions, and a rough calculation of dietary iron absorption was made. The 4 individuals were then phlebotomized until iron deficiency was produced. Calculations could then be made to determine the extent to which excretion and absorption had contributed to the regaining of a normal iron balance. The evidence suggested that the iron stores had been reconstituted through absorption much more easily than they had been reduced through excretion. So again it appears that there is no effective mechanism for rapidly reducing excessive stores.

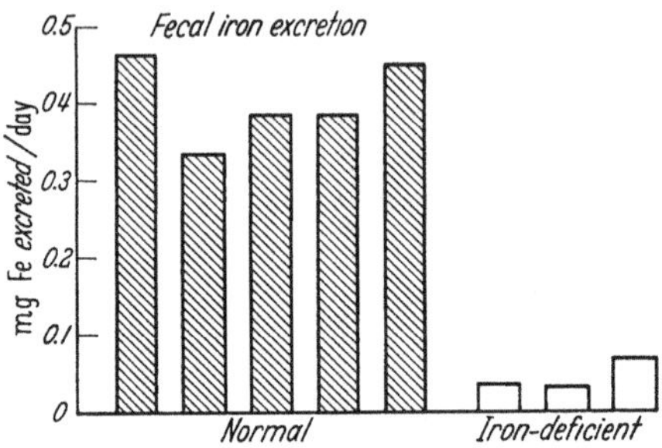

Fig. 4. Fecal iron excretion as calculated from radio-iron loss [from DUBACH et al. (*6*)]

Table 1. *Regulation of body iron stores* (figures in mg.)

	Depletion (2 subjects)	Overload (2 subjects)
Existing stores	(1,250)	(1,250)
Alteration	—1,250	+1,400
Initial size	0	2,650
Recovery after 2 years	1,300	2,100
Total balance	+1,300	— 550
Daily balance	+ 2.2	— 1.0
Absorption	3.0	0.6
Excretion	0.8	1.2

In pathologic states of negative iron balance, *bleeding* occupies a dominant position. Only bleeding appears to be responsible for a negative iron balance in excess of 2 mg./day, and since the diet can generally supply this amount and more, blood loss is the usual reason for iron-deficiency anemia after childhood. The causes of bleeding are too numerous to mention, but the delicate mucosa of the gastro-intestinal tract and uterus should be singled out as particularly vulnerable. Menorrhagia and gastro-intestinal bleeding frequently escape detection. We were embarrassed to find that, among the adult patients with iron-deficiency anemia on whom we took careful histories and whose stools we tested for occult blood, at least one-third had pathologic bleeding which had at first escaped detection. Worthy of particular mention, because of its uniqueness, is bleeding into the pulmonary alveoli. Iron so deposited is not reclaimed by the body, and one finds pulmonary siderosis associated with iron deficiency.

Other varieties of iron loss are more restricted and are thus not in themselves a cause of iron deficiency. One consists of protein leaks, as in nephrosis or perhaps protein-losing gastro-enteropathies. Since the molecular weight of transferrin is only about 90,000, it is to be expected that it may resemble albumin in the ease with which it traverses damaged blood vessels. Losses of iron bound to transferrin have been reported as amounting to up to 1 mg. (*3*). Finally, iron-laden cells may be desquamated from the body. THIRAYOTHIN and CROSBY (*27*) have emphasized the possible importance of reticulo-endothelial cells migrating from the intestinal villi into the lumen of the gut.

The multiple mechanisms which may be involved in iron loss, and their complexity, are well illustrated by the intestinal tract. There is a daily exfoliation of perhaps 50 g. of epithelial cells. Their iron may be derived both from absorption – which means that the iron in question therefore really never gets into the body – and from iron transported to these cells from transferrin. The iron-containing macrophages, which appear to migrate into the intestinal lumen from the villi, may also either have derived their iron from the influx of absorbed iron or may carry out iron which has been within the body. Another source of iron is loss of blood into the feces, which has been variably estimated at from 0.1 to 1.2 mg./day (*7*, *24*). Secretions may also contain some iron, and of these bile is probably the most important. Bile contains approximately 0.1 mg. iron/100 ml. (*15*, *28*) and probably more in hemolytic anemia (*12*). Its iron content is not greatly increased in experimental iron overload. Reabsorption of some of the iron lost into the gut probably occurs to further complicate the picture.

Further discussion of the complexities of evaluating iron losses would serve little purpose. Rather we would hope to formulate a general statement of iron losses and their nature. These might best be tabulated into 3 general categories:

(1) Iron losses through protein leaks, bile, and other secretions. These appear to be limited to less than 1 mg./day and may therefore be disregarded.

(2) Placental transport of iron, which in late pregnancy may exceed the amount of iron absorbed from a poor diet, i.e. 3 or 4 mg./day.

(3) Loss of body cells. It is this category which is largely responsible for a negative iron balance. The tissues of high iron content are the erythrocytes and reticulo-endothelial cells, which normally contain over 80% of body iron and have an iron concentration of about 1,000 μg./g. of tissue. In the normal individual other body tissues contain perhaps 5 to 10 μg. of iron/g. of tissue. This hundredfold difference places cellular losses in perspective. Desquamation losses amounting to perhaps 50 to 60 g. of low-iron tissues may then account for the normal male loss of 0.6 mg./day. This amount may further vary, as the iron content of such cells is altered in iron deficiency and iron overload, over a range of perhaps 2 mg. While the exact figure is a matter of opinion, there is no convincing evidence that physiologic or pathologic losses other than those involving red-cell iron and placental transit can exceed this figure.

Finally, it has been possible to manipulate iron losses by removing erythrocytes, since in the replacement of the lost blood by new cells, iron is withdrawn from tissue stores. Iron losses produced by phlebotomy in the patient with idiopathic hemochromatosis amount to 30 mg./day or more. Recently, with the development of chelating agents, a new mechanism of iron excretion has become available. A chelating agent such as desferrioxamine appears to compete with transferrin for iron on the surface of parenchymal and reticulo-endothelial cells in patients with iron overload. Urinary iron losses achieved by the use of such agents amount to approximately 15 mg./day over long periods of time. Thus, there are two therapeutic devices for implementing the very restricted capacity of the body to lose iron.

Summary

Available evidence indicates a highly restricted iron loss, amounting to approximately 0.6 mg./day in normal man and to double or triple this in woman during her reproductive period. Basal iron losses in man are largely due to exfoliated cells. While there is evidence of modest alterations in iron loss in parallel with the total-body iron content, this range appears small. The only demonstrated pathologic mechanism of quantitative importance in implementing iron loss is red-cell or hemoglobin loss. Therapeutic means of releasing iron from the body in iron overload include phlebotomy and treatment with chelating agents.

Zusammenfassung

Die vorhandenen Daten ergeben einen sehr geringen täglichen Eisenverlust beim Normalen, der beim Mann ungefähr 0,6 mg. und bei der Frau während der Zeugungsperiode etwa das Zwei- bis Dreifache beträgt. Der hauptsächliche regelmäßige Eisenverlust erfolgt durch Zellabschilferung. Zwar liegen Hinweise dafür vor, daß geringe Abweichungen in der Eisenabgabe in Beziehung zum gesamten Eisenbestand stehen, doch dürfte der dafür in Betracht kommende Bereich nur sehr eng sein. Der einzige sicher nachgewiesene pathologische Mechanismus, der quantitativ für das Auftreten einer negativen Eisenbilanz ins Gewicht fällt, ist ein Verlust von Erythrozyten oder von Haemoglobin. Aderlaß und die Anwendung von spezifischen Komplexbildnern sind die heute verfügbaren Maßnahmen, um übermäßig im Organismus gespeichertes Eisen zu entfernen.

Résumé

L'élimination quotidienne de fer est très limitée, s'élevant approximativement à 0,6 mg. par jour chez l'homme normal et à deux ou trois fois plus chez la femme en période d'activité génitale. Les pertes de base de fer chez l'homme sont en grande partie dues à l'exfoliation cellulaire. Bien qu'il existe de discrètes variations dans l'élimination du fer, parallèlement à la charge totale de fer de l'organisme, cette marge de variations est étroite. Le seul mécanisme pathologique démontré ayant une certaine importance quantitative dans l'accroissement des pertes de fer est la perte d'hématies ou d'hémoglobine. Les possibilités thérapeutiques d'enlever le fer d'un organisme en hypersidérose comprennent les saignées et les agents chélatants.

References

1. Bothwell, T. H., and C. A. Finch: Iron Metabolism. Little, Brown & Co., Boston, 1962, p. 126. — 2. Bothwell. T. H., and C. A. Finch: Iron Metabolism. Little, Brown & Co., Boston, 1962, p. 308. — 3. Cartwright, G. E., C. J. Gubler, and M. M. Wintrobe: J. Clin. Invest. (U.S.A.) **33**, 685 (1954). — 4. Chappelle, E., B. W. Gabrio, A. R. Stevens, Jr., and C. A. Finch: Amer. J. Physiol. **182**, 390 (1955). — 5. Consolazio, C. F., L. O. Matoush, R. E. Nelson, R. S. Harding, and J. E. Canham: J. Nutrit. (U.S.A.) **79**, 407 (1963). — 6. Dubach, R., C. V. Moore, and S. T. Callender: J. Laborat. Clin. Med. (U.S.A.) **45**, 599 (1955). — 7. Ebaugh, F. G., T. Clemens, G. Rodnan, and R. E. Peterson: Amer. J. Med. **25**, 169 (1958). — 8. Fenillen, Y. M., and M. Plumier: Acta paediatr. (Sweden) **41**, 138 (1952). — 9. Finch, C. A.: J. Clin. Invest. (U.S.A.) **38**, 392 (1959). — 10. Frenchman, R., and F. A. Johnston: J. Amer. Diet. Ass. **25**, 217 (1949). — 11. Gisinger, E., and H. Puxkandl: Wien. Zschr. inn. Med. **9**, 491 (1955). — 12. Hawkins, W. B., and P. F. Hahn: J. Exper. Med. (U.S.A.) **80**, 31 (1944). — 13. Hussain, R., V. N. Patwardhan, and S. Sriramachari: Indian J. Med. Res. **48**, 235 (1960). — 14. Ingalls, R. L., and F. A. Johnston: J. Nutrit. (U.S.A.) **53**, 351 (1954). — 15. Jasinsky, B., and O. Roth: Larvierte Eisenmangelkrankheit. Benno Schwabe & Co., Basle, 1954. — 16. Johnston, F. A.: Amer. J. Clin. Nutrit. **6**, 136 (1958). — 17. Little, A. G., Jr., M. H. Power, and E. G. Wakefield: Ann. Int. Med. (U.S.A.) **23**, 627 (1945). — 18. McCance, R. A., and E. M. Widdowson: Lancet (G.B.) **233**, 680 (1937). — 19. McCance, R. A., and E. M. Widdowson: Nature (G.B.)

152, 326 (1943). — 20. MILLIS, J.: Med. J. Australia **1951/II**, 874. — 21. PLOTNER, K.: 5. Kongreß der Europäischen Gesellschaft für Hämatologie, Springer, Berlin/Göttingen/Heidelberg, 1956, p. 164. — 22. PRICE, D. C., S. H. COHN, L. R. WASSERMAN, P. G. REIZENSTEIN, and E. P. CRONKITE: Blood (U.S.A.) **20**, 517 (1962). — 23. RANKIN, G. L. S., N. VEALL, R. G. HUNTSMAN, and J. LIDDELL: Lancet (G.B.) **1962/I**, 567. — 24. ROCHE, M., M. E. PEREZ-GIMENEZ, M. LAYRISSE, and E. DIPRISCO: J. Clin. Invest. (U.S.A.) **36**, 1183 (1957). — 25. SAITO, H., T. S. SARGENT, G. PARKER, and J. H. LAURENCE: Abstract. Soc. of Nuclear Med., June 26, 1963. — 26. STEVENS, A. R., Jr., P. L. WHITE, D. M. HEGSTED, and C. A. FINCH: J. Biol. Chem. (U.S.A.) **203**, 161 (1953). — 27. THIRAYOTHIN, P., and W. H. CROSBY: J. Clin. Invest. (U.S.A.) **41**, 1206 (1962). — 28. VANNOTTI, A., and A. DELACHAUX: Iron Metabolism. Grune & Stratton, New York, 1949.

Discussion

BEUTLER: I have been quite interested, Dr. FINCH, in information of the type which you cited on the decrease in the iron loss in iron deficiency. I have sometimes used this as evidence that there may be a decrease in tissue-iron enzyme content. On the other hand, the concept you introduced — that some of this iron loss might be due to loss of reticulo-endothelial cells, which are relatively heavily laden with iron, or of red blood cells — is also a real possibility that ought to be considered. I wonder whether we have any knowledge as to the relative proportions in which what you refer to as iron-rich and iron-poor cells are present among the desquamated cells in the gastro-intestinal tract or in the sweat.

NAJEAN: Could I ask Dr. FINCH if the urinary excretion of iron represents free iron or transferrin-bound iron? I ask this question because I tried to measure the urinary excretion of iron by an isotope technique which gives only the transferrin-bound iron excreted by the kidney. I don't know if this represents the total amount of iron excreted per day or only a part of it.

PETERS: What would be, approximately, the total daily iron loss in a normal rat, a normal dog, or a normal rabbit? How much iron is, in fact, lost in the urine in severe cases of the nephrotic syndrome? What is the degree of saturation of urinary transferrin?

POLLYCOVE: I should like to agree with, and emphasise, Dr. FINCH's statement that blood loss is almost always the aetiologic basis of iron-deficiency anaemia, and I would add that even in children and infants this is also usually the case. Several years ago, HOAG, WALLERSTEIN, and myself[1] studied a number of infants in the first year of life with iron-deficiency anaemia of under 9 g. Hb./100 ml. By labelling circulating cells with radio-iron and collecting all stools for 30 days we demonstrated that within one month a gastro-intestinal blood loss equivalent to more than 4.5—18% of the blood volume occurred. In iron-deficient adult patients who, as Dr. FINCH mentioned, have been repeatedly examined and in whom many tests for occult blood in the stools, as well as X-ray examinations, have yielded negative findings, it is frequently concluded that blood loss is not a significant aetiologic factor in the development of the anaemia. Nevertheless, with but one exception, all such cases which we investigated by means of radio-iron and stool collection or whole-body counting showed a blood loss sufficient to account for the existing iron-deficiency anaemia. A reduction in iron absorption large enough to result in moderate to severe iron-deficiency anaemia in the absence of blood loss is a very rare occurrence in the United States.

Though it is true that over a year is required for approximation of uniform labelling of body iron in humans, and that PRICE et al.[2], using a whole-body

---

[1] HOAG, M. S., R. O. WALLERSTEIN, and M. POLLYCOVE: Pediatrics (U.S.A.) **27**, 199 (1961).

[2] PRICE, D. C., S. H. COHN, L. R. WASSERMAN, P. G. REIZENSTEIN, and E. P. CRONKITE: Blood (U.S.A.) **20**, 517 (1962).

counter, have reported a surprisingly high "normal" radio-iron loss of 0.0014 per day during the first 20—100 days after ingestion of radio-iron, a good estimate of the daily iron loss can nevertheless be obtained with the whole-body counter if the relationship of counting efficiency to body radio-iron distribution is taken into account. Using this approach, SAITO and his associates[1] in our laboratory have made serial measurements for almost a year in 10 normal volunteers, as shown in Fig. 1. The measured fractional rate of loss of body radio-iron was not more than 0.0003 per day. When this daily fractional loss is related to a labelled

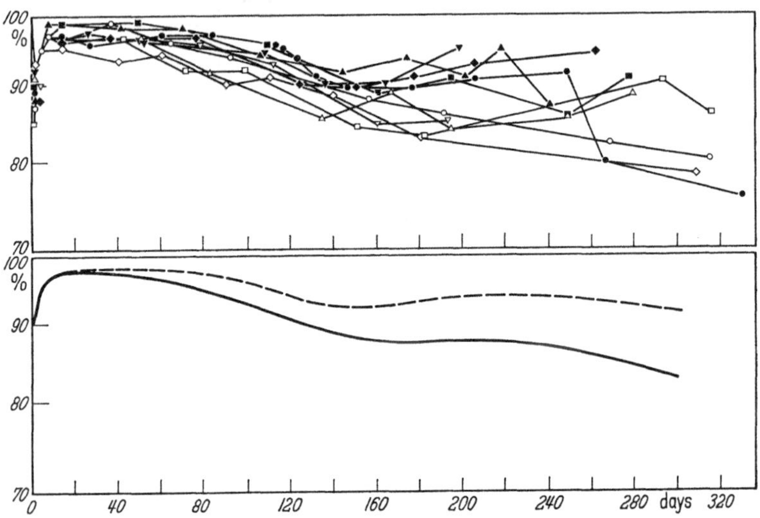

Fig. 1. Total radio-iron in 10 normal subjects measured with a whole-body counter after a single intravenous injection of 20 μc. plasma transferrin-bound radio-iron. The counting rate obtained 5 min. after injection is taken as 100%. ——— average of the experimental data obtained in 10 normal subjects. - - - - - - calculated counting rate in the absence of radio-iron loss, showing the changes resulting from the movement of radio-iron through the marrow and its distribution between blood and storage iron

iron pool of 3,000 mg. (2,400 mg. haemoglobin iron measured by red-cell volume, haemoglobin, and haematocrit determinations, plus 600 mg. labelled miscible storage iron as estimated by FINCH), an iron loss of not more than 0.9 mg./day is obtained. This is in reasonable agreement with absorption measurements performed in these same subjects (9% of a 4 mg. dose of elemental iron, or an expected value of less than 1.35 mg./day from 15 mg. of *dietary* iron per day) as well as with the absorption measurements of other investigators and the older chemical iron-balance studies.

Comparison of the initial distribution of radio-iron between circulating haemoglobin (90%) and non-haemoglobin iron (10%), and the distribution of stable iron in haemoglobin (67%) and non-haemoglobin iron (33%), may

[1] SAITO, H., T. SARGENT III, H. PARKER, and J. H. LAWRENCE: Univ. of Calif. Lawrence Radiation Laboratory Semiannual Report, Biology and Medicine, U.C.L.R.L. 10683, 32 (1962); J. Nuclear Med., in press (1964).

be used to estimate that almost uniform mixing would require 4 generations of red cells or approximately 470 days (assuming a similar 90/10 redistribution of radio-iron after erythrocyte death, erythrophagocytosis, and re-entry of radio-iron into the plasma; $0.9^4 = 0.66$ in haemoglobin). This delay in the mixing of radio-iron, however, may introduce a smaller error into the calculation of iron loss than might be expected, since stool and urine collections in two subjects, shown in Fig. 2, suggest that more than two-thirds of the daily iron loss (0.65 mg./day) occurs via blood loss from the gastro-intestinal tract.

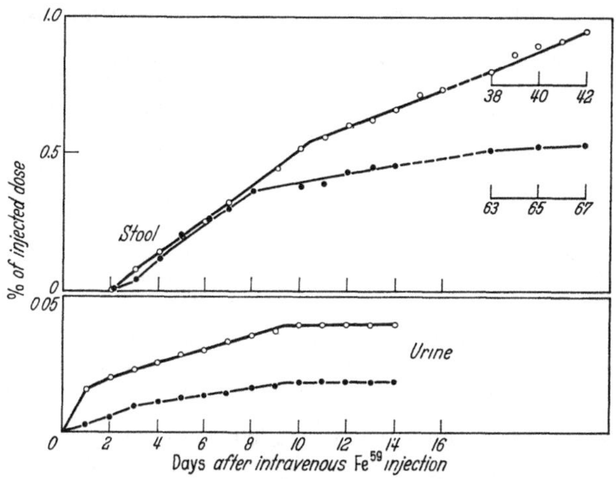

Fig. 2. Cumulative excretion in stool and urine of Fe^{59} injected intravenously in two of the normal subjects shown in Fig. 1

TUBIANA: I already mentioned during the discussion of Dr. MOORE's paper that we have observed in small animals (mice and rats) what we call an intestinal cycle of iron[1], i.e. after intravenous injection of radioactive iron there is a very rapid appearance of iron both in the intestinal mucosa and in the lumen of the intestine. This phenomenon is by no means negligible, since, only 10 minutes after injection of radioactive iron bound to transferrin, 5% of this iron is already mixed with the contents of the gut. Do you think that such a rapid phenomenon can be explained in terms of cell desquamation? Alternatively, do you think that it is due to the transfer of transferrin with radioactive iron or to an active transfer of iron to the cell mucosa and the lumen? The amount of radioactive iron present in the lumen of the gastro-intestinal tract a few hours after intravenous injection is greater than the faecal excretion. It thus seems probable that part of this iron is reabsorbed in the gastro-intestinal tract. Do you think that in man this phenomenon of secretion-reabsorption might partly explain the way in which the amount of iron present in the body is regulated?

MOORE: Dr. FINCH, how did you obtain the figure of 1.8 mg. iron as the estimate for the average daily iron "cost" of pregnancy? It seems a reason-

[1] TUBIANA, M., and E. FRINDEL: Rev. franç. étud. clin. biol. **6**, 276 (1961).

able and entirely acceptable estimate to me, but at the same time, when I have tried to analyse the data recorded in the literature, I have been struck by the fact that the variation must be very great. Isn't it perhaps a mistake to give the impression that a pregnancy costs every woman this much iron? In some instances the iron "cost", over and above what would have been lost in menses, might be almost negligible, whereas some other pregnant women might lose even more iron than you postulate.

STURGEON: I should like to make a comment on Dr. POLLYCOVE's remarks about iron loss in children. The data he cited for the average iron loss in children with iron-deficiency anaemia of severe degree may be representative of such a population. There is, however, considerable evidence that in every infant with iron-deficiency anaemia there is an increase in the permeability of the gastro-intestinal mucosa. We have found that the average patient of this kind shows a decrease in the serum protein concentration, which reverts to normal in response to iron therapy. Also, investigators who have done intestinal permeability experiments with I^{131}-polyvinylpyrrolidone have observed increased permeability in such patients. The anaemia in those infants who actually show a blood loss may therefore not be due to the loss of blood, but may be a symptom of the secondary increase in intestinal permeability rather than the initial cause. The fact that with therapy the vast majority of such infants get well and stay well seems to favour this interpretation.

FINCH: This discussion has served to indicate that there are plenty of good leads that deserve to be looked into; at the same time, it has also revealed the rather embarrassing limitation of our present knowledge on certain aspects of iron loss.

Dr. BEUTLER raised the question as to the nature of the cells in sweat. Dr. HOSAIN found that most of these cells were epithelial cells which should have been of low iron content. More detailed examination has not shown any significant amount of ferritin in these cells. There is always the possibility that some of the iron may be from external contamination.

To answer Dr. NAJEAN's query, I'm afraid I don't have specific information on the nature of the iron in the urine, but I would suppose that for the most part the iron is not bound to transferrin; for example, after a dose of iron by mouth, the urinary iron excretion increases appreciably, and the amount of iron thus excreted would seem to be in excess of the transferrin protein expected in normal urine.

The answer to Dr. PETERS' question about the amount of transferrin iron which may appear in the urine is contained in a portion of my paper which I did not have time to read; it works out at as much as 1 mg./day. I am afraid I cannot comment on the amount of iron lost by the different species of animals mentioned. The percentage lost by mice, which is the only species of animal we have studied over long periods, is greater than in man, but I do not know whether the body iron turnover has been measured in any other species.

The problem of the iron balance in infancy is one that certainly deserves more attention. It is a problem complicated by the fact that the infant loses large amounts of iron into his own body as he grows. So he not only has the possibility of an external but also of an internal iron loss. The iron balance in pregnancy must of necessity be variable. The infant's body iron will be directly related to its weight, the mean being about 280 mg. iron; it will therefore vary, depending on the child's degree of maturity at birth. However, one can argue that the loss of iron to the foetus occurring in pregnancy is one of the most precisely defined losses, if one limits consideration to the known size of the infant. But one should not overlook the reverse consideration, i.e. that of the size of the mother in comparison with the baby, because in some regions where the average woman may weigh 90 pounds the foetus is still the same size. This represents, relatively speaking, a far greater maternal iron loss. The only real variability in maternal iron loss beyond the size of the infant and mother must relate to blood loss at the time of delivery.

Finally, the question of the intestinal cycling of iron raised by Dr. TUBIANA is a very complex one, which I had hoped to avoid by putting particular emphasis on the total iron balance.

The chemical basis of chelation

By

J. Schubert

Introduction

The period when the 19th century merged into the 20th coincided with the introduction of revolutionary concepts and discoveries in science whose impact is still being felt — relativity, the quantum theory, and Gibbsian thermodynamics, to name only a few. During these brief but spectacularly fruitful years were also evolved the coordination theory of Alfred Werner, which now dominates inorganic chemistry, and Paul Ehrlich's chemotherapy, which laid the foundations for drug therapy in modern medicine.

The apparently unrelated work and ideas of Werner and Ehrlich have now become closely interwoven, as evidenced by the enormous expansion of investigations on the role of coordination chemistry in biology and medicine. A tangible link between the research of Werner and Ehrlich was already established in 1912, when Paul Karrer, then a young inorganic chemist in Werner's institute in Zurich, went to Frankfurt to work in Ehrlich's laboratories. It was there that Karrer introduced his associates to the then little-known theories of coordination chemistry (*9*).

The first deliberate use of metal-complexing agents for the treatment of heavy-metal poisoning was made in 1940 when Peters, Stocken, and Thompson (*13*) developed 2,3-dimercaptopropanol (B.A.L.) to treat the harmful effects of arsenic poisoning caused by arsenical war gases. It is interesting to note that Ehrlich also tried to make less toxic complex compounds of arsenic for use in the treatment of syphilis. The application of synthetic non-toxic chelating agents in medicine received a great impetus with the introduction by Bersworth in the 1940's of the universal chelating agent, ethylene-diamine tetra-acetic acid (E.D.T.A.). The past few years have seen the introduction of a chelating agent possessing a remarkably high relative affinity and specificity under physiological conditions for a single cation, i.e. trivalent iron. This low-toxicity chelating agent, desferrioxamine, which was developed by PRELOG (*14*) and his associates in Zurich and by the CIBA group in Basle, opens up new vistas in the medical treatment of heavy-metal poisoning.

The fact that more has now become known about the reactions of synthetic chelates with metals has also led to an improved understanding of the structure and function of naturally occurring chelates in the plant and animal world.

Besides the many books and articles that have been published dealing with the basic chemical and physical nature of chelation, the implications of chelation as regards the biological sciences have also been the subject of special conferences whose proceedings have likewise been published (*5*, *8*, *19*).

It is the purpose of this paper to present a simple yet quantitative method for evaluating the relative stabilities of metal chelates under physiological conditions. The method enables one to assess the effects of interfering or competing cations or anions, whether these be simple ions with or without chelating action or polymers such as proteins. This covers more ground than might at first be imagined, because it involves studying such properties of metals as hydrolysis, their accessibility to the action of chelating agents, the formation of polynuclear and insoluble species, and the rates of interaction between a chelating agent and different forms of metallic salt.

The so-called physiological conditions usually refer to an aqueous system having a pH of 7.25, various proteins, and a free calcium-ion concentration of about 10^{-3}M. In fact, however, depending on whether one is dealing with blood, discrete parts of organs, or certain subcellular fractions, the pH conditions and the concentrations of ions and polymeric materials may vary considerably. Nevertheless, in dealing with the interactions of polyvalent metals and chelating agents, the pH is one variable which can be, and indeed always should be, included when evaluating the stability of a chelate *in vivo* and the state of the metallic ion itself. The conventional stability constants as employed in physical chemistry serve as a basis for calculating the relative stability of chelates under a given set of conditions. On the other hand, numerous examples will be provided showing that the conventional stability constants may fail to indicate the true order of stability of chelates under physiological conditions and, in fact, may be entirely misleading.

Basic concepts

This section briefly reviews certain definitions and conventions customarily employed in the chemistry of chelates. Further details are to be found in numerous publications, among which the books of MARTELL and CALVIN (*11*) and CHABEREK and MARTELL (*3*) and the articles by SCHWARZENBACH (*25*, *26*) and RINGBOM (*17*) are especially useful.

All metallic ions in aqueous solutions are hydrated; hence, strictly speaking, no simple metallic ions exist in aqueous solution. The water molecules in the hydration shell can be replaced by other molecules or ions – the *ligands* – thus forming a complex ion. The maximum number of ligands bound by the metallic ion is its *coordination number*. If the ligand links several metallic ions – the so-called bridging reaction – *polynuclear species* are formed. Depending on the metallic ion and its concentration, polynuclear species may immediately precede the formation of precipitates.

The reaction between a ligand, L, and a metallic ion, M, is usually simplified by omitting the charges and solvent molecules. Accordingly, complexing reactions with *monodentate* ligands, i.e. ligands which combine at one point with the metal, form a series of complexes as the concentration of L increases to a maximum:

$$M \overset{L}{\rightleftharpoons} ML \overset{L}{\rightleftharpoons} ML_2 --\rightarrow ML_n .$$

Under a given set of conditions only one species, say ML, may predominate.

There exist as many stability or *formation constants* as there are complexes, as, for example:

$$K_1 = \frac{[ML]}{[M][L]} : K_2 = \frac{[ML_2]}{[ML][L]} : K_n = \frac{[ML_n]}{[ML_{n-1}][L]} , \qquad (1)$$

where the brackets represent molar concentrations.

The overall constants, β, or *stability products* are also employed:

$$\beta_n = \frac{[ML_n]}{[M][L]^n} . \qquad (2)$$

Thus

$$\beta_1 = K_1 \qquad (3)$$

$$\beta_2 = K_1 K_2 \qquad (4)$$

$$\beta_n = K_1 K_2 \cdots K_n . \qquad (5)$$

Polynuclear complexes are also formed stepwise and are expressed as:

$$mM + nL \rightleftharpoons M_m L_n . \qquad (6)$$

The value for the stability constant depends on the nature of the ligand which displaces the water molecules surrounding the metallic ion. Simple monodentate ligands such as acetate, chloride, or ammonia satisfy one coordination site of a metal cation. They generally form charged complex ions soluble in water. A bidentate molecule, such as hydrazine, H_2N-NH_2, can satisfy two sites simultaneously, but not with one cation because of strain. Hence, hydrazine may link two metal cations, and so on, until an infinite three-dimensional polynuclear lattice is produced. Such ligands are called *lattice-building* ligands (*25*). Included in this category are OH^-, $CO^=$, and $PO_4^=$.

When polydentate ligands combine with a metal to form strain-free heterocyclic rings, the resulting structure is called a *chelate*, a term suggested by MORGAN and DREW (*12*) in 1920.

"The adjective 'chelate', derived from the great claw or 'chela' ('chely') of the lobster and other crustaceans, is suggested for these caliper-like groups which function as two associating units and fasten on to the central metallic atom so as to produce heterocyclic rings . . ."

The chelate effect

An important characteristic of chelates is that their stability is greater than that of the corresponding complex formed with monodentate ligands. The increase in stability resulting from the formation of a chelate ring is called the *chelate effect*. Thermodynamically, the chelate effect arises from the fact that the formation of a chelate ring involves a greater positive entropy change. Since the bonds attaching the metal to the ligand are almost the same, the enthalpy change, ΔH, is nearly the same, whether the complex MA_2 or the chelate 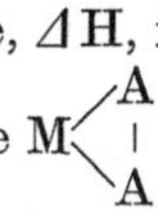 is formed.

A practical example of the chelate effect is found in the case of desferrioxamine, which can be viewed as a chelating agent constructed by linking together three molecules of a derivative of hydroxamic acid, 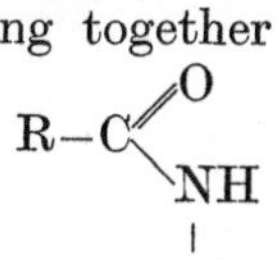 into a single unit through the nitrogen. Hydroxamic acid forms strong complexes with ferric iron. It is of interest to compare the stability constants of the complexes formed stepwise with acetylhydroxamine with the stability constant of the closely corresponding chelate of desferrioxamine.

Let L^- represent the anion of acetylhydroxamine. Then, from the work of SCHWARZENBACH and associates (*27*), the formation constants are as follows:

$$Fe^{+3} + L^- \rightleftharpoons FeL^{+2};\ \log. K_1 = 11.4 \qquad (7)$$

$$FeL^{+2} + L^- \rightleftharpoons FeL_2^+;\ \log. K_2 = 9.7 \qquad (8)$$

$$FeL_2^+ + L^- \rightleftharpoons FeL_3;\ \underline{\log. K_3 = 7.2} \qquad (9)$$

$$\log.\ \beta_3 = 28.3\,.$$

In the case of desferrioxamine, H.D.F.O.$^{-2}$, the corresponding reaction for chelate formation is:

$$Fe^{+3} + H.D.F.O.^{-2} \rightleftharpoons Fe(H.D.F.O.)^+;\ \log.\ K = 30.6\,. \qquad (10)$$

The net result is an increase of 2.3 log. units in log. K as a consequence of chelate ring formation.

As has been pointed out (*26*), the largest chelate effect (2–3 units in log. K) occurs with the formation of the smallest ring which is free of strain; this usually means five-membered rings. Under certain conditions, as for example when the chelate ring has double bonds, the six-membered ring may be more stable. In the case of four, seven, or eight-membered rings, little or no chelate effect is generally observed, because the greater probability of forming rings is offset by the ring strain, or, in thermodynamic terms, ΔH has become more positive. In the case of ions like Ag^+ and Hg^{+2}, even five-membered rings are strained, because these ions prefer linear arrangements.

The formation of chelate rings results in a greater stability against dissociation by dilution. For example, the stability against dissociation of the complex FeL_3 of acetylhydroxamine varies with the third power of the ligand concentration, in contrast to a first-power dependence in the case of the desferrioxamine chelate. Let us consider the fraction of ferric iron bound by these agents present in excess relative to iron at a concentration of 10^{-4} molar of ligand:

For acetylhydroxamine we have:

$$\frac{[FeL_3]}{[Fe]} = 10^{28.3} \times (10^{-4})^3 = 10^{16.3}, \qquad (11)$$

whereas for desferrioxamine we have:

$$\frac{[Fe_{(H.D.F.O.)}]}{[Fe]} = 10^{30.6} \times 10^{-4} = 10^{26.6}. \qquad (12)$$

Hence, the fraction of iron bound by desferrioxamine is relatively independent of dilution.

Design of chelating agents

It is of interest to consider some of the factors which enter into the design of chelating agents along the lines discussed by SCHWARZENBACH (*25*). A universal chelating agent, i.e. one which will react strongly with most metals, would have to contain oxygen atoms. In such a case, the oxygen of the water molecules in the hydration shell of the cation will be replaced by the oxygen ligand atoms of the complexing agent. Of the oxygen-containing groups, the acetate ion is known to form complexes – albeit weak ones – with nearly all metals. The tying together of carboxyl groups by carbon atoms is not very successful, because, except for oxalic acid, it is not possible to form five-membered rings. Oxalic acid suffers from the disadvantage that there is no possibility of attaching more ligand atoms.

Let us consider the following anions:

$$\begin{array}{l} CH_2-COO^- \\ | \\ CH_2 \\ | \\ CH_2-COO^- \end{array} \qquad\qquad \begin{array}{l} CH_2-COO^- \\ | \\ NH \\ | \\ CH_2-COO^- \end{array}$$

Glutarate Iminodiacetate

The introduction of a basic nitrogen able to donate electrons to metals in an α-position to the carboxyl groups brings the two carboxyl groups into the correct position to form strain-free chelate rings. The stability of the complexes is thus enormously increased. Two of the best structures conceivable are:

$$\begin{array}{l} CH_2-N(CH_2COO^-)_2 \\ | \\ CH_2-N(CH_2COO^-)_2 \end{array} \qquad\qquad N(CH_2COO^-)_3$$

Ethylene-diamine tetra-acetate Nitrilo-acetate

There exist many instances, especially in biological systems, in which less universality and more specificity are desired in a chelating agent. In such cases one may exploit different properties such as: (1) the variation in stability with pH; (2) the use of ligand atoms which react with fewer cations, e.g. sulphur, which reacts strongly with lead ions and shows practically no reaction with calcium; and (3) special geometrical arrangements which are particularly favourable to a restricted number of cations.

Relative orders of stability

The relative thermodynamic stability of metallic cations has been expressed in terms of many empirical rules. Unfortunately, numerous exceptions occur, although in some cases the rules apply remarkably well. Thus, for example, the equilibrium constants for the bivalent transition elements follow the so-called Irving-Williams order:

$$Mn^{+2} > Fe^{+2} > Ca^{+2} > Ni^{+2} < Cu^{+2} > Zn^{+2},$$

in which a maximum stability is reached with cupric ion. This order holds good for practically all ligands. Occasional exceptions do occur, however, e.g. when comparing over-all constants for six-coordinate complexes as measured by β_6. In this case, cations which usually have a coordination number of four are at a disadvantage.

The Irving-Williams order is related to the fact that the entropies for complex formation are essentially constant in this series, so that the formation constants correspond to the order of the ΔH values. The radii of these transition-metal cations decrease from Mn^{+2} to Cu^{+2} and increase again with Zn^{+2}, as does also the ionisation potential.

Another order which holds very well for simple electrostatic reasons is that of the alkaline earth cations:

$$Ca^{+2} > Sr^{+2} > Ba^{+2} > Ra^{+2}.$$

It is important to note that, as the differences in the thermodynamic stability between these cations diminish, the absolute values for the stability constant decrease. This means that, for practical purposes, only a small probability exists that a chelating agent will be formed having a high affinity for Sr^{+2} (say, log. $K > 6$) and, at the same time, having a much lower affinity for Ca^{+2}.

It is beyond the purpose of this paper to describe in greater detail empirical and theoretical data on the chemical aspects of chelation. However, further information is given in many of the papers presented at this Symposium and in the general references cited earlier (*3*, *26*). For those interested in an excellent and comprehensive treatment of chelation in terms of ligand field theory, the book by Cotton and Wilkinson (*4*) is highly recommended. A short but valuable account of coordination compounds, which emphasises the biological importance and role of ligand field theory, is given by Williams (*30*).

The effective formation constant and side-reaction coefficients

In order to estimate the absolute and relative degree to which a complexing agent may interact with different metallic ions under physiological conditions, it may be necessary to consider several equilibrium constants. Such calculations have been made for systems in which injected chelating agents have been used to remove radio-elements from animals (*7*, *20*). An elegant way in which the calculations can be simplified to make them more readily applicable to biological and medical systems can be adapted from those developed for use in analytical chemistry by RINGBOM (*16*, *17*), who simplified the method as introduced by SCHWARZENBACH. The method is especially applicable to systems involving the use of strong chelating agents which generally form predominantly 1:1 chelates.

Let us consider the formation constant for the chelate ML:

$$K_{ML} = \frac{[ML]}{[M][L]} . \qquad (13)$$

In point of fact, the concentration of each of the components is rarely represented by the stoichiometric concentrations. For example, the actual concentration of M may be diminished by the formation of hydroxide complexes such as M(OH) and $M(OH)_2$, while the concentration of L may be diminished because of incomplete dissociation of the acid H_mL, that is to say, because of competition from H^+. Furthermore, the concentration of 1:1 chelates as represented by ML may be greater when the possibility of acid or basic complexes such as [MHL] and [M(OH)L] is considered. In the body, other ions, such as calcium ions, compete against L for M.

The effective constant is defined as:

$$K_{eff} = K_{(ML)'M'L'} = \frac{[ML']}{[M'][L']} , \qquad (14)$$

where [ML′] represents the sum of concentration of all species containing M and L in the molar ratio 1:1, as, for example:

$$[(ML)'] = [ML] + [MHL] + [MOHL] + \ldots \qquad (15)$$

Similarly, [M′] is the concentration of the free metallic ion and of all of its metallic ions in solution which have not reacted with L, but which have reacted with anions and complexing ligands, as, for example:

$$[M'] = [M] + [M(OH)] + [MA] + \ldots \qquad (16)$$

Finally, [L′] is the concentration of the free ligand and the concentration of all species combined with other cations, β, and not specifically combined with the given metal:

$$[L'] = [L] + [HL] + [H_2L] + [BL] + \dots \quad (17)$$

The effective constant is handled in the same way as ordinary equilibrium constants, and one does not need to know the exact nature of the species contributing to M and L and ML. However, all these definitions are useless unless one can obtain in a simple manner the numerical value of the effective constant. For this purpose, alpha coefficients or the so-called side-reaction coefficients are employed, which afford a measure of the extent of side reactions. For ML, M, and L, these are defined as follows:

$$\alpha_{ML} = \frac{[(ML')]}{[ML]} \quad (18)$$

$$\alpha_{M} = \frac{[M']}{[M]} \quad (19)$$

$$\alpha_{L} = \frac{[L']}{[L]} \,. \quad (20)$$

If the reactions take place without interference or competing reactions, then the alpha values are unity, i.e.:

$$[(ML')] = [ML];\ [M'] = [M];\ [L'] = [L]. \quad (21)$$

The effective constant is calculated from the alpha values on the basis of the simple definition:

$$K_{eff} = K_{(ML')\,M'\,L'} = \left(\frac{\alpha_{ML}}{\alpha_M\,\alpha_L}\right) K_{ML}, \quad (22)$$

so that, if no interference or competition reactions are involved:

$$K_{eff} = K_{ML}\,. \quad (23)$$

There exists an important simplifying rule (*16*) for calculating over-all alpha coefficients when at least one alpha term is a large one, namely: *the over-all alpha coefficients can be taken to be approximately equal to the sum of the individual coefficients.* For example, assuming that in a system there are, apart from L, several ligands, L_1, L_2, etc., competing for the metallic ion M, this means that:

$$\alpha_M = \alpha_{M(L_1)} + \alpha_{M(L_2)} + \cdots \quad (24)$$

and, likewise, if several cations interfere, B_1, B_2, which may include H^+, then:

$$\alpha_L = \alpha_{L(B_1)} + \alpha_{L(B_2)} + \cdots \quad (25)$$

Usually one of the alpha terms predominates, so that the other terms can be dropped.

Numerical values for alpha are obtained from known equilibrium constants as compiled in many general references and, in particular, in the comprehensive tables of BJERRUM, SCHWARZENBACH, and SILLÉN (*2*). Typical equations for calculating alpha are as follows:

(1) For a disturbing ligand, A, that forms complexes with M:

$$\alpha_{M(A)} = 1 + [A]\,K_{MA} + [A]^2 K_{MA_2} + \ldots \qquad (26)$$

(2) For disturbing cations, B, where B can also be H^+:

$$\alpha_{L(B)} = 1 + [B]\,K_{BL} + [B]^2 K_{B_2L} + \ldots \qquad (27)$$

(3) When acid complexes are formed:

$$\alpha_{ML(H)} = 1 + [H]\,K^{H}_{MHL} + \ldots, \qquad (28)$$

where K^{H}_{MHL} is the constant for the dissociation of a proton from the complex MHL.

Numerical calculations

Proton-ligand interaction ($\alpha_{L(H)}$)

Let us now consider calculations involving three chelating agents, which are widely used in biology and medicine, and which have been employed in attempts to modify iron metabolism. The chelating agents are ethylene-diamine tetra-acetic acid (E.D.T.A.), diethylene-triamine penta-acetic acid (D.T.P.A.), and desferrioxamine (H.D.F.O.) (Table 1).

Table 1. *Acid dissociation constants of three chelating agents*[1,2]

Reaction	Log. K for each step			Over-all log. β		
	D.T.P.A.	E.D.T.A.	H.D.F.O.	D.T.P.A.	E.D.T.A.	H.D.F.O.
$H + H_4L \rightleftharpoons H_5L$	1.79	—	—	27.95	—	—
$H + H_3L \rightleftharpoons H_4L$	2.56	2.00	—	26.16	21.09	—
$H + H_2L \rightleftharpoons H_3L$	4.42	2.67	8.39	23.60	19.09	27.12
$H + HL \rightleftharpoons H_2L$	8.76	6.16	9.03	19.18	16.42	18.73
$H + L \rightleftharpoons HL$	10.42	10.26	9.70	10.42	10.26	9.70

[1] The tabulated constants are taken from tables in reference *2* for D.T.P.A. and E.D.T.A. and are for 25° and $\mu = 0.1$ and 20° and $\mu = 0.1$, respectively. Those for desferrioxamine (H.D.F.O.) are taken from reference *27* and are for 20° and $\mu = 0.1$

[2] Desferrioxamine is treated as a tribasic acid, since the fourth hydrogen is very tightly bound with a log. K > 11.

From equation (*27*) the values of $\alpha_{L(H)}$ for each of the chelating agents have been calculated for pH's from 0 to 12 from the constants listed in Table 1. The data are presented in the form of a graph in Fig. 1. Since the principal ligand-binding metal is the fully dissociated form, L, it can be seen that the actual concentrations of L vary precipitously with the pH. Thus, at pH 7 the concentration of H.D.F.O.⁼ available to react with M is actually about one-millionth of the stoichiometric concentration of desferrioxamine (log. $\alpha_{L(H)} = 6.1$)!

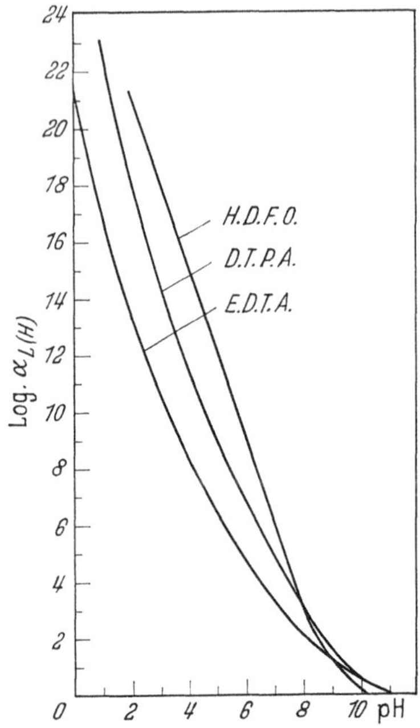

Fig. 1. Variation of the log. of the side-reaction coefficient for hydrogen-ion interference with pH for the free ligands of three chelating agents

Hydroxide-metallic ion interaction ($\alpha_{M(OH)}$) and the mononuclear barrier

The competition of hydroxide ion versus the chelating ligand for a metallic ion is a very important consideration when dealing with readily hydrolysable cations. The formulation of polynuclear complexes with hydroxide complicates the calculations. The systems in which polynuclear formation leads to precipitates are dealt with later. The problem, however, is how to ascertain whether soluble polynuclear complexes are formed. From the work of SILLÉN and his school (*17*, *28*) it appears that the average number of OH^- bound per metallic ion is independent of the metallic ion concentration if only mononuclear complexes are formed. As a general rule, the concentration of polynuclear complexes decreases on dilution. At some particular dilution a "mononuclear wall" is reached, so that below this critical metal concentration one is dealing only with mononuclear complexes. Some cations, like thorium and uranyl, do not appear to form mononuclear complexes, but dissociate directly into metallic ions.

In the case of Fe^{+3} the mononuclear barrier occurs at a concentration of less than $10^{-3.7}$M. Consequently, since the concentration of free Fe^{+3} is very low in biological systems, one can regard

Fe^{+3}, at least in circulating fluids, as forming mononuclear complexes with hydroxide ion. For purposes of calculation, let us consider the formation of $\alpha_{M(OH)}$ for the cations of Cu^{+2}, Fe^{+2}, and Fe^{+3} as a function of pH. From equation (26) we can write:

$$\alpha_{M(OH)} = 1 + [OH]\,K_{M(OH)} + [OH]^2\,K_{M(OH)_2}. \qquad (29)$$

Table 2. *Logarithmic stability products of hydroxy complexes*[1,2]

Metal	$K_{M(OH)}$	$K_{M(OH)_2}$	$K_{M_2(OH)_2}$
Fe(III)	11.0	21.7	25.1
Fe(II).	4.5	—	—
Cu(II).	6.0	—	17.4

[1] The data are taken from the article by RINGBOM (*17*), in which the references to the original literature are cited.

[2] The constants listed were determined at 25° C. with $NaClO_4$ as neutral electrolyte at an ionic strength of 3.

From these $\alpha_{M(OH)}$ values and the constants listed in Table 2 the curves in Fig. 2 were plotted. Note that only in the case of Fe(III) does OH^- interfere appreciably. At pH 7 the $\alpha_{Fe(OH)} = 10^8$, while that for Cu(II) and Fe(II) is still unity. It is apparent that chelates of Fe(III) at neutral pH must overcome strong competition from OH^-, so that the effective constant could be less than that of Cu(II) chelates, even though the latter may possess a much smaller conventional stability constant, as we shall see later.

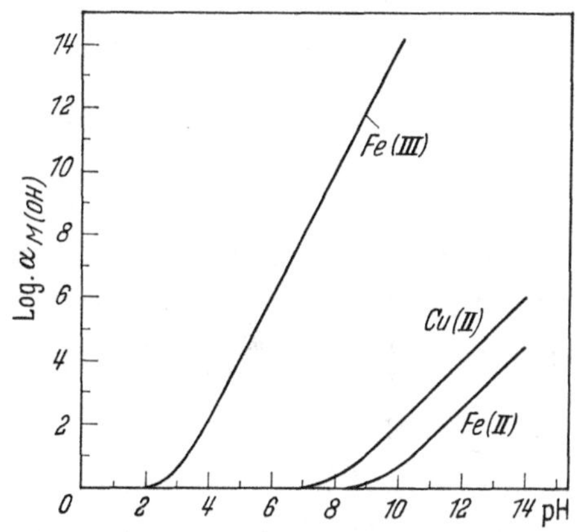

Fig. 2. Variation of the log. of the side-reaction coefficient for hydroxide interference with pH for three metallic ions

Calcium ion competition

When evaluating the *in vivo* stability of a metal chelate, it is always necessary to consider the competition of calcium ion. Blood, for example, contains about 10^{-3} M of Ca^{++}, and it strives to maintain this level, since a decrease in the level might lead to death from hypocalcaemia. Obviously, a chelating agent having a small affinity for Ca^{++} is preferable. Otherwise, in view of the relatively high concentration of free Ca^{++}, the metallic component of a chelate present in the serum might become partly or completely replaced by calcium. Whether the competition from Ca^{++} is sufficient to overcome the competition from H^{+1} for the chelating agent must be considered in a biological system.

Table 3. *Side-reaction coefficients of calcium ion for chelating agents*[1]

Chelating agent	Log. K_{CaL}	$\alpha_{L(Ca)}$
D.T.P.A. . .	10.1	7.1
E.D.T.A. . .	10.6	7.6
H.D.F.O. . .	3.2	0.15

[1] Calculated from equation (30). The constants of log. K_{CaL} are for 20° and $\mu = 0.1$, and [Ca] is taken to be 10^{-3} M.

The $\alpha_{L(Ca)}$ can be calculated from equation (27). Since only the 1:1 complex is important, the following relationship is used:

$$\alpha_{L(Ca)} = 1 + [Ca]\, K_{CaL}\,. \qquad (30)$$

The resulting values for $\alpha_{L(Ca)}$ are tabulated in Table 3. In the light of Fig. 1 and in view of the rule expressed in equations (24) and (25), it can be concluded that $\alpha_{L(Ca)}$ becomes dominant over $\alpha_{L(H)}$ for E.D.T.A. above a pH of 5 and for D.T.P.A. above a pH of 6. However, it plays no role in the case of H.D.F.O. until a pH of > 9 is reached.

Effective constants for Fe (II), Fe (III), and Cu (II)

The relative stability *in vivo*, in terms of K_{eff}, of the chelates formed between D.T.P.A., E.D.T.A., and H.D.F.O. and the three

Table 4. *Formation constants utilised for the calculation of effective constants*[1]

Metallic ion	Log. K_{ML}			Log. K^{H}_{MHL}			Log. K^{OH}_{MOHL}		
	D.T.P.A.	E.D.T.A.	H.D.F.O.	H-D.T.P.A.	H-E.D.T.A.	H_2-D.F.O.	(OH)-[2] D.T.P.A.	(OH)-[3] E.D.T.A.	(OH) H.D.F.O.
Fe(II)	16.7	14.3	11	5.2	2.79	unstable	5.0	4.9	—
Fe(III)	27.4	25.1	30.6	3.6	1.36	0.94	4.1	6.5	$<10^{-11}$
Cu(II)	20.5	18.8	14.1	5.0	3.00	9.08	—	—	$<10^{-11}$
Ca	10.6	10.7	2.6	6.4	3.1	—	—	—	—

[1] The data listed were obtained or calculated from data in references *2, 3, 15, 17*, and *27*, and are all for conditions of $\mu = 0.1$ and 20°, except in the case of D.T.P.A. in which they were obtained at 25°.

[2] The constants for the formation of $(OH)_2$-D.T.P.A. for Fe(II) and Fe(III) are 9.4 and ~ 6, respectively.

[3] The constants for the formation of $(OH)_2$-E.D.T.A. for Fe(II) and Fe(III) are 9.0 and 11.0, respectively.

metallic ions Fe^{+2}, Fe^{+3}, and Cu^{+2} have been calculated as a function of pH. The conventional stability constants used for calculating the necessary side-reaction coefficients, apart from those listed in Tables 1–3, are tabulated in Table 4.

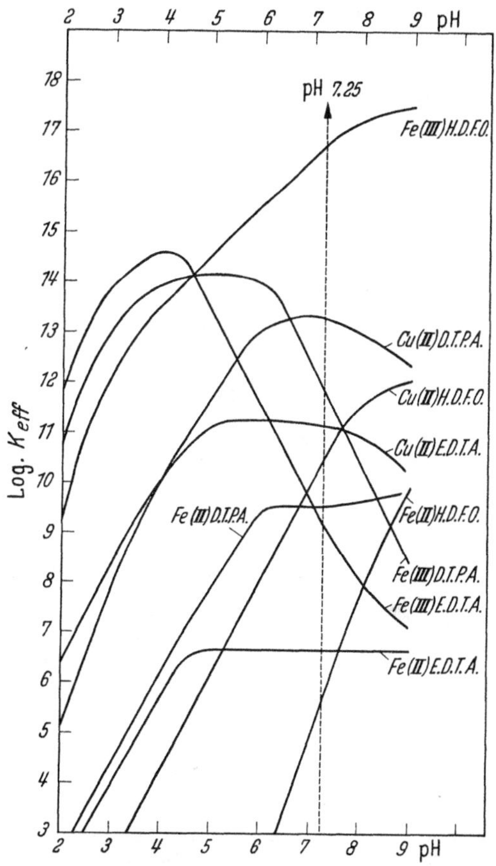

Fig. 3. Variation of the log. of the effective constants with pH for Fe(III), Fe(II), and Cu(II). In the calculations the following side-reaction coefficients were taken into account: $\alpha_{L(H)}$, $\alpha_{L(Ca)}$, $\alpha_{M(OH)}$, $\alpha_{ML(H)}$, $\alpha_{ML(OH)}$

The effective constants have been calculated by taking into account interferences from H^+, Ca^{++}, and OH^-, that is to say, $\alpha_{L(H)}$, $\alpha_{L(Ca)}$, and $\alpha_{M(OH)}$. Also included are the effects of the formation of acid complexes, MHL, and basic complexes, M(OH)L, i.e.

$\alpha_{ML(H)}$ and $\alpha_{ML(OH)}$. The resulting K_{eff}'s are presented graphically in Fig. 3. Several important observations are worth noting. Thus, at pH 7.25, the Cu-E.D.T.A. chelate is more stable than that of Fe(III)-E.D.T.A., despite the fact that the conventional stability constant (log. $K_{Fe\,E.D.T.A.} = 25.1$ as compared to log. $K_{Cu\,E.D.T.A.} = 18.8$) is over a million times stronger. At pH 4, Fe(III)-H.D.F.O. is weaker than the corresponding E.D.T.A. or D.T.P.A. complexes. However, at pH 7.25, Fe(III)-H.D.F.O. stands in a class by itself, revealing an unprecedented specificity for a chelating agent *in vivo* at neutral pH. Another interesting finding is the superiority of D.T.P.A. over E.D.T.A. for Fe(III) under a neutral pH. The conclusions derived from K_{eff} are in agreement with experimental observations on the relative degree to which these chelating agents enhance the excretion of ferric ion as described in the work of several investigators.

A summary of the relative order of stability of the various chelates, as revealed by the effective constants, is given in Table 5. The orders are calculated for three pH ranges covering the regions of biological interest.

Table 5. *Relative stability*[1] *of the chelates of* Fe(II), Fe(III), *and* Cu(II), *as a function of* pH

D = D.T.P.A, E = E.D.T.A. H = H.D.F.O.

pH = 4.0
$Fe^{III}E > Fe^{III}D > Fe^{III}H >> CuD, CuE >> Fe^{II}D > Fe^{II}E >> CuH >> Fe^{II}H$
pH = 7.25
$Fe^{III}H >> CuD > Fe^{III}D > CuE > CuH > Fe^{II}D > Fe^{III}E >> Fe^{II}E > Fe^{II}H$
pH = 9.0
$Fe^{III}H >> CuH > CuD >> CuE > Fe^{II}H, Fe^{II}D > Fe^{III}D > Fe^{III}E > Fe^{II}E$

[1] The orders are obtained from Fig. 3. Where the stability of a metal chelate in terms of K_{eff} is at least 1,000 times, i.e. 3 log. units, greater than that of its neighbour, this is indicated by the two "greater than" (>>) signs.

It is interesting to include the relative stabilities of different metallic ions for the much-used chelating agent E.D.T.A. when corrections for $\alpha_{L(H)}$, $\alpha_{M(OH)}$, and $\alpha_{ML(H)}$ are made. The results are summarised in Table 6. It may be noted that Cu(II) and especially Ni(II) form the most stable chelates at pH 7 and that above this pH, Ni is slightly more stable than Cu. At pH 9, for example, the effective constants for Ni-E.D.T.A. and Cu-E.D.T.A. are 16.9 and 16.4 log. units, respectively. Experimentally it has been observed that injected E.D.T.A. is particularly successful in promoting the excretion and countering the toxic action of nickel and that it has no effect on mercury.

Table 6. *Relative stability of the chelates formed by E.D.T.A. with different metallic ions*[1]

pH = 4.0 $Fe^{+3} >> Hg > Cu$, $Ni > Pb > Zn$, Cd, $Co > Al > Mn$, $Fe^{+2} >> Ca > Sr$
pH = 7 Cu, $Ni > Fe^{+3} > Pb > Zn$, Cd, $Co > Fe^{+2} > Mn$, $Hg >> Al > Ca > Sr$
pH = 9 $Ni > Cu > Zn$, Co, $Cd > Pb$, $Fe^{+3} > Fe^{+2}$, $Mn > Ca > Hg > Sr > Al$

[1] The relative orders are derived from the effective constants which included the effects of interferences from OH^-, H^+, and acid and basic complexes.

Mobilisation of insoluble deposits of metals

Owing to the formation of precipitates with anions such as phosphates, and the formation of polynuclear species, polyvalent metals such as Fe(III) become incorporated as insoluble deposits within the tissues. A decrease in pH in these cases usually enhances the solubility by decreasing the concentration of the precipitating anions. However, as regards *in vivo* conditions, it is not feasible to induce significant changes in pH for the purpose of enhancing solubility.

Iron is stored in insoluble forms, predominantly as the hydroxide in the proteins ferritin and haemosiderin. According to HARRISON (p. 47) the ferric hydroxide accounts for up to about 40% of the weight of the ferritin molecule.

What is the degree to which solubilisation through chelate formation can occur in response to administration of a chelating agent? Assuming that contact between the chelating agent and the insoluble material is made, it is interesting to estimate the effective constants for the reaction between a chelating agent and an insoluble metallic salt. We will ignore for the moment the fact that the rate of reaction of polynuclear species with a chelating agent is generally much slower than with mononuclear species. The calculation is made using equations as presented by REILLY et al. (*15*) (see also reference *3*, p. 183 *et sqq.*).

The effective equilibrium constants for the reaction between the chelating agents and the insoluble hydroxides at pH 7 are summarised in Table 7. The following equations were used for the calculations:

Bivalent cation

$$\log. K_{eff} = [\log. K_{ML} + 28] - [pK_{sp} + \log. \alpha_{L(H)} + 2\,pH]. \quad (31)$$

Trivalent cation

$$\log. K_{eff} = [\log. K_{ML} + 42] - [pK_{sp} + \log. \alpha_{L(H)} + 3\,pH]. \quad (32)$$

Table 7. *Effective equilibrium constants*[1] *for the reaction between metal hydroxides and chelating agents at* pH 7

Hydroxide	Solubility product[2] pK_{sp}	Log. K_{eff} [3]		
		D.T.P.A.	E.D.T.A.	H.D.F.O.
$Fe(OH)_2$ . . .	15	11 (9.6)	10 (6.7)	4 (4.9)
$Fe(OH)_3$ . . .	37	5 (12.3)	5 (9.6)	8 (16.5)
$Cu(OH)_2$ . . .	19	11 (13.4)	11 (11.2)	3 (10.1)

[1] The equilibrium constants were calculated from equations (31) and (32).

[2] The solubility products were obtained from reference *3*, p. 446.

[3] The values of log. K_{eff} for the soluble or circulating forms of the same metals as shown in Fig. 3 are given in brackets. It should be noted that the log. K_{eff} for the circulating forms includes corrections for $\alpha_{L(Ca)}$.

H.D.F.O. is clearly superior to D.T.P.A. and E.D.T.A. for dissolving insoluble iron hydroxide. It is also apparent that the effectiveness of the reaction between desferrioxamine and insoluble Fe(III) is much less than in the case of the soluble forms. This fact – coupled with the slower rate of reaction with insoluble forms, and the probability that the concentration of injected H.D.F.O. capable of contacting the insoluble iron salts is less than that available for the circulating form – means that, by and large, the removal of excess deposits of iron in the body will be a slow process.

The slowness with which insoluble deposits of metallic salts are solubilised by a chelating agent has interesting consequences. For example, following injection of a chelating agent into an animal containing extraneous or excessive amounts of a metallic ion, a sharp increase in the urinary excretion of the metal may be observed.

In those cases in which *circulating* metallic ions are chelated and excreted, the relatively increased urinary excretion levels show a day-to-day decline in response to daily administration of a chelating agent, i.e. as the available metal in circulation diminishes. However, in the case of insoluble deposits of the same metallic ion, an opposite pattern emerges in which, following daily injections of a chelating agent, the urinary excretion rises with each successive day. In the latter case, the slow dissolution and depolymerisation of the polynuclear species is responsible for the pattern of the response. These phenomena have been described elsewhere in more detail together with experimental evidence relating to the metallic ions of thorium (*23*) and plutonium (*24*).

The distinctive pattern of urinary excretion of insoluble polynuclear species of a metal present in the tissues, as contrasted with the labile circulating mononuclear species, provides an experimental means for determining whether a chelating agent is removing metal from the circulation or from tissue deposits. Moreover, the point at which the response becomes characteristic of circulating metallic ions may indicate either that the excessive tissue deposits have been depleted, or that the metal-storage disease is of a particularly refractory type, i.e. resistant to the action of chelating agents, or that the remaining deposits are inaccessible. It is well known that freshly precipitated hydroxides are more soluble than those of longer standing. For example, aged ferric hydroxide has a solubility product four times less than the freshly precipitated forms (*1*). Be that as it may, the eventual decrease in the apparent efficiency with which a chelating agent removes metal is a normal phenomenon characteristic of any extraction process, whether occurring in a test-tube or in the body.

Transferrin and the effective constant

The use of side-reaction coefficients offers a convenient means of evaluating the potential interferences from several components of a system. In this connection, let us consider the effect of the binding of iron by transferrin. The problem here is to evaluate $\alpha_{M(P)}$, where P represents the protein anion. The value of $\alpha_{M(P)}$ in relation to $\alpha_{M(OH)}$ is important where it is desired to include the transferrin protein interference in the effective equilibrium constants for different chelating agents.

Transferrin comprises 2 to 4% of the plasma protein and, according to WESTERFELD (*29*), it contains all of the approximately 0.1 mg.% of plasma Fe. It is estimated (*18*, *29*) that under normal physiological conditions a third to a half of the transferrin molecule's capacity for iron is utilised. Iron overload leading to saturation of transferrin results in toxic effects as the excess iron leaves the bloodstream and enters the tissues.

In these cases where transferrin is saturated, it is not necessary to include the protein as a ligand competing for iron. Under normal circumstances or in iron-deficiency states, however, it is interesting to determine the degree to which an injected chelating agent is capable of removing transferrin-bound iron.

Transferrin (TF) has a molecular weight of about 90,000. The molar concentration of TF in the blood ranges from about 1 to 4 × 10^{-5}M. The iron in the plasma is present in a concentration of about 2 × 10^{-5}M and is considered to be entirely bound by transferrin. According to SALTMAN (*18*), TF has two binding sites for iron, one with a $K_{M(TF)} = 10^{29}$ and the other with a $K_{M(TF)} = 10^{27}$. Assuming an average concentration of TF = 2 × 10^{-5}M and using the value of 10^{27} for the formation constant, the side-reaction coefficient is:

$$\alpha_{M(TF)} = 1 + [TF]\,K_{M(TF)} = 2 \times 10^{22}. \tag{33}$$

Since $\alpha_{M(TF)}$ is far larger than $\alpha_{M(OH)}$ for Fe(III), we can disregard the latter in accordance with the rule of additivity of the alphas. Hence, from the logarithmic form of equation (14), and assuming that $\alpha_{ML(H)}$ and $\alpha_{ML(OH)}$ are unity:

$$\log. K_{eff} = \log. K_{ML} - [\log. \alpha_{M(TF)} + \log. \alpha_{L(H)}]. \tag{34}$$

We find for desferrioxamine that:

$$\log. K_{eff} = 30.6 - [21.7 + 6.1] = \sim 2.8. \tag{35}$$

Therefore:

$$K_{eff}\ (\text{Fe-H.D.F.O.}) = \sim 10^{3}.$$

The usual dose of H.D.F.O. injected into patients is about 500 mg. and, assuming equal distribution in 5 litres of blood and no excretion, the peak concentration would reach about 10^{-4}M. Hence the ratio of bound to free cation would be:

$$\frac{[\text{Fe(H.D.F.O.)}]}{[\text{Fe}]} = K_{eff}\ \text{H.D.F.O.} = \sim 10^{-1}. \tag{36}$$

This means that roughly 10% of the iron bound to transferrin would be removable by H.D.F.O*. Although this is a comparatively small percentage, if the removal of iron from TF is viewed as a multi-stage extraction process, then, by maintaining a sustained concentration of H.D.F.O. with the aid of repeated injections, it should be possible to remove a significant quantity of iron from

* On the basis of new data it must be concluded that the recalculated effective constant indicates that little or no iron can be removed by H.D.F.O. from transferrin. The Fe(III)-transferrin binding constants have now been reported to be 27.7 and 30.2 in log. units (*4a*). These data, together with PETERS' statement (p. 519) that the desferrioxamine "space" is equivalent to more than 50% of total body-weight, mean that less than 1% of the iron bound to transferrin is calculated to be removable by H.D.F.O. under equilibrium conditions.

TF. If the binding constants of Fe(III) are less than reported, and if the concentration of TF is reduced, then proportionally more Fe(III) could be mobilised by H.D.F.O. from TF. In normal individuals, up to 3 and 4 mg. of iron can be removed daily following administration of H.D.F.O. (MOESCHLIN, p. 528, 541). Since in normal subjects about 35 mg. of iron enter and leave the plasma each day (POLLYCOVE, p. 158), a good fraction of the roughly 3 mg. of iron removed by H.D.F.O. could be derived from this source.

In the case of E.D.T.A. and D.T.P.A. the values of K_{eff} ($\sim 10^{-3}$ and $10^{-0.6}$, respectively, as compared with $\sim 10^3$ for H.D.F.O.) are too small, from which it may be concluded that the usual *in vivo* concentrations of D.T.P.A. and E.D.T.A. are insufficient to effect significant removal of Fe(III) from TF. However, in *in vitro* systems, where far stronger concentrations of chelating agents can be employed, some removal could be obtained with much higher levels of D.T.P.A. or E.D.T.A.

In the test-tube, iron can be removed from TF easily and completely at pH $\sim$ 6 in the presence of an Fe(II)-selective chelating agent, such as o-phenanthroline, and with simultaneous reduction of Fe(III) to Fe(II) by $Na_2S_2O_4$ or cysteine (*29*). However, *in vivo*, such drastic conditions are not possible. Whereas Cu reacts with TF, it is easily replaced by Fe at neutral pH.

Ferritin and the mononuclear barrier

It would appear that the iron present in protein, such as ferritin, can be removed directly from tissue deposits. In view of the fact that the K_{eff} of H.D.F.O. is $\sim 10^8$ for such deposits of iron, it is reasonable to expect some depletion of these naturally insoluble iron hydroxides. In this connection it should be mentioned that iron phosphates are more soluble than iron hydroxides (*2*).

It has been pointed out that, above a concentration of $10^{-3.7}$M, ferric ion forms polynuclear hydroxide complexes which precede the formation of the insoluble hydroxide. In order for Fe^{+3} to penetrate the small volumes (HARRISON, p. 50) within the ferritin molecule, a "squeezing out" of water molecules must occur. Consequently, the molar concentration of Fe^{+3} will rapidly exceed the mononuclear barrier, so that precipitation occurs. Thus, ferritin can be visualised as a polymer, the structure of which is so contrived as to enable it to store, mechanically, as much iron as possible though the simple process of providing a three-dimensional network within whose pores or channels the concentration of Fe^{+3} exceeds the mononuclear barrier.

Discussion

There is no doubt that the most practical method for estimating the relative performance of chelating agents *in vivo* is by use of the effective equilibrium constants in which, as a minimum, the effects of interferences from OH^-, H^+, Ca^{++}, and the formation of acid and basic complexes are included. It is true that this does not allow for competitive effects from protein, but these can be included if the molar concentration and formation constants are known. However, for a given metal ion, reacting with a series of chelating agents, the effective constant still offers the best relative method for correlating and anticipating the experimental results. It is obvious that the conventional stability constants can be misleading and may even suggest behaviour which is actually the opposite of that observed. For example, from the conventional constants it might be expected that E.D.T.A. would prove useful in the treatment of mercury poisoning, but this is not the case. The effective constant, on the other hand, predicts the inertness of E.D.T.A. towards Hg *in vivo*. On the whole, the effective constant correctly predicts the relative excretion of metals by a given agent. The effective constant also explains why E.D.T.A. reacts more strongly at neutral pH with Cu(II) than with Fe(III), despite the fact that the conventional stability constant of the latter is more than a million times stronger than that of Cu(II). That the conventional stability constants follow the relative order of effectiveness of E.D.T.A., H.D.F.O., and D.T.P.A. towards Fe(III) at neutral pH is a coincidence. As for the relative stabilities of the Fe(III) chelates of H.D.F.O., D.T.P.A., and E.D.T.A. at lower pH's – an important factor when interpreting the breakdown of a metal chelate in the kidney – the conventional stability constant gives the wrong order.

The relative *in vivo* effectiveness of different chelating agents with respect to a given metal can be determined directly by ultrafiltration techniques (*10*). Thus, following administration of the chelating agent to an experimental animal, the individual tissues can be removed at a given time and either homogenised with saline solution before subjecting them to low-pressure ultrafiltration, or else cut into small pieces and ultrafiltered without addition of saline. Such techniques allow a practical comparison of the efficiency of different chelating agents under conditions in which the biological, metabolic, and chemical factors are automatically accounted for, so to speak.

It does not necessarily follow, of course, that when the effective constant for two metallic ions is the same in the case of a given chelating agent, the *in vivo* response of the metals in terms of their degree of mobilisation and toxicity will be equivalent. While additional terms can be added to the side-reaction coefficients, the accessibility *in vivo* of each metal to the chelating agent may differ appreciably. Each metal has a distinctive pattern of distribution within the tissues; moreover, though the gross tissue distributions may appear similar, the intracellular distributions may, and often do, differ considerably. Consequently, apart from the chemical factors, such as the pH, which influence the metabolism of metal chelates, the biological factors must also be considered. Even here, however, the fact that two metals may possess identical effective stability constants for a given chelating agent can offer certain worthwhile clues: for example, if the two metals in question show differing responses *in vivo*, the difference is probably due mainly to biological and metabolic rather than to simple chemical factors.

Esterification to render chelating agents more capable of penetrating tissues has sometimes proved useful, as shown by CATSCH (*8*, p. 206). Another approach has involved the use of metabolic inhibitors – themselves devoid of chelating action – to induce the tissues to produce excessive amounts of a naturally occurring chelating agent. This has been demonstrated (*6*) in the case of experimental lead poisoning, in which the injection of small non-lethal amounts of sodium fluoro-acetate caused tissue such as that of the spleen to increase its production of citric acid to 20 times the normal level, with the result that local tissue concentrations of up to 5×10^{-3} M occurred.

A great deal of experimental evidence has accumulated over the years which shows that the toxicity of metals can sometimes be enhanced by the use of chelating agents. The reason for this appears to lie in the fact that a chelating agent can also make a metal available or distribute it to sites normally inaccessible to it.

It is worth mentioning that the treatment of chronic metal poisoning need not necessarily require the use of chelating agents which form soluble metal chelates. Instead, one can use chelating dyestuffs which form insoluble polychelates *in situ* and thus inactivate a metal without mobilising it. The greater effectiveness of dyestuffs as compared with simple chelating agents in the treatment of experimental beryllium poisoning has been demonstrated (*21*).

Another potentially useful application of chelation to medicine is the use of chelating agents to control the distribution of a metal within the body. Since the tissue distribution of polynuclear complexes is a function of particle size, it is possible to exercise control over this factor by altering the concentration ratio of the chelating agent to the metal (*21*).

Reference should also be made to the selective stabilisation by chelating agents of different oxidation states of metals with variable valence. Many examples are available (*22*), especially in the case of reactions involving oxygenation. One interesting example concerns the stabilisation of ferrous ions against radiation-induced oxidation by the use of a ferrous-preferring chelating agent, whereas the use of a ferric-preferring chelating agent promotes the radiation-induced oxidation of ferrous ion. Hence, by controlling the type and concentration of a chelating agent, it is possible to regulate the degree of reduction or oxidation of a metallic ion in response to ionising irradiation. Similarly, by the use of suitable concentrations of E.D.T.A., the copper-catalysed destruction of ascorbic acid can be inhibited or promoted.

The presumed role of copper (*22*) offers an interesting example of a chelating action in radiobiology. Chemical protective agents, such as the mercaptans, dithiols, dithiocarbamates, cyanides, and azides, complex or chelate perferentially with cuprous copper, whereas chemical sensitising agents, such as the α-alkyl alanines and quinoids, favour cupric copper. Consequently, apart from effects on the cell nucleus, it has been postulated that retardation of the oxidising action of acutely lethal doses of ionising irradiation could result from chemical stabilisation of critical Cu(I) sites, whereas corresponding reactions involving Cu(II) would enhance oxidation of Cu(I). Let us consider in this connection such well-known protective agents as the mercapto-alkylamines, which have the general formula:

$$\begin{array}{lcl} CH_2 & —(CH_2)_n— & CH_2 \\ | & & | \\ SH & & NH_2 \end{array}$$

These compounds show high protective activity when n has values of 0 and 1, but not when n has other values. It is significant that only the compounds in which $n = 0$ and $n = 1$ can form stable five and six-membered chelates capable of stabilising Cu(I).

Similarly, remarkable correlations between radio-protective ability and structures capable of chelating cuprous copper have been observed in the case of dozens of compounds as described in a forthcoming monograph (*22*).

Summary

Basic concepts of chelate chemistry are reviewed, including a discussion of the chelate effect, especially in relation to desferrioxamine. Also stressed and illustrated are problems relating to the mechanism of action of chelating agents *in vivo* from the chemical, metabolic, and cellular aspects.

Detailed consideration is given to the problem of estimating the stability *in vivo* of metal chelates. Simple, quantitative methods are described by which it is possible to evaluate the relative effectiveness of chelating agents in promoting the excretion of metallic ions and in the treatment of metal poisoning.

Two examples are given: one in which the metallic ions are in the circulation and the other in which they are present as insoluble deposits in the tissues. In both instances the concept of the effective constant is introduced; this enables one to assess the degree to which interfering cations and anions affect the *in vivo* efficiency of the chelating agents administered. The conventional stability constants are shown to be unreliable and may be misleading when employed to estimate the relative stabilities of metal chelates *in vivo*.

In order to obtain numerical values for the effective constant, use is made of the so-called alpha or side-reaction coefficients, which give a direct measure of the extent of side reactions caused, for example, by competition of H^+ and Ca^{++} against a metallic ion, M, for the chelating agent, L, or by OH^- competition for the metallic ion (hydrolytic reactions). The effective constant is calculated from the α-values as included in the definition of the effective constant:

$$K_{\text{eff}} = \left(\frac{\alpha_{\text{ML}}}{\alpha_{\text{M}}\alpha_{\text{ML}}}\right) K_{\text{ML}}\,.$$

An important rule exists for simplifying the calculations when several interfering ions must be considered, namely: the over-all alpha coefficients can be taken as being approximately equal to the sum of the individual coefficients. Usually one of the alpha terms predominates, so that the other terms can be dropped.

Three important chelating agents, ethylene-diamine tetra-acetic acid (E.D.T.A.), diethylene-triamine penta-acetic acid (D.T.P.A.), and desferrioxamine (H.D.F.O.) are considered with particular reference to their interactions with Fe(III), Fe(II), and Cu(II). The effective constants are calculated as a function of pH by taking into account interferences from H^+, Ca^{++}, and OH^- and the formation of acid and basic complexes. The results are in full agreement with experimental observations on the effectiveness or lack of effectiveness of these chelating agents in promoting the excretion of metallic ions and in the treatment of metal poisoning. Thus, at pH 7.25 the Cu-E.D.T.A. chelate is more stable than that of Fe(III)-E.D.T.A., despite the fact that the conventional stability constant of the iron chelate is more than a million times greater than that of the corresponding copper chelate. At pH 7.25 the Fe(III)-H.D.F.O. chelate is in a class by itself, revealing an unprecedented specificity for Fe(III), though at pH 4 it is weaker than the corresponding E.D.T.A. and D.T.P.A. chelates.

Another example of the application of the effective constant is in the action of E.D.T.A. on mercury. Although the conventional stability constant of Hg-E.D.T.A. is nearly 22 log. units, its effective constant is one of the smallest. Consequently the failure of E.D.T.A. to afford protection against mercury poisoning becomes quite clear.

The ability of chelating agents to remove transferrin-bound iron is evaluated by reference to the effective constant and the known concentration of transferrin in the blood and its binding constant for iron(III). According to the calculations, following injection of H.D.F.O. in man, less than 10% of the transferrin-bound iron is transferred to H.D.F.O. at a given time. In the case of E.D.T.A. and D.T.P.A. as well the effective constants are too small to permit any removal of iron from the protein *in vivo*.

The mechanism of action of the iron-storage protein is evaluated by introducing the concept of the mononuclear barrier. It is known that the formation of polynuclear complexes with the hydroxide ion precedes the formation of insoluble compounds. However, the concentration of polynuclear species decreases with dilution, and at a particular dilution a "mononuclear wall" is reached, with the result that below this critical metal concentration one is dealing only with mononuclear species. With Fe(III) the mononuclear barrier occurs below $10^{-3.7}$ M. It is concluded that ferritin functions as a polymer, whose structure is contrived to store as much iron as possible. This it does by providing a three-dimensional network containing such small pore or channel volumes that the entering iron ions must give up part of their water of hydration. Thus, the concentration of iron increases to the point where the mononuclear barrier is exceeded.

Zusammenfassung

Es wird eine Übersicht über die Grundlagen der Chemie der Komplexbildner gegeben, unter besonderer Berücksichtigung der Eigenschaften von Desferrioxamin. Probleme, die im Zusammenhang mit dem Wirkungsmechanismus der Komplexbildner *in vivo* stehen, werden im Hinblick auf chemische, metabolische und zelluläre Aspekte erörtert.

Die Frage der Bestimmung der Stabilität von Metallkomplexen *in vivo* wird im einzelnen besprochen. Einfache quantitative Methoden werden diskutiert, mit deren Hilfe es möglich ist, die relative Wirksamkeit von Komplexbildnern im Hinblick auf die Förderung der Ausscheidung von Metallionen und bei der Behandlung von Intoxikation mit Metallen zu bestimmen.

Zwei Beispiele werden im einzelnen erläutert — eines, bei dem die Metallionen im Blut kreisen, das andere, bei dem sie in unlöslicher Form im Gewebe abgelagert sind. Für beide Fälle wird der Begriff der effektiven Konstante diskutiert, die ein Urteil erlaubt, in welchem Maße interferierende Kationen und Anionen die *in vivo*-Wirkung eines gegebenen Komplexbildners beeinflussen. Die üblichen Stabilitätskonstanten sind in dieser Hinsicht nicht zuverlässig und können sogar irreführend sein, wenn man sie für die Bestimmung der relativen Stabilität von Metallkomplexen *in vivo* benutzt.

Um zahlenmäßige Werte für die effektive Konstante zu erhalten, bedient man sich der sogenannten alpha- oder Nebenreaktionskoeffizienten, die ein direktes Maß für den Grad der kompetitiven Nebenreaktionen geben. So können für den Komplexbildner, L, H^+ und Ca^{++} mit einem Metallion, M, konkurrieren, oder auch OH^- mit einem Metallion (hydrolytische Reaktionen). Die effektive Konstante wird berechnet aus den alpha-Werten, die sich aus der Definition der effektiven Konstante ergeben:

$$K_{eff} = \left(\frac{\alpha_{ML}}{\alpha_M \alpha_{ML}}\right) K_{ML} .$$

Wenn verschiedene, miteinander interferierende Ionen vorliegen, kann die Berechnung in folgender Weise vereinfacht werden: Die gesamten alpha-Koeffizienten können annähernd mit der Summe der Einzelkoeffizienten gleichgesetzt werden. Im allgemeinen überwiegt einer der alpha-Werte, so daß die anderen zu vernachlässigen sind.

Drei wichtige Komplexbildner, Aethylendiamin-tetraessigsäure (EDTA), Diaethylentriamin-pentaessigsäure (DTPA) und Desferrioxamin (HDFO) werden im Hinblick auf ihre Reaktion mit Fe^{++}, Fe^{+++} und Cu^{++} behandelt. Die effektiven Konstanten werden berechnet als eine Funktion des pH unter Berücksichtigung der Einwirkung von H^{+}, Ca^{++} und von OH^{-} und der Bildung saurer und basischer Komplexe. Die Ergebnisse stimmen überein mit experimentellen Beobachtungen über die Wirksamkeit oder Unwirksamkeit der genannten Komplexbildner im Hinblick auf die Ausscheidung der Metallionen und auf die Behandlung von Metallintoxikationen. So ist bei einem pH von 7,25 der Cu-EDTA Komplex stabiler als der entsprechende Fe^{+++}-EDTA Komplex, obwohl die konventionelle Stabilitätskonstante des Eisenkomplexes mehr als eine Million mal größer ist als diejenige des entsprechenden Kupferkomplexes. Bei einem pH von 7,25 steht der Fe^{+++}-HDFO Komplex in einer Gruppe für sich und zeigt eine Spezifität für Fe^{+++}, die nicht vorherzusehen war, während der Komplex bei pH 4 schwächer als die entsprechenden EDTA und DTPA Komplexe ist.

Ein anderes Beispiel für die Anwendungsmöglichkeiten der effektiven Konstante ist die Wirkung von EDTA auf Quecksilber. Trotz der Tatsache, daß die übliche Stabilitätskonstante von Hg-EDTA nahezu 22 Zehnerpotenzen beträgt, ist ihre effektive Konstante eine der schwächsten. Daraus erklärt sich das Versagen von EDTA bei der Behandlung einer Quecksilbervergiftung.

Die Fähigkeit der Komplexbildner, an Transferrin gebundenes Eisen zu entfernen, wird mit Hilfe der effektiven Konstante und der bekannten Konzentration von Transferrin im Blut sowie seiner Bindungsfähigkeit für dreiwertiges Eisen bestimmt. Entsprechend diesen Berechnungen werden beim Menschen nach Injektion von HDFO weniger als 10% des an Transferrin gebundenen Eisens zu einem bestimmten Zeitpunkt auf HDFO übertragen. Auch für EDTA und DTPA sind die effektiven Konstanten zu klein, um Eisen aus seiner Eiweißbindung *in vivo* zu entfernen.

Der Wirkungsmechanismus der Eisenspeicherung an Eiweiß wird durch Einführung des Begriffes der mononukleären Schranke bestimmt. Es ist bekannt, daß die Bildung polynukleärer Komplexe mit dem Hydroxydion der Bildung unlöslicher Verbindungen vorausgeht. Die Konzentration polynukleärer Komplexe nimmt jedoch bei Verdünnung ab und erreicht schließlich eine „mononukleäre Schranke". Unterhalb dieser kritischen Metallkonzentration liegt nur noch ein mononukleärer Komplex vor. Mit Fe^{+++} tritt die mononukleäre Schranke unterhalb einer Konzentration von $10^{-3.7}$ M auf. Es wird geschlossen, daß Ferritin als ein Polymer wirkt, dessen Struktur es ermöglicht, so viel Eisen wie möglich zu speichern. Dies wird durch eine dreidimensionale Netzstruktur erreicht, die sehr kleine Poren oder Kanäle enthält, so daß die eintretenden Eisenionen einen Teil ihres Hydratationswassers abgeben müssen. Auf diese Weise steigt die Konzentration von Eisen bis zu einem Punkt an, an dem die mononukleäre Schranke überschritten wird.

Résumé

Les concepts fondamentaux de la chimie des agents chélatants sont passés en revue, comprenant une discussion sur l'effet chélateur, en particulier en ce qui concerne la desferrioxamine. Les problèmes en relation avec le mécanisme d'action des agents chélatants *in vivo* sont également soulignés et illustrés des points de vue chimique, métabolique et cellulaire.

Des considérations détaillées sont données sur le problème de l'évaluation de la stabilité *in vivo* des agents chélateurs des métaux. Des méthodes quantitatives simples sont décrites qui permettent d'évaluer l'efficacité relative des agents chélatants quant à leur effet de stimulation de l'excrétion des ions métalliques et dans le traitement des intoxications par les métaux.

Deux exemples en sont donnés: l'un, dans lequel les ions métalliques sont dans la circulation, l'autre, dans lequel les ions métalliques existent sous forme de dépôts insolubles dans les tissus. Dans ces deux exemples la notion de constante d'efficacité est introduite; ceci permet d'apprécier à quel degré l'interférence des cations et anions influe sur l'efficacité *in vivo* des agents chélatants administrés. Les constantes conventionnelles de stabilité ne donnent pas une image fidèle et peuvent conduire à des erreurs si on les emploie pour estimer les stabilités relatives *in vivo* des complexes de chélateurs liés au métal.

Afin d'obtenir des valeurs numériques de la constante d'efficacité, on utilise les coefficients dits alpha ou de réaction collatérale, ce qui donne une mesure directe de l'importance des réactions collatérales provoquées, par exemple, par la compétition des ions H^+ et Ca^{++} avec un ion métallique M pour l'agent chélatant, L, ou par la compétition des ions OH^- pour l'ion métallique (réaction d'hydrolyse). La constante d'efficacité est calculée à partir des valeurs alpha telles qu'elles sont comprises dans la définition de la constante d'efficacité:

$$K_{\text{eff}} = \left(\frac{\alpha_{ML}}{\alpha_M \alpha_{ML}}\right) K_{ML}\,.$$

Il existe une règle importante pour simplifier les calculs quand on doit considérer plusieurs ions qui interfèrent, à savoir: l'ensemble des coefficients alpha peut être considéré approximativement égal à la somme des coefficients pris isolément. Habituellement l'un des termes alpha domine, de sorte qu'on peut négliger les autres.

Trois agents chélatants importants, l'acide éthylène-diamine tétra-acétique (E.D.T.A.), l'acide diéthylène-triamine penta-acétique (D.T.P.A.) et la desferrioxamine (H.D.F.O.) sont envisagés, en particulier en ce qui concerne leur réaction avec le Fe^{+++}, le Fe^{++}, et le Cu^{++}. Les constantes d'efficacité sont calculées en fonction du pH en considérant les interférences à partir des ions H^+, Ca^{++} et OH^-, et la formation de complexes acides et basiques. Les résultats sont en parfait accord avec les observations expérimentales sur l'efficacité ou l'inefficacité de ces agents chélatants quant à l'accélération de l'excrétion des ions métalliques et quant au traitement de l'intoxication aux métaux. Ainsi, à pH 7,25 le complexe d'E.D.T.A. et de Cu est plus stable que le complexe d'E.D.T.A. et de Fe^{+++}, en dépit du fait que la constante de stabilité conventionnelle pour le complexe de fer est plus d'un million de fois plus élevée que celle du complexe de cuivre. A un pH de 7,25, le complexe de H.D.F.O. et de Fe^{+++} constitue une classe à part, car il comporte une spécificité sans précédent pour le Fe^{+++}, bien qu'à un pH de 4, il soit plus faible que les complexes correspondants d'E.D.T.A. et de D.T.P.A.

Un autre exemple de l'application de la constante d'efficacité est l'action de l'E.D.T.A. sur le mercure. Bien que la constante de stabilité conventionnelle du complexe E.D.T.A. de mercure soit près de 22 unités log., sa constante d'efficacité est l'une des plus petites. En conséquence, l'incapacité de l'E.D.T.A. d'assurer une protection contre l'intoxication au mercure s'explique parfaitement.

La capacité des agents chélatants de déplacer le fer lié à la transferrine est évaluée au moyen de la constante d'efficacité et de la concentration connue de la transferrine dans le sang ainsi que de sa capacité de fixation du Fe^{+++}. Selon les calculs, chez l'homme, moins que 10% du fer lié à la transferrine passe à un moment donné sur l'H.D.F.O. après injection de celle-ci. Aussi dans le cas de l'E.D.T.A. et du D.T.P.A., les constantes d'efficacité sont trop petites pour permettre *in vivo* un déplacement du fer de la protéine.

Le mécanisme d'action de la protéine de stockage du fer est déterminé par la notion de barrière mononucléaire. On sait que la formation de complexes polynucléaires avec les ions hydroxydes précède la formation de composés insolubles. Cependant, la concentration des espèces polynucléaires décroît avec la dilution, et pour une dilution donnée le "mur mononucléaire" est atteint, avec comme résultat que, en dessous de cette concentration critique en métal, on n'a plus affaire qu'à des espèces mononucléaires. Avec le Fe^{+++}, la barrière mononucléaire se place au dessous de $10^{-3,7}$ M. On en conclut que la ferritine fonctionne comme un polymère, dont la structure est adaptée pour stocker autant de fer que possible, ce qu'elle fait en fournissant un réseau à trois dimensions contenant des pores et des défilés de si petit volume que les ions fer qui y pénètrent doivent abandonner une partie de leur eau d'hydratation. Ainsi, la concentration de fer augmente jusqu'au point où la barrière mononucléaire est dépassée.

References

1. Biederman, G., and P. Schindler: Acta chem. Scand. **11**, 731 (1957). — 2. Bjerrum, J., G. Schwarzenbach, and L. G. Sillén: Chem. Soc. London, Spec. Publ. No. 6 (1957); *ibid.* Spec. Publ. No. 7 (1958). — 3. Chaberek, S., and A. E. Martell: Organic Sequestering Agents. John Wiley & Sons, New York, 1959. — 4. Cotton, F. A., and G. Wilkinson: Advanced Inorganic Chemistry. Interscience Publishers, New York, 1962. — 4a. Davis, B., P. Saltman, and S. Benson: Biochem. Biophys. Res. Commun. (U.S.A.) 8, 56 (1962). — 5. Fredrick, J. F. (Editor): Chelation Phenomena. Ann. N. Y. Acad. Sc. 88, 281 (1960). — 6. Fried, J. F., M. W. Rosenthal, and J. Schubert: Proc. Soc. Exper. Biol. Med. (U.S.A.) **92**, 331 (1956). — 7. Heller, H. J.: Some Aspects of Chelation Chemistry. In: Diagnosis and Treatment of Radioactive Poisoning. International Atomic Energy Agency, Vienna, 1963. — 8. Johnson, L. A., and M. J. Seven (Editors): Biological Aspects of Metal-Binding. Fed. Proc. (U.S.A.) **20**, Suppl. No. 10, Part II (1961). — 9. Karrer, P.: Personal communication to the author, dated 11th January, 1960. — 10. Lindenbaum, A., and J. Schubert: Nature (G.B.) **187**, 575 (1960). — 11. Martell, A. E., and M. Calvin: Chemistry of the Metal Chelate Compounds. Prentice-Hall, Inc., New York, 1952. — 12. Morgan, G. T., and H. D. K. Drew: J. Chem. Soc. (G.B.) **117**, 1456 (1920). — 13. Peters, R. A., L. A. Stocken, and R. H. S. Thompson: Nature (G.B.) **156**, 601 (1945). — 14. Prelog, V.: Pure and Appl. Chem. (G.B.) **6**, 327 (1963). — 15. Reilly, C. N., R. W. Schmidt, and F. S. Sadek: J. Chem. Educ. (U.S.A.) **36**, 555 (1959). — 16. Ringbom, A.: J. Chem. Educ. (U.S.A.) **35**, 282 (1958). — 17. Ringbom, A.: Complexation Reactions. In: Treatise on Analytical Chemistry. Part I, Vol. 1, Chapter 14. Ed. by I. M. Kolthoff, P. J. Elving, and E. B. Sandell: The Interscience Encyclopedia, Inc., New York, 1959, p. 543. — 18. Saltman, P.: Fed. Proc. (U.S.A.) **20**, Suppl. No. 10, 95 (1961). — 19. Seven, M. J., and L. A. Johnson (Editors): Metal-Binding in Medicine. Lippincott, Philadelphia, 1960. — 20. Schubert, J.: Ann. Rev. Nuclear Sc. (U.S.A.) **5**, 369 (1959); Schubert, J.: Fed. Proc. (U.S.A.) **20**, Suppl. No. 10, 219 (1961). — 21. Schubert, J., and A. Lindenbaum: Ref. 19, p. 68. — 22. Schubert, J.: Copper and Peroxides in Radio-

biology and Medicine. Thomas, Springfield, Ill. (in press). — 23. SCHUBERT, J., and J. F. FRIED: Nature (G.B.) **185**, 551 (1960); FRIED, J. F., and J. SCHUBERT: Radiol. Res. (U.S.A.) **15**, 227 (1961). — 24. SCHUBERT, J., J. F. FRIED, M. W. ROSENTHAL, and A. LINDENBAUM: Radiol. Res. (U.S.A.) **15**, 220 (1961). — 25. SCHWARZENBACH, G.: The Analyst. J. Soc. Anal. Chem. (G.B.) **80**, 713 (1955). — 26. SCHWARZENBACH, G.: The General, Selective, and Specific Formation of Complexes by Metallic Cations. In: Advances in Inorganic Chemistry and Radiochemistry. Vol. 3. Ed. by H. J. EMELÉUS and A. G. SHARPE. Academic Press Inc., New York, 1961, p. 257. — 27. SCHWARZENBACH, G., and K. SCHWARZENBACH: Helvet. chim. acta **46**, 1390 (1963); ANDEREGG, G., F. L'EPLATTENIER, and G. SCHWARZENBACH: Helvet. chim. acta **46**, 1400 (1963); Helvet. chim. acta **46**, 1409 (1963). — 28. SILLÉN, L. G.: Acta chem. Scand. **8**, 299 (1954); Recueil trav. chim. Pays-Bas **75**, 705 (1956). — 29. WESTERFELD, W. W.: Fed. Proc. (U.S.A.) **20**, Suppl. No. 10, 158 (1961). — 30. WILLIAMS, R. J. P.: Fed. Proc. (U.S.A.) **20**, Suppl. No. 10, 5 (1961).

Discussion

EICHHORN: Dr. SCHUBERT, it strikes me that perhaps the most difficult part of the calculation of this effective constant is the problem of determining, under any set of physiological conditions, which metals in what concentrations, and which ligands in what concentrations, must be considered. So I wonder if you could give one example, without calculations, to show how one takes these factors into account.

PETERS: There are quite a few questions which I hesitate to ask, because I fear I am one of those medical doctors to whose calculating abilities you were referring! First question: In your calculations you assumed that desferrioxamine was distributed in blood water. This is not quite justifiable, since the space of distribution is nearly equal to the total body water. A change in the assumed plasma concentrations of desferrioxamine by one decimal order of magnitude would result. How would your data be influenced by this change, which, as I realise, is small in the field of physical chemistry? — Second question: Your calculations are based on stability constants which are equilibrium constants. Now, what evidence is there that under biological conditions an equilibrium in the system desferrioxamine + iron $\rightleftharpoons$ ferrioxamine is ever reached? — Third question: You referred repeatedly to the concentration of free ferric ions in the plasma, which is actually extremely small — so small that you could, perhaps, be justified in assuming an activity coefficient of 1.0. There is, however, little evidence from biological experiments that desferrioxamine actually interacts with free ferric ions in the plasma. Would not rather small changes in the assumed free ferric ion concentration cause rather large changes in your results?

PRELOG: In the examples given by Dr. SCHUBERT the stability constants of transferrin complexes should really be included in calculations of "effective" dissociation constants for blood plasma. For the transferrin-iron(III) complex, the high stability constant $K = 10^{30}$ is given in the literature[1]. One should also not forget that transferrin in normal blood is only half-saturated with iron(III) ion. Thus, transferrin is a very important competitor and should not be disregarded. As the stability constants for complexes of other biologically important ions with transferrin and with other protein components of blood plasma are practically unknown, I believe that realistic calculations of "effective" dissociation constants are not possible at present.

CLETON: Dr. SCHUBERT, how long does it take for transferrin and desferrioxamine to reach equilibrium in iron exchange? Do you think that such a state of equilibration would ever occur *in vivo*, considering the rapidity with which desferrioxamine is excreted?

SCHUBERT: Let me first answer Dr. EICHHORN's question. You use the side-reaction coefficients, α, as described in my paper. As a minimum you should include the competitive effects of OH^-, H^+, and Ca^{++} under physio-

[1] DAVIS, B., P. SALTMAN, and S. BENSON: Biochem. Biophys. Res. Commun. (U.S.A.) 8, 56 (1962).

logical conditions. The required data are obtained from tables available in the literature and cited in my paper.

As to the other question which Dr. PETERS asked about the distribution of iron, the volumes I used for iron distribution were plasma volumes. However, I want to emphasise that the calculations give a *relative* measure of the efficiency of different chelating agents with respect to a given metal. This partially answers Dr. PRELOG's question as well, because for a given metal the unknown competitive factors have identical α-values, regardless of the chelating agent. The effective stability is a far more practical measure than the absolute stability constant, as shown in Fig. 3 of my paper (p. 479), from which it will be seen that, depending on the pH, the relative effectiveness of a given chelating agent may be completely the reverse of what one would expect from the absolute constant. One can estimate the relative effect of transferrin on the effective constant when the concentration of transferrin and its binding constant for iron are known. These calculations are not quite so theoretical as they may appear; they are, in fact, used very practically in analytical chemistry in connection with complexometric titration techniques.

As far as equilibration rates are concerned, I have not worked with desferrioxamine — but I do believe, and I have been told, that the amount of iron removed *in vivo* approaches the theoretical amount on a millimol-for-millimol basis. For practical purposes I regard an *in vivo* removal of 20% or more as being sufficiently complete. This would indicate that the reaction is very rapid. Insofar as competition by transferrin for iron is concerned, it is known that transferrin binds most of the plasma iron. However, from a consideration of the molar concentration of transferrin ($\sim 3 \times 10^{-5}$M) and its binding constants for iron, it may be estimated that desferrioxamine can still remove some plasma iron *in vivo*. In any case, the exclusion of the side-reaction coefficient for transferrin in the evaluation of the effective constant does not alter the conclusions as to the relative effectiveness of different chelating agents for a given metal under physiological conditions. Knowing the concentration of transferrin and the appropriate binding constant for iron — which involves knowledge of the degree of saturation — one can include them in the evaluation of the effective constant. However, if you want to know the actual fraction of iron that will be removed from a given tissue, one of the best ways to determine it is to remove the tissue after injection of a chelating agent, homogenise it, dialyse the prepared tissue suspended in the serum against serum, and thus discover the amount of iron actually removed. This does not involve any calculation, but just a straightforward measurement under physiological conditions.

Introduction to the General Discussion

By

B. Dreyfus

In introducing the general discussion, I should like first of all to make a few comments on the treatment of iron deficiency and on the papers of Dr. Undritz and Dr. Figueroa.

I am particularly interested in so-called masked iron deficiency, since it is not yet perfectly clear to me as to how the diagnosis can be established. Masked iron deficiency is characterised by normal haemoglobin values and by signs and symptoms such as fatigue, headache, dyspnoea, koilonychia, atrophy of various mucous membranes, etc. These, as Dr. Beutler has shown, are probably related to a deficiency of iron-containing enzymes such as cytochrome C. The most important point is that they can be relieved by means of iron therapy. But this raises the question as to how such states are to be recognised and correctly treated, particularly since not only the haemoglobin values are normal but also, in many cases, the plasma iron and – or so I understand – the iron-binding capacity as well. Perhaps, as has been indicated by studies with radioactive iron, increased absorption from the gut and possibly increased incorporation of iron into the red cells might provide some helpful clues in this connection. The same may apply to haemosiderin in the bone marrow, i.e. it is conceivable that in such cases Perls' staining might show that in the erythroblasts, as well as in the reticulo-endothelial cells, iron is greatly reduced or even absent, whereas the plasma iron remains normal and no alteration occurs in haemoglobin formation.

Alternatively, as Dr. Beutler has pointed out, it may be that, in cases where an initial study of the blood reveals apparently normal haemoglobin values, a subsequent improvement in the haemoglobin concentration offers the best and simplest criterion on which to base a correct diagnosis.

Another question I should like to raise is: how are we to explain the fact that many of the signs and symptoms allegedly due to depletion of tissue iron are quite unusual in severe iron-deficiency anaemia, even of long duration? Dr. Undritz's observations on so-called physiological anaemia in infants and children strike me as being of great importance in this context. I should like to know whether he noted an improvement in the haemoglobin values in response to iron therapy in all the cases he studied. Is this improvement in the haemoglobin values regarded, as I believe it should be, as being characteristic of iron deficiency and, if so, are there no other ways of proving this, as in the case of masked iron deficiency?

With regard to treatment, I think everyone will agree with Dr. FIGUEROA's conclusion that, in view of the possibility of severe toxic or allergic reactions, parenteral iron therapy in any form should be resorted to only in very specific cases in which it is clearly indicated, oral treatment being employed in all other cases.

The work done by Dr. FINCH a few years ago has convincingly demonstrated the need for eliminating excess iron in haemochromatosis. Unfortunately, as Dr. FINCH and Dr. MOORE have already pointed out in this Symposium, since healthy individuals excrete such very small quantities of iron, there is no physiological mechanism of iron excretion which can be stimulated for therapeutic purposes. There are, in fact, only two physiopathological means by which the organism rids itself of excessive iron, namely repeated blood loss and chronic haemoglobinuria.

It is obvious that only the first of these two processes can be recommended as a form of treatment. But venesection, though most useful in idiopathic haemochromatosis, may provoke undesirable effects in secondary haemochromatosis of the kind seen in cirrhosis of the liver and in the course of anaemia, i.e. hypochromic hypersideraemic anaemia, including thalassaemia major, and particularly aplastic or refractory varieties. The introduction of chelating agents may therefore constitute a most important advance in this field; and in this connection I think we can derive a good deal of hope from the paper by Dr. SCHUBERT.

General Discussion

BEUTLER: Perhaps Dr. UNDRITZ will not mind if I discuss in part the questions which Dr. B. DREYFUS raised about the diagnosis of masked iron deficiency, since I have been quite interested in this problem. Unfortunately, in very many of the observations which have been made over the past century, no diagnostic techniques were employed. What was done was simply that iron was administered to a chronically fatigued woman; if she improved, then a diagnosis of iron deficiency was considered to have been confirmed. More recently, other means have been used to diagnose iron deficiency in these patients. The plasma iron and iron-binding capacity in such cases is not always normal. It is sometimes normal and sometimes abnormal. A considerable number of these patients do have a low plasma iron and an elevated iron-binding capacity. Dr. VERLOOP, for example, has published a series of 10 or 15 such cases in which this fact was well documented[1]. The method on which we rely most heavily in the patients with a normal plasma iron and iron-binding capacity is investigation of the bone-marrow iron. Bone-marrow iron estimations, however, do leave something to be desired. It is my concept that, when a patient begins to lose body iron, the body iron is first mobilised from the stores, and the storage depots become depleted — or nearly so — before there is loss of either haemoglobin or enzyme iron. Unfortunately, we have no way of distinguishing clinically between that point in the development of iron depletion when the iron depots are empty and that point at which not only are the iron depots empty, but there is also a small loss of either haemoglobin or enzymes. To do this, we have to perform measurements of other iron compounds in our patients, such as measurements of cytochrome oxidase, cytochrome C, aconitase, and so forth. The success in doing this has been quite limited in man, and what success there has been, has been on a laboratory scale and is not clinically practical.

Radio-iron turnover and incorporation studies have been found to be no more sensitive than measurement of the plasma iron levels. Thus, there is at present no satisfactory solution to the problem of diagnosing masked iron deficiency — assuming, of course, that such a state does in fact exist.

KATZ: I should like to point out that it is perhaps not desirable to use a chelating substance which has the ability to remove iron from transferrin *in vivo*. Some years ago, JANDL and his coworkers[2] showed that, when sufficiently high concentrations of E.D.T.A. are used in systems of reticulocytes and transferrin, there is a marked decrease in the uptake of iron by the reticulocytes. Presumably the E.D.T.A.-iron complexes are not able to enter the developing red cells. Therefore, if the chelating agent is sufficiently powerful to remove iron from circulating transferrin, it may very seriously interfere with normal iron kinetics and may compromise haemoglobin production.

FINCH: I should like to express my concern that we should define iron supply in proper terms. Stores have not been shown to be related to the supply

[1] VERLOOP, M. C., J. E. MEEUWISSEN, and E. W. BLOKHUIS: Brit. J. Haemat. **4**, 70 (1958).

[2] JANDL, J. H., J. K. INMAN, R. L. SIMMONS, and D. W. ALLEN: J. Clin. Invest. (U.S.A.) **38**, 161 (1959).

of iron to the body cells, whereas there is quite a lot of evidence that the plasma iron levels are of considerable significance in this connection.

A saturation of transferrin of above 15% appears to be critical to the marrow, and presumably other tissues have other critical levels.

FIGUEROA: I have not been very much concerned with bone-marrow depression by desferrioxamine B, as I believe that most of the patients in whom this drug is indicated are not making very much blood.

KATZ: I was talking about the use of excessively powerful chelating substances in haemochromatosis, where marrow function is normal. Under such circumstances sideropenic anaemias may be produced.

POLLYCOVE: I want to emphasise Dr. FINCH's point, which is also well supported by the work of JANDL and KATZ[1], namely, that the transfer of iron to red cells is dependent upon an adequate iron saturation and concentration of transferrin in the plasma. Our iron-kinetic studies and the investigations of marrow sideroblasts by BAINTON and FINCH[2] indicate that, unless the iron saturation of plasma transferrin is decreased considerably below the lower limits of normal, immature red cells will not be deprived of an adequate supply of iron. Consequently, I believe that, in the presence of normal iron saturation of transferrin, one does not get a latent or masked iron-deficiency anaemia that can be improved by administering iron. Recently, WALLERSTEIN and his colleagues[3], in the course of a study on two normal subjects as they were systematically venesected, carried out serially complete haematologic blood measurements, measured the plasma iron concentrations, and stained the bone marrow for haemosiderin. They found unequivocal evidence in both subjects that the most sensitive indicator of iron depletion was the decrease in the plasma iron concentration and transferrin saturation; these decreased considerably before they could observe any diminution in marrow haemosiderin. As Dr. FINCH said, I think it is desirable to focus attention upon the supply and transport mechanisms.

BEUTLER: I should like to comment further on the relative importance of serum iron values and stainable bone-marrow iron in the diagnosis of iron deficiency. I quite agree with Dr. FINCH and Dr. POLLYCOVE that when the plasma iron is normal there ought to be an adequate supply of iron to the erythroid tissue, and therefore there should not be any iron-deficiency anaemia. I do not know why this is not the case, but I must state that, when we have performed careful studies of plasma iron and bone-marrow iron, we have found that patients with normal plasma iron, but without bone-marrow iron, have responded to iron therapy. This has been true not only in our experience, but also in that of other investigators, e.g. Dr. ZIZZA[4]. I therefore consider the method of stainable bone-marrow iron estimation, which was introduced by Dr. FINCH, to be a very important haematologic determination. Why should normal plasma iron values be encountered in patients with iron-deficiency anaemia? It could be that this is due to technical errors in performing serum iron determinations. However, I doubt this. I think that our laboratory is quite accurate in doing such iron determinations. It is possible that we set the lower limit of plasma iron at the wrong level, or perhaps it has something to do with diurnal variations in the plasma

---

1 JANDL, J. H., and J. H. KATZ: J. Clin. Invest. (U.S.A.) **42**, 314 (1963).
2 BAINTON, D. F., and C. A. FINCH: Amer. J. Med. (in press, 1964).
3 WALLERSTEIN, R. O.: Personal communication.
4 ZIZZA, F., and N. BLOCK: Acta haemat. (Switz.) **25**, 1 (1961).

iron levels, so that the supply to the bone marrow is not continuously adequate. But, in the light of experience, I would have to maintain that there are patients who have iron-deficiency anaemia and who nevertheless have a normal plasma iron — at least as shown by a single determination in our laboratory.

SCHAPIRA: You said that the plasma iron was normal, but if you try to repeat the estimation after the treatment, the iron value may become higher, because there is a big dispersion of normal values, and what seems to be normal may be abnormally low.

BEUTLER: No, I think this is a very good point, but we have taken as the lower level of normal for plasma iron something of the order of 70 to 80 μg. %. However, we have not re-determined plasma iron after iron therapy. I think Dr. STURGEON has done something of that sort in pregnancy.

STURGEON: Several years ago I reported on results of a rather extensive study of this nature, both in pregnant women and in their offspring, the latter through 18 months of age. The data from the infants are in essential agreement with those presented by Dr. UNDRITZ. In the women the haematocrit, haemoglobin, and red blood counts were determined and the erythrocyte constants calculated. Serial serum iron, iron-binding capacity, serum copper, and free erythrocyte protoporphyrin determinations were also made. Fifty of the women took large doses of oral iron; a similar group was given 1,000 mg. of saccharated iron oxide intravenously in the first trimester of pregnancy or shortly thereafter; and a third group of 50 served as controls. The usual pattern of shift toward iron deficiency, as noted by Dr. VENTURA many years ago[1], was observed. With administration of supplementary iron, the shift was less marked, particularly with the intravenous preparation. However, under no circumstances did the mean values fall within the normal range, except for free erythrocyte protoporphyrin. I concluded from this that the pattern of iron deficiency was due only in part to the lack of iron and that it was also attributable to some more fundamental change in iron distribution which takes place during pregnancy[2].

POLLYCOVE: I think that whenever there is an increased erythropoietic demand for iron there will be an increase in the removal of iron from the plasma, and under these circumstances the plasma iron concentration will decrease, even though the iron stores may be entirely normal. The decreased plasma iron concentration makes possible the transfer of iron from the stores to the red cells at the required increased rate. The abnormally low plasma iron concentration does not necessarily signify that the patient is iron deficient; in the absence of infection, inflammation, malignancy or necrosis, which stimulate the reticulo-endothelial system, and in the presence of adequate iron stores, the low concentration of plasma iron indicates that the erythropoietic removal of plasma iron exceeds the rate at which iron would enter the plasma if the plasma iron concentration were normal.

FINCH: It is important to have some way of defining impairment of marrow function due to iron deficiency. One can point out that in certain conditions the reticulo-endothelial cell and the plasma iron go in different directions; but, as far as we can tell, impaired haemoglobin synthesis due

[1] VENTURA, S., and A. KLOPPER: J. Obstetr. Gynaec. Brit. Empire 58, 173 (1951).

[2] STURGEON, P.: Brit. J. Haemat. 5, 31 (1959).

to iron deficiency will be found only with a depression in transferrin saturation to below 15%. We recently did a study on pregnancy in which we attempted to identify iron-deficient patients according to their transferrin saturation in response to iron, and we were satisfied that their response did correspond to the prediction based on the plasma measurement. We bled a number of subjects and followed their transferrin, their plasma iron, and also their ability to respond by making new red cells. Again it was the percent saturation of transferrin which seemed best to indicate the point at which erythropoiesis was impaired.

VENTURA: I agree completely with Dr. POLLYCOVE's and Dr. FINCH's opinion on the value of the plasma transferrin — and especially its degree of saturation — in the diagnosis of early iron-deficiency states. I think this is also borne out by the results of research LARIZZA and I[1] did while working on the pathogenesis of hookworm anaemia.

Some patients with hookworm infestation, but without any pathological changes in their serum iron, transferrin, or haemoglobin values, were subjected to weekly removal of 50—75 ml. blood. The first value to show a modification of statistical significance was the degree of transferrin saturation. Only later did a decrease in serum iron and, finally, in haemoglobin occur.

---

[1] LARIZZA, P., and S. VENTURA: L'Anemia da Anchilostoma. Studio Patogenetico. Tipografia Libro, Pavia, 1950.

A pharmacological comparison of the binding of iron and other metals

By

J. Tripod

The use of chelating agents to bind certain metals and metalloids and to eliminate them for therapeutic purposes has become such a vast problem during the past ten years or so that it is impossible to review this topic in summary fashion, particularly if the biochemical, pharmacological, and toxicological implications are to be considered as well. It has now become a common practice to employ chelating agents, such as E.D.T.A., D.T.P.A., and E.D.D.H.A. [ethylene-diamine tetra-acetic acid, diethylene-triamine penta-acetic acid, and ethylene-diamine di-(o-hydroxyphenyl-acetic) acid], in order to promote the excretion of various metallic ions, and the biological and therapeutic properties of these agents have already been described in detail and summarised by various authors (*3, 13, 18, 22, 29*). There are also other "minor" chelating agents, e.g. penicillamine (*2, 25, 27, 38*), chlortetracycline, and oxytetracycline (*1, 19*), which for quite some time now have been known to display an affinity for certain metallic ions – including particularly Cu, Pb, and Mg in the case of penicillamine.

Meanwhile, however, desferrioxamine (Desferal) – obtained from the sideramine ferrioxamine, a metabolite of *Streptomyces pilosus* Ettlinger et al. (*6*) – has appeared on the scene; this new substance, the pharmacological properties of which have recently been reviewed (*34, 35, 36*), shows a remarkably strong specific affinity for ionic iron (*27, 32, 33, 34, 36*) and has therefore been employed as a specific in a wide variety of primary and secondary forms of haemochromatosis (*15, 16, 17, 23, 27, 39*).

In this connection, it would be interesting to compare the biological properties displayed by desferrioxamine with those of chelating agents such as E.D.T.A. But a detailed study of this kind would be beyond the scope of this Symposium; and a review of the problem would of necessity be incomplete in many respects, because sometimes, although a number of systematic data are perhaps available on – to take only two aspects – the biological and pharmacological properties of a chelating agent such as E.D.T.A.,

D.T.P.A., etc., the corresponding data may be lacking in the case of desferrioxamine, and *vice versa*. For various reasons of this nature, all that can be presented here are some experimental observations which, though they may serve as a basis of comparison and should help to differentiate more clearly between the two types of substance, constitute but a few elements in the mosaic of chelation with particular reference to iron. A systematic comparison, including also other recent chelating agents such as D.T.P.A. or E.D.D.H.A., would certainly have added further information on which to base a differentiation, but would have exceeded the present scope of our possibilities.

Be that as it may, E.D.T.A. (*3*, *4*, *18*, *22*, *29*) displays a variable affinity for a whole series of ions, including particularly metallic ions such as Zn (*18*, *26*), Mn (*10*), Cu (*13*, *29*, *30*, *37*), and Pb (*13*), as well as for rare and radioactive elements (*7*, *12*, *13*, *14*, *29*). It also has an affinity for Fe (*8*, *9*, *11*, *13*, *28*, *29*, *34*), in which we are especially interested here, because – as we have already seen – the most distinctive feature of desferrioxamine is its very strong affinity for this element. Hence, it is particularly interesting to differentiate between desferrioxamine and E.D.T.A. on the basis of the following points:

1. Their detoxicating potency with respect to iron and other metals under various experimental conditions.
2. Their effect on the elimination of iron.
3. Their influence on the urinary excretion of other metals.

These, of course, are only a few aspects of the problem of chelation. They are of quite considerable practical importance, however, since they are closely related to the phenomena of intoxication and/or poisoning due to metals, to the problem of eliminating excessive accumulations of metallic elements in the organism, and to the pathology and treatment of such conditions.

1. Detoxication of various metals by means of desferrioxamine and E.D.T.A.

Both desferrioxamine and E.D.T.A. have their own particular stability constants, which express the ratio between the concentration of the dissociated and the non-dissociated complex; the greater the stability of the complex, the higher the stability constant. Besides iron, the metals selected for study were Cu, Mn, Ni, and Zn, whose toxicity can easily be determined under certain experimental conditions. The respective stability constants are given in Table 1.

These physico-chemical constants, determined *in vitro*, show that the affinity of desferrioxamine for iron is considerably more specific than for the other metals listed and also appreciably greater than that of E.D.T.A.

Table 1. *Stability constants for desferrioxamine and E.D.T.A. with respect to various metallic ions*

Metallic ion	Desferrioxamine (*27*)	E.D.T.A. (*3, 18, 20, 22*)
Mn^{2+}	—	10^{14}
Fe^{3+}	10^{31}	10^{25}
Cu^{2+}	10^{14}	10^{18}
Ni^{2+}	10^{10}	10^{18}
Zn^{2+}	10^{11}	10^{16}

1.1 Detoxication in vitro. If we examine the detoxication of these metals *in vitro* by desferrioxamine and E.D.T.A., determining – in the mouse, for example – the acute oral toxicity of $FeSO_4$, $MnCl_2$, $CuSO_4$, $NiCl_2$, and $ZnSO_4$ when employed either alone or after mixing and incubating them *in vitro* at 37° for 2 hours with desferrioxamine, we obtain the results shown in Fig. 1. The acute

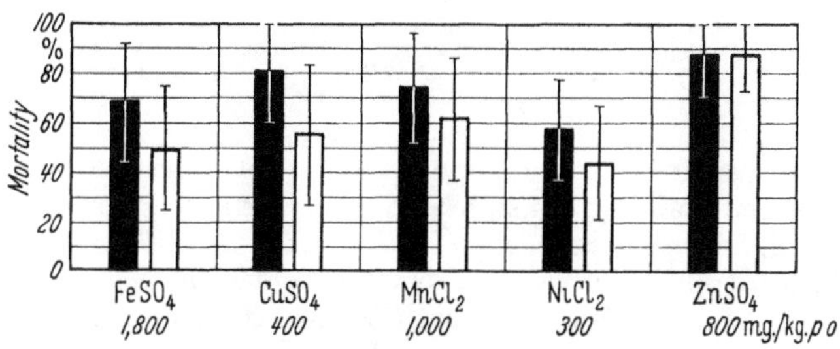

Fig. 1. Desferrioxamine, when previously mixed *in vitro* with various metals, causes very little decrease in their acute toxicity in the mouse. Ordinate: mortality of the animals in % ($n = 16-24$). $P = 0.05$[1]. ■ Metal alone p.o. □ Metal + desferrioxamine 2,000 mg./kg.p.o.

toxicity of $FeSO_4$, 1,800 mg./kg. p.o. (18% solution), is not significantly reduced by incubation with desferrioxamine, 2,000 mg./kg. p.o. (20% solution), and the same applies to the acute toxicity of $CuSO_4$, 400 mg./kg. p.o. (4% solution), $MnCl_2$, 1,000 mg./kg. p.o. (10% solution), $NiCl_2$, 300 mg./kg. p.o. (3% solution), and $ZnSO_4$, 800 mg./kg. p.o. (8% solution). This is in spite of the fact that desferrioxamine reacts with these metals *in vitro* to form red ferrioxamine with $FeSO_4$ (*5, 6*), a green complex with $CuSO_4$, a yellowish complex with $MnCl_2$, a dark-blue complex with $NiCl_2$, and a brownish complex with $ZnSO_4$.

[1] We are indebted to Dr. W. STAMM for the statistical analysis of these and of the other results given in this paper.

After having been incubated with these metals in the same concentrations, E.D.T.A. in a dose of 1,000 mg./kg. p.o. (10% solution) diminishes only the acute toxicity of $MnCl_2$ and – to a significant degree – that of $NiCl_2$. On the other hand, the toxicity of $FeSO_4$, $CuSO_4$, and $ZnSO_4$ is if anything increased (Fig. 2). E.D.T.A. reacts to form a brown complex with $FeSO_4$, a blue complex with $CuSO_4$, a green complex with $NiCl_2$, and a precipitate with $MnCl_2$.

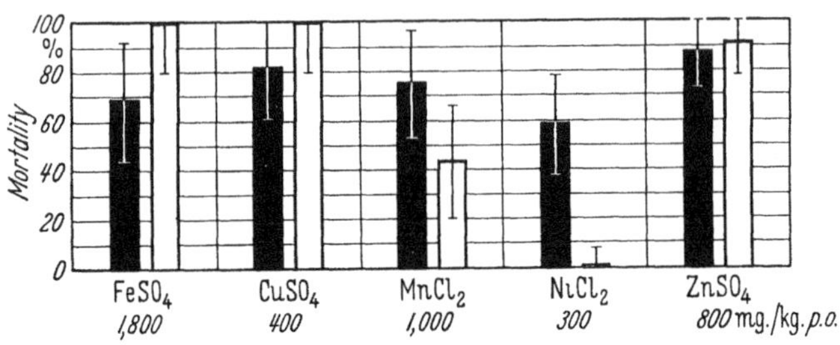

Fig. 2. In the mouse, E.D.T.A., after having been mixed with various metals *in vitro*, diminishes the acute toxicity of Mn and particularly Ni, but not that of Fe, Cu, or Zn. Ordinate: mortality of the animals in % (n = 16—24). P = 0.05. ■ Metal alone p.o. □ Metal + E.D.T.A. 1,000 mg./kg. p.o.

These results clearly demonstrate that it is impossible on the basis of the stability constants to predict the degree to which a metal will be detoxicated, even *in vitro*, since the stability constants would lead one to expect a greater activity on the part of desferrioxamine and E.D.T.A. with respect to iron, for example, whereas this is not the case. In fact, the reactions which desferrioxamine and E.D.T.A. undergo *in vitro* with these metals transform their physico-chemical properties to such an extent that their absorption is basically modified; this may be due to peculiarities in the kinetics of these reactions *in vitro*, to competitive mechanisms in the organism which cause a shift in the affinity of the chelating agent towards other ions (Na, K, Mg, and especially Ca, etc.), or simply to the formation *in vitro* of metallic complexes which become either less readily absorbable (Fe with desferrioxamine, Mn and Ni with E.D.T.A.) or, alternatively, more readily absorbable (Fe, Cu, or Zn with E.D.T.A.), etc.

1.2 Detoxication in vivo. Whatever the explanation may be, even more interest attaches in this connection to an examination of the detoxication *in vivo* of similar doses of these same metals under the influence of identical doses of desferrioxamine or E.D.T.A. For this purpose, we determined in the mouse the acute oral toxicity of

$FeSO_4$ (1,800 mg./kg.), $CuSO_4$ (400 mg./kg.), $MnCl_2$ (1,000 mg./kg.), $NiCl_2$ (300 mg./kg.), and $ZnSO_4$ (800 mg./kg.).

In parallel series of experiments, other animals were treated orally with desferrioxamine (2,000 mg./kg.) either immediately or 30, 60 or 120 minutes after the administration of the metallic salt.

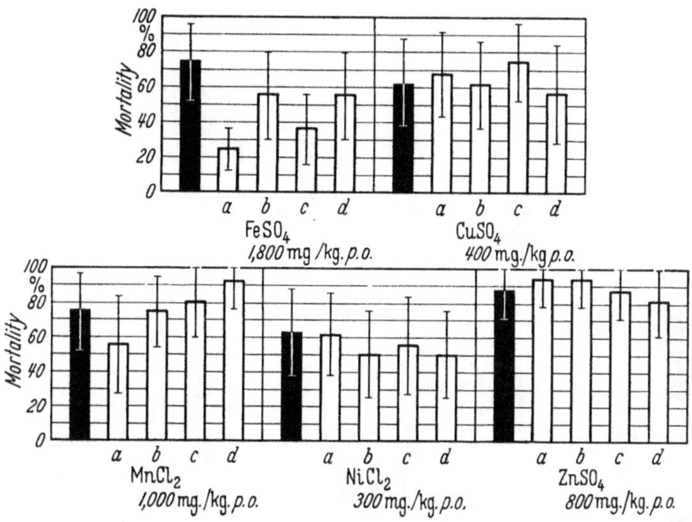

Fig. 3. Administered orally to mice, desferrioxamine affords partial protection against acute oral poisoning with Fe, particularly if given immediately after the Fe; but it has no influence on poisoning due to Cu, Mn, Ni, or Zn. Ordinate: mortality of the animals in % ($n = 16$). $P = 0.05$. ■ Metal alone □ Metal + desferrioxamine 2,000 mg./kg. p.o., *a* immediately, *b* after 30 min., *c* after 60 min., and *d* after 120 min.

The results obtained, which are outlined in Fig. 3, show that only $FeSO_4$ is detoxicated to any significant extent by desferrioxamine, particularly when the latter is given immediately after the ferric salt. The protection afforded against such acute poisoning diminishes successively in relation to the time elapsing between the administration of the salt and of the desferrioxamine – a fact which suggests that the desferrioxamine and the $FeSO_4$ probably become bound to each other chiefly in the gastro-intestinal tract. No significant modification in the toxicity of $CuSO_4$, $MnCl_2$, $NiCl_2$, or $ZnSO_4$ occurs in response to desferrioxamine.

In a second series of tests conducted in exactly the same manner, E.D.T.A. (1,000 mg./kg.) was employed orally instead of desferrioxamine; the results, as summarised in Fig. 4, show that E.D.T.A. is unable to protect the animals against poisoning due to $FeSO_4$,

$CuSO_4$, or $MnCl_2$, regardless of the time elapsing between the administration of the metallic salt and of the chelating agent. On the other hand, E.D.T.A. does afford protection against poisoning with $ZnSO_4$ and especially $NiCl_2$.

In a third series of experiments, desferrioxamine was administered subcutaneously in a dose of 1,000 mg./kg. in order to determine whether it was also capable of affording protection once it had

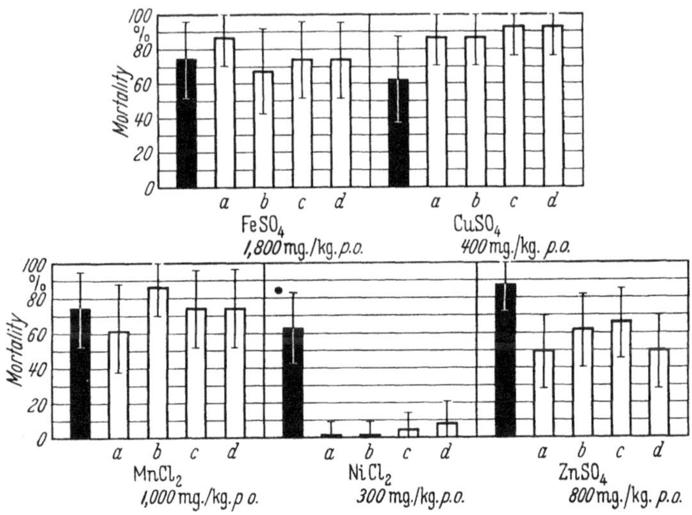

Fig. 4. Administered orally, E.D.T.A. does not protect the mouse against acute oral poisoning with $FeSO_4$, $CuSO_4$, or $MnCl_2$, but does afford protection in the case of $ZnSO_4$ and especially $NiCl_2$. Ordinate: mortality of the animals in % (n = 16—24). P = 0.05. ■ Metal alone □ Metal + E.D.T.A. 1,000 mg./kg. p.o.; *a*—*d* as in Fig. 3

already become distributed in the organism. The technicalities of the experiment were otherwise the same as for the first series of experiments. Fig. 5 shows that the protective effect of desferrioxamine does not manifest itself until an interval of 30 minutes has elapsed between the oral administration of $FeSO_4$ and the subcutaneous administration of desferrioxamine, i.e. not until the desferrioxamine has become distributed throughout the organism. The desferrioxamine is also still capable of protecting the animal against iron poisoning after 60 and 120 minutes, i.e. when both the ferric salt and the desferrioxamine are already in the organism. On the other hand, under these conditions, desferrioxamine is once again unable to afford any protection against poisoning caused by $CuSO_4$, $MnCl_2$, $NiCl_2$, or $ZnSO_4$.

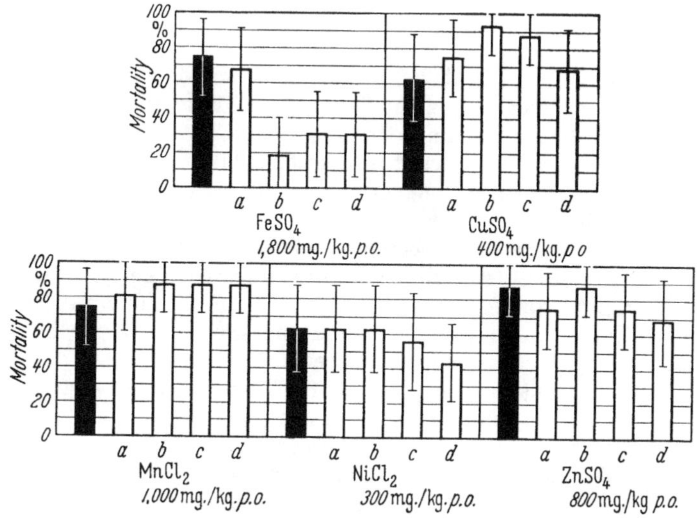

Fig. 5. Administered subcutaneously, desferrioxamine still protects the mouse against acute oral poisoning with $FeSO_4$ after a certain interval. But it has no influence on poisoning due to various other metals. Ordinate: mortality of the animals in % ($n = 16$). $P = 0.05$. ■ Metal alone □ Metal + desferrioxamine 1,000 mg./kg.s.c.; *a*—*d* as in Fig. 3

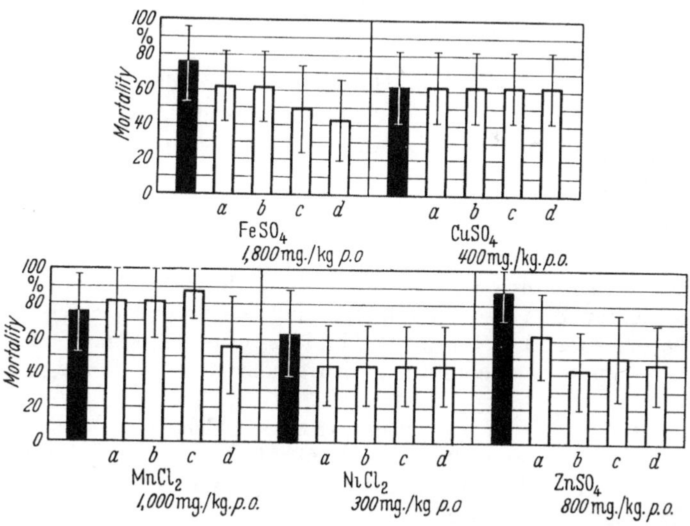

Fig. 6. Administered subcutaneously, E.D.T.A. protects the mouse against acute oral poisoning with $FeSO_4$ and particularly $ZnSO_4$, but only after a certain interval. On the other hand, E.D.T.A. has no influence on poisoning due to $CuSO_4$, $MnCl_2$, or $NiCl_2$. Ordinate: mortality of the animals in % ($n = 16$—24). $P = 0.05$. ■ Metal alone □ Metal + E.D.T.A. 250 mg./kg. s. c.; *a*—*d* as in Fig. 3

In the fourth series of experiments, conducted in exactly the same manner as the previous series, E.D.T.A. was given subcutaneously in a dose of 250 mg./kg. instead of desferrioxamine. Here, slight protection against $FeSO_4$ poisoning was observed, although it was not significant after 120 minutes, whereas in the case of $ZnSO_4$ poisoning significant protection was afforded from 30 minutes onwards. Neither the acute toxicity of $CuSO_4$ nor that of $MnCl_2$ or $NiCl_2$ is significantly reduced by E.D.T.A. (Fig. 6).

These four series of experiments *in vivo* clearly demonstrate that desferrioxamine protects the animal only against Fe poisoning, but not against poisoning due to Cu, Mn, Ni, or Zn. This protective effect against iron poisoning is not due simply to a mechanism whereby Fe and desferrioxamine become bound to each other in the digestive tract, but suggests that the iron becomes neutralised and/or bound to desferrioxamine during the process of its distribution throughout the organism. As for E.D.T.A., this chelating agent affords protection only against poisoning with Ni and Zn in the digestive tract, and against Fe and more expecially Zn once the latter have already become distributed in the organism. For the rest, E.D.T.A., whether administered orally or subcutaneously, is inactive against poisoning with Cu or Mn.

Here again, these differences between the properties of desferrioxamine and E.D.T.A. can be ascribed to one or more of the following factors:

a) The kinetics of the reactions between metallic salts and desferrioxamine or E.D.T.A. vary from case to case, quite apart from the differences in the stability constants to which reference has already been made.

b) The reaction between the metallic salt on the one hand and desferrioxamine or E.D.T.A. on the other leads to the formation of more or less dissociated complexes, the solubility, and hence the gastro-intestinal absorption of which, is different. But the solubility of these complexes, and the way in which they become bound to the plasma and tissue proteins, may also be very different as compared with the situation in the digestive tract.

c) The kinetics of absorption, transportation, and elimination are different for each metallic salt; hence, the time intervals required for detoxication may also be different, as in the case, for example, of desferrioxamine and E.D.T.A. administered subcutaneously.

d) Each chelating agent, in turn, has its own particular fate, enabling it to exert its more or less specific effects for a period of time which varies depending upon its absorption, fixation, and elimination.

e) Finally, these observations are also subject to another important pharmacological factor, i.e. the dosage. The doses of desferrioxamine administered by the oral route are, in fact, twice as high as those of E.D.T.A., but represent for desferrioxamine 1:6 and for E.D.T.A. 1:3 of the acute LD_{50} in mice (13,500 mg./kg. p.o. for desferrioxamine and 3,000 mg./kg. p.o. for E.D.T.A.). On the other hand, the doses of desferrioxamine administered subcutaneously are four times higher than those of E.D.T.A., but are roughly equitoxic, because they are equivalent to 1:1.6 of the acute LD_{50} for desferrioxamine in the mouse (1,600 mg./kg.) and to 1:1.8 of the acute LD_{50} for E.D.T.A. (455 mg./kg.). These are relatively high doses which one cannot raise much higher, particularly by the subcutaneous route, for fear of encountering the toxic effects which desferrioxamine and especially E.T.D.A. are liable to produce at such levels. This quantitative aspect of the problem, i.e. the relationship between specific effect and toxicity, is by no means a negligible factor from the point of view of a general comparison between these two substances, E.D.T.A. being roughly four times more toxic than desferrioxamine both by the subcutaneous and by the oral route.

These observations serve to supplement what was already known about the protection afforded by desferrioxamine in acute experimental poisoning with ionic iron (*23*, *27*, *36*), since they show that this protection applies specifically to iron, but does not include other elements such as Cu, Mn, Ni, or Zn. In addition, they reveal that the protection afforded under comparable circumstances by a chelating agent such as E.D.T.A. is not particularly satisfactory in the case of Fe and, though better with regard to Zn and Ni, is virtually nil in respect to Cu and Mn – as has already occasionally been indicated under other experimental conditions (*5*, *18*, *27*, *29*, *31*). In view of the frequency with which iron preparations are employed in certain countries, and of the correspondingly high incidence of iron poisoning, the observations outlined here may well have some practical bearing on the therapeutic use of desferrioxamine.

Finally, these observations demonstrate that it is impossible to predict detoxication *in vivo* on the basis of stability constants or tests conducted *in vitro*, because there are too many biological factors which intervene to modify the latter beyond recognition.

2. Effect of desferrioxamine and E.D.T.A. on the elimination of iron

The specific affinity of desferrioxamine for Fe can also be demonstrated by studying the elimination of iron. Laboratory animals have virtually no iron depots, and the task of inducing haemosiderosis in such animals – for example, post-haemolytic (*24*) or feed-induced (*21*) haemosiderosis in the rat – is far too problematical and complicated for the screening of iron-chelating agents. Nevertheless, we have found that in the dog, for example, desferrioxamine *per se* does considerably increase urinary iron excretion when given orally or subcutaneously (*33*). In the rabbit, it is necessary to give a simultaneous iron load in order to obtain better evidence of the affinity which desferrioxamine displays for this metal, and to have a simple method by which this property can be biologically titrated (*27*, *32*, *33*, *34*, *35*, *36*).

Under these experimental conditions, desferrioxamine – given, for example, in doses of 50 mg./kg. s.c. — substantially increases the urinary excretion of iron; the same applies to E.D.T.A., which, when administered in the same doses, exerts an effect both quantitatively and qualitatively similar to that of desferrioxamine, particularly as regards duration of action (Fig. 7).

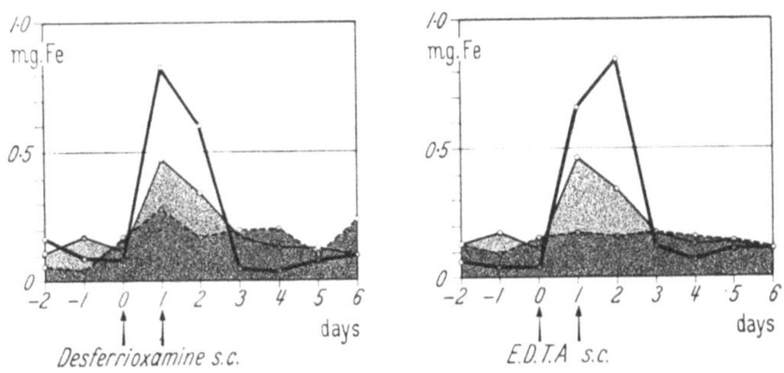

Fig. 7. Following an intramuscular load of Fe, desferrioxamine and E.D.T.A. increase urinary iron excretion in the rabbit. Ordinate: urinary iron excretion in mg. daily. Abscissa: days. ——— Fe^{III}, 2 × 50 mg./kg. i.m. (12); – – – Desferrioxamine or E.D.T.A., 2 × 50 mg./kg. s.c. (6); ——— Desferrioxamine or E.D.T.A., 2 × 50 mg./kg. s.c. + Fe^{III}, 2 × 50 mg./kg. i.m. (6).
The figures in brackets indicate the number of animals per experiment

From this comparison between the effects of desferrioxamine and E.D.T.A. on urinary iron excretion, the following conclusions can be drawn:

a) Neither the administration of iron nor of desferrioxamine or E.D.T.A. are in themselves sufficient to produce a significant increase in urinary iron excretion; to exploit the affinity for iron which desferrioxamine and E.D.T.A. display, it is necessary to have an overload of iron. In other words, both of the two agents probably rely upon the same mechanism for mobilising the iron added to the organism, irrespective of whether the iron is in free or bound form. But it is difficult for them to mobilise iron other than that originating from the overload, i.e. iron which is bound to ferritin, haemosiderin, transferrin, etc. In these experiments, in fact, it would appear that desferrioxamine and E.D.T.A. merely attract the iron of which there is an artificial excess. Moreover, as we have already seen, the same applies to pathological accumulations of iron. This suggests the existence of various types of iron in the organism, which do not react in the same way to chelating agents, the latter in their turn displaying differing degrees of affinity for iron.

b) Finally, from the pharmacological aspect, and bearing in mind its toxicity by the subcutaneous route, desferrioxamine has a very high index of 1:80 for its effect on the elimination of iron. This is a much more favourable index than that of E.D.T.A., which works out at about 1:9 for the subcutaneous route.

3. Action of desferrioxamine and E.D.T.A. on the urinary excretion of other metals

From the previous series of tests it is apparent that both desferrioxamine and E.D.T.A. cause a very substantial increase in the elimination of iron when administered to animals, particularly under certain experimental conditions. In view of the physicochemical properties and especially the stability constants of desferrioxamine and E.D.T.A., it is important in this connection to know whether they also enhance the excretion of other metalloids, metals, and trace elements. Systematic comparisons recently undertaken (*32*, *34*, *36*) indicate that this is not so, at least as regards many of these other metals, etc. As for the metals to which reference has already been made earlier, including particularly Cu, Mn, Ni, and Zn, experiments were performed to determine their 48-hour urinary excretion in groups of 6 rabbits which were given desferrioxamine or E.D.T.A. in daily injections of 50 mg./kg. s.c. for 2 days without having previously received an overload of the metal in question. The metals in the urine were determined using a continuous-arc spectrograph and X-ray fluorescence[1]. The results

[1] We should like here to express our thanks to Drs. M. Brandenstein, H. Keberle, R. Müller, and W. Rockenbauer for carrying out the determinations.

obtained, as outlined in Fig. 8, show that in the same group of animals there was some increase in urinary iron excretion, as already described above, in response both to desferrioxamine and to E.D.T.A. As for Cu and Ni, these metals could not as a rule be traced in the urine in these experiments, and their urinary excretion was not affected by either desferrioxamine or E.D.T.A. The situation was quite different, however, with respect to Mn and especially Zn, of which small quantities are normally present in the urine. Desferrioxamine had no influence whatsoever on their urinary excretion, whereas E.D.T.A. provoked a marked increase in the excretion of Mn and particularly Zn.

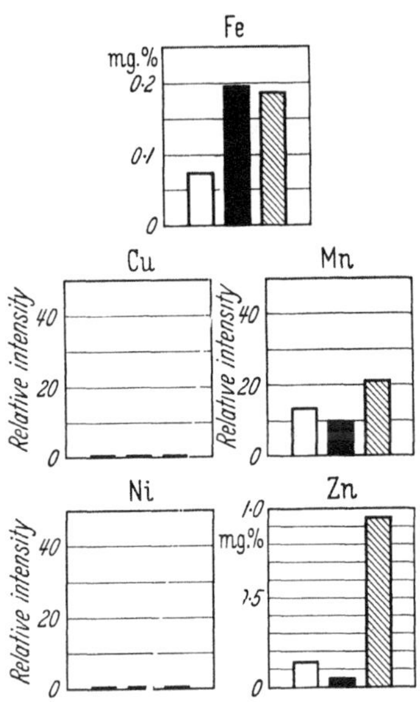

Fig. 8. In the normal rabbit, desferrioxamine affects only the excretion of Fe, whereas E.D.T.A. enhances the urinary excretion of Fe, Mn, and particularly Zn, but not that of Cu or Ni. Ordinate: 48-hour urinary excretion of the metal ($n = 6$). □ Controls, ■ Desferrioxamine, ▨ E.D.T.A.

These tests reveal that desferrioxamine has a predilection for iron only, whereas E.D.T.A. also shows an affinity for Mn and especially Zn. This entirely confirms the observations previously mentioned, at least as regards the two elements Mn and Zn. The biological importance of Mn is a subject about which more is now beginning to be discovered; for example, this metal is known to activate various enzymes (*10*, *13*) and has also been identified as an aetiological factor in certain forms of Parkinsonism (*7*, *10*). Zn, too, appears to play an important role in connection with certain enzymes and with pancreatic function (*13*); its urinary excretion is considerably increased following treatment with E.D.T.A. for certain types of hypercholesteraemia (*26*) and sclerodermia (*18*).

Desferrioxamine displays an affinity for iron only, and the selectivity of its action is much greater than that of E.D.T.A. when the two substances are administered in comparable doses – doses which, from the point of view of equitoxicity are, as we have already seen, some ten times more favourable in the case of desferrioxamine.

Summary

The observations reported here show that the detoxicating properties of desferrioxamine *in vitro*, and particularly *in vivo*, are confined to iron, whereas E.D.T.A. detoxicates Mn and particularly Ni *in vitro*, and Ni, Zn, and Fe under certain conditions *in vivo*. Both agents in the rabbit also promote the urinary excretion of iron, in addition to which E.D.T.A. enhances the urinary excretion of Mn and especially Zn. Thus, despite their stability constants *in vitro*, E.D.T.A. shows a polyvalent action, whereas, even under a wide range of experimental conditions, desferrioxamine does not.

These various effects are subject to a large number of biological factors whose mutual interaction may modify not only the gastro-intestinal absorption and transportation of a metal, but also its fixation to the proteins and/or tissues and its elimination, particularly via the kidneys. Added to this is the fact that each reaction has its own particular kinetics, that the processes by which metals become bound to proteins are susceptible to competitive influences, that other chelating mechanisms intervene, and that the chelating agents themselves are metabolised in different ways. All these factors, whether in cases of acute accidental poisoning or of more or less chronic intoxication, are responsible for pathological deposition of a metal with resultant functional impairment; they are also responsible for elimination of the metal with corresponding therapeutic results. In addition, it must be borne in mind that the circumstances differ each time depending on the metal and on the chelating agent, and that the situation also varies depending on whether it is a question of an endogenous or exogenous element slowly accumulated in the organism or, alternatively, an acute accidental or artificial intoxication of the type which can also be induced experimentally in animals.

The fact that desferrioxamine has an almost exclusive affinity for iron and a very low toxicity makes it a particularly interesting therapeutic agent for use in mobilising the iron stored in the organism. Desferrioxamine differs from a chelating agent such as E.D.T.A., which also displays an affinity for other metals and is more toxic.

Zusammenfassung

Aus den mitgeteilten Befunden geht hervor, daß sich die entgiftende Wirkung von Desferrioxamin *in vitro* und besonders *in vivo* auf Eisen beschränkt, während E.D.T.A. *in vitro* Mangan und besonders Nickel entgiftet, ein Effekt, der sich unter bestimmten Bedingungen *in vivo* auch auf Zink und Eisen erstreckt. Beide Chelatbildner fördern beim Kaninchen die Eisenausscheidung im Urin, jedoch begünstigt E.D.T.A. zusätzlich die Elimination von Mangan und Zink. Trotz der *in vitro* bestimmten Stabilitätskonstanten zeigt somit E.D.T.A. eine polyvalente Wirkung, während dies für Desferrioxamin, selbst unter ganz verschiedenen experimentellen Bedingungen, nicht zutrifft.

Für alle *in vivo* erhobenen Befunde ist eine Vielzahl biologischer Faktoren maßgebend, deren Wechselwirkung nicht nur die gastrointestinale Resorption und den Transport eines Metalles verändern kann, sondern auch seine Bindung an Eiweiß oder Gewebe oder seine Ausscheidung, besonders diejenige durch die Nieren. Hinzu kommt die für jede einzelne Reaktion besondere Kinetik, eine kompetitive Beeinflussung in bezug auf die Bindung an Eiweiß, andere Chelatwirkungen und der eigene Stoffwechsel der Komplexbildner. Das Zusammenwirken aller dieser Faktoren, unabhängig davon, ob es sich um eine akute oder um eine mehr oder weniger chronische Vergiftung handelt, äußert sich in der pathologischen Ablagerung eines Metalles, die mehr oder weniger schwere funktionelle Störungen zur Folge hat; außerdem sind diese Faktoren für die Ausscheidung und die sich daraus ergebenden therapeutischen Konsequenzen verantwortlich, wobei die Verhältnisse für jedes Metall und jeden einzelnen Chelatbildner verschieden liegen. Die Situation ändert sich auch je nachdem, ob es sich um ein endogenes oder exogenes Element handelt, das sich langsam im Organismus akkumuliert, oder um eine akute akzidentelle oder experimentelle Intoxikation, wie sie zum Beispiel im Tierversuch hervorgerufen wird.

Die Tatsache, daß Desferrioxamin eine nahezu ausschließliche Affinität für Eisen und eine niedrige Toxizität besitzt, läßt es besonders als einen therapeutisch anwendbaren Komplexbildner interessant erscheinen, der für die Mobilisierung von Speichereisen im Organismus verwendet werden kann. In dieser Hinsicht unterscheidet sich Desferrioxamin von Chelatbildnern vom Typus des E.D.T.A., die auch eine hohe Affinität zu anderen Metallen haben und außerdem toxischer sind.

Résumé

Les observations rapportées ici montrent clairement que le pouvoir détoxifiant *in vitro*, mais surtout *in vivo*, de la desferrioxamine est limité à Fe, tandis que celui de l'E.D.T.A. *in vitro* s'adresse à Mn et surtout à Ni, ou dans certaines conditions *in vivo* à Ni, Zn et Fe. Ces deux agents activent en outre l'élimination urinaire de Fe chez le lapin, et l'E.D.T.A. le fait en plus pour Mn et surtout Zn, montrant ainsi une polyvalence dont la desferrioxamine est dépourvue dans toute une série de conditions expérimentales, en dépit de leurs constantes de stabilité *in vitro*.

Ces phénomènes *in vivo* sont en effet soumis à un nombre élevé de facteurs biologiques, qui, par leur interaction réciproque, modifient la résorption gastro-intestinale, le transport, la fixation protéinique et/ou tissulaire et l'élimination surtout rénale de l'un ou l'autre métal. Il s'y ajoute encore la cinétique particulière de chaque réaction, des compétitions pour les liaisons protéiniques, l'intervention d'autres mécanismes chélateurs et les métabolismes différents des chélateurs en eux-mêmes. La combinaison de tous ces facteurs, qu'il s'agisse d'un empoisonnement aigu accidentel ou d'une intoxication plus ou moins chronique, s'exprime par des dépôts pathologiques avec leurs conséquences fonctionnelles plus ou moins graves, ainsi que par des éliminations plus ou moins influençables au point de vue thérapeutique, la situation étant chaque fois différente selon le métal et le chélateur envisagé. Cette situation varie aussi beaucoup selon qu'il s'agit d'un élément endogène ou exogène lentement accumulé dans l'organisme, ou au contraire d'une intoxication artificielle et/ou accidentelle aiguë, telle qu'elle existe aussi expérimentalement chez l'animal.

L'affinité quasi exclusive de la desferrioxamine pour le fer, ainsi que sa toxicité très basse, en font un agent thérapeutique particulièrement intéressant pour mobiliser le fer de l'organisme. La desferrioxamine diffère donc d'un chélateur tel que l'E.D.T.A., dont l'affinité s'étend simultanément à d'autres métaux et qui est en outre plus toxique.

References

1. ALBERT, A.: Nature (G.B.) **172**, 201 (1953). — 2. APOSHIAN, H. V.: In: Metal-Binding in Medicine. Lippincott, Philadelphia/Montreal, 1960, p. 290.

— 3. BERSIN, T.: Schweiz. med. Wschr. 83, 608 (1953). — 4. BERSIN, T., A. MÜLLER, and H. SCHWARZ: Arzneimittel-Forsch. (G.) **4**, 199 (1955). — 5. BEUTLER, E., V. F. FAIRBANKS, and J. L. FAHEY: Clinical Disorders of Iron Metabolism. Grune & Stratton, New York/London, 1963. — 6. BICKEL, M., E. GÄUMANN, W. KELLER-SCHIERLEIN, V. PRELOG, E. VISCHER, A. WETTSTEIN, and H. ZÄHNER: Experientia (Switz.) **16**, 129 (1960). — 7. BRIEGER, H.: In: Metal-Binding in Medicine. Lippincott, Philadelphia/Montreal, 1960, p. 200. — 8. CLETON, F. J.: Synthetic Chelating Agents in Iron Metabolism. Thesis, Leyden, 1962. — 9. CLETON, F., A. TURNBULL, C. A. FINCK, L. THOMPSON, and J. MARTIN: J. Clin. Invest. (U.S.A.) **42**, 327 (1963). — 10. COTZIAS, G. C., D. C. BORG, and A. J. BERTINCHAMPS: In: Metal-Binding in Medicine. Lippincott, Philadelphia/Montreal, 1960, p. 50.— 11. FIGUEROA, W. G.: In: Metal-Binding in Medicine. Lippincott, Philadelphia/Montreal, 1960, p. 146. — 12. FOREMAN, H.: In: Metal-Binding in Medicine. Lippincott, Philadelphia/Montreal, 1960, p. 160. — 13. GOODMAN, L. S., and A. GILMAN: The Pharmacological Basis of Therapeutics. Macmillan, New York, 1960. — 14. GREENBERG, J., and H. C. DUDLEY: In: Metal-Binding in Medicine. Lippincott, Philadelphia/Montreal, 1960, p. 245. — 15. HEILMEYER, L.: Münch. med. Wschr. **104**, 157 (1962). — 16. HEILMEYER, L.: Med. Klin. (G.) **57**, 121 (1962). — 17. HEILMEYER, L.: 19th International Congress of Haematology, Mexico, 1962. — 18. HÖSLI, P.: Arzneimittel-Forsch. (G.) **10**, 65, 177 (1960). — 19. ISHIDATE, M., and T. SAHAGUCHI: Pharmaceut. Bull. (Jap.) **3**, 147 (1955). — 20. JOHNSON, L. A., and M. J. SEVEN: In: Metal-Binding in Medicine. Lippincott, Philadelphia/Montreal, 1960, p. 225. — 21. KINNEY, T. D., N. KAUFMAN, and J. V. KLAVINS: Nature (G.B.) **195**, 604 (1962). — 22. MARTELL, A. E., and M. CALVIN: Chemistry of Metal Chelate Compounds. Prentice Hall Inc., New York, 1952. — 23. MOESCHLIN, S., and U. SCHNIDER: 19th International Congress of Haematology, Mexico, 1962. — 24. MORGAN, E. H.: J. Path. Bact. (G.B.) **84**, 65 (1962). — 25. OHLSSON, W. T. L.: Brit. Med. J. **1962/I**, 1454. — 26. PERRY, H. M., and G. H. CAMEL: In: Metal-Binding in Medicine. Lippincott, Philadelphia/Montreal, 1960, p. 209. — 27. Round-table Discussion: 30. Jahresversammlung d. Schweiz. Ges. f. Inn. Med., Lugano. Schweiz. med. Wschr. **82**, 1295 (1962). — 28. SALTMAN, P., and P. J. CHARLEY: In: Metal-Binding in Medicine. Lippincott, Philadelphia/Montreal, 1960, p. 241. — 29. SEVEN, M. J., and L. A. JOHNSON: In: Metal-Binding in Medicine. Lippincott, Philadelphia/Montreal, 1960, p. 225. — 30. SHIELDS, G. S., H. MARKOWITZ, G. E. CARTWRIGHT, and M. M. WINTROBE: In: Metal-Binding in Medicine. Lippincott, Philadelphia/Montreal, 1960, p. 259. — 31. SIMPSON, K., and A. BLUNT: Lancet (G.B.) **1960/II**, 1120. — 32. TRIPOD, J., and H. KEBERLE: Helvet. med. acta **29**, 674 (1962). — 33. TRIPOD, J., and H. KEBERLE: Helvet. physiol. pharmacol. acta **20**, 291 (1962). — 34. TRIPOD, J., H. KEBERLE, and K. SCHMID: 19th International Congress of Haematology, Mexico, 1962. — 35. TRIPOD, J.: Nouv. rev. franç. hémat. **3**, 1 (1963). — 36. TRIPOD, J.: Schweiz. med. Wschr. **93**, 969 (1963). — 37. UZMAN, L. L.: In: Metal-Binding in Medicine. Lippincott, Philadelphia/Montreal, 1960, p. 269. — 38. WALSHE, J. M.: In: Metal-Binding in Medicine. Lippincott, Philadelphia/Montreal, 1960, p. 265. — 39. WÖHLER, F.: 19th International Congress of Haematology, Mexico, 1962.

Discussion

HEILMEYER: I have one question. Patients whom we had given prolonged treatment with E.D.T.A. have not infrequently complained of bone pain, due presumably to decalcification; but we have not had this trouble with desferrioxamine. How much is known about the excretion of calcium in the stools and urine following lengthy treatment with E.D.T.A.?

PETERS: I should like to present a few data on the distribution and renal excretion of desferrioxamine and its iron chelate, which may have some bearing on its therapeutic application.

When we first attempted to elucidate the mechanism of the renal excretion of desferrioxamine with H. KEBERLE, H. BRUNNER, and K. SCHMID, it proved extremely difficult to maintain stable and measurable plasma concentrations,

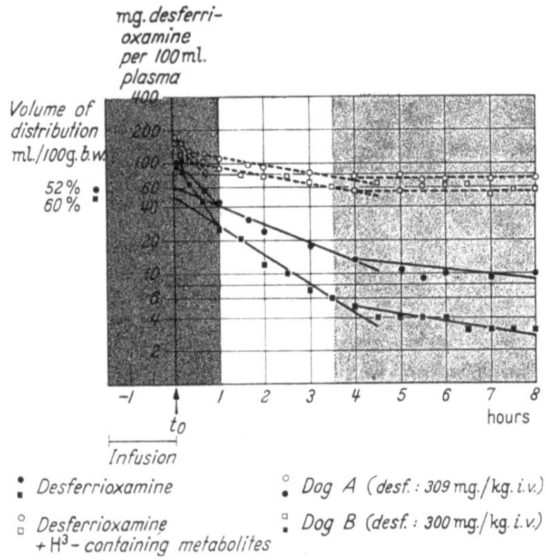

Fig. 1. Plasma concentrations of desferrioxamine B in nephrectomised dogs, expressed as mg. of the free base per 100 ml. plasma, after the administration of a large dose containing a small amount of tritium-labelled desferrioxamine B. 90 minutes were necessary for the intravenous infusion of the large dose in order to avoid a fall in blood pressure; 10% of the total dose was infused within the first 30 minutes, and 40% within the first hour. Volumes of distribution were calculated for t_0. The uninterrupted lines show concentrations measured chemically; the interrupted lines show concentrations computed from c.p.m.

even when a very rapid renal excretion was assumed to occur. This difficulty was due to two particularities which are clearly seen in experiments on acutely nephrectomised dogs (Fig. 1). When unlabelled and tritium-labelled desferrioxamine were injected simultaneously in these animals, a comparison of concentrations, measured either chemically or as total radioactivity, showed that desferrioxamine is *metabolised* very rapidly. Its biological half-life in the nephrectomised dog is approximately one hour. By extrapolating the plasma concentration to t_0 from the straight line which describes the fall in the plasma concentration presumably due to metabolic destruction, we found a desferrioxamine *"space" of 52—60%* of the total body-weight. This means that desferrioxamine either penetrates uniformly into a large number of body cells or is concentrated to an unknown extent in some body cells before being metabolised.

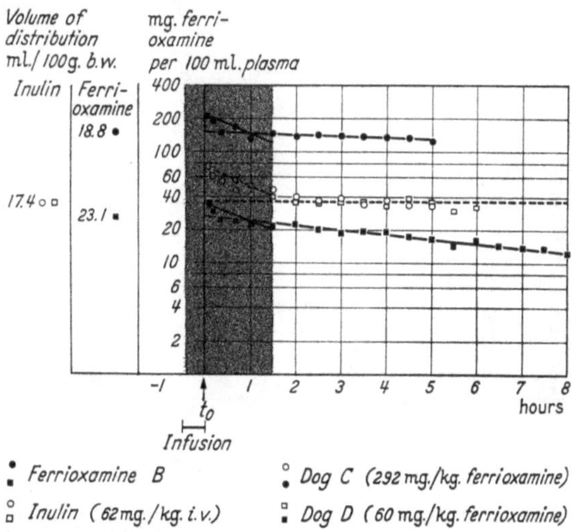

Fig. 2. Plasma concentrations of ferrioxamine B (and of inulin), expressed as mg. of the free base per 100 ml. of plasma, after the intravenous infusion of a single dose in nephrectomised dogs. 30 minutes were needed for the infusion of the whole dose without inducing a major fall in blood pressure. Volumes of distribution were calculated for t_0. The uninterrupted lines show concentrations measured chemically; the interrupted lines show concentrations computed from c.p.m.

When desferrioxamine is chelated with iron, its fate in the organism becomes very different from that of the original compound (Fig. 2). The resulting ferrioxamine is apparently not metabolised. A very slow fall in initially low plasma concentrations in the nephrectomised dog is presumably due to biliary excretion of ferrioxamine. Desferrioxamine, on the other hand, is not excreted into the bile before being metabolised to as yet unidentified compounds. The ferrioxamine "space" in nephrectomised dogs was equal to 19—23% of the body-weight and was thus just a little larger than the inulin space.

The mechanism of the renal excretion of the two compounds also differs markedly. In rats, desferrioxamine is clearly excreted by tubular secretion (Fig. 3), limited by a Tm (maximal transport capacity) which is reached at plasma concentrations of around 100 mg. % of the free base. Since even high plasma concentrations of desferrioxamine did not markedly depress C_{PAH}, the secretory mechanism may be different from that responsible for the secretion of p-aminohippurate, phenol red, etc. In dogs, similar excretory patterns were observed; there may, however, be an additional mechanism of tubular reabsorption in this species. Metabolic destruction, as well as the rapid renal elimination, may explain why it is sometimes so difficult to secure a therapeutic response to desferrioxamine.

The renal excretion of ferrioxamine is somewhat less rapid. In the dog, there is no evidence for tubular secretion, since the clearance ratio $C_{\text{ferrioxamine}}/C_{\text{inulin}}$ oscillated around 1.0. In the rat, ferrioxamine is reabsorbed at low plasma concentrations.

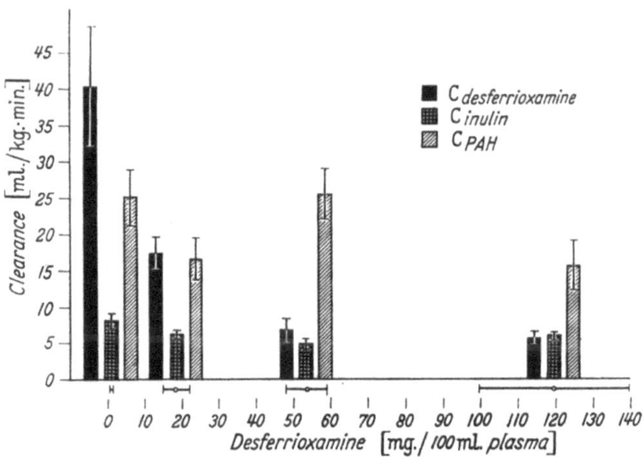

Fig. 3. Renal clearances of desferrioxamine B, inulin, and p-aminohippurate, measured simultaneously in rats at different plasma concentrations of desferrioxamine. Columns are means with ± S.E. indicated by vertical lines with brackets. Each group of three columns represents values from a group of 11—20 male rats. Plasma concentrations of desferrioxamine are also shown as means (periods) with ± S.E. indicated by horizontal lines with brackets. Clearance values are conventionally given as ml./kg. body-weight · minute

To sum up, the desferrioxamine "space" is nearly equal to total body water, and the iron-free compound is excreted by tubular secretion as well as by filtration, while ferrioxamine, the iron chelate, is limited to the extracellular space and does not appear to be secreted by renal tubular cells.*

Vannotti: In relation to the very interesting paper by Dr. Tripod I should like to draw attention to the fact that the iron excretion may vary

* *Addendum:* These conclusions are not substantially modified by our recent finding (H. Keberle) that the method used for estimating desferrioxamine in these experiments actually measured the sum of the concentrations of desferrioxamine and one of its metabolites. This metabolite is a carboxylic acid formed by removal of a free terminal amino group and subsequent oxidation of —CH_2 to —COOH. The metabolite binds iron and yields an iron complex having the same absorption characteristics as ferrioxamine. The renal excretory pattern of the iron-free metabolite in the dog appears to be similar to that of desferrioxamine.

in its response to desferrioxamine in patients not suffering from severe siderosis of the tissues. I can illustrate this by reference to some tests which we carried out as follows.

We gave patients Fe^{59} by mouth and followed up the absorption and excretion for 12 days, measuring the amount of Fe^{59} in the stools and urine and the amount of non-radioactive iron in the urine once a day, as well as the serum iron and serum Fe^{59} every other day. After the first period we again gave the same quantity of Fe^{59} by mouth and made the same determinations in the blood, stools, and urine for 12 days under daily treatment with 1,000 mg. Desferal intramuscularly.

Table 1 gives the data on three cases, each of which showed a different response. In the first case, we observed during the treatment with Desferal an increase in the absorption of Fe^{59} from the intestine and in the excretion of iron in the urine. This corresponds to the usual effect of desferrioxamine seen in normal subjects.

Table 1. *Differences in the intestinal absorption and urinary excretion of iron in 3 patients after receiving, firstly, an oral dose of Fe^{59} and, secondly, the same oral dose of Fe^{59} + daily doses of 1,000 mg. Desferal i.m. for 12 days*

	Serum iron. Mean value (μg. %)	Intestinal absorption of Fe^{59} in % of dose administered (measured for 12 days)	Variation in intestinal absorption of Fe^{59} (in % as compared with Fe^{59} absorption before Desferal)	Urinary excretion of Fe^{59}. Average/24 hours in % of dose administered (measured for 12 days)	Urinary excretion of non-radioactive iron. Mean value (μg./24 hrs)
			Differences given in %		
First case					
Before Desferal treatment	50	22.50		0.25	
After Desferal treatment	—	58.10	*+ 158.0*	0.63	
				+ 152.0	
Second case					
Before Desferal treatment	141	19.70		0.25	
After Desferal treatment	—	9.50	*— 51.8*	0.51	
				+ 104.0	
Third case					
Before Desferal treatment	156	5.20		0.27	253—259
After Desferal treatment	—	19.90	*+ 283.0*	0.27	1,062
				0	*+ 310*

In the second case — a patient with mild hypersideraemia — we observed a decrease in Fe^{59} absorption during Desferal treatment (—51.8%), but at the same time an increase in Fe^{59} excretion in the urine (+ 104%).

In the third case — one of cirrhosis with hypersideraemia — we found a significant increase in iron absorption under treatment with Desferal

(+283%), but no increase in Fe^{59} excretion in the urine; however, the total iron excretion in the urine was markedly increased (+310%).

These three examples show that desferrioxamine may vary in its effect on the absorption and urinary excretion of iron, depending on the type of case with which one is dealing. As a rule, we find that an acute increase in urinary iron excretion in response to treatment with Desferal leads to an increase in the intestinal absorption of iron. On the other hand, in some cases, even though Desferal enhances the urinary excretion of iron, no increase in iron absorption occurs.

Finally, we have cases, such as patients with cirrhosis, in which Desferal does not provoke an increase in the urinary excretion of Fe^{59}, but in which it does remove non-radioactive iron from the tissues; here, the absorption of Fe^{59} is increased. In these cases we have to admit that the newly absorbed iron is not eliminated, whereas the old storage iron is. It is difficult at the moment to explain these differing responses to desferrioxamine treatment, but we propose to try in the future to clarify this problem, especially with regard to cases of liver cirrhosis and iron-deficiency anaemia.

Schubert: You mentioned, Dr. Tripod, that the toxicity of E.D.T.A. was greater than that of desferrioxamine. I was wondering whether you were comparing the toxicity of the sodium or of the calcium salt of E.D.T.A. with desferrioxamine. The toxicity of E.D.T.A. relative to desferrioxamine should be based on the calcium-sodium salt of E.D.T.A. In the case of desferrioxamine, the binding of calcium is too small to make any difference.

I think one can lay down a few general rules relating to the fact that in certain cases the administration of chelating agents causes an increase in the amounts of metal deposited in certain tissues such as the bone marrow. This usually happens with metals which are very highly toxic and which coincidentally often very readily form insoluble hydroxides. Chelating agents may solubilise these metals from one tissue and deposit the metal in another tissue in amounts greater than would occur without treatment. As a general rule, when evaluating the effect of a chelating agent on the distribution or toxicity of hydrolysable metals, the results obtained will depend on the chemical and physical state of the metallic salt being tested. This, I think, explains why some people may report that E.D.T.A., for example, reduces the toxicity of metals such as lead or iron, whereas others may report an enhanced toxicity.

Cleton: I want to raise the point about the distribution of chelating agents in the body. We have done some experiments with C^{14}-labelled D.T.P.A. in rabbits, and we found a distribution space similar to that which you mentioned for ferrioxamine. We are concerned with the finding that the distribution space is larger than the extracellular compartment, but not as large as the total body water. I wonder whether the distribution of chelating agents over the various organs is uniform and whether these compounds concentrate on the cell membranes.

Secondly, I should like to confirm the observation of Dr. Heilmeyer concerning bone pains in patients after administration of E.D.T.A. We have seen one patient who had severe pains in all limbs, starting four hours after an E.D.D.H.A. infusion and associated with high fever for a period of about 12 hours.

Hallberg: We have done some studies concerning the factors influencing the acute oral toxicity of iron in mice; for this purpose we labelled the oral dose with Fe^{59}. We found that the toxicity was related not only to the amount absorbed, but also to the rate at which the iron was absorbed. I think that the rate of iron absorption is a factor which should be taken into consideration when discussing the effect of chelating agents on oral iron toxicity.

Peters: As far as our experiments are concerned, the distribution could not possibly have been influenced by the kidneys. The distribution experiments were done in nephrectomised animals.

Najean: Could you tell me, Dr. Tripod, if desferrioxamine is able to mobilise thorium from the liver?

Figueroa: Dr. Heilmeyer asked whether desferrioxamine administration resulted in calcium excretion in the urine. Table 2 shows the results of a calcium-balance study in a patient with primary haemochromatosis. You can see that, on a diet of 885 mg. calcium per day, the patient in this particular control period had average daily stool values of 781 mg. and average urinary calcium values of 104 mg. daily, and he was in balance during this period. We then gave him 600 mg. desferrioxamine B for 4 days (800 mg. on the fifth day). As you can see, the urinary calcium excretion remained approximately the same (102 mg.). As a matter of fact, during this particular period, the patient showed a positive balance and was retaining 66 mg./day. I think that on the basis of a 5-day calcium balance one cannot draw any definite conclusions as to whether the retention of some 300 mg. calcium over a period of 5 days is of significance. The period is too short.

Table 2. *Calcium balance during intravenous treatment with desferrioxamine B*

	Calcium content in mg./day				
	Days	Diet	Stool	Urine	Balance
Control period	10	885*	781*	104*	In balance
Desferrioxamine B 600 mg./day	5	885	717	102	+ 66 mg./day
Recovery	5	885	777	94	+ 14 mg./day

* Average per day, ashed specimens.

Table 3. *Urinary calcium excretion after intravenous treatment with desferrioxamine B*

Day	mg.	Diluent	24-hour urinary calcium in mg.
1	600	Normal saline	107
2	600	Normal saline	116
3	600	Normal saline	106
4	600	5% Glucose	91
5	800	5% Glucose	93

Then we took 5 days during which we gave desferrioxamine B (Table 3). As you can see, 600 mg. of the drug was administered in normal saline on day 1, 2, and 3. During these three days, the urinary calcium excretion amounted to 107, 116, and 106 mg., respectively. When we infused the desferrioxamine B in 5% glucose, the urinary calcium excretion dropped to 91 and 93 mg. These findings seem to bear out observations made in the dog and in man that calcium excretion in the urine is fairly closely related to the sodium content of the urine[1,2]. I feel that if you are going to study calcium excretion in the urine you must pay particular attention to how much sodium you are giving and how much sodium is coming out. If you do this, I think it will show that the effect of Desferal on urinary calcium excretion is probably bound up with the variation in sodium.

TRIPOD: Dr. FIGUEROA has told Dr. HEILMEYER just what I was also going to say about the excretion of calcium after desferrioxamine. We have carried out experiments on the calcium, sodium, and magnesium excretion in the rabbit, and the fact that desferrioxamine does not influence their excretion is very important.

With regard to the toxicity of E.D.T.A. in relation to the binding of metals, I fully agree with what Dr. SCHUBERT has said. But the conditions are very different depending on whether you have an acute poisoning of the animal, as we had in this sort of experiment, or whether you have a subchronic or chronic intoxication. The fate of the metal and of the chelating agents, the rate of absorption and the elimination through the kidney, etc. are decisive factors.

As for the question of the distribution of desferrioxamine in the body or in the cells, I think Dr. PETERS has given you all the answers.

Dr. HALLBERG has emphasised the importance of the rate of absorption. I believe that, besides the experimental conditions, the choice of animal species is important, and our experiments were done on rats. But I think that, if the same intoxication studies had been done in mice instead of in rats, we should perhaps have observed a different pattern of activity with these chelating agents.

Finally, in reply to Dr. NAJEAN, I'm afraid I don't know anything about the possible chelation of thorium by desferrioxamine.

---

[1] KLEEMAN, C. R., J. BOHANNAN, D. BERNSTEIN, and M. H. MAXWELL: Clin. Res. (U.S.A.) **11**, 88 (1963).

[2] WALSER, M., and A. A. BROWDER: J. Clin. Invest. (U.S.A.) **38**, 4104 (1959).

Treatment of primary and secondary haemochromatosis and acute iron poisoning with a new, potent iron-eliminating agent (desferrioxamine B)

By

S. Moeschlin and U. Schnider

The purpose of this paper is to study the clinical value of a new and potent specific iron-eliminating agent (desferrioxamine B) in cases of *chronic iron overload* (primary and secondary haemochromatosis) and to determine experimentally its clinical importance in *acute iron poisoning*.

In primary haemochromatosis the excessive amounts of stored iron could, until recently, only be eliminated by venesection. Secondary haemochromatosis in sideroachrestic anaemia, aplastic anaemia (transfusions), thalassaemia major, and sickle-cell anaemia remained an unsolved problem. Different chelating agents had been tried, but had proved unsatisfactory, either because they caused toxic side reactions or because they also eliminated other essential oligometals, such as copper or magnesium. The recent discovery of desferrioxamine B can therefore be considered a significant therapeutic advance.

I. Chemical properties and methods of administration

a) Chemical properties of desferrioxamine B. In the CIBA Laboratories in Basle, and at the Department of Organic Chemistry of the Swiss Federal Institute of Technology, Bickel and coworkers (*1*) succeeded in obtaining desferrioxamine B by starting from an iron (Fe^{+++})-containing substance belonging to the group of "siderochromes" and subsequently splitting the iron molecule.

Desferrioxamine B is a water-soluble substance featuring three molecules of trihydroxamic acid (cf. p. 76), and it reacts slightly with alkali. It has a molecular weight of 597, and one molecule binds 1 M Fe^{+++} ions, i.e. 100 weight units of desferrioxamine B bind 9.35 weight units of Fe^{+++} in the form of an octahedral iron complex, the reddish-coloured ferrioxamine, which is water-soluble and can therefore be excreted by the kidneys.

Table 1. *Stability constants of different desferrioxamine B-metal complexes, compared with the corresponding figures for E.D.T.A. and D.T.P.A.* (kindly supplied by Prof. SCHWARZENBACH, Institute of Physics, University of Zurich)

Metallic ion	Desferrioxamine	E.D.T.A.	D.T.P.A.
Mg^{2+}	10^4	10^9	10^9
Ca^{2+}	10^2	10^{11}	10^{10}
Sr^{2+}	10	10^9	10^{10}
Fe^{3+}	10^{31}	10^{25}	10^{29}
Co^{2+}	10^{11}	10^{16}	10^{19}
Ni^{2+}	10^{10}	10^{19}	10^{20}
Cd^{2+}	10^8		
Zn^{2+}	10^{11}		

Binding capacity with transferrin and ferritin. Because the stability constant of $10^{30.7}$ [BICKEL et al. (*1*)] is higher than that for transferrin (10^{25-29}), it is theoretically possible to withdraw all the iron from transferrin by the use of desferrioxamine. Moreover, for the same reason, transferrin is unable to withdraw iron from the ferrioxamine molecule, as shown by NIELSEN (*2*).

When washed erythrocytes and haemolysed erythrocytes are incubated in a desferrioxamine solution, *no binding of haemoglobin iron occurs* [KEBERLE (*3*)]. WÖHLER (*4*) was able to demonstrate experimentally that desferrioxamine is actually capable of eliminating iron from iron proteins, such as transferrin, in the serum and from ferritin in the tissues, leading to the formation of ferrioxamine (cf. p. 76); he found that the iron complex, i.e. ferrioxamine, was excreted in the urine on the first day of administration in quantities equivalent to 50–90% of the dose administered. However, in bone marrow removed by aspiration and washed several times with distilled water, MANN and MAIER (*5*) were unable to eliminate iron from haemosiderin by the use of desferrioxamine.

Solubility. The solubility of *desferrioxamine hydrochloride* in water at 20° C. is 4.8%. That of *desferrioxamine methane-sulphonate* is more than 25%.

Stability. In a buffer solution of pH 6.1, desferrioxamine remains stable for 84 hours. At a pH of 1.1 it decomposes slowly, i.e. at a rate of 10% in 14 hours. Incubated with gastric juice of pH 2.5 at 37° C., it disintegrates at a rate of 4% per hour.

b) Determination of ferrioxamine in urine and body fluids [modified method of KEBERLE (*3*)]. Ferrioxamine is first extracted with the aid of benzyl alcohol. The alcohol is then diluted with ether and extracted with water, ferrioxamine remaining in the aqueous phase. An aliquot of this aqueous phase is then ashed and the amount of iron determined. From the concentration of iron, the amount of ferrioxamine can then be determined. The iron in the urine is always present in the form of ferrioxamine iron and gives the urine a characteristic salmon colour.

c) Determination of desferrioxamine in urine. Two portions of the same urine are tested. In the first, ferrioxamine is extracted with benzyl alcohol as described above. In the second portion, immediately before extraction an excess of $FeCl_3$ is added, causing the desferrioxamine to become transformed into ferrioxamine. If there is already some desferrioxamine in the urine, the salmon colour due to the presence of ferrioxamine will be more intense. The two portions are then compared colorimetrically and the difference between the two noted; from this difference, the amount of desferrioxamine present can be calculated.

d) Determination of iron in body fluids and tissues [modified method of KEBERLE (*3*)]. After ashing and transformation of the ionic iron into a coloured complex, determination is carried out by means of the colorimeter. Alpha-alpha-dipyridyl and alpha-alpha-tripyridyl are recommended for formation of the complex, because they are able to bind the Fe^{+++} ion, thereby giving rise to an intense red colour. The stability of this complex is largely determined by the pH of the solution. A sample of urine, body fluid, or tissue is then placed in a small Kjeldahl flask and mixed with sulphuric acid and nitric acid. The fluid is then decolorised with hydrogen peroxide and bisulphite, diluted with water, and neutralised with ammonia and paranitrophenol. The Fe^{+++} is then transformed to Fe^{++} by the application of hydroquinone, and finally coloured with orthophenanthroline.

e) Clinical application of desferrioxamine. Desferrioxamine was supplied to us in 1961 by CIBA in Basle, first in the form of desferrioxamine hydrochloride and later as desferrioxamine methane-sulphonate. Both substances were dissolved in distilled water and given by intramuscular injection or by drip infusion mixed with physiological saline, glucose, or laevulose. In some cases, and in our experimental trials, desferrioxamine (dissolved in distilled water) was also administered orally.

f) Experimental evaluation of desferrioxamine therapy in acute iron poisoning of guinea-pigs.

Technique. Ferrous sulphate. In the initial trials, the LD_{50} for guinea-pigs of 250–500 g. body-weight was established at 1–1.2 g. $FeSO_4$ plus 7 H_2O/kg. body-weight, and the LD_{100} at 1.6–1.8 g./kg.

body-weight. $FeSO_4$ plus 7 H_2O containing 199.8–200.8 mg. iron/g. ferrous sulphate was dissolved in distilled water and stabilised by the addition of 2.5% ascorbic acid. The solutions were freshly prepared every day.

Desferrioxamine was administered in the form of a 10% solution in distilled water and the dose calculated per kg. body-weight for each animal before injection. One g. $FeSO_4$ plus 7 H_2O contains approximately 200 mg. iron. 100 mg. desferrioxamine is capable of binding 9.3 mg. iron. Thus, 2,140 mg. desferrioxamine is theoretically required to neutralise 1 g. ferrous sulphate. In practice, however, the dose needed is significantly higher.

II. Clinical observations

Iron excretion in normal subjects. Three persons received 1,200 mg. desferrioxamine daily i.m. in two divided injections. The daily excretion of iron in the urine, which normally does not exceed 0.5 mg., rose to 2.5–3 mg. on the second and third day and then slowly decreased to 1–2 mg. daily on the following days.

Single injection studies in normal subjects (6). Following the injection of 500 mg. desferrioxamine i.m., in the normal subject, there is an increase in total iron excretion in the 24-hour urine from an average of 0.125 mg. to an average of 0.8 mg. By such a procedure it may be possible to develop a test which will help to distinguish between persons with normal iron stores and those patients with iron overload in whom a similar dose of desferrioxamine may cause the 24-hour urinary iron excretion to rise to 4–12 mg.

III. Haemochromatosis

A. Primary haemochromatosis

Case 1: P. L., 52-year-old male. This patient was discovered to be suffering from advanced hereditary familial haemochromatosis in 1956; he was treated by means of periodic venesection until 1958, when oesophageal haemorrhage occurred, necessitating a portacaval shunt. However, severe myocardial damage and liver cirrhosis due to chronic iron poisoning persisted and gradually worsened, leading to death from heart failure following influenza in the spring of 1962.

Because of the patient's serious general condition, complicated by water retention, only short periods of desferrioxamine infusion were tried. Nevertheless, a *striking influence on urinary iron excretion was observed.* The first treatment with desferrioxamine was given at a dosage of only 200 mg. daily, administered by drip infusion in physiological saline (diabetes!). This initial dosage, which subsequently proved to be too small, nevertheless induced an iron excretion of 5–7.3 mg. daily. Later we also gave the preparation intramuscularly. A second period of treatment in March 1962, with 1,200 mg. daily, given in three divided doses of 400 mg. i.m., increased the urinary iron excretion to 23.5 mg. daily (Fig. 1).

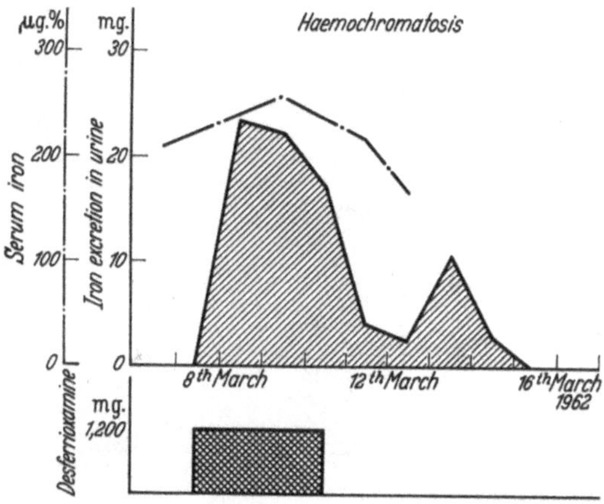

Fig. 1. *Advanced familial haemochromatosis.* P. L., 52-year-old male. Despite the severity of the disease and the fact that the patient received only 4 days' treatment, 23.5—17 mg. iron was excreted daily.Dosage: 1,200 mg. desferrioxamine daily, in a 5% laevulose drip infusion. Because of the patient's poor general condition (severe hepatic insufficiency and heart failure) the treatment was not continued. The renewed rise in urinary iron excretion 4 days after the last infusion can probably be accounted for in terms of impaired renal function (water retention)

B. Secondary haemochromatosis

1. In sideroachrestic anaemia

Case 2: L. G., 35-year-old male. Anaemia was first discovered in 1955 and was thought to be of the thalassaemia minor type. In 1961, the patient was admitted for the first time to our hospital and a diagnosis of typical sideroachrestic anaemia was made: high serum iron (235 μg. %), normal to increased erythrocyte survival time, low reticulocyte counts, and in the bone marrow an increase in basophilic erythroblasts (75 erythroblasts per 100 white cells), with many typical sideroblasts (80—90%). The haemoglobin was 6.4 g. with a colour index of 0.81, and the leucocyte count was 3,800. The blood smear showed pronounced anisocytosis as well as some elliptocytes and target cells. The liver (16 cm.) and spleen (14 cm.) were enlarged and showed deposits of pigment typical of haemochromatosis, both the liver-biopsy specimen and the smear obtained by puncture of the spleen yielding a positive reaction when stained for iron. Starch-block electrophoresis showed no pathological haemoglobins and no increase in haemoglobin A_2 (E). Pyridoxine, vitamin B_{12}, and folic acid treatment elicited no clinical response.

Treatment (Fig. 2). Desferrioxamine therapy was started in October 1961 and has continued since. During his stay in hospital, the patient received 1,200 mg. daily, given in three divided doses of 400 mg. each i.m. The serum iron concentration reflected the *mobilising effect of desferrioxamine* on the iron deposits; it rose from 260 to 398 μg. % and then decreased again after high urinary iron excretion levels had been maintained for some time. The

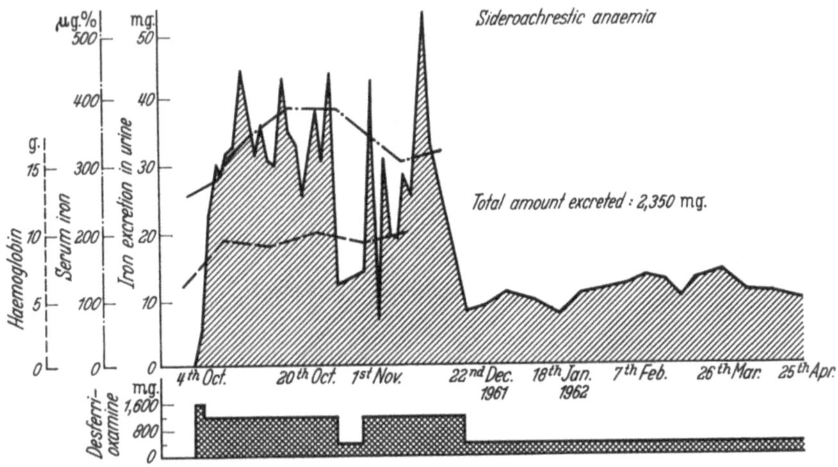

Fig. 2. *Secondary haemochromatosis due to sideroachrestic anaemia*. L. G., 35-year-old male. Dosage: 1,200 mg. daily during hospitalisation, and 400 mg. daily i.m. after the patient's discharge from hospital. Note the initial mobilising effect of desferrioxamine on the iron, the serum concentration of which rose from 260 to 398 μg. %, and the striking effect on the haemoglobin (which in 3 months rose from 6.4 g. to 9.8 g.). Treatment has now been continued for over 2 years

urinary iron excretion rose to a maximum of 54 mg. daily during hospitalisation and fluctuated between 8.3 and 14.5 mg. daily thereafter. By 25th April 1962, i.e. over a period of 7 months, a total of 2,350 mg. iron had been eliminated in the urine, and by 15th June the total had risen to 3,050 mg. No side effects have been noted. The patient has been on full-time work since February 1962 and has been giving himself one intramuscular injection of 400 mg. daily since 22nd December 1961. He feels normal and looks healthy again. By 1st February 1963, a total of 7,348 mg. iron had been excreted in the urine. Fig. 2 also demonstrates the striking effect of the treatment on the haemoglobin, which in 3 months rose from 6.4 g. (October 1961) to 9.8 g. (January 1962); by January 1963, it had reached 10 g. In response to 400 mg. desferrioxamine daily, urinary iron excretion still averages 12.5 mg.

These cases of anaemia associated with iron overloading, in which severe haemochromatosis usually proved fatal at one time, seem to offer one of the most promising indications for desferrioxamine.

2. In aplastic anaemia (transfusion haemochromatosis)

Case 3: K. F., 71-year-old male. In 1959, the patient was found to be suffering from severe hyperchromic anaemia, which persisted for 3 years and resulted in an almost complete arrest of erythrocyte maturation [only a few large basophilic erythroblasts in the bone marrow and few, if any, reticulocytes (0—2%)]; the thrombocyte count was also low (92,000), but there was no leucopenia (9,200) and no pathological forms. All treatment proved unavailing (vitamin B_{12}, folic acid, vitamin B_6, cortisone, methyltestosterone, etc.); transfusions were therefore started and have since had to be given every two weeks. The serum iron (180 μg. %) was elevated from the very beginning. Here also, the incorporation of iron into the haemoglobin seemed to be inhibited by an enzymatic defect. The serum iron slowly rose to 320 μg. % in the spring of 1962.

Liver biopsy revealed marked steatosis, with incipient siderosis and fibrosis. However, the Bromsulphalein retention was normal (4.5%) as were also the results of other liver tests. The E.S.R. was always high (57/97 Westergren), and electrophoresis showed an increased gamma-globulin of 29.6%. The results of the last blood count were as follows: Hb. 4.2 g., R.B.C. 2.4 mill., colour index 0.96, reticulocytes 0.1%, W.B.C. 7,400, 5.5% stab forms, 53.5% segmented, 6.8% eosinophils, 13.5% monocytes, 21% lymphocytes, and 75,000 thrombocytes.

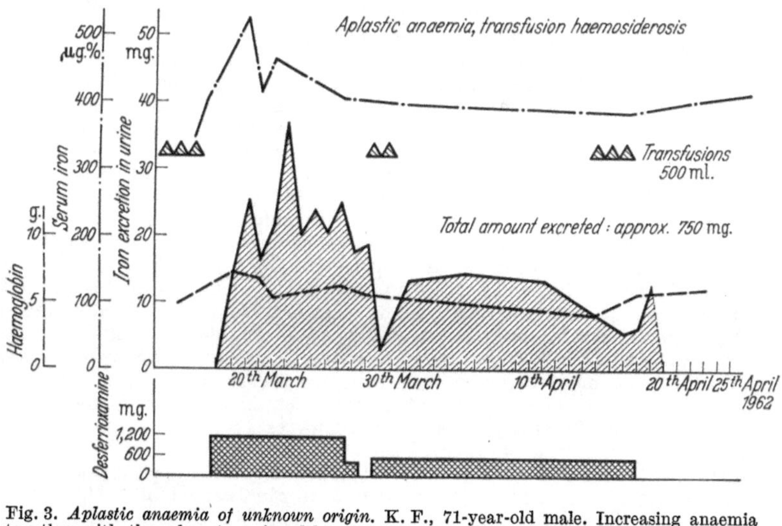

Fig. 3. *Aplastic anaemia of unknown origin.* K. F., 71-year-old male. Increasing anaemia together with thrombocytopenia, although no leucopenia developed over a period of 3½ years. Treatment with desferrioxamine was started with daily injections of 1,200 mg. i.m. (3 daily injections of 400 mg.), reduced later to 600 mg. daily. The serum iron rose from 320 to 500 μg. % and the urinary excretion of iron to a maximum level of 38.9 mg./day

Treatment (Fig. 3). Treatment with desferrioxamine was commenced in March 1962 with 1,200 mg. daily, given i.m. in 3 divided doses, and was later continued on an ambulatory basis with 600 mg. daily, dissolved in 10 ml. distilled water and injected i.m. once daily. The effect of desferrioxamine in mobilising the iron deposits in the body is shown by the increase in the serum iron, which initially rose from 320 to over 500 μg. % and then oscillated around 400 μg. %. The iron excretion in the urine rose promptly to a maximum of 38.9 mg./day. In 40 days, 750 mg. iron was eliminated. After an interruption of 5 months, the patient went back to work again. No side effects were noted.

Another patient (B.F., 65-year-old female) was suffering from *aplastic anaemia* (now under treatment) probably as the result of treatment for syphilis with arsenical preparations (Salvarsan). After two years of transfusion therapy, the patient shows only slight incipient secondary haemochromatosis. In response to desferrioxamine, administered in a dosage of 500 mg. 3 times daily, the serum iron rose from 158 to 264 μg. %; urinary iron excretion amounted to 6.24 mg. on the 1st day, 18 mg. on the 2nd day, and 16.8 mg. on the 3rd day, after which it became stabilised at an average of 12.5 mg. daily.

3. In thalassaemia and in severe haemolytic anaemia

Case 4: F. T., 8-year-old boy. Family history: Both parents of Italian origin. Personal history: At the age of 3 months, anorexia, splenomegaly, anaemia with 2.2 mill. erythrocytes and many erythroblasts. At 6 months, thalassaemia major was diagnosed. The haemoglobin fell to 3.5 g. and transfusions, at intervals of 2—3 weeks, were started because of severe fatigue. At the age of 2 years, the enlarged spleen was removed. Slight improvement. At 3 years, Prof. MARMON in Genoa found the following blood values: Hb. 6 g., reticulocytes 124‰, erythrocytes 2.6 mill., osmotic resistance 0.36—0.20, erythroblasts 220, bilirubin 1.7 mg. %. Transfusions had to be continued, because otherwise the haemoglobin remained below 4 g. The patient was admitted to our hospital on 24th July 1962.

Findings: Body-weight 21.2 kg. Typical haemochromatosis, skin greyish-brown. Liver enlarged (10 cm.), biopsy was refused. Blood findings: Haemoglobin 6 g. %, reticulocytes 0.3%, erythroblasts 178/200 white cells. Erythrocytes 1.9 mill., colour index 1.0. Severe anisochromasia, anisocytosis, poikilocytosis, many target cells. Leucocytes 148,000 with 1% myelocytes, 3.5% stab forms, 19% segmented, 4.5% eosinophils, 1% basophils, 10.5% monocytes, 58.5% lymphocytes. Thrombocytes 110,000. Sternal marrow: Enormous hyperplasia (4—5 times the normal) of the erythropoietic system with many immature basophilic erythroblasts. Many macrophages with ferritin and haemosiderin. *Haemoglobin electrophoresis:* Hb. A_2 2.1%, Hb. F 5.6%, typically increased, no abnormal haemoglobin. Glucose-6-phosphate-dehydrogenase normal. Protein 8.2 g. %. Immuno-electrophoresis normal. Serum iron 216 μg. %! Electrocardiogram: no pathological findings. Liver tests normal. Urinary sediment: no haemosiderin, no free haemoglobin.

Treatment (Fig. 4). The patient was given 400 mg. desferrioxamine for 10 days, followed by 200 mg. daily i.m. The serum iron rose to 250 μg. % and urinary iron excretion to 12–17 mg. daily, falling to 5–7 mg. when the dosage was reduced to 200 mg. desferrioxamine. In 60 days a total of 360 mg. iron was excreted. Desferrioxamine was then withdrawn. From 17th December 1962 onwards, the patient received continuous treatment with 200 mg.

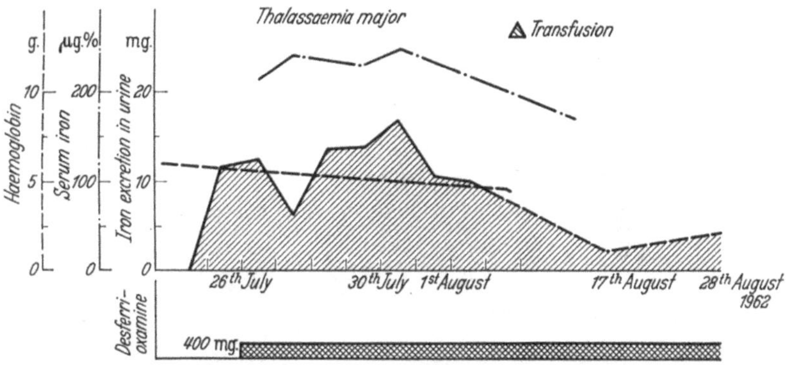

Fig. 4. ***Haemochromatosis in severe thalassaemia major.*** F. T., 8-year-old boy of Italian parentage. The child was splenectomised at 2 years and had always had a very low haemoglobin of 3.5–4 g. Following transfusions, typical haemochromatosis developed. Desferrioxamine treatment was instituted with 400 mg. i.m. daily, reduced to 200 mg. daily for out-patient therapy. Urinary iron excretion varied between 12 and 17 mg. daily in response to 400 mg. desferrioxamine and between 5 and 7 mg. in response to 200 mg.

desferrioxamine i.m. (except on Sundays), in response to which 180 mg. iron was eliminated in the urine in 30 days. Under intermittent therapy until 18th January 1963, a total of 675 mg. iron was eliminated in 90 days. The child's general condition gradually improved, but not the anaemia. Treatment has been continued for 15 months.

Case 5: W. A., 53-year-old housewife. No record of anaemia in the family. At the age of 28 years, splenectomy because of haemolytic anaemia. At the age of 46 years, diabetes set in, and haemochromatosis slowly developed. Transfusions were started in 1958 because of pronounced, refractory anaemia, despite slight reticulocytosis of 4.6%.

Findings in 1962: Greyish-brown and yellow discoloration. Skin biopsy revealed haemochromatosis. Heart enlarged and severe electrocardiographic changes. Pretibial oedema. Liver enlarged (17 cm.), increased resistance. Liver biopsy: severe haemochromatosis with incipient cirrhosis. Electrophoresis: dysproteinaemia of the gamma type. Takata slightly positive. Serum iron 195 μg. %, bilirubin 1.32 mg. %. Reticulocytes normal, 0.9%, but with pronounced increases during haemolytic crises. Haemoglobin fluctuating between 6 and 12.5 g. Severe anisocytosis. Colour index 0.96.

Leucocytes 9,600, differential count normal, numbers of erythroblasts with striking nuclear pyknosis and karyorrhexis. Sideroblasts slightly increased, but to a lesser degree than in sideroachrestic anaemia. Some ferritin and haemosiderin macrophages. Coombs' test, direct and indirect, negative. No cold or warm agglutination. No haemosiderin in the urinary sediment.

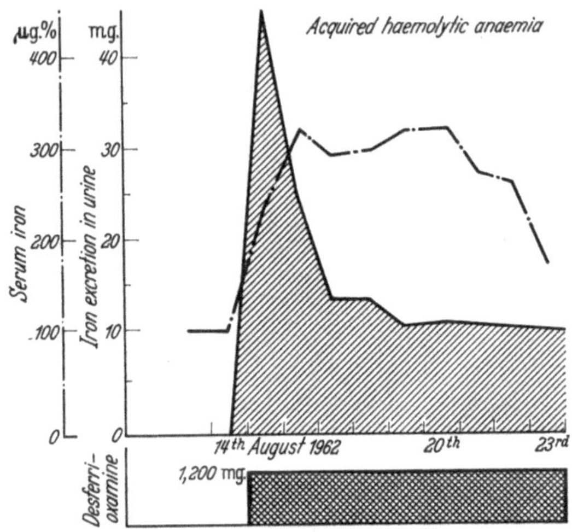

Fig. 5. *Haemochromatosis in severe haemolytic anaemia of unknown origin.* W. A., 53-year-old housewife. Haemolytic anaemia of long standing, marked haemochromatosis, and diabetes. Desferrioxamine treatment was started with 1,200 mg. daily i.m. The serum iron rose from 100 to 310 µg. %. Urinary iron excretion reached a maximum of 45 mg. daily and then decreased to about 10 mg. daily

Treatment (Fig. 5). Desferrioxamine therapy was started with 1,200 mg. daily i.m. (in two injections of 600 mg. each). The serum iron rose from 100 to 310 µg. %. Urinary iron excretion reached a maximum of 45 mg. daily and then decreased to about 10 mg. daily. It was not possible to continue the treatment at home because of lack of cooperation on the patient's part.

4. In secondary haemochromatosis due to toxic haemolytic anaemia following abuse of phenacetin

Case 6: S. H., 55-year-old female. This patient was suffering from typical *interstitial nephritis* following phenacetin abuse of 25 years' duration [MOESCHLIN (*6*)]. The skin showed the greyish-brown colouring characteristic of chronic phenacetinism. Since 1956, marked renal insufficiency had been evident. Although in February 1962 the blood urea nitrogen was only slightly elevated (53 mg. %), the urea clearance was found to be significantly pathological (40.5%), with marked impairment of concentrating ability (maximum specific gravity 1012). The haemoglobin was 12.5 g., with 12% reticulocytes and an elevated serum iron of 180 µg. %. The bone marrow showed typical evidence of iron loading, with many haemosiderin macrophages and an increase in erythropoiesis due to the haemolytic effect of the chronic phenacetin intake [Moeschlin (*6*)].

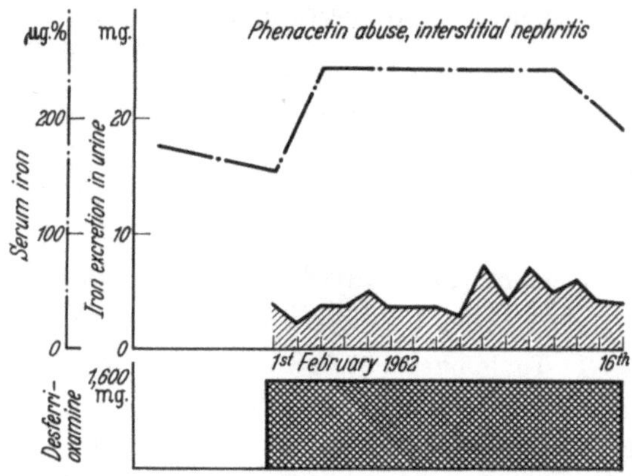

Fig. 6. ***Interstitial nephritis caused by chronic abuse of phenacetin.*** S. H., 55-year-old female. Pronounced haemosiderin deposits in the sternal marrow, slight anaemia, marked reticulocytosis, brownish-grey discoloration of the skin, and interstitial nephritis. Desferrioxamine treatment was tried for 15 days. Despite the high dosage of 1,600 mg. i.m., only small amounts of iron, not exceeding 7.8 mg. daily, were excreted. Although the desferrioxamine mobilised iron from the deposits (the serum iron rose from 180 to 240 μg. %), urinary iron excretion remained low, presumably because of impaired renal function

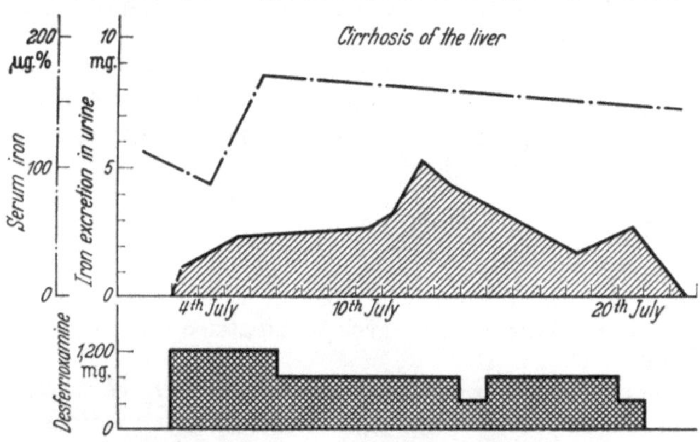

Fig. 7. ***Secondary haemochromatosis in alcoholic cirrhosis.*** R. W., 66-year-old male. Despite treatment with desferrioxamine, urinary iron excretion remained low, not exceeding 5 mg. daily. Biopsies revealed that the iron in the liver and sternal marrow was present chiefly in the form of haemosiderin. As renal function was already impaired, it is difficult to determine whether the low iron excretion was due to renal insufficiency rather than to the fact that haemosiderin is more difficult to mobilise than ferritin.

Treatment (Fig. 6). To establish whether in this form of secondary haemochromatosis iron could be mobilised from the large haemosiderin deposits and excreted despite severe renal damage, a high daily dose of 1,600 mg. desferrioxamine i.m. was given for 16 days. Despite the size of the dose, only small amounts of iron were excreted, i.e. never more than 7.8 mg./day. During treatment, the serum iron rose from 180 μg. % to 240 μg. %. In spite of this mobilising effect, urinary iron excretion remained low, presumably because of impaired renal function. Similar low urinary excretion levels were observed in a patient (Case 7) with secondary haemochromatosis associated with alcoholic cirrhosis, who also showed marked renal impairment (Fig. 7).

IV. Experimental results in acute iron poisoning with ferrous sulphate in guinea-pigs

1. Toxic effects of $FeSO_4$ in guinea-pigs

The signs we observed in experimental poisoning of guinea-pigs closely resembled those of the biphasic clinical picture. In the first phase the animals became weak and often showed paralysis of the legs. In addition, they frequently passed greenish-black diarrhoeal stools. Death often followed tonic-myoclonic convulsions. Such animals as survived the first phase subsequently died in severe shock within 12–24 hours.

Pathology. The gastric mucosa of the animals poisoned in this way showed swelling and haemorrhagic erosion. Histological examination revealed infiltration of leucocytes and diffuse impregnation of the mucosa and blood vessels with iron pigments. The liver showed central necrosis and fatty infiltration of the hepatic cells. Haemorrhagic effusions were also found in the pleura and in the lungs.

2. Therapeutic effect of desferrioxamine

To evaluate the therapeutic effect of desferrioxamine, we divided our experiments into four groups and attempted to answer four questions:

a) What effect, if any, does desferrioxamine have when given orally, in a dose of 2,000 mg./kg. body-weight, immediately after ferrous sulphate in a dose of 1.2 g./kg. body-weight?

b) How great is the protective and therapeutic effect of desferrioxamine when administered at different intervals?

c) In guinea-pigs receiving an LD_{100} dose of 1.8 g. ferrous sulphate per kg., will a high dose of desferrioxamine, i.e. 2,500 mg./kg., still have some effect?

d) How does the effect of desferrioxamine compare with that of the old method using sodium bicarbonate?

a) *First group (LD_{50} followed immediately by desferrioxamine)*

2,000 mg. desferrioxamine per kg. body-weight was given immediately after the administration of 1.2 g. ferrous sulphate per kg. (= LD_{50}) by stomach tube. As shown in Fig. 8 (extreme left), all the animals survived.

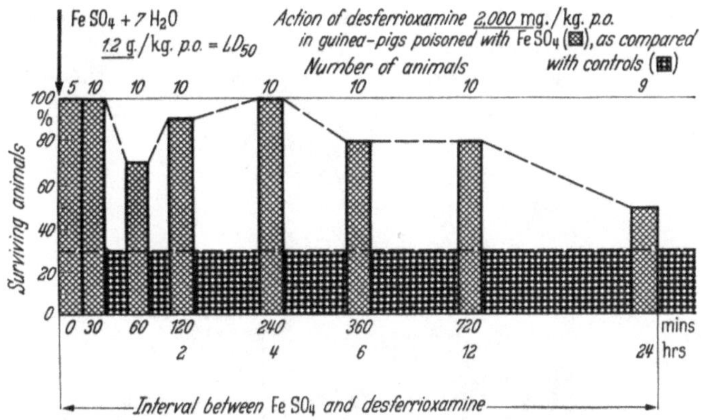

Fig. 8. *Experimental ferrous-sulphate poisoning.* Chart showing survival rates for guinea-pigs following ingestion of 1.2 g./kg. ferrous sulphate (LD_{50}) administered by stomach tube. Desferrioxamine, in a dosage of 2,000 mg./kg. body-weight, was given at intervals ranging from immediately after ingestion of the ferrous sulphate to 24 hours after. The controls showed a survival rate of only 30% (lower shaded portion), whereas the survival rates for the treated animals are represented by the columns. Given within up to 4 hours after ingestion of the iron, desferrioxamine prevented death in 70 to 100% of the animals

b) *Second group (LD_{50} followed by desferrioxamine at varying intervals of time)*

When the desferrioxamine was given after 30 minutes the survival rate was 100%, as compared with 70% after 60 minutes, 90% after 2 hours, 100% after 4 hours, 80% after 6 hours, and 80% after 12 hours. Beyond 24 hours, treatment with desferrioxamine exerted no detectable effect (Fig. 8, extreme right). In the control group (Fig. 8, lower shaded portion), 70% of the animals died during the first 12 hours.

c) *Third group (LD_{100} followed by desferrioxamine at varying intervals of time)*

In this group, 1.8 g. ferrous sulphate per kg. body-weight (= LD_{100}) was administered, followed by desferrioxamine in a dose of 2,500 mg./kg. (Fig. 9). *In response to the LD_{100}, all the untreated animals died in the first phase of poisoning,* whereas a high proportion of the treated animals survived; when the desferrioxamine was administered simultaneously with the ferrous sulphate, 70%

survived; when it was given after an interval of 30 minutes, 60% survived, as compared with 60% after one hour and only 20% after two hours.

d) *Control group (LD_{100} together with sodium bicarbonate as antidote)*

10 ml. of 5% sodium bicarbonate per kg., given simultaneously with the ferrous sulphate by stomach tube, failed to save any of the animals. All 10 animals died within 12 hours (Fig. 9, extreme right) and showed no difference as compared with another control group which received no treatment at all.

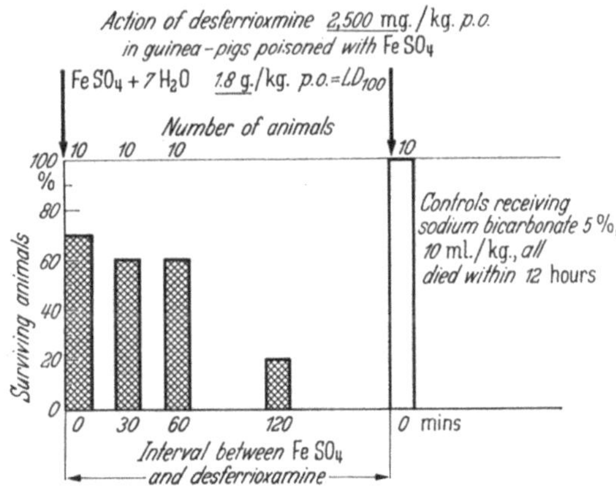

Fig. 9. *Experimental ferrous-sulphate poisoning with LD_{100}*. Survival rates of guinea-pigs poisoned with ferrous sulphate in a dosage of 1.8 g./kg. (LD_{100}). Desferrioxamine was given in a dosage of 2,500 mg. by stomach tube at various time intervals after administration of the ferrous sulphate. 60% of the animals could be saved if the desferrioxamine was given within one hour after the ferrous sulphate, whereas later no significant effect was observed. Sodium bicarbonate was completely ineffective (right column)

Discussion

I. Treatment with desferrioxamine in haemochromatosis

The clinical results which treatment has so far yielded in 8 cases of haemochromatosis (1 primary and 7 secondary forms), 7 of which are reported here and have been followed up for periods of up to 17 months, have clearly demonstrated that desferrioxamine B is the most potent and specific iron-eliminating agent known to date, particularly with regard to secondary haemochromatosis.

As the preparation was at first available only in limited quantities, clinical evaluation was reserved for typical cases of chronic iron overloading which could also be followed up over a prolonged period. Before discussing our results we should like to summarise our experience with respect to the dosage and methods of administration of this new drug.

1. Methods of administering desferrioxamine

Orally. The absorption of desferrioxamine itself from the gastro-intestinal tract amounts at the most to only 15% of the dose administered [TRIPOD and KEBERLE (*7*), WÖHLER (*4*), KELLER (*8*)]. The high price of this compound, which, like certain antibiotics, has to be prepared from streptomyces cultures, does not yet permit its use in clinical trials for the chronic inhibition of nutritional iron uptake by the gastro-intestinal tract – for instance, in polycythaemia vera or primary haemochromatosis. Since desferrioxamine is unable to remove iron from haemoglobin, it cannot block the intestinal absorption of nutritional haemoglobin iron when administered orally, nor can it block that of nutritional myoglobin iron (*7*). However, other forms of nutritional iron (*8*, *14*), such as liver iron for example, may be bound by desferrioxamine if the latter is given by mouth immediately or shortly after the intake of food. Orally administered desferrioxamine can therefore be expected also to prove of value in acute iron poisoning, which will be discussed later.

Intramuscularly. Our own investigations, as well as those of others (*8*, *9*, *10*), would appear to suggest that the best method for clinical administration is by intramuscular injection, the daily dose of desferrioxamine being given in two injections of 400 to 600 mg. each, dissolved in 10 ml. distilled water. The injections are well tolerated locally and produce no known side effects.

Intravenously. The drug can also be given by intravenous drip infusion in physiological saline or isotonic glucose (after first being dissolved in distilled water). Clinical studies by various investigators ("Round-Table Discussion", held in Lugano in May 1962) have shown that about the same effect on urinary iron excretion can be obtained by either route, i.e. intramuscular or intravenous, using the same dosage.

2. Dosage

The ideal dosage is between 800 and 1,200 mg. daily. A further increase in dosage produces no corresponding increase in iron excretion. This is consistent with the data on the iron-binding capacity of desferrioxamine, which cannot be stepped up beyond a certain point. In fact, only 25–30% of the dose of desferrioxamine administered becomes bound to iron. However, a certain "overdose" appears to be necessary in order to mobilise the iron stores in haemochromatosis, and possibly also in order to inhibit tubular reabsorption.

3. Side effects

Until now, no side effects have been observed with desferrioxamine, either in our cases or in patients treated by other workers. Experimental studies on the excretion of other elements (sodium, potassium, calcium, and the trace elements: magnesium, copper, chrome, nickel, aluminium, and manganese) have been undertaken by BICKEL et al. (*1*, *9*) and by TRIPOD (*10*). The results obtained have shown that the effect on the excretion of such elements is minimal; in particular, desferrioxamine – unlike the versenate derivatives – does not enhance excretion of the essential oligometals Cu, Zn, and Mg. In clinical studies, no significant increase in copper excretion was found by RISSEL and SCHNACK (*11a*, *11b*), or in zinc excretion by TRIPOD (*10*). It can thus be assumed that desferrioxamine has no side effects worthy of note, whereas it has a very distinct elective affinity for body iron, forming a non-toxic complex, ferrioxamine, which is easily excreted by the kidney without damaging the renal tissues. No albuminuria or urea could be demonstrated. Allergic drug reactions are liable to occur with any preparation, but so far, though several thousand injections have been administered, only one patient [MANN and MAIER (*5*)] with alcoholic cirrhosis has shown what may possibly have been an allergic reaction after intravenous injection of desferrioxamine.

It might have been thought that patients treated with desferrioxamine run a risk of developing anaemia. This, however, is not the case in haemochromatosis patients; on the contrary, we and others have actually observed an improvement in the haemoglobin levels in some cases, cf. Case 2, for example, in Fig. 2. KELLER (*8*) has demonstrated that in anaemia the iron uptake is not decreased if desferrioxamine is given.

4. Iron mobilisation, the serum iron level, and iron excretion

As will be seen from the figures reproduced in this paper, the serum iron concentration increases in the first few days owing to the mobilisation of iron from the deposits in the tissues, i.e. mainly from ferritin and transferrin and probably to a lesser extent from haemosiderin; the serum iron concentration then slowly decreases in the following weeks, but does not usually decline to pre-treatment levels.

A rise in urinary iron excretion sets in shortly after the first injection of desferrioxamine and leads to a distinct reddish coloration of the urine reminiscent of the colour of *vin rosé*. If this discoloration occurs, it may be concluded that the patient is excreting iron at the rate of some 10–30 mg./24 hours. In secondary haemochromatosis the iron excretion may rise to between 25 and 54 mg. daily in response to intramuscular injections of 600 mg. desferrioxamine twice daily. In primary haemochromatosis the iron excretion may be less pronounced, i.e. 15–25 (–30) mg. daily (cf. Case 1, Fig. 1). In normal individuals, judging from our experience, the excretion does not normally rise above 2, or at the most, 4 mg. daily.

5. Clinical indications and effects of treatment

a) Primary hereditary haemochromatosis

Our own experience of this indication is very limited, because we have had occasion to treat only one patient for a short period. However, good results with desferrioxamine in the long-term treatment of primary haemochromatosis have been reported by WÖHLER (*12*), HEILMEYER (*13*), FREY (*14*), MANN and MAIER (*5*), and RISSEL and SCHNACK (*11a, 11b*). Urinary iron excretion in this disease does not usually rise as high as in secondary haemochromatosis, i.e. it varies between 15 and 25 mg. daily. Thus, venesection, if performed at weekly intervals, is still able to eliminate more iron (i.e. 200–250 mg. per 500 ml. blood); here, desferrioxamine may accordingly be reserved for patients with concurrent anaemia or for combination with venesection in very serious advanced cases. Theoretically, it should also be possible, with daily oral doses of about 2,000 mg. desferrioxamine, partially to block the intestinal absorption of nutritional iron, though not of nutritional haemoglobin iron; this has been demonstrated by KELLER (*8*), using radioactive iron in human subjects, and by KEBERLE (*15*) in experiments on rabbits. This method, however, is of no practical value in primary haemochromatosis, because larger amounts of iron can be eliminated by combining venesection with intramuscular injections of desferrioxamine.

b) Secondary haemochromatosis

The most important indication for the clinical use of desferrioxamine is *secondary haemochromatosis*, a form of chronic iron overloading usually due to increased haemoglobin destruction or to transfusion therapy in cases of aplastic anaemia. Until now, there has been no solution to the problem of treating secondary haemochromatosis as encountered in sideroachrestic anaemia, aplastic anaemia (transfusions), severe thalassaemia major, and sickle-cell anaemia.

Sideroachrestic anaemia. This type of anaemia, characterised by the presence of many typical sideroblasts in the bone marrow, had previously been described under various names, but was recognised as a special clinical entity in 1956 by BJÖRKMAN (*16*) in Sweden and was further investigated by HEILMEYER (*17*) and his co-workers in Germany. In this form of anaemia, the iron uptake is sometimes increased and – owing probably to an enzymatic defect that has yet to be identified – the incorporation of iron in the protoporphyrin is disturbed. Hence, after some years, even without transfusions, iron overloading (i.e. secondary haemochromatosis) develops. This clinical syndrome of sideroachrestic anaemia has recently (1961) been reviewed in the U.S.A. by BYRD and COOPER (*18*) under the name of "hereditary iron-loading anaemia with secondary haemochromatosis". In our experience, a distinction can be drawn between two different forms. The first corresponds to the type described by BYRD and COOPER (*18*) and starts in childhood or between the ages of 20 and 30 years, as in our Case 2 mentioned above; it may finally lead to death from severe haemochromatosis. The second is an acquired form, occurring particularly in older women, and tends to run a milder and more benign course. Pyridoxine has proved of no value in our patients, but it may be helpful in some cases. The nature of this type of anaemia is still obscure. The hereditary or acquired disorder seems to involve an enzymatic defect, the erythrocytes being unable to utilise the readily available iron and porphyrin precursors in a normal manner [HEILMEYER (*17*), BYRD and COOPER (*18*)].

The striking results obtained with desferrioxamine in Case 2, which have been maintained continuously from October 1961 until now, offer new hope with regard to the treatment of this disease in the future. The patient, who was unable to do a proper day's work before receiving desferrioxamine treatment, has now been working full-time for one year and looks healthy. He continues to give himself an intramuscular injection of 400 mg. desferrioxamine once a day. No side effects have appeared, although treatment has been in progress for over 2 years. This case clearly illustrates what can be done today for such patients with the aid of desferrioxamine. In this particular instance bone-marrow and liver biopsies have revealed no striking change due to the iron overload. However, we know that up to at least 30–70 g. iron have to be retained before severe histological changes develop in patients with haemochromatosis. Treatment will therefore probably have to be continued over an even longer period. At all events, one may be satisfied that the haemochromatosis appears at least to have been arrested. *Early treatment would seem to be essential for other cases of sideroachrestic anaemia.*

Aplastic anaemia with secondary haemochromatosis due to multiple transfusions. We have already seen that in Case 3 the severe aplastic anaemia was associated with almost complete arrest of erythrocyte maturation and with disappearance of the erythroblasts, which had gradually become more and more marked over a period of 3 years. The haemoglobin could be maintained only by transfusions at fortnightly intervals. All cases of this kind requiring continuous transfusion therapy develop severe secondary haemochromatosis, which may cause clinical symptoms after 2 to 3 years and become dangerous after 4 to 6 years, leading eventually to death from general and, particularly, hepatic and myocardial haemochromatosis. The results obtained in Case 3, as illustrated in Fig. 3, show that one may be able completely to offset the abnormal iron overloading in these patients by continuous or even intermittent therapy with desferrioxamine. On the basis of the amount of blood transfused and the daily iron excretion in the urine it is possible to calculate the daily dose of desferrioxamine required for each case. In this way, any further increase in the degree of secondary haemochromatosis can be arrested in all patients with severe aplastic anaemia receiving transfusions. Our patient needs an intramuscular injection of 400 mg. desferrioxamine every second day to eliminate the additional iron which he is receiving in the transfusions. As the preparation is still expensive, such calculations are also important in order to avoid an unnecessarily high dosage of desferrioxamine. The same treatment may also be essential for the so-called Blackfan-Diamond form of aplastic anaemia occurring in children.

Severe thalassaemia and severe acquired haemolytic anaemia of alternative origin. Case 4 (Fig. 4) demonstrates the marked increase in daily iron excretion of up to 12–15 mg. which can be obtained with 400 mg. desferrioxamine i.m. in severe thalassaemia major. This boy, though only 8 years of age, is already suffering from severe haemochromatosis, and it is known that many of these patients (homozygous forms) die at the early age of 18 to 22 years from severe myocardial damage due to the haemochromatosis. It may be possible to prevent this in future by early and continuous treatment with desferrioxamine. The drug may also prove useful in certain cases of severe secondary haemochromatosis associated with haemolytic anaemia, as in Case 5.

In a case of chronic phenacetin abuse, which is still a problem in Switzerland [MOESCHLIN (*6*)], the haemolytic action of this compound had given rise to secondary haemochromatosis. Here, we found very low iron-excretion levels, despite a very high daily dose of 1,600 mg. desferrioxamine for 16 days (Case 6, Fig. 6). It is difficult to determine whether the low rate of iron excretion was due to renal impairment [so-called "interstitial phenacetin nephritis", MOESCHLIN (*6*)] or to the fact that in these cases the iron is stored mainly in the form of haemosiderin, which is probably not so easily mobilised by desferrioxamine as ferritin (cf. the incubation studies with washed marrow specimens carried out by MANN and MAIER (*5*) and already mentioned above). The fact that the serum iron rose from 180 to 240 μg. % would rather seem to suggest that the patient's failure to excrete larger quantities of ferrioxamine was due to impairment of renal function.

Similar low excretion levels were also found in a patient with secondary haemochromatosis associated with primary alcoholic cirrhosis (Fig. 7), a complication not uncommon among the many cases of alcoholic cirrhosis encountered in Switzerland.

II. Treatment with desferrioxamine in acute accidental iron poisoning

In our experimental studies on guinea-pigs we have attempted to assess the value of desferrioxamine for the treatment of accidental iron poisoning in children. At this point, it may be worth recalling some of the more important aspects of this accidental poisoning.

Every haematologist knows that acute iron poisoning in children due to accidental ingestion of iron tablets (usually prescribed for the sideroanaemic mother) has hitherto presented an unsolved therapeutic problem. Many children, in fact, die each year from this type of poisoning. In 1954, BIRK and STALLARD (*19*) reviewed 80 cases from the literature, many of which involved children between the ages of 1 and 3 years. Since then, numerous individual reports have been published [THOMSON (*20*), SPENCER (*21*), SHEPHERD (*22*), and others]. The majority of cases are due to poisoning with ferrous sulphate [BIRK (*19*) and others]. Unfortunately, some of the iron preparations on sale are sugar-coated and attractively coloured. *Every doctor prescribing iron tablets should warn his patients of the serious consequences which may result from not keeping the tablets under lock and key.*

Clinical signs and symptoms. Acute iron poisoning is generally characterised by a *biphasic* course extending over 24 hours [THOMSON (*20*), SPENCER (*21*)].

In the *first phase*, i.e. 30 to 120 minutes after ingestion, severe vomiting of black, haemorrhagic fluid occurs, accompanied by severe gastric pain and often blackish diarrhoeal stools. Profound shock then develops. Approximately $^1/_4$ of the cases die in this first phase. In the others, the patient improves slightly and then enters the *second phase* after about 20 hours. This is characterised by sudden collapse, Cheyne-Stokes breathing, convulsions, and sometimes toxic hepatitis. If the patient overcomes this phase, pyloric stenosis due to cicatrisation [ELLIOT-SMITH (*23*), ROSS (*24*), SHEPHERD (*22*), CROSSKEY (*25*)] may develop.

The serum iron rises quickly to toxic levels (BIRK has reported one case with 4,000 μg. %!). The alkali-binding capacity is markedly reduced.

It may be concluded that acute iron intoxication *acts mainly in two ways*: firstly, it causes corrosion of the gastro-intestinal tract, primarily of the stomach and ileum [see also the experimental investigations of REISSMANN et al. (*26a, 26b*)]; secondly, the excess iron which is absorbed affects the nervous system, causing severe toxic damage, perhaps through an enzyme-blocking effect [SPENCER (*21*), MOESCHLIN (*27a, 27b*)].

Lethal dose. The lethal dose for children between 1 and 3 years is about 3 to 10 g. ferrous sulphate, i.e. 15–50 tablets of 0.2 g. HOPPE (*28*) has calculated from the literature that the lethal dose is 900 mg./kg. body-weight.

From the results of our experiments (Figs 8 and 9) it is evident that, provided treatment with desferrioxamine (2,000 mg./kg.) is initiated immediately or within half an hour, acute ferrous-sulphate poisoning in guinea-pigs can be cured (100% survival with LD_{50} and 80% survival with LD_{100}), even when a comparatively high dose of ferrous sulphate is administered. If treatment is not given until after 6 or 12 hours, 80% of the animals survive. After 24 hours no significant effect can be demonstrated. From calculations of the iron content it would appear that 2,568 mg. desferrioxamine is required to neutralise the ferrous sulphate. However, the smaller doses used by us also afforded good protection.

On the basis of animal experiments it seems highly probable that in man a beneficial effect could also be obtained by administering a high dose of desferrioxamine as soon as possible after ingestion of ferrous sulphate. Even after a delay of some hours, one would probably still be able to achieve a protective effect. It must be admitted, of course, that results based on animal experiments can never be directly applied to man. Nevertheless, the striking results obtained in the LD_{100} experiments, i.e. with 1.8 g. ferrous sulphate and 2,500 mg. desferrioxamine per kg. *strongly suggest that in man also a good and even life-saving effect may be expected if desferrioxamine treatment is instituted without delay.*

Dosage of desferrioxamine in acute iron poisoning in children

In the light of the above-mentioned experiments and the fact that 2,140 mg. desferrioxamine is able to bind about 1 g. ferrous sulphate (i.e. about 200 mg. iron), it may be concluded that in a child poisoned with 3 to 4 g. ferrous sulphate, at least 8,000 mg. desferrioxamine would be necessary to neutralise the ingested iron in the stomach and upper intestinal tract. On the basis of our experiments we would accordingly recommend the following procedure:

Prevention and treatment of acute iron poisoning

1. Prevention

a) Never use or prescribe sugar-coated or coloured iron tablets!

b) Always warn the patient of the consequences of iron poisoning in children, stressing that the tablets should be kept under lock and key. Avoid the use of ferrous sulphate!

2. Treatment

a) **Gastric lavage** should be undertaken only if the child is seen in the first hour following ingestion of the tablets and if no severe shock is present. Wash with small amounts of physiological saline, i.e. 100 ml. per portion (100 mg. desferrioxamine in 500 ml. physiological saline), and place the patient in the shock position or side position to avoid aspiration.

b) **Enteral administration of the antidote.** The patient should immediately be given by stomach tube 8,000–12,000 mg. desferrioxamine dissolved in distilled water (10 ml. per 2,000 mg.), in order to neutralise the iron in the gastro-intestinal tract.

c) **Parenteral administration of the antidote.** To counteract the toxic effect of the excessive iron absorbed, immediately infuse 2,000 mg. desferrioxamine in 5% laevulose solution. Continue this dose for the next two days.

d) **Treatment for shock** should, if necessary, be given with plasma, pressor agents, and corticosteroids. Prophylactically, an intravenous drip infusion should always be instituted, so as not to lose time in case of sudden shock.

Summary

1. An account is given of clinical and experimental results obtained with a new and potent iron-binding substance (desferrioxamine B = Desferal) which is capable of forming a water-soluble non-toxic iron complex (ferrioxamine) that is excreted by the kidneys.

2. Desferrioxamine is non-toxic and has so far shown no side effects. Very little of the drug is absorbed enterally, but it can be given intravenously by drip infusion or preferably by intramuscular injection (twice daily). Desferrioxamine does not enhance the excretion of other oligometals (Zn, Cu, etc.).

3. *Dosage.* To achieve a high degree of iron mobilisation from the iron stores, leading to a rise in the serum iron concentration and to a subsequent marked increase in urinary iron excretion, the optimum dose is 1,000 to 1,200 mg. daily, given in the form of intramuscular injections of 500 mg. each, twice daily, or by intravenous drip infusion in physiological saline or glucose. For maintenance treatment, 500 mg. daily is sufficient in many cases.

4. *Iron excretion.* In normal individuals the urinary iron excretion rises to 2—3 mg. daily in response to desferrioxamine, whereas in patients with haemochromatosis up to 20—40 (—50) mg. iron may be excreted daily. Thus, with continuous treatment for a period of one year, up to 7—18 g., and sometimes even more, can be eliminated.

5. Clinical data on various patients treated with desferrioxamine have been presented. Desferrioxamine is today the treatment of choice for:

Secondary haemochromatosis in:

a) aplastic anaemia (transfusion haemosiderosis)

b) sideroachrestic anaemia

c) thalassaemia major (severe cases in children)

d) severe sickle-cell anaemia

e) severe Marchiafava syndrome

f) severe chronic acquired haemolytic anaemia with severe haemochromatosis.

In *primary haemochromatosis*, more iron can be eliminated by venesection than with desferrioxamine; the latter can therefore be reserved for anaemic patients or for combined treatment with venesection in advanced cases.

6. *Experimental work on the treatment of acute iron poisoning* in guinea-pigs has been described, showing that desferrioxamine yields excellent results (100% survival with LD_{50} and approx. 80% with LD_{100}) if administered by stomach tube up to $^1/_2$—2 hours following ingestion of ferrous sulphate. It is therefore suggested that, in children suffering from accidental iron poisoning, a dose of 8,000—12,000 mg. desferrioxamine in distilled water should be administered as soon as possible after ingestion of the poison, and that 2,000 mg. may at the same time be given intramuscularly or intravenously.

Zusammenfassung

1. Es wird eine Übersicht über klinische und experimentelle Befunde gegeben, die mit einem neuen, für Eisen spezifischen Komplexbildner (Desferrioxamin B = Desferal) erhoben wurden. Desferrioxamin bildet einen

wasserlöslichen, nicht toxischen Eisenkomplex (Ferrioxamin), der durch die Nieren ausgeschieden wird.

2. Desferrioxamin ist untoxisch und hat bisher nicht zu schwerwiegenden Nebenwirkungen geführt. Die Substanz wird nur in geringen Mengen durch den Darm resorbiert. Sie kann entweder intravenös in Form einer Dauertropfinfusion oder vorzugsweise intramuskulär (zweimal täglich) gegeben werden. Desferrioxamin fördert nicht die Ausscheidung von anderen Metallen (Zn, Cu, etc.).

3. *Dosierung.* Um eine möglichst hochgradige Mobilisierung von Eisen aus den Depots zu erreichen, die zu einem Anstieg der Serumeisenkonzentration und in der Folge zu einer stark vermehrten Ausscheidung von Eisen im Urin führt, ist eine Dosierung von 1'000—1'200 mg./Tag optimal. Sie wird entweder in Form von zwei intramuskulären Injektionen zu je 500 mg. oder durch intravenöse Infusion in physiologischer Kochsalzlösung oder Glukose gegeben. Für die Erhaltungsbehandlung genügen in den meisten Fällen 500 mg. täglich.

4. *Eisenausscheidung.* Beim Normalen steigt die tägliche Eisenausscheidung im Urin nach Gabe von Desferrioxamin auf 2—3 mg. an, während Patienten mit Haemochromatose täglich 20—40 (—50) mg. Eisen ausscheiden können. Durch eine Dauerbehandlung während einer Zeitspanne von einem Jahr können auf diese Weise 7—18 g. Eisen, gelegentlich sogar mehr, eliminiert werden.

5. Es werden klinische Befunde mitgeteilt, die an verschiedenen mit Desferrioxamin behandelten Patienten erhoben wurden. Desferrioxamin ist heute das Mittel der Wahl für die Behandlung der *sekundären Haemochromatose* im Verlaufe von:

a) aplastischer Anaemie (Transfusionshaemosiderose)
b) sideroachrestischer Anaemie
c) Thalassaemia major (schwere Fälle bei Kindern)
d) schwerer Sichelzellanaemie
e) schwerem Marchiafava Syndrom
f) schwerer erworbener chronischer haemolytischer Anaemie mit Haemochromatose.

Bei *primärer Haemochromatose* kann durch Aderlaß mehr Eisen entfernt werden als durch Desferrioxamin; das letztere kann daher für anaemische Patienten reserviert bleiben oder kommt bei fortgeschrittenen Fällen für eine kombinierte Behandlung zusammen mit Aderlaß in Betracht.

6. Experimentelle Arbeiten über die Behandlung akuter Eisenvergiftung beim Meerschweinchen werden besprochen. Daraus geht hervor, daß mit Desferrioxamin sehr gute Resultate erzielt werden können, wenn es durch die Magensonde $^1/_2$—2 Stunden nach Einnahme von Eisensulfat gegeben wird (100% überleben nach Gabe der LD_{50} und ungefähr 80% nach Gabe der LD_{100}). Es wird daher vorgeschlagen, daß bei Kindern mit akuter Eisenvergiftung Dosen von 8'000—12'000 mg. Desferrioxamin in destilliertem Wasser so rasch wie möglich nach der Aufnahme des Eisens oral verabreicht werden, und daß 2'000 mg. gleichzeitig entweder intramuskulär oder intravenös injiziert werden.

Résumé

1. L'auteur donne un compte-rendu des résultats cliniques et expérimentaux qu'il a obtenus avec une nouvelle et puissante substance chélatrice du fer (la desferrioxamine B = Desféral) qui est capable de former avec ce métal un complexe soluble non toxique (ferrioxamine) excrété par les reins.

2. La desferrioxamine n'est pas toxique et jusqu'à présent n'a provoqué aucun effet secondaire. Le produit n'est que très peu absorbé par voie digestive, mais il peut être administré en perfusion intra-veineuse ou de préférence par voie intramusculaire (deux fois par jour). La desferrioxamine ne renforce pas l'excrétion d'autres oligo-éléments (Zn, Cu, etc.).

3. *Posologie.* Pour obtenir un haut degré de mobilisation du fer de ses dépôts avec élévation de la concentration du fer dans le sérum, et par voie de conséquence une élimination urinaire notablement accrue, la dose optimum est de 1.000 à 1.200 mg. par jour, administrée sous forme d'injections intramusculaires de 500 mg. chaque, deux fois par jour, ou en perfusion intraveineuse dans du sérum physiologique salé ou glucosé. Pour le traitement d'entretien, 500 mg. par jour sont suffisants dans la plupart des cas.

4. *Excrétion du fer.* Chez le sujet normal l'excrétion urinaire du fer sous desferrioxamine s'élève à 2 à 3 mg. par jour, tandis que chez les malades présentant une hémochromatose, cette excrétion peut atteindre 20, 40, (50) mg. par jour. Ainsi, avec un traitement continu pendant une période d'un an, 7 à 18 g., et quelquefois plus, de fer peuvent être éliminés.

5. Des observations cliniques de divers malades traités par la desferrioxamine ont été présentées. La desferrioxamine est actuellement le traitement de choix dans:

Les hémochromatoses secondaires

a) des anémies aplastiques (hémosidérose transfusionnelle)
b) des anémies sidéro-achrestiques
c) des thalassémies majeures (cas sévères chez les enfants)
d) des anémies graves à hématies falciformes
e) des syndromes de Marchiafava graves
f) des anémies hémolytiques chroniques acquises graves avec hémochromatose importante.

Dans *l'hémochromatose primaire,* on peut éliminer plus de fer par les saignées que par la desferrioxamine; cette dernière peut donc être réservée au traitement des malades anémiques ou utilisée en association avec les saignées dans les cas avancés.

6. *Des travaux expérimentaux sur le traitement de l'intoxication aiguë au fer* chez le cobaye ont été présentés, montrant que la desferrioxamine donne d'excellents résultats (100% de survies avec la DL_{50} et approximativement 80% avec la DL_{100}) lorsqu'elle est administrée par sonde gastrique jusqu'à $^1/_2$ heure à 2 heures après l'ingestion de sulfate ferreux. On peut donc conseiller d'administrer chez les enfants présentant une intoxication accidentelle au fer une dose de 8.000 à 12.000 mg. de desferrioxamine dans de l'eau distillée aussitôt que possible après l'ingestion du toxique, et 2.000 mg. en même temps par voie intramusculaire ou intra-veineuse.

Acknowledgement

The authors would like to express their thanks to CIBA Limited, Basle, for kindly supplying them with desferrioxamine and for the titration of different samples.

References

1. Bickel, H., E. Gäumann, W. Keller-Schierlein, V. Prelog, E. Vischer, A. Wettstein, and H. Zähner: Experientia (Switz.) **16**, 129 (1960). — 2. Nielsen, J. B.: In: Round-Table Discussion: Schweiz. med. Wschr. **92**, 1295 (1962). — 3. Keberle, H.: Personal communication

(CIBA Limited, Basle, Switzerland). — 4. WÖHLER, F.: In: Round-Table Discussion. Schweiz. med. Wschr. **92**, 1295 (1962). — 5. MANN, M., and C. MAIER: In: Round-Table Discussion: Schweiz. med. Wschr. **92**, 1295 (1962). — 6. MOESCHLIN, S.: Klinik und Therapie der Vergiftungen. 3rd Ed. Georg Thieme, Stuttgart 1959, p. 378-401 (an English edition is now in press, Grune & Stratton Inc., New York 1963). — 7. TRIPOD, J., and H. KEBERLE: Helvet. physiol. pharmacol. acta **20**, 291 (1962). — 8. KELLER, H. M.: In: Round-Table Discussion: Schweiz. med. Wschr. **92**, 1295 (1962). — 9. BICKEL, H.: In: Round-Table Discussion. Schweiz. med. Wschr. **92**, 1295 (1962). — 10. TRIPOD, J.: In: Round-Table Discussion. Schweiz. med. Wschr. **92**, 1295 (1962). — 11a. RISSEL, E., and H. SCHNACK: In: Round-Table Discussion. Schweiz. med. Wschr. **92**, 1295 (1962). — 11b. RISSEL, E., and H. SCHNACK: Wien. klin. Wschr. **74**, 577 (1962). — 12. WÖHLER, F.: Med. Klin. (G.) **57**, 1370 (1962). — 13. HEILMEYER, L.: In: Round-Table Discussion. Schweiz. med. Wschr. **92**, 1295 (1962). — 14. FREY, F.: In: Round-Table Discussion. Schweiz. med. Wschr. **92**, 1295 (1962). — 15. KEBERLE, H.: In: Round-Table Discussion. Schweiz. med. Wschr. **92**, 1295 (1962). — 16. BJÖRKMAN, S. E.: Blood (U.S.A.) **11**, 250 (1956). — 17. HEILMEYER, L.: Med. Klin. (G.) **57**, 121 (1962). — 18. BYRD, R. B., and T. COOPER: Ann. Int. Med. (U.S.A.) **55**, 103 (1961). — 19. BIRK, R. E., and S. K. STALLARD: J. Pediatr. (U.S.A.) **45**, 164 (1954). — 20. THOMSON, J.: Brit. Med. J. **1947**/I, 640. — 21. SPENCER, I. O. B.: Brit. Med. J. **1951**/II, 1112. — 22. SHEPHERD, J.: Brit. Med. J. **1955**/II, 418. — 23. ELLIOT-SMITH, A., and P. A. DAVIES: Brit. Med. J. **1954**/I, 156. — 24. ROSS, F. G. M.: Brit. Med. J. **1953**/II, 1200. — 25. CROSSKEY, P. H.: Brit. Med. J. **1952**/II, 285. — 26a. REISSMANN, K. R., J. BOLEY, G. F. CHRISTIANSON, and M. H. DELP: J. Laborat. Clin. Med. (U.S.A.) **43**, 572 (1954). — 26b. REISSMANN, K. R., T. J. COLEMAN, B. S. BUDAI, and L. R. MORIARTY: Blood (U.S.A.) **10**, 35 (1955). — 26c. REISSMANN, K. R., and T. J. COLEMAN: Blood (U.S.A.) **10**, 46 (1955). — 27a. MOESCHLIN, S.: Klinik und Therapie der Vergiftungen. 3rd Ed. Georg Thieme, Stuttgart, 1959, p. 110 (an English edition is now in press, Grune & Stratton Inc., New York, 1963). — 27b. MOESCHLIN, S.: In: Round-Table Discussion. Schweiz. med. Wschr. **92**, 1295 (1962). — 28. HOPPE, J. O.: Amer. J. Med. Sc. **230**, 491 (1955).

The treatment of haemochromatosis with desferrioxamine

By

F. Wöhler

Hitherto, venesection has had to be regarded as the method of choice for treating haemochromatosis. Now, however, we have another means of withdrawing iron from the human organism. The great advantage of this new method over venesection is that it can also be employed in cases of transfusion haemosiderosis, haemolytic anaemia, and sideroachrestic anaemia, as well as in the many different forms of secondary siderosis.

The method consists of administering a hydroxamic acid compound, known as desferrioxamine B hydrochloride. Attempts to remove iron ions from the organism with the aid of chelating agents were undertaken as far back as 1952 (Figueroa et al., Palmieri et al., Gisinger et al., Foreman et al., etc.). The drugs used were di-oxyethylglycine, ethylene-diamine tetra-acetic acid, and B.A.L. Recently, use has been made of diethylene-triamine penta-acetic acid (D.T.P.A.) (Fahey et al., Finch et al., etc.). We ourselves have also employed this substance, but it was not successful in long-term therapy because of toxic side effects.

Desferrioxamine is a naturally occurring substance which is formed from *Actinomycetes*. It belongs to the category of siderochromes which are able to form brownish-red complexes with trivalent iron. The siderochromes can be divided into two main groups: the so-called sideromycins, which are iron-containing antibiotics, and the sideramines, which possess growth-promoting properties and specifically antagonise the antibacterial effect of the sideromycins.

The desferrioxamine in which we are interested here is the iron-free parent substance of ferrioxamine, a member of the sideramine group. Desferrioxamine is a filamentous trihydroxamic acid derivative which forms an octahedral complex with an Fe^{+++} ion. The long chain of desferrioxamine coils itself round the iron atom so that the latter becomes thoroughly embedded. 100 mg. desferrioxamine B hydrochloride is capable, theoretically, of binding 9.3 mg. Fe^{+++} ions. This complex, composed of iron and hydroxamic acid, has a molecular weight of 613 and can therefore pass very easily through the kidney. The stability constant of the Fe^{+++} complex is $10^{30.7}$ and is thus somewhat higher than that of transferrin (10^{27} and 10^{29}), which possesses two binding centres. The stability constants for alkaline earths are lower than in the case of E.D.T.A. (for calcium 1.7×10^2 and for magnesium 2×10^4). This also explains why desferrioxamine does not exert any untoward effects on the serum electrolytes, even when administered for periods of more than two years.

Investigations to date have shown that other heavy-metal ions, including particularly trace elements, are not affected by desferrioxamine. Consequently, it appears certain that the drug displays a selective effect on the iron proteins in the organism.

Ferrioxamine was prepared in a pure condition, defined, and synthesised in the Research Laboratories of CIBA, Basle (BICKEL, GÄUMANN, KELLER-SCHIERLEIN, PRELOG, VISCHER, WETTSTEIN, and ZÄHNER; BICKEL, HALL, KELLER-SCHIERLEIN, PRELOG, VISCHER, and WETTSTEIN; VISCHER).

Originally, we attempted to use ferrioxamine in the treatment of iron-deficiency anaemias. Despite the administration of extremely large doses, however, neither the haemoglobin nor the erythrocyte level rose; on the other hand, one finding that did strike us as interesting was the brief rise in the serum iron which occurred. To obtain information about the metabolism of iron in the body, radioactive ferrioxamine was administered intravenously. As Fig. 1 shows, some 90% of the labelled ferrioxamine was already excreted in the urine on the first day – a finding which, with slight deviations, was recorded time and again in repeated studies. By the third day only very small amounts of ferrioxamine could still be detected. In the serum, an activity of some 20% was found 5 minutes after the injection of ferrioxamine, but this activity rapidly declined thereafter, amounting to only about 2% after 24 hours. After 72 hours, activity could no longer be demonstrated in the serum. Admittedly, considerable activity was detected over the liver, spleen, and sacrum after only 5 minutes, but a massive decline set in subsequently. Repetition of these tests invariably yielded results which were, in principle, identical. On each occasion, between 80% and 90% of the injected amount of ferrioxamine labelled with Fe^{59} was recovered in the urine within the first 3 days.

In order to obtain more information about the distribution and behaviour of ferrioxamine in the organs, radioactive ferrioxamine was administered to rats and the activity in the organs determined. The activity in various organs rose to maximum levels within only 5 minutes and then, in some cases, fell away considerably after only 20 minutes (Table 1). This pattern is most pronounced in the case of the liver. The rise in activity in the lung 20 minutes after injection and the rapid fall to 0.76% in this organ

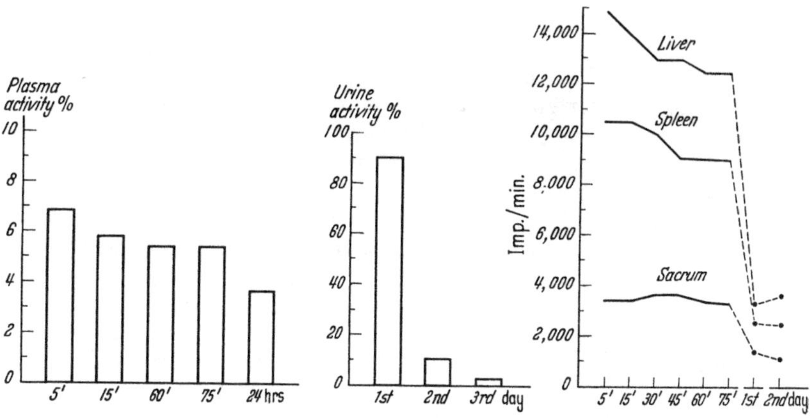

Fig. 1. Distribution of radioactive ferrioxamine B in the organism (intravenous injection of 30 μc. ferrioxamine labelled with Fe^{59})

Table 1. *Radioactive ferrioxamine in the organs of the rat in terms of the time elapsing after injection of 15 μc.* Fe^{59} (values expressed in % of the amount injected and calculated per gramme of tissue)

Organs	After 5 min.	After 20 min.	After 24 hrs
Liver	4.47	2.63	0.15
Spleen	2.82	1.56	1.30
Kidney	1.96	1.38	0.80
Heart	2.20	0.82	0.99
Lung	2.05	5.32	0.76
Bone marrow (thigh)	2.50	1.50	1.12
Thigh muscle	0.43	0.30	0.36
Thymus	2.49	2.10	2.00
Stomach	1.70	1.29	0.60
Duodenum	0.85	1.29	1.52
Small intestine	0.67	0.88	0.78
Large intestine	0.63	0.65	0.68
Abscess	1.50	1.40	1.88
Skin	0.22	0.30	0.15

(Mean values for groups of 5 animals each)

within 24 hours are probably to be ascribed to the ferrioxamine circulating in the blood. Of importance is the fact that the bone marrow does not show such a marked loss of activity as, for instance, the liver, although the spleen, too, a typical iron-depot organ, apparently retains ferrioxamine. Surprisingly enough, the same is also true of the thymus. As for the intestinal tract, it is interesting to compare the values after 24 hours with the initial levels. Whether the relatively high concentration of ferrioxamine in the intestinal mucosa can be interpreted as indicating a genuine excretion of the drug must remain a moot point since, for technical reasons, the activity in the faeces was not accurately determined. It may be pointed out, furthermore, that in accordance with our earlier findings, radioactive ferrioxamine was enriched in inflamed tissue (subcutaneous abscess).

On the whole, then, the ferrioxamine molecule was relatively quickly eliminated in these rat experiments, as also in the previously described injection test in human beings.

Since the Fe^{+++} complex could pass so easily through the kidney and since the parent substance was evidently a potent Fe^{+++} complex former, I was prompted to use the iron-free hydroxamic acid compound, desferrioxamine B hydrochloride, for the first time as a means of eliminating iron from the organism. Experiments were conducted initially on animals (rabbits). Following the intravenous injection of 20 mg. ferrum vitis (ferric saccharate complex), the organ iron concentration rose. Subsequent infusion of 1 g. desferrioxamine over a period of 4 hours led to an appreciable fall in the concentration of organ iron in the test animals as compared with the controls. The difference was least marked in the kidney, because renal excretion was still not completed 12 hours after the infusion, and a relatively large amount of iron was therefore still present in the kidney.

Simultaneous determination of the ferritin iron and of the haemosiderin iron in these rabbit experiments revealed that in the organs the ferritin iron, which is apparently more readily available, is surrendered almost completely to the desferrioxamine (Fig. 2). Following the administration of ferric saccharate complexes (ferrum vitis) or sorbitol iron, the concentration of ferritin and haemosiderin iron in the liver, spleen, and kidney invariably rose. Even though, as exact quantitative determinations showed, the mass of the mobilised iron came from the haemosiderin, the ferritin iron was none the less almost completely eliminated. It may thus be concluded that both fractions of depot iron surrender their iron to desferrioxamine in the cells. Since ferritin can release its entire content of iron, the actual turnover of depot iron between ferritin and haemosiderin is probably also increased, i.e. the apoferritin that is produced will endeavour to take up the haemosiderin iron present, thus intensifying the breakdown of the haemosiderin. Determination of serum iron in the rabbit before and after administration of desferrioxamine in these experiments clearly showed that the serum iron level rose during the mobilisation of

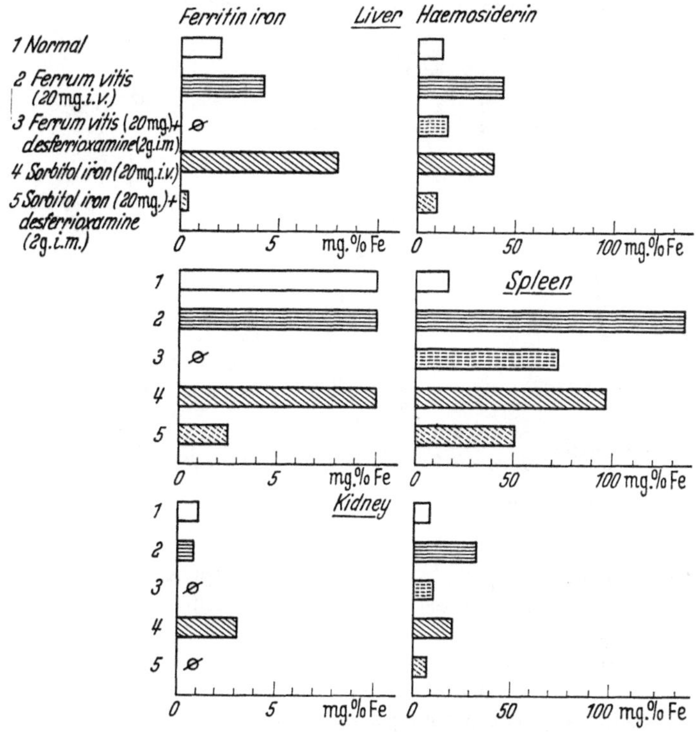

Fig. 2. Ferritin and haemosiderin iron in various organs of the rabbit following administration of ferrum vitis (20 mg. i.v.), sorbitol iron (20 mg. i.v.), and desferrioxamine (2 g. i.m.)

the depot iron. This finding was considerably more marked in human beings.

When the iron-free hydroxamic acid compound, desferrioxamine B, was administered to normal test subjects, the serum iron level regularly rose depending upon the amount injected, and more iron was subsequently excreted in the urine. If iron was given orally at the same time, iron excretion did not show any substantial increase, although the serum iron levels were somewhat higher (Fig. 3).

In response to desferrioxamine the urine turns salmon-pink in colour, the degree of the discoloration depending on the amount of iron that has been removed. This salmon-pink colouring is due to ferrioxamine.

Paper-chromatographic studies of urine and bile showed that the desferrioxamine-iron complex could be demonstrated only in the urine. Hence, none is excreted via the bile. The unidimensional

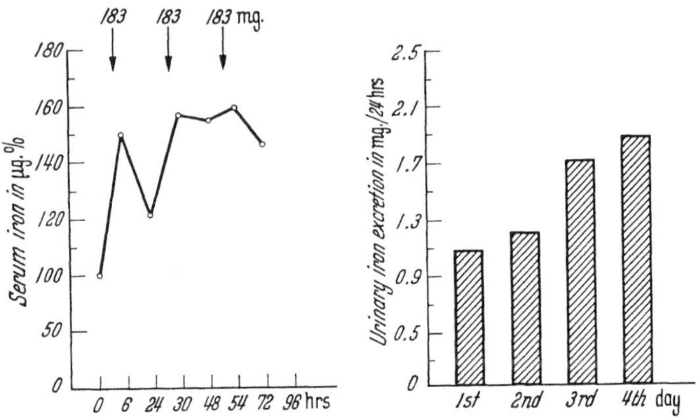

Fig. 3. Serum iron level and urinary iron excretion following administration of desferrioxamine in a normal subject (306 mg. Fe^{+++} daily by mouth)

chromatograms reveal that, as was to be expected, the desferrioxamine-iron complex possesses the same characteristic properties as ferrioxamine.

That desferrioxamine charged with iron and circulating in the blood is in fact responsible for the rise in serum iron usually observed following administration of the substance is evidenced by the ease with which the hydroxamic acid and iron complex can be removed from the serum by dialysis; the values for actual transferrin iron are then considerably lower.

It seems particularly interesting to note that, where the serum iron levels are very high, transferrin can take up iron ions from ferrioxamine until it (i.e. transferrin) is completely saturated – a finding which was confirmed by appropriate *in vitro* dialysis tests with pure ferrioxamine and iron-free transferrin. This result should not be considered surprising, because the stability constants for desferrioxamine and transferrin differ only slightly. However, it would appear that iron ions can only be transferred from ferrioxamine to transferrin if the desferrioxamine is saturated to the maximum of its binding capacity. On the other hand, this process easily explains why we have never observed any case of anaemia occurring in the course of desferrioxamine treatment. Apparently, therefore, despite the mobilisation of iron, there is still sufficient iron available for erythropoiesis. However, one must also bear in mind the possibility that the desferrioxamine-iron complex may donate its iron directly to the erythroblasts for haem synthesis.

From which iron-containing proteins does desferrioxamine take up iron? An exact answer to this question was obtained in dialysis tests. If pure, iron-free transferrin is introduced into a dialysis tube and ferrous sulphate into the external fluid, the ferrous sulphate will diffuse through the membrane and saturate the transferrin.

If desferrioxamine is now added and, after an incubation period of about 6 hours at room temperature, dialysis is performed against flowing distilled water, the quantity of iron removed practically attains the theoretical binding capacity of desferrioxamine. Similar results were obtained with human haemosiderin and ferritin (man and horse). This means that desferrioxamine is capable of separating and absorbing iron from all iron-bearing proteins in the organism (Table 2). Similarly, the ability of desferrioxamine to take up iron can also be demonstrated in normal organs and in organs rich in iron.

Table 2. *Dialysis tests with transferrin, ferritin, and haemosiderin following the addition of desferrioxamine*

Substance	Concentration inside *before* dialysis	Concentration inside *after* dialysis	Iron taken up by desferrioxamine
Transferrin (human) + 20 mg. desferrioxamine	225 mg. = 280.5 μg. Fe	34 μg. Fe (225 mg.)	246.5 μg. Fe
Ferritin (human) + 20 mg. desferrioxamine	20 mg. = 4.8 mg. Fe	3.63 mg. Fe	1.170 mg. Fe
Haemosiderin (human) + 20 mg. desferrioxamine	20 mg. = 7.1 mg. Fe	5.358 mg. Fe	1.742 mg. Fe
Ferritin (horse) + + 20 mg. desferrioxamine	20 mg. = 4.2 mg. Fe	2.77 mg. Fe	1.43 mg. Fe

About two years ago we began to introduce desferrioxamine into therapy. I should now like to give you a survey of 40 treated cases, including 13 of primary haemochromatosis, in 8 of which definite evidence of heredity was found. Our material also comprises 2 cases of thalassaemia, 2 of pulmonary haemosiderosis, 7 of cirrhosis, 1 of Blackfan-Diamond anaemia in a four-year-old boy, 2 of sideroachrestic anaemia with extremely severe siderosis, 7 of transfusion siderosis, and 2 of Marchiafava-Micheli anaemia.

The results of the treatment can be judged to some extent from the iron-excretion tables. In one case, iron excretion rose after a

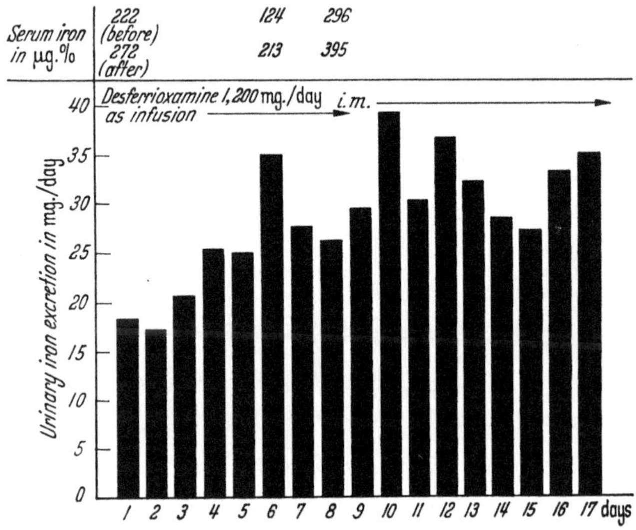

Fig. 4. Urinary iron excretion following administration of desferrioxamine in a patient with haemochromatosis

certain period to 80 mg. daily in the course of the first few months, but then diminished to levels of about 30 mg. daily (Fig. 4). In this patient, approximately 18 g. iron has so far been eliminated in the space of one year. The same level of iron excretion was attained in a second case of hereditary haemochromatosis over a period of 14 months. Liver-biopsy studies revealed an extremely severe degree of siderosis prior to treatment. After treatment, quite a considerable decrease in histochemically demonstrable liver iron had occurred[1]. The iron had largely disappeared from the cells of

[1] Grateful acknowledgement is made here to Dr. W. Creutzfeld, who performed the liver biopsies, and to Dr. E. Grundmann, who carried out the histochemical examinations at the Institute of Pathology, University of Freiburg.

both parenchymal and connective tissue. Similar startling improvements were achieved in other patients as well.

One impressive clinical feature of the treatment was that the dark coloration of the patient's skin often began to disappear after only 2–3 weeks. Examination of excised portions of skin in these cases tended to show a reduction in the melanin content of the basal layer rather than a definite decrease in iron; in this

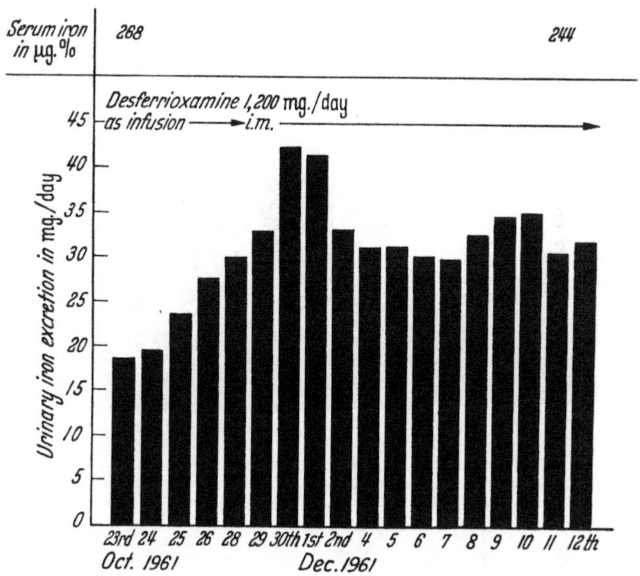

Fig. 5. Urinary iron excretion following administration of desferrioxamine in a case of thalassaemia

connection, it must be borne in mind that desferrioxamine may display a catalytic effect here, since adrenaline may fail to be oxidised via adrenochrome to melanin in the presence of Fe^{+++} ions. The rapid subjective improvement of the patients was also most striking, although in many cases the laboratory findings did not improve until some considerable time had elapsed.

Very good results were obtained in two cases of thalassaemia. The urinary iron-excretion figures in one of the cases are illustrated in Fig. 5; altogether, 14 g. iron has been removed from this female patient to date. Liver-biopsy studies showed that there has also been a marked reduction in haemosiderin iron in the liver of this patient. Similarly, we were also able to achieve a very good iron-excretion level of 30 mg. daily in two patients with Marchiafava-Micheli anaemia and severe transfusion haemosiderosis, who were given 500 mg. desferrioxamine twice daily by subcutaneous injection. The treatment had no effect on the basic illness – which, of course, was only to be expected. The improvement in the siderosis in these two cases was, however, most impressive.

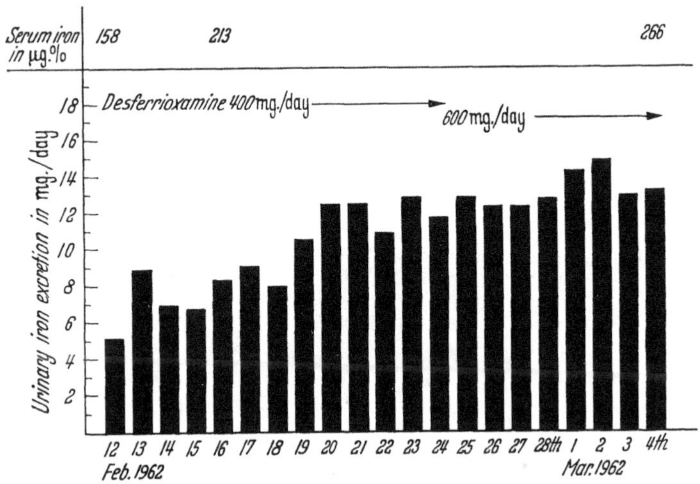

Fig. 6. Urinary iron excretion following administration of desferrioxamine in a 4-year-old boy with Blackfan-Diamond anaemia

We likewise administered desferrioxamine intramuscularly to a four-year-old boy with Blackfan-Diamond anaemia who had been receiving transfusions of between 200 and 300 ml. blood every 3 weeks since his third month of life. As can be seen, iron excretion was very satisfactory in this case as well. Even now, 7 months after the beginning of treatment, daily excretion levels of some 12–14 mg. are still being recorded (Fig. 6).

Understandably enough, patients who have already undergone successful venesection therapy display lower daily iron-excretion levels in response to desferrioxamine. In such cases smaller doses of desferrioxamine can be given. We have also observed lower iron-excretion levels in patients with hepatic cirrhosis and siderosis of the liver (Fig. 7). Here, it is impossible to determine the extent to which the low iron-excretion levels are due to the severe cirrhotic changes and the impaired blood flow, or to the type of haemosiderin deposited. It is very probable that the lower iron-excretion levels observed in such patients, as compared with cases of haemochromatosis, are primarily due to the fact that they store less iron; moreover, bearing in mind the distribution pattern of ferrioxamine in the body of the rat (5% for the liver), it may well be that this is perhaps a question of the balance between the iron content of the liver and the elimination time of desferrioxamine.

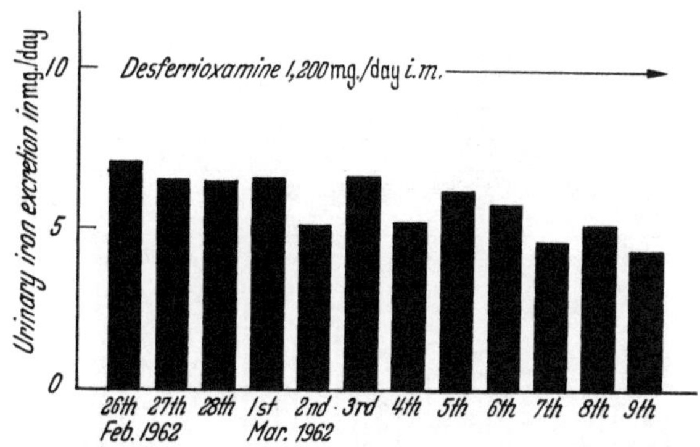

Fig. 7. Urinary iron excretion following administration of desferrioxamine in a case of liver cirrhosis

Finally, I should like to mention the iron-excretion levels obtained in a case of essential pulmonary haemosiderosis, in which up to 10 mg. iron was eliminated daily. Owing to pulmonary haemorrhages, however, the treatment had to be discontinued in order to prevent an additional drain on the body's iron depots with resultant iron deficiency (Fig. 8).

Desferrioxamine medication, like venesection, still possesses one unsatisfactory feature, namely that increased quantities of dietary iron are constantly being absorbed during the treatment. The increase in iron absorption from the gastro-intestinal tract observed during treatment with desferrioxamine is due to the fact that more iron is being eliminated from the organism. Even if this increased amount of absorbed iron were to be bound and excreted by the desferrioxamine circulating in the body, an attempt should obviously be made to block iron absorption from the gastro-intestinal tract.

We therefore carried out tests with desferrioxamine B with the aim of preventing the absorption of inorganic and dietary iron by binding the latter in the gastro-intestinal tract. A radioactive desferrioxamine and Fe^{+++} complex was fed to rabbits by stomach tube, and it was found that this complex was not absorbed. No specific activity could be demonstrated in the animals' serum after either 4 or 12 hours.

To find out whether the absorption of iron can be blocked in the gastro-intestinal tract in human beings, we administered reduced iron to normal test subjects. The serum iron level and urinary iron excretion were measured before and after administration of the

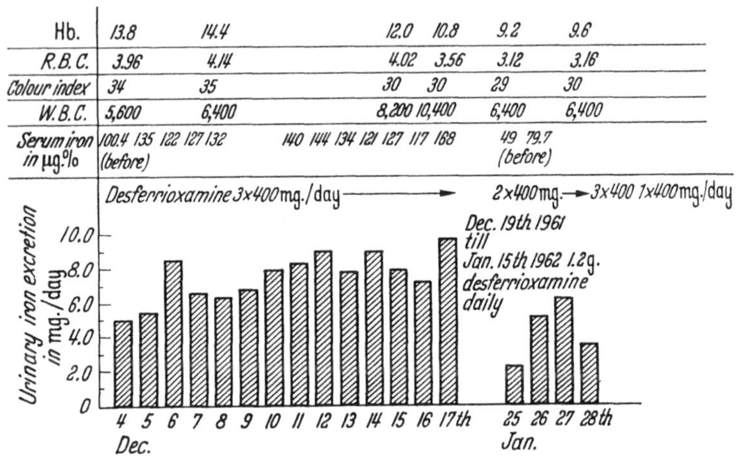

Fig. 8. Blood picture and urinary iron excretion during desferrioxamine treatment in a case of pulmonary haemosiderosis

reduced iron with and without desferrioxamine. Whenever reduced iron was given alone, the serum iron rose as expected, whereas when desferrioxamine was given simultaneously, this rise did not occur (Fig. 9).

As when desferrioxamine was administered alone, a slight excretion of iron in the urine was observed, but it did not exceed 1 mg. despite the massive doses of reduced iron. From these tests it may be concluded that the iron was bound in the gastro-intestinal tract and could no longer be absorbed. However, a small amount of the desferrioxamine – the exact quantity cannot be determined with certainty – was undoubtedly absorbed, leading to the increase in iron excretion as well as to the decrease in transferrin iron.

When ferrous sulphate was administered by mouth to healthy subjects it was also found that, whereas the serum iron level rose in response to ferrous sulphate alone, no such rise occurred when desferrioxamine was given at the same time. On the contrary, there was quite a marked decrease in the serum iron level in subjects receiving ferrous sulphate plus desferrioxamine (Fig. 10), a decrease

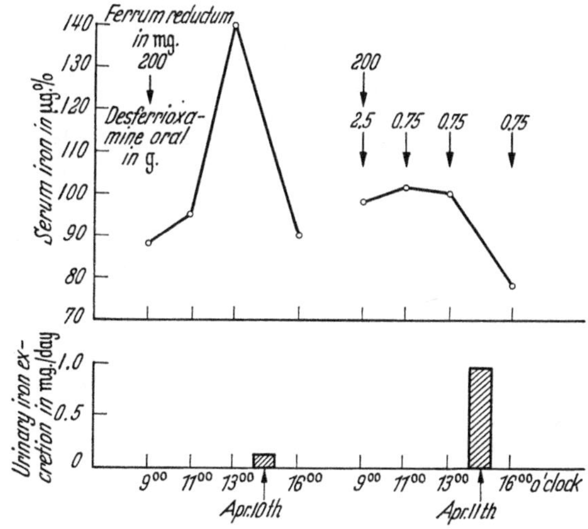

Fig. 9. Serum iron levels and urinary iron excretion in response to oral administration of reduced iron with and without desferrioxamine

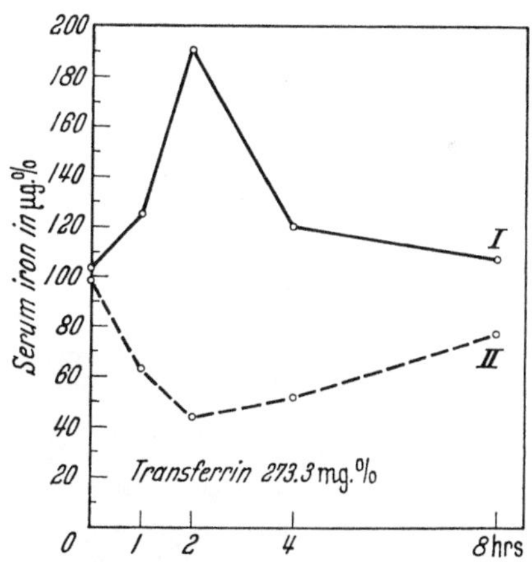

Fig. 10. Serum iron levels in healthy subjects after oral administration of 20 mg. ferrous sulphate = 7 mg. Fe^{++} ions (I) and 20 mg. ferrous sulphate + 1 g. desferrioxamine (II)

which we think may be due to the fact that part of the desferrioxamine administered is absorbed and reduces the amount of transferrin iron.

In order to determine whether desferrioxamine is also capable of blocking the absorption of inorganic iron contained in the food, test subjects were given biscuits to eat which contained ferrum reductum as well as ferrous sulphate. Here, once again, the serum iron level rose, whereas when desferrioxamine was given at the same time, it failed to rise or even showed a decrease. From these results it may be inferred that desferrioxamine is able to bind inorganic iron in the gastro-intestinal tract and that the ferrioxamine molecule cannot be absorbed. Both Keller (personal communication) and Moeschlin have obtained similar results.

The question as to the absorption of inorganic iron in patients with haemochromatosis seemed a difficult one to answer, because it is known that in most cases of this kind the iron-binding capacity is fully exploited, with the result that the serum iron levels show no further increase in response to oral absorption tests. For this reason, we employed both non-radioactive and radioactive iron

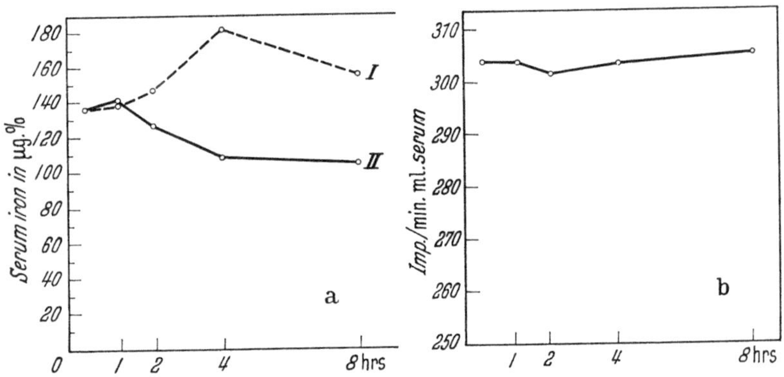

Fig. 11. a) Serum iron level in a case of haemochromatosis after oral administration of 20 mg. ferrous sulphate = 7 mg. F^{++} ions (I) and 20 mg. ferrous sulphate + 2 g. desferrioxamine (II). b) Serum iron level in the same patient after oral administration of 20 mg. ferrous sulphate (Fe^{59}) + 2 g. desferrioxamine

in our studies. The findings obtained showed that, depending on their initial serum iron levels, patients with haemochromatosis showed a more or less significant increase in serum iron following administration of ferrous sulphate, although the increase was less pronounced than in normal subjects (Figs 11 a, b and 12). When desferrioxamine was administered simultaneously, a slight fall in the serum iron level was noted, as in the case of healthy subjects. When the radioactivity in the serum following administration of radioactive ferrous sulphate (20 mg. ferrous sulphate = 20 $\mu c. Fe^{59}$)

plus desferrioxamine was investigated in 12 patients with haemochromatosis, the number of impulses/min. measured in the serum was practically identical with the initial value and no significant increase could be detected.

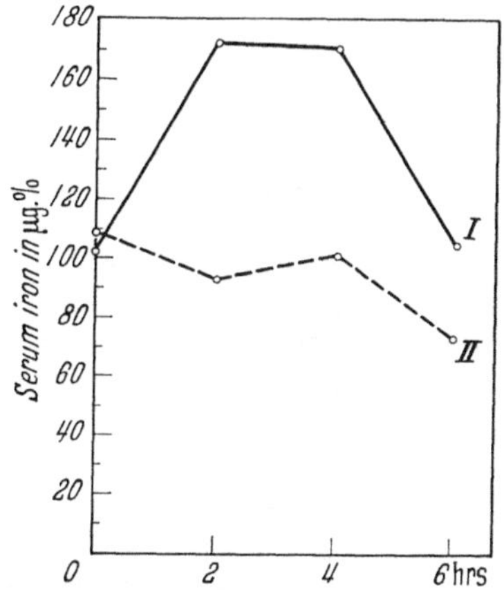

Fig. 12. Serum iron level in a healthy subject after ingestion of 100 g. of pig's liver (= 42 mg. iron) (I) and 100 g. of pig's liver + 1.5 g. desferrioxamine (II)

Having succeeded in demonstrating by means of these tests that desferrioxamine is definitely capable of preventing the absorption of inorganic iron, we then studied its effect on the absorption of genuine dietary iron (haemosiderin and ferritin iron, as well as haemoglobin iron, etc.). For this purpose, 10 healthy subjects were given either 100 g. of pig's liver (corresponding to 42 mg. iron) or 120 g. of pure black-pudding with the skin removed (iron content: 21 mg.) with and without desferrioxamine. As shown in Fig. 12, the administration of liver is followed by a corresponding rise in the serum iron level, but not when desferrioxamine is given at the same time. Similar results were obtained with black-pudding (Fig. 13). It would therefore appear that desferrioxamine is capable of blocking and preventing the absorption not only of inorganic iron but also of iron ions from haemosiderin, ferritin, haemoglobin, and other organic compounds.

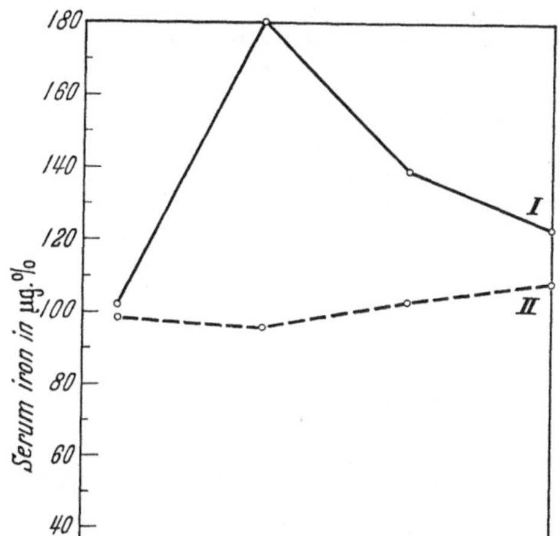

Fig. 13. Serum iron level in a healthy subject after ingestion of 120 g. of pure black-pudding (= 21 mg. iron) (I) and 120 g. of pure black-pudding + 1.5 g. desferrioxamine (II)

The possibility of blocking iron absorption with the aid of desferrioxamine may well have an extremely important bearing on the treatment of patients with haemochromatosis as well as of their children, in whom hypersideraemia is due to an hereditary factor. Desferrioxamine would, in fact, seem to provide an effective means by which to prevent the development of haemochromatosis.

To sum up, the combined parenteral and oral administration of desferrioxamine makes it possible both to remove iron from the human organism and to prevent iron from being absorbed. Such combined treatment appears to offer an ideal approach to the management of haemochromatosis in the future.

Summary

A new method of treating iron-storage diseases is reported. The method is based on the principle that iron ions in the organism can be specifically bound by desferrioxamine, a hydroxamic acid compound, and then, owing to the low molecular weight of the resultant complex, eliminated via the kidney. Other trace elements are not affected by desferrioxamine. Experimental data are given on iron excretion in animals, as well as on the extent to which desferrioxamine removes iron from transferrin, ferritin, and haemosiderin. In patients suffering from iron-storage diseases, iron-excretion levels of up to 80 mg. daily have been recorded, with an average of about 30 mg. daily. The patients treated comprised cases of primary and secondary haemochromatosis, sideroachrestic anaemia, Blackfan-Diamond anaemia, liver cirrhosis, and pulmonary haemosiderosis. Since desferrioxamine also inhibits enteral absorption of iron, the most effective treatment would seem to consist in administering the drug both intramuscularly or subcutaneously (500 mg. twice daily) and orally in the form of capsules to be taken with meals (250 mg. 3 times daily).

Zusammenfassung

Es wird über eine neue Möglichkeit der Behandlung von Eisenspeicherkrankheiten berichtet. Das Prinzip besteht darin, daß Eisenionen im Organismus spezifisch durch Desferrioxamin, eine Hydroxamsäureverbindung, gebunden werden. Der dabei entstehende niedermolekulare Komplex ist gut wasserlöslich und wird durch die Nieren ausgeschieden. Andere Spurenelemente werden durch Desferrioxamin nicht gebunden. Es werden experimentelle Befunde über die Eisenausscheidung nach Gabe von Desferrioxamin mitgeteilt sowie quantitative Angaben über das Ausmaß, in dem Desferrioxamin Eisen aus Transferrin, Ferritin und Haemosiderin löst. Beim Menschen mit pathologischer Eisenspeicherung kann die tägliche Eisenausscheidung Werte von 80 mg. erreichen, bei einem Durchschnittswert von etwa 30 mg. Es wurden Patienten mit primärer und sekundärer Haemochromatose, sideroachrestischer Anaemie, Blackfan-Diamond Anaemie, Leberzirrhose und pulmonaler Haemosiderose behandelt. Da Desferrioxamin auch in der Lage ist, die enterale Resorption von Eisen zu hemmen, dürfte die zweckmäßigste Art der Behandlung von Eisenspeicherkrankheiten in der gleichzeitigen intramuskulären oder subkutanen (500 mg. 1—2 mal täglich) und oralen Verabreichung (in Form von Kapseln à 250 mg. 3 mal täglich) von Desferrioxamin bestehen.

Résumé

L'auteur expose une nouvelle méthode de traitement des hypersidéroses, basée sur le principe de la fixation spécifique des ions fer de l'organisme par la desferrioxamine, un acide hydroxamique, suivie de l'élimination par le rein du complexe formé, grâce à son faible poids moléculaire. Les autres oligo-éléments ne sont pas touchés par la desferrioxamine. Des données expérimentales sont rapportées sur l'excrétion du fer chez l'animal, ainsi que sur la question de savoir dans quelle mesure la desferrioxamine est capable de capter le fer de la transferrine, de la ferritine et de l'hémosidérine. Chez l'homme présentant une hypersidérose pathologique, des taux d'excrétion allant jusqu'à 80 mg. par jour ont été enregistrés, avec une moyenne d'environ 30 mg. par jour. Les cas traités comprenaient des cas d'hémochromatose primaire et secondaire, d'anémie sidéro-achrestique, d'anémie de Blackfan-Diamond, de cirrhose hépatique et de cirrhose pulmonaire. Puisque la desferrioxamine inhibe également l'absorption intestinale du fer, il semble que le traitement le plus utile serait d'administrer le produit à la fois par voie intramusculaire ou sous-cutanée (500 mg. deux fois par jour) et par voie orale sous forme de capsules à prendre au cours des repas (250 mg. trois fois par jour).

References

Bickel, H., E. Gäumann, W. Keller-Schierlein, V. Prelog, E. Vischer, A. Wettstein, and H. Zähner: Experientia (Switz.) **16**, 129 (1960). — Bickel, H., G. E. Hall, W. Keller-Schierlein, V. Prelog, E. Vischer, and A. Wettstein: Helvet. chim. acta **18**, 261 (1960). — Cleton, F. J., W. D. Noyes, A. Turnbull, and C. A. Finch: Clin. Res. (U.S.A.) **9**, 91 (1961). — Fahey, J., J. Princiotto, C. Rath, and M. Rubin: Clin. Res. (U.S.A.) **8**, 52 (1960). — Figueroa, W. G., and S. G. Tuttle: Clin. Res. (U.S.A.) **9**, 92 (1961). — Foreman, H.: In: Seven's and Johnson's Metal-Binding in Medicine. Lippincott, Philadelphia, 1960, p. 82. — Gisninger, E., and H. Puxkandl: Wien. Zschr. inn. Med. **36**, 491 (1955). — Moeschlin, S., et al.: Schweiz. med. Wschr. **92**, 1295 (1962). — Palmieri, A., and S. Giacca: Arch. Maragliano pat. (It.) **11**, 993 (1955). — Rubin, M., and J. V. Princiotto: Ann. N. Y. Acad. Sc. **88**, 450 (1960). — Vischer, E.: Chemie des Desferrioxamin B. Meeting of clinical investigators held at CIBA Limited, Basle, 1961. — Wöhler, F.: Klinisch-experimentelle Ergebnisse mit Desferrioxamin. Meeting of clinical investigators held at CIBA Limited, Basle, 1961. — Wöhler, F.: Proceedings of the 8th Congress of the European Society of Haematology. Karger, Basle/New York, 1961, p. 244. — Wöhler, F.: Therapie der Haemochromatose. 8. Deutsche Haematologen-Tagung, Wiesbaden, 1962. — Wöhler, F.: Med. Klinik (G.) **57**, 1370 (1962). — Wöhler, F.: Acta haemat. (Switz.) **30**, 65 (1963).

Evaluation of trisodium calcium diethylene-triamine penta-acetate in hemochromatosis and transfusion hemosiderosis

By

I. B. Brick and C. E. Rath

Iron excess in the body with iron deposition in the parenchyma of many organ systems, as in idiopathic hemochromatosis and transfusion hemosiderosis, may lead to eventual tissue damage, manifested by altered organ function and fibrosis. This tends to increase with the passage of time. Appreciation of this problem has led to therapeutic efforts to remove iron from the body in an attempt to arrest or reverse the course of these iron-storage diseases. Repeated phlebotomy has been demonstrated to be the most effective method of iron removal and is now accepted as the treatment of choice in most cases of hemochromatosis. However, in some patients, repeated phlebotomies may be impractical. Advanced liver disease with anemia or concurrent coronary insufficiency, for example, may make repeated phlebotomies inadvisable in hemochromatosis. Transfusion hemosiderosis, usually associated with severe anemia, presents the same problem. As an alternative means of removing iron from the organs, chelation has been used, particularly since this method would appear to be especially suited to the complications mentioned.

By this approach a chelating compound is introduced into the body, where it forms an iron-chelate complex. This complex is then excreted in the urine. Foreman and co-workers (*1*) reported that the urinary excretion of iron in rats can be increased by the intraperitoneal administration of such a chelate (Fe^3-specific). However, clinical experiences with chelates have not been too rewarding to date. Ohlsson and collaborators (*2*) obtained less than 3 mg. iron per 24 hours in the urine after British anti-lewisite therapy. Others (*1–6*), using disodium calcium ethylene-diamine tetra-acetate (E.D.T.A.) and related compounds, have recovered up to 10.5 mg. iron per 24 hours when the agent was administered intravenously. In contrast, about 250 mg. iron can be removed in a single phlebotomy.

The search for more effective iron chelates has been guided by several biochemical and physiologic considerations: (1) no known chelate will remove iron from the plasma iron-binding protein (I.B.P.) at pH 7.4 (*7*); (2) the iron-chelate bond must be strong enough to be maintained in the presence of the competing plasma iron-binding protein; (3) the iron-chelate complex should be completely excreted; (4) the chelate should be non-toxic.

An agent structurally similar to E.D.T.A., i.e. trisodium calcium diethylene-triamine penta-acetate (D.T.P.A.) is shown in Fig. 1. It does not yield iron to the plasma iron-binding protein *in vitro* at

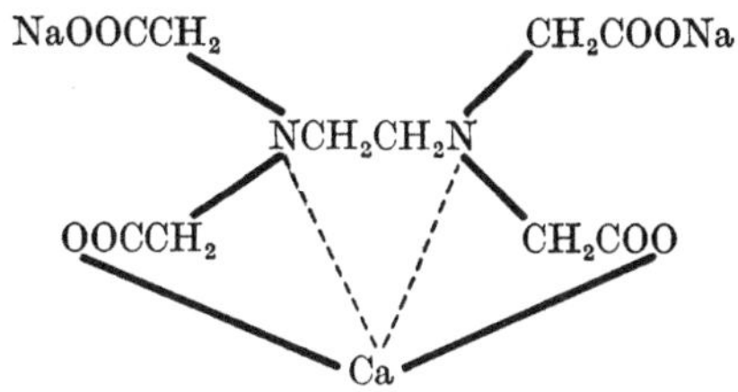

Disodium calcium ethylene-diamine tetra-acetate

(E.D.T.A.)

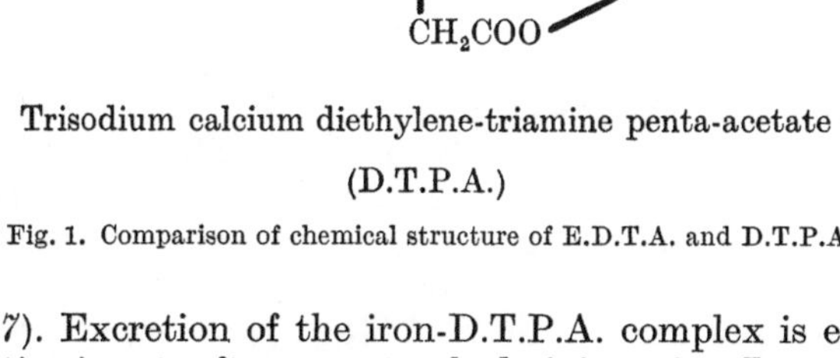

Trisodium calcium diethylene-triamine penta-acetate

(D.T.P.A.)

Fig. 1. Comparison of chemical structure of E.D.T.A. and D.T.P.A.

pH 7.4 (*7*). Excretion of the iron-D.T.P.A. complex is essentially quantitative in rats after parenteral administration. In comparison, the excretion of iron-E.D.T.A. is approximately 70% under the same circumstances (*8*). Finally, animal studies with D.T.P.A. have revealed no gross or histological signs of toxicity (*8*). This evidence suggested that D.T.P.A. might be effective in mobilizing iron in humans. Clinical trials were then undertaken and the experience obtained has been sufficiently encouraging (*9*) to justify continuing studies with this substance in iron-storage diseases.

Methods and materials

All of the laboratory procedures in this study were performed in the laboratories of the Hematology Division, Georgetown University, Washington, D.C., under the direction of one of the authors (C. E. RATH).

Serum and urine iron levels were determined by the method of RAMSAY (*10*), slightly modified as follows: the reagent used consisted of 500 mg. 222 tripyridine, 500 mg. hydroxylamine HCl, 23.52 ml. 36% acetic acid, and 34.12 g. sodium acetate hydrate (National Formulary granular). The mixture is brought to 500 ml. with iron-free water, mixed well, and heated at 50 to 70° C. until a drop of oily reagent is formed at the bottom of the flask. The supernatant is then decanted into an iron-free flask and stored in the dark at room temperature. It is stable for at least three to four weeks. RAMSAY's improved technique is then followed (*10a*). Protein precipitated by heating the serum samples is removed by centrifugation at 3,500 r.p.m. for 15 minutes. The same procedure is followed for the urine iron determinations with two further modifications: (a) tubes containing the urine samples and reagent mixture are heated in a boiling water bath for 15 minutes instead of 5 to 10 minutes; (b) urine turbidity varies and is difficult to eliminate without removing the iron and the sample at the same time; therefore the unknown sample is read against a water blank in the Coleman Junior spectrophotometer at 520 mμ, and from this reading both a reagent blank and a "urine blank" (urine sample plus reagent mixture less tripyridine) are subtracted.

In the studies of the patients, the unsaturated iron-binding capacity (U.I.B.C.) of the serum was determined by the method of RATH and FINCH (*11*). Body iron stores were estimated by bone-marrow aspiration (*12*) in all cases and by liver biopsy. D.T.P.A. was administered intravenously over a three-hour period as a 25% solution of the trisodium monocalcium salt diluted in 500 ml. 5% dextrose in water. The chelate was given intramuscularly as a 25% solution without further dilution. Twenty-four hour urine collections were made in iron-free equipment.

Results

For the purposes of this discussion, hemochromatosis is defined as extensive intracellular iron deposition with fibrosis in the liver.

The term hemosiderosis refers to iron deposition, intracellular or otherwise, without fibrosis or other evidence of structural damage to the liver.

In 15 cases with hemochromatosis, all proven by liver biopsy, chelate studies with D.T.P.A. have been done. The results in several of these patients are shown in Tables 1–5.

Table 1 demonstrates, in a patient with fully developed hemochromatosis, a repeatedly increased excretion of urinary iron on consecutive days when the chelate was given either intramuscularly or intravenously. Also to be noted is the fact that, despite the reduction of iron stores by concurrent phlebotomies, 10 months after the first series of chelate administration, increased iron excretion continued.

Table 1. *Hemochromatosis*

Name	Date	Phlebotomy data	Chelate administered	Iron excretion (mg.)	Serum iron (μg./100 ml.)	U.I.B.C.
J. D.	18/4/60	16/10/59 to 18/1/63 cumulative: 164		0.03	a.m. 207	0
	19/4/60			1.00	p.m. 192	0
	20/4/60		1.5g. D.T.P.A. i.v.	3.30		
	21/4/60		1.0g. D.T.P.A. i.m.	5.20		
	22/4/60		1.0g. D.T.P.A. i.m.	3.50		
	23/4/60		2.5g. D.T.P.A. i.v.	7.70		
	24/4/60		1.0g. D.T.P.A. i.m.	3.60		
	25/4/60		1.0g. D.T.P.A. i.m.	3.20		
	26/4/60		1.0g. D.T.P.A. i.m.	2.90		
	27/4/60		1.0g. D.T.P.A. i.m.	3.70		
	13/2/61				215	0
	14/2/61		2.5g. D.T.P.A. i.v.	3.70	103	100
	15/2/61		1.0g. D.T.P.A. i.m.	2.40	68	150
	16/2/61			0.20	71	100
	17/2/61				149	50

The patient reported in Table 2 had hemochromatosis with portal hypertension and was studied after an episode of gastrointestinal hemorrhage. While initially the iron excretion was quite marked (6.3 mg. Fe in the 24-hour period after 2.5 g. D.T.P.A. intravenously), the excretion of iron lessened as the iron stores became diminished by phlebotomies. Thus, 21 months later, when the serum iron was normal, the same dose of chelate resulted in only a small increase in iron excretion.

The patient reported in Table 3 is a sibling of the patient shown in Table 2. At the time the chelate was used, the iron stores were

Table 2. *Hemochromatosis*

Name	Date	Phlebotomy data	Chelate administered	Iron excretion (mg.)	Serum iron (μg./100 ml.)	U.I.B.C.
P. H.	18/10/60				265	0
	19/10/60	30/6/59 to	2.5g. D.T.P.A. i.v.	0.20	265	0
	20/10/60	2/11/62		6.30	268	0
	21/10/60	total: 72	1.0g. D.T.P.A. i.m.	0.10		
	22/10/60			1.90		
	13/2/61			0.80	153	150
	14/2/61		2.5g. D.T.P.A. i.v.	1.10	177	150
	15/2/61		1.0g. D.T.P.A. i.m.	0.90	225	50
	16/2/61			0.60	306	0
	17/2/61				319	0
	9/7/62			0.10		
	10/7/62			0.04	88	200
	11/7/62		2.5g. D.T.P.A. i.v.	0.30		
	12/7/62			0.30		

judged to be relatively normal, as shown by a marked diminution of iron in marrow and liver biopsies in comparison with the initial findings approximately 5 years before the chelate was administered. Thus, the increases in iron excretion after the chelate was given were quite modest, albeit three to seven times greater than during control periods.

Table 3. *Hemochromatosis*

Name	Date	Phlebotomy data	Chelate administered	Iron excretion (mg.)	Serum iron (μg./100 ml.)	U.I.B.C.
J. H.	18/2/61	8/8/55 to		0.70	87	0
	19/2/61	30/9/58	2.5g. D.T.P.A. i.v.	1.00	89	50
	5/3/62	total: 64		0.30		
	6/3/62			0.40		
	7/3/62			0.20		
	8/3/62		2.5g. D.T.P.A. i.v.	1.90	81	0
	9/3/62			0.10		
	10/3/62			0.10		
	11/3/62			0.10		
	12/3/62				130	0
	13/3/62				159	0
	18/4/63				210	0
	22/4/63			0.30		
	23/4/63			0.20		
	24/4/63		1.0g. D.T.P.A. i.m.	1.50	157	0
	26/4/63			0.20	151	0

Table 4 demonstrates a case of hemochromatosis in which the chelate was given before phlebotomy. An increased dose (2.5 g.) given the day after a 1.0 g. dose of D.T.P.A., both intravenously, resulted in an almost threefold increase in the excretion of iron.

Table 4. *Hemochromatosis*

Name	Date	Phlebotomy data	Chelate administered	Iron excretion (mg.)	Serum iron (μg./100 ml.)	U.I.B.C.
J. T.	28/9/60			0.40		
	29/9/60	23/9/60 to	1.0g. D.T.P.A. i.v.	15.40	157	0
	30/9/60	19/3/63	2.5g. D.T.P.A. i.v.	44.60	152	0
	1/10/60	total: 76		0.10		
	2/10/60			0.10		
	3/10/60		2.5g. D.T.P.A. i.v.	41.50	120	0

This was not uniformly the case, however, as Table 5 demonstrates. This patient was suffering from hemochromatosis and had increased iron stores after 81 phlebotomies. However, the increased dose did not result in an excretion of iron greater than that produced by the lesser dose.

Table 5. *Hemochromatosis*

Name	Date	Phlebotomy data	Chelate administered	Iron excretion (mg.)	Serum iron (μg./100 ml.)	U.I.B.C.
M. W.	16/5/60	From 1956 to 1960		0.06		
	1st 12hrs 17/5/60	cumulative: 81	1.0g. D.T.P.A. i.v.	4.00		
	2nd 12hrs 17/5/60			1.20		
	18/5/60			0.20		
	19/5/60		1.0g. D.T.P.A. i.v.	3.20	176	0
	20/5/60		2.5g. D.T.P.A. i.v.	1.30	154	0

In Table 6 are listed the data of a patient with transfusion hemosiderosis secondary to thalassemia major. Marked increases in iron excretion were noted after administration of the chelate similar to those obtained in patients with hemochromatosis.

Some tentative conclusions can be drawn from the data presented. Iron excretion tended to increase as the dose of chelate was raised from 0.5 to 1.0 g. However, there was considerable variation in the amount of iron obtained with both the 1.0 and 2.5 g. infusions. Higher doses of D.T.P.A. (2.5 and 3.0 g.) did not result in uniformly increased amounts of urinary iron.

Table 6. *Transfusion hemosiderosis*

Name	Date	Phlebotomy data	Chelate administered	Iron excretion (mg.)	Serum iron (μg./100 ml.)	U.I.B.C.
A. G.	26/12/61	0			195	0
	27/12/61			0.04		
	28/12/61			0.03		
	29/12/61			0.04		
	30/12/61			0.02	211	0
	31/12/61		1.0g. D.T.P.A. i.v.	9.90		
	1/1/62			0.07		
	2/1/62			0.03		
	3/1/62			0.06		
	4/1/62			0.04		
	5/1/62		1.0g. D.T.P.A. i.v.	15.00	203	0
	6/1/62			0.03	171	0
	7/1/62			0.08		
	8/1/62		1.0g. D.T.P.A. i. m.	3.40		
	9/1/62		1.0g. D.T.P.A. i. m.	13.10		
	10/1/62			0.40		
	11/1/62			0.40		
	12/1/62			0.10		
	13/1/62			0.07		
	14/1/62			0.07		
	15/1/62			0.06		
	16/1/62		0.5g. D.T.P.A. i.m.	10.00		
	17/1/62			0.10		
	18/1/62		1.0g. D.T.P.A. i.v.	4.00		
	19/1/62			0.02		
	20/1/62			0.20		
	21/1/62			0.20		
	22/1/62			0.20		

In several patients the major portion of the iron was removed in the first 12 hours. In one such patient, 42.0 mg. was removed in 24 hours, 36.6 mg. being removed in the first 12 hours. Equivalent amounts of urinary iron were found after both intramuscular and intravenous administration, and there was no indication of a decrease in iron excretion after repeated doses of the chelate.

Toxic reactions to the drug were mild. Nausea, vomiting, and mild diarrhea were encountered intermittently in a few patients, but these symptoms could not always be definitely related to the D.T.P.A. There was no persistent local reaction to the intramuscular injections. The pain with the injections was considered by the patient to be the equivalent to that experienced with intramuscular procaine penicillin. In a few patients soft stools were noted on the day of administration of the drug, but no frank diarrhea occurred in any of these patients.

Blood counts, urinalyses, and blood urea nitrogen levels were unaffected by administration of the drug. The changes in the prothrombin time (Quick) and serum calcium before and after intravenous chelate are shown in Fig. 2. Although the D.T.P.A. was given in the form of the monocalcium salt, there was no consistent effect on serum calcium. The greatest change (a rise from 10.4 to 13.2 mg. per 100 ml.) occurred after a 4 g. infusion of D.T.P.A. This was the largest amount of chelate given in a 24-hour period. Prothrombin times were in general increased after D.T.P.A., but the increase never exceeded 2 seconds, even when the initial value was abnormal.

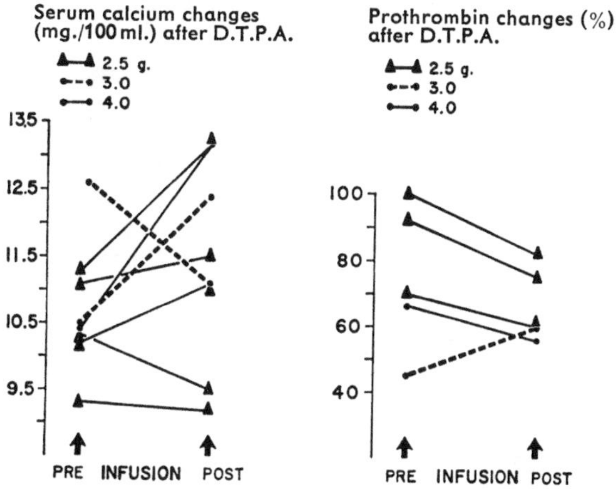

Fig. 2. Pre- and post-infusion levels of calcium and prothrombin after varying intravenous doses of D.T.P.A.

Discussion

The data presented indicate that significant amounts of iron can be removed from the body by the use of D.T.P.A. In one patient, 225 mg. iron was removed with four separate doses of D.T.P.A., totalling 14.5 g. Over a longer period, 17 doses, totalling 22.5 g., resulted in the removal of 660.7 mg. iron. These figures compare well with the 250 mg. iron removed with one pint of blood and are much greater than results reported with other chelating agents. Although it is noted that there is a decreased level of urinary iron excreted after repeated daily infusions, the iron excretion seems to depend upon the amount of the available iron stores, and when there are such stores available, excretion of iron appears satisfactory. In addition, neither local nor systemic toxicity were observed after repeated parenteral injections of D.T.P.A.

It is interesting that in our patients there was no correlation between iron excretion after D.T.P.A. administration and the serum iron level. Furthermore, D.T.P.A. will not remove iron from the iron-binding protein *in vitro* at pH 7.4, and it seems unlikely that it would do so *in vivo*. Although the exact mechanism of iron removal by chelation is unknown, it seemed most likely that storage iron is the source of the iron excreted, since it was in this area that the patients differed most.

Table 7. *Correlation of iron stores with iron excretion*

Patient	Estimated body iron stores	Iron excretion after initial 2.5 g. D.T.P.A. (mg.)
W. D.*	4+	42.0
P. M.	4+	30.4
P. H.	3+	22.4
R. D.*	2+	7.0
H. D.*	2+	2.4
W. W.	1+	0.3
L. D.	0	0.8

* Siblings

The induced iron excretion varied directly in proportion to the estimated iron stores. Comparing the effects of the initial 2.5 g. dose of D.T.P.A., the normal subject and the non-anemic iron-deficient subject show no increase in iron excretion. Patients with moderate increases in their iron stores had modest increases in iron excretion (2.4 and 7.0 mg.), and the patients with the most marked increases in their iron stores excreted as much as 42.0 mg. iron. Table 7 illustrates this point.

On the basis of these clinical observations, the following hypothesis is suggested. Parenterally administered chelate is carried in the circulation to iron-storage sites. Here, the calcium in the chelate is replaced by iron. This newly formed iron-chelate complex continues in the circulation until it reaches the kidneys and is then excreted in the urine. Free filtration at the glomerulus, because of the small molecular size of D.T.P.A. (molecular weight 497), is assumed.

In this study, D.T.P.A. administration resulted in a far greater excretion of iron than that obtained with comparable doses of E.D.T.A. The explanation for this may lie in two important biochemical differences between these compounds First, their relative affinity for iron differs. The absolute value for the iron-binding strength of D.T.P.A. has been listed at $10^{28.6}$ in comparison with $10^{25.1}$ for E.D.T.A. (*13*). It has also previously been noted (*7*) that when Fe^{59}, combined with chelate, was administered parenterally to animals, urine iron recovery was only about 70% of the injected dose with E.D.T.A., in contrast to the 90–100% recovery with D.T.P.A. Thus, Fe^{59}-E.D.T.A. may lose some of its attached iron as it passes through the animal, resulting in less efficient iron excretion. It is also possible that a given amount of D.T.P.A. would actually chelate more iron from body stores than would the same amount of E.D.T.A., because of this difference in binding strength.

The clinical application of D.T.P.A. in hemochromatosis is, of course, not yet defined, and further studies must be done. Although intravenous administration is cumbersome, the intramuscular route offers obvious advantages. Our data indicate that absorption from the intramuscular site is complete in that iron excretion was equivalent when the same dose of D.T.P.A. was given intramuscularly and intravenously. The drug may offer some real promise in those cases of iron-storage disease where phlebotomy is contraindicated and may also be used to supplement phlebotomy and thus reduce the treatment period necessary. In the average case of hemochromatosis, 2 to 3 years of weekly phlebotomy may be required to eliminate the excess iron.

Summary

Results of parenteral administration of the chelate trisodium calcium diethylene-triamine penta-acetate (D.T.P.A.) in patients with iron-storage disease are reported. D.T.P.A., given intravenously in doses of 2.5 to 4.0 g., resulted in iron-excretion levels of up to 109 mg. for 24 hours in patients with clinical hemochromatosis. Control subjects showed no increase in urinary iron after the chelate was given.

There was little, if any, clinical toxicity and no significant effects on hemogram, urinalyses, blood urea nitrogen, or serum calcium. Prothrombin times were only slightly prolonged. Comparable iron excretion occurred after intravenous and intramuscular administration of D.T.P.A.

The amount of iron excreted in various subjects correlated best with the estimated iron stores. The hypothesis is advanced that parenterally administered D.T.P.A. is carried in the circulation to iron storage sites, where the calcium in the chelate is exchanged for iron; the resultant iron complex continues in the circulation and is excreted in the urine.

The increased efficiency of D.T.P.A. over E.D.T.A. is discussed. Clinical application of D.T.P.A. is not yet established, but the results reported here suggest a possible role as a supplement to phlebotomy in the treatment of hemochromatosis and as an alternative therapy for individuals with iron-storage disease who could not undergo phlebotomy.

Zusammenfassung

Es wird über Ergebnisse nach parenteraler Anwendung des Trinatrium-Calcium Komplexes von Diäthylen-triamin-penta-azetat (D.T.P.A.) bei

Patienten mit Eisenspeicherkrankheiten berichtet. Bei Patienten mit Haemochromatose führt D.T.P.A. in Dosen von 2,5—4,0 g. intravenös zu einer Eisenausscheidung bis zu 109 mg. innerhalb von 24 Stunden. Bei Kontrollpersonen fand sich nach Gabe des Komplexbildners keine Zunahme von Eisen im Urin.

Toxische Symptome waren entweder gering oder überhaupt nicht nachweisbar, ebenso fand sich kein Einfluß auf Haemogramm, Harnzusammensetzung, Blutharnstoff oder Serumcalcium. Die Prothrombinzeit war nur unbedeutend verlängert. Die Eisenausscheidung nach intravenöser und intramuskulärer Gabe von D.T.P.A. war ähnlich.

Die ausgeschiedene Eisenmenge zeigte bei den verschiedenen Patienten eine gute Korrelation mit den geschätzten Eisenspeichern. Es ist zu vermuten, daß parenteral gegebenes D.T.P.A. mit dem Blut in die Eisenspeicher gelangt, wo dann Calcium gegen Eisen ausgetauscht wird; der so gebildete Eisenkomplex bleibt zunächst im Blut und wird dann durch die Niere eliminiert.

Die gegenüber E.D.T.A. gesteigerte Wirksamkeit von D.T.P.A. wird besprochen. Die klinischen Anwendungsmöglichkeiten von D.T.P.A. sind zwar noch nicht zu beurteilen, jedoch sprechen die mitgeteilten Befunde dafür, daß das Präparat entweder zusätzlich zur Aderlaßtherapie der Haemochromatose eine Rolle spielen könnte oder daß es sie bei Patienten mit anderen Eisenspeicherkrankheiten, bei denen ein Aderlaß nicht in Betracht kommt, ersetzen kann.

Résumé

Les résultats de l'administration parentérale de calcium trisodium diéthylène-triamine penta-acétate (D.T.P.A.) chez des malades en hypersidérose sont rapportés. Le D.T.P.A. administré par voie intra-veineuse à des doses de 2,5 à 4,0 g. provoque une excrétion du fer atteignant 109 mg. par 24 heures chez des malades présentant des signes cliniques d'hémochromatose. Les sujets témoins n'ont montré aucun accroissement du fer urinaire après l'administration du chélateur.

Il n'a été noté que peu ou pas de toxicité clinique et aucune modification notable de la formule sanguine, des urines, de l'urée et du calcium sérique. Seul le temps de prothrombine s'est montré légèrement allongé. Les éliminations du fer sont comparables après administration intra-veineuse ou administration intramusculaire du D.T.P.A.

Les quantités de fer excrétées chez les différents sujets ont été plutôt en rapport avec l'importance supposée des dépôts de fer. On avance l'hypothèse que le D.T.P.A. administré par voie parentérale est véhiculé par la circulation jusqu'au lieu de dépôt du fer, que le calcium du chélateur s'échange avec le fer et que le complexe formé reste dans le torrent circulatoire d'où il est excrété par les urines.

La supériorité d'efficacité du D.T.P.A. sur l'E.D.T.A. est discutée. Les applications cliniques du D.T.P.A. ne sont pas encore bien établies, mais les résultats rapportés ici laissent supposer un intérêt possible en tant que thérapeutique adjuvante des saignées dans le traitement des hémochromatoses, ou comme traitement de remplacement chez les sujets en hypersidérose chez lesquels les saignées sont contre-indiquées.

References

1. Foreman, H., R. Huff, J. Oda, and J. Garcia: Proc. Soc. Exper. Biol. Med. (U.S.A.) **79**, 520 (1952). — 2. Ohlsson, W. T., G. T. Kullendorff, and K. L. Wungberg: Acta med. Scand. **145**, 410 (1953). — 3. Finch,

S. C., and C. A. FINCH: Medicine (U.S.A.) **34**, 381 (1955). — 4. WISHINSKY, H., T. WEINBERG, E. M. PREVOST, B. BURGIN, and M. J. MILLER: J. Laborat. Clin. Med. (U.S.A.) **42**, 550 (1953). — 5. SEVEN, M. J., H. GOTTLIEB, H. L. ISRAEL, J. G. REINHOLD, and M. RUBIN: Amer. J. Med. Sc. **228**, 646 (1954). — 6. GREENWALT, T., and V. E. AYERS: Amer. J. Clin. Path. **25**, 266 (1955). — 7. RUBIN, M., J. HOULIHAN, and J. V. PRINCIOTTO: Proc. Soc. Exper. Biol. Med. (U.S.A.) **103**, 663 (1960). — 8. RUBIN, M., and J. V. PRINCIOTTO: Ann. N. Y. Acad. Sc. (in press). — 9. FAHEY, J. L., C. E. RATH, J. V. PRINCIOTTO, I. B. BRICK, and M. RUBIN: J. Laborat. Clin. Med. (U.S.A.) **57**, 436 (1961). — 10. RAMSAY, W. N. M.: Biochem. J. (G.B.) **53**, 227 (1953). — 10a. RAMSAY, W. N. M.: Biochem. J. (G.B.) **57**, 17 (1954). — 11. RATH, C. E., and C. A. FINCH: J. Clin. Invest. (U.S.A.) **28**, 79 (1949). — 12. RATH, C. E., and C. A. FINCH: J. Laborat. Clin. Med. (U.S.A.) **33**, 81 (1948). — 13. CHABEREK, S., and A. E. MARTELL: Organic Sequestering Agents. John Wiley & Sons, New York, 1959, pp. 572, 580.

Introduction to the General Discussion

By

C. Albahary

Now that we have reached the general discussion on the treatment of siderosis, I should like briefly to show you some results which my colleagues and I obtained when we experimented with various forms of treatment at the St. Denis Hospital.*

The drugs we employed comprised D.T.P.A. (given by direct intravenous administration), occasionally oral penicillamine, and more often desferrioxamine. The latter was almost always given

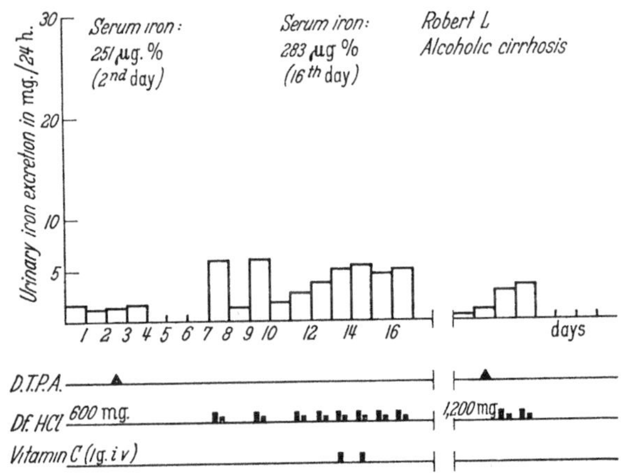

Fig. 1. Siderosis in a male patient suffering from alcoholic cirrhosis. Note that doses of 1,200 mg. desferrioxamine hydrochloride (Df. HCl) did not prove more effective than doses of 600 mg.

by the intramuscular route, not only because this is easier, but also because it is our impression that desferrioxamine is more active when injected i.m. than when infused i.v.

The following figures illustrate the results obtained in some of the 24 patients whom we have so far treated. As will be seen from these figures, D.T.P.A. was employed only for the purpose of a

* The chemical determinations were kindly performed by N. Phu-Lic [Laboratory of Toxicology, Faculté de Pharmacie (Prof. Truhaut)].

one-day test; it was given in a dose of 1 to 2 g. in one or two intravenous injections, and was never administered by slow intravenous infusion. With regard to the use of desferrioxamine, I should perhaps point out that, unfortunately, we were not able to treat patients with this drug for as long as we should have preferred, because from time to time we ran out of supplies. In the present series, the longest period of treatment with desferrioxamine is, in fact, only 26 days.

In Fig. 1 we have a case of alcoholic cirrhosis associated with siderosis. Here, it can be seen that, in a dose of 1,200 mg., desferrioxamine hydrochloride was not more effective than when given in a dose of 600 mg. In contrast to this case, the patient in Fig. 2, who was also suffering from siderosis due to alcoholic cirrhosis, showed a much better response to 1,200 mg. desferrioxamine hydrochloride. Normally, the urinary iron excretion in cases of this type does not show such a pronounced rise and does not exceed 10 mg./24 hours.

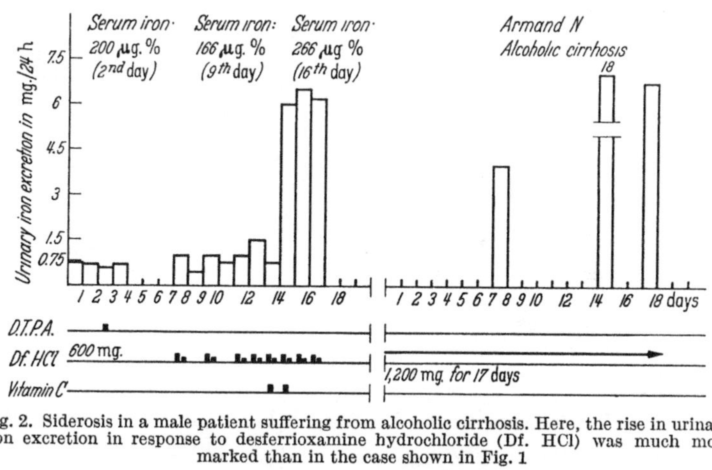

Fig. 2. Siderosis in a male patient suffering from alcoholic cirrhosis. Here, the rise in urinary iron excretion in response to desferrioxamine hydrochloride (Df. HCl) was much more marked than in the case shown in Fig. 1

Fig. 3 shows the results of treatment with desferrioxamine in a case of idiopathic haemochromatosis. Here, the drug was employed in the form of the methane sulphonate (Desferal), administered in a dosage of 1,000 mg. in two daily injections; in addition, two doses of desferrioxamine hydrochloride were given by mouth as supplementary treatment. Other patients treated in the same way showed an increase in urinary iron excretion of roughly the same degree or even a little higher.

Fig. 4 illustrates the response to treatment in a 61-year-old woman with pancytopenia and post-transfusional haemochromatosis. Here, depression of bone-marrow function was particularly severe. In a second case of post-transfusional haemochromatosis with pancytopenia, the patient, a 54-year-old man, responded with a daily iron excretion of up to 26 mg. Another female patient with

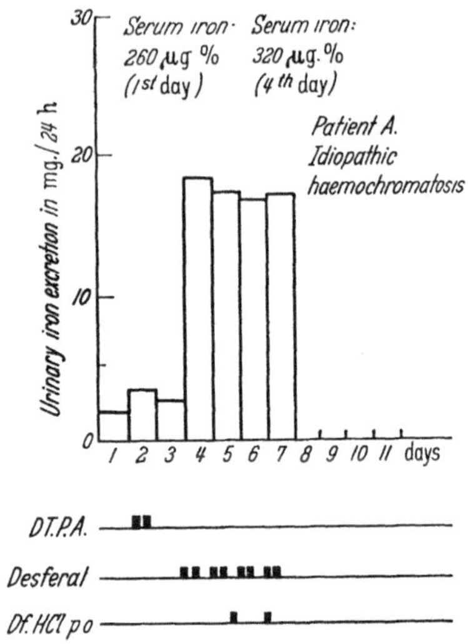

Fig. 3

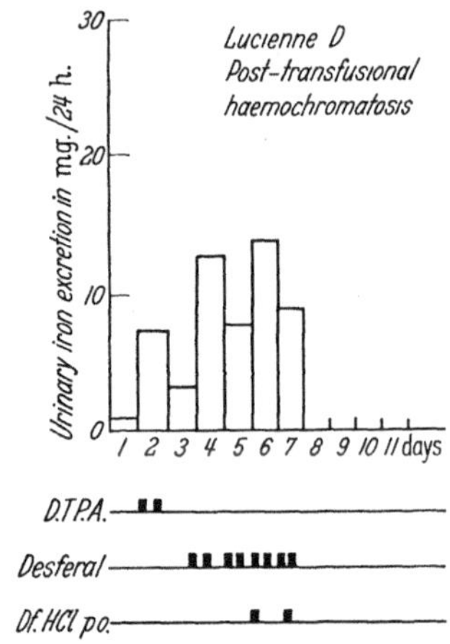

Fig. 4

Fig. 3. Idiopathic haemochromatosis in a 27-year-old patient. In addition to 2 doses of D.T.P.A., the patient received Desferal in a dosage of 1,000 mg. in two daily injections, as well as two oral doses of desferrioxamine hydrochloride

Fig. 4. Post-transfusional haemochromatosis in a 61-year-old woman with pancytopenia characterised by particularly severe depression of bone-marrow function. Same treatment as for the patient shown in Fig. 3

post-transfusional haemochromatosis received more prolonged treatment with desferrioxamine in the form of the hydrochloride; it will be noted that, when the drug was given by intravenous infusion, it did not produce a greater increase in urinary iron excretion than when administered intramuscularly (Fig. 5).

A 39-year-old woman suffering from thalassaemia major with secondary haemochromatosis responded to daily doses of only 500 mg. Desferal with a urinary iron excretion of almost 20 mg./24 hours (Fig. 6). I understand from Dr. PATHÉ in Grasse, who kindly supplied the data for this case, that the patient is now excreting up to 38 mg./24 hours on a daily dosage of 1,000 mg. Desferal.

Figs 7a–c show a case of refractory anaemia with secondary haemochromatosis in a 44-year-old woman, upon whom a report

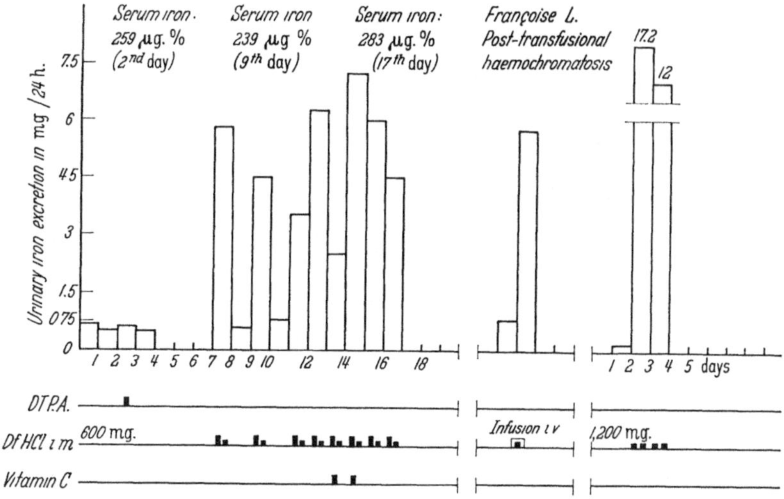

Fig. 5. Post-transfusional haemochromatosis in a female patient. Note that intravenous infusion of desferrioxamine hydrochloride did not produce a greater increase in urinary iron excretion than in response to intramuscular injection

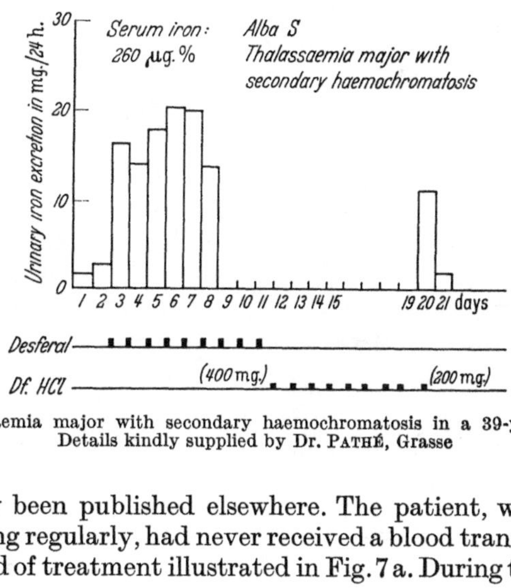

Fig. 6. Thalassaemia major with secondary haemochromatosis in a 39-year-old woman. Details kindly supplied by Dr. PATHÉ, Grasse

has already been published elsewhere. The patient, who was still menstruating regularly, had never received a blood transfusion prior to the period of treatment illustrated in Fig. 7a. During the 3 months preceding each of the courses of treatment shown in Figs 7b and 7c she had been given only 4 litres of blood.

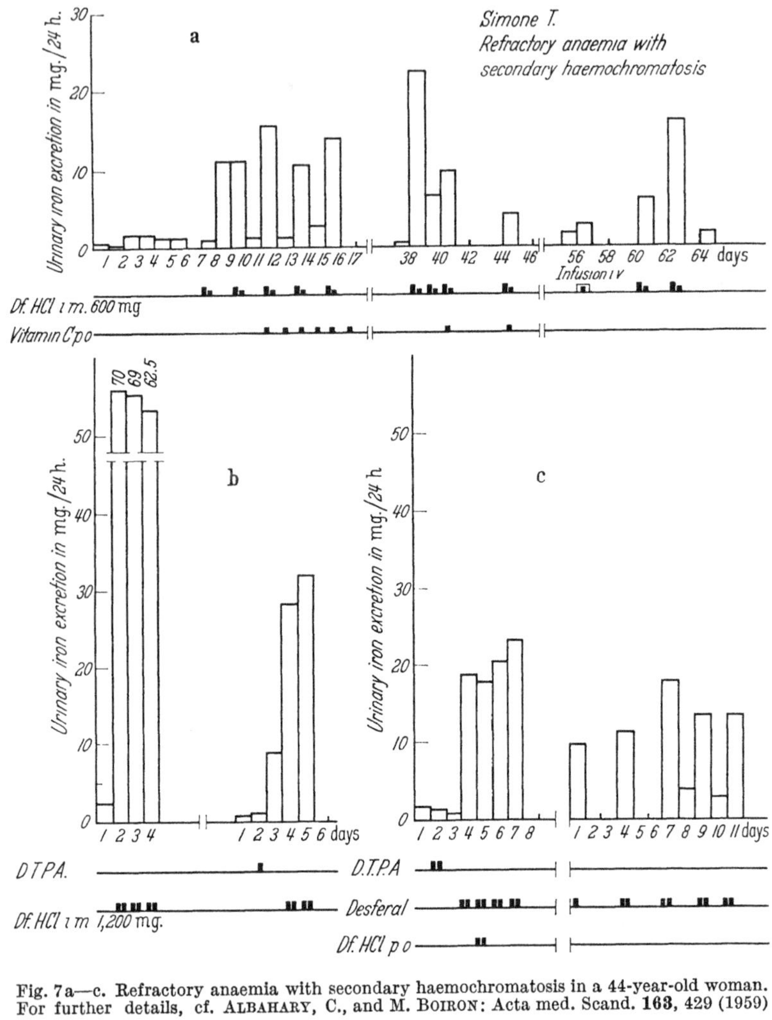

Fig. 7a—c. Refractory anaemia with secondary haemochromatosis in a 44-year-old woman. For further details, cf. ALBAHARY, C., and M. BOIRON: Acta med. Scand. **163**, 429 (1959)

The only further comment I should like to make on these cases is that, except for the last case illustrated in Figs 7a–c, the results obtained – though quite good – are not as striking as some of those reported by other investigators. On the other hand, our patients have undergone only rather short periods of treatment. I should perhaps add that my attempts to treat patients suffering from occupational pulmonary siderosis have been a complete failure. However, from the chemical aspect, this type of localised siderosis is of course different from the classic form of generalised siderosis with which we are primarily concerned here.

Now, with your permission, I should like to raise a few practical points for discussion.

In the first place, may I ask Dr. Brick and Dr. Figueroa whether they think that D.T.P.A. really is a suitable chelating agent for use in a daily dose of 3 to 4 g. in the long-term management of siderosis? I raise this question because it has been our experience in Paris that intramuscular injections of D.T.P.A. are too painful to be used regularly. I also think that slow intravenous infusions are probably more effective than rapid intravenous injections of 1 g. each. I have often been disappointed at the poor results I have obtained when I carried out my one-day test with 1 g. D.T.P.A. given by rapid intravenous injection*, although on the other hand this same test has proved highly satisfactory in cases of lead poisoning. However, I hesitate to resort to another type of administration or to employ daily over a prolonged period such large doses as have been mentioned in this Symposium. In this connection, I should like to know whether anyone has any views on the possible risk of Zn depletion, as well as damage to the renal tubules, in response to such massive treatment with D.T.P.A. or with E.D.T.A.

I would at all events suggest that D.T.P.A. might perhaps usefully be combined over short periods with desferrioxamine or, alternatively, with venesection in cases of idiopathic haemochromatosis that are resistant to desferrioxamine.

I should be interested to hear from Dr. Moeschlin and Dr. Wöhler whether, in their experience, there is any delay in the onset of effect of desferrioxamine and, if so, whether in cases where the effect is delayed one might achieve increased activity by raising the dosage and then possibly lowering it again afterwards. Another question I should like to ask is: do you frequently encounter tolerance to desferrioxamine, i.e. does the drug's effect tend to wear off after several months of treatment with the result that larger and larger doses have to be given or that the treatment has to be aban-

* Meanwhile, I have had much better results with tests in which either two daily intravenous injections of 1 g. were given or 2 g. administered during a 3-hour infusion.

doned? Do you think, as I do, that, where maintenance therapy is required, treatment can justifiably be restricted – without any serious loss of effectiveness – to one injection of 1,000 or 2,000 mg. every 10 to 15 days? It seems to me that this would not only be desirable from the psychological point of view, but that it might also provide an opportunity for the readily mobilisable iron to become reconstituted from the iron deposits in the tissues.

Is it possible that desferrioxamine has a fairly rapid effect in mobilising and eliminating the iron stored in the liver and pancreas and that this might account for the relief from hepatalgia noted in some patients and for the sometimes surprisingly prompt improvement in diabetes? I should also like to know if anyone has an explanation to offer for the fact that, apart from patients who have recently been subjected to venesection, one also sometimes encounters cases of idiopathic haemochromatosis which prove refractory to desferrioxamine from the very start. I have run up against this unexpected resistance to treatment in a case of secondary siderosis as well.

Another point I would mention is that, in my opinion, the degree of saturation of transferrin is not sufficient evidence on which to predict the success or failure of treatment with desferrioxamine. For example, in a case sent to me by Dr. J.-C. DREYFUS there was no response to desferrioxamine, although the patient – the son of a person with idiopathic haemochromatosis – showed the complete biological picture of the disease. In another apparently similar case, however, treatment was not a failure. Dr. J.-C. DREYFUS thinks that the lack of response to chelating agents in such cases is due simply to the fact that very little iron storage has yet occurred. I do not entirely agree with this view; I believe there must be some other explanation for the complete lack of effect of the drug – possibly its rapid destruction in the plasma or elsewhere.

May I ask if anyone has had any personal experience of the use of desferrioxamine in iron poisoning in man, from which we might be able to determine how much of the drug should be administered at once by mouth? I suspect that one would probably have to give not less than 15 to 20 g. (after first having induced the patient to vomit), as well as 2 or 3 g. parenterally.

My next question concerns the side effects of desferrioxamine. I know of only one instance – a very complex case reported by MAIER at the Round-Table Discussion in Lugano – in which thrombocytopenia may possibly have been attributable to the drug. I myself have observed one minor complication in a patient receiving desferrioxamine, i.e. cystalgia and dysuria; this makes me think that, in cases where a good response is achieved in terms of urinary iron excretion, the urine may contain not only ferrioxamine but also some mineral iron.

I should like to ask Dr. TRIPOD whether he thinks that desferrioxamine, when administered by mouth, really exerts a protective effect against normal alimentary iron, and that oral treatment with the drug might therefore be useful in idiopathic haemochromatosis.

Finally, one last question: is there any hope of finding in the near future a new form of desferrioxamine which is active by mouth in all types of siderosis? This would certainly be the best method of treatment, because it would be the simplest.

General Discussion

HEILMEYER: Particularly interesting are the results of treatment with desferrioxamine in sideroachrestic anaemias. Originally, when we began with this therapy, we merely hoped to be able to diminish the severe siderosis of the organs. We were therefore surprised to find that the drug also influenced porphyrin metabolism. As Fig. 1 impressively demonstrates, the pathological increase in coproporphyrin and protoporphyrin in the erythrocytes, as well as the increased delta-aminolaevulinic acid in the urine, practically reverted to normal. At the same time, an increase in haemoglobin and in the number of erythrocytes was observed. The iron withdrawn in about 3 months amounted to approximately 4.5 g. For the 10 months during which we treated the patient it totalled 11.3 g.

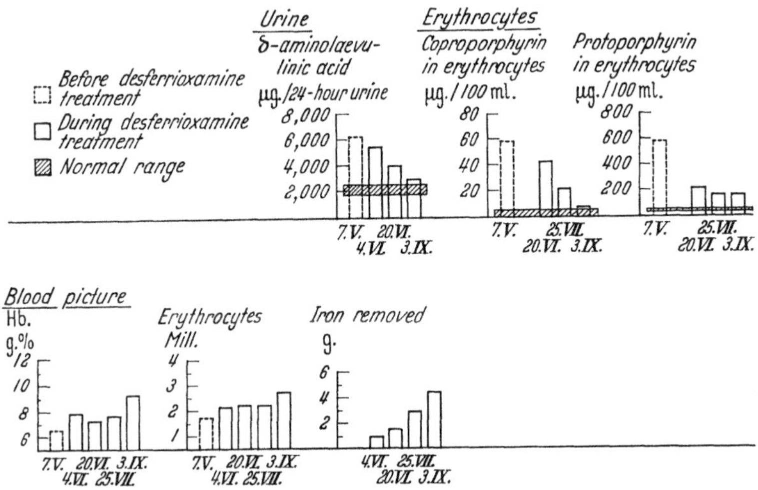

Fig. 1. Behaviour of the porphyrins in the erythrocytes and urine during treatment with desferrioxamine in a case of sideroblastic anaemia

In another case (Fig. 2), the patient, aged 57 years, was also suffering from acquired sideroblastic anaemia; the results of treatment were the same as in the case previously mentioned. The urinary excretion of delta-aminolaevulinic acid, porphobilinogen, uroporphyrin, and coproporphyrin, which had been very high prior to treatment, returned almost to normal; particularly significant, however, is the fact that the erythrocytes showed a normal amount of coproporphyrin and a low content of protoporphyrin. At the same time, the blood picture underwent a slight improvement. The iron withdrawn during the period of clinical observation amounted to approximately 1.4 g. We have seen similar responses in cases of porphyria cutanea tarda.

What is the explanation for these effects? From investigations by BISHOP and BETHELL[1] it is known that increased deposition of iron in the cell has an undesirable effect on haem synthesis, and studies by BROWN[2], as well as further investigations undertaken by myself and CLOTTEN[3], have shown that delta-aminolaevulinic acid dehydrase is inhibited — possibly because the SH groups are blocked. GIBSON and co-workers[4] have arrived at the same results. On the other hand, it seems to be certain that the deposition of iron in the mitochondria can cause them to become severely damaged (BESSIS[5]).

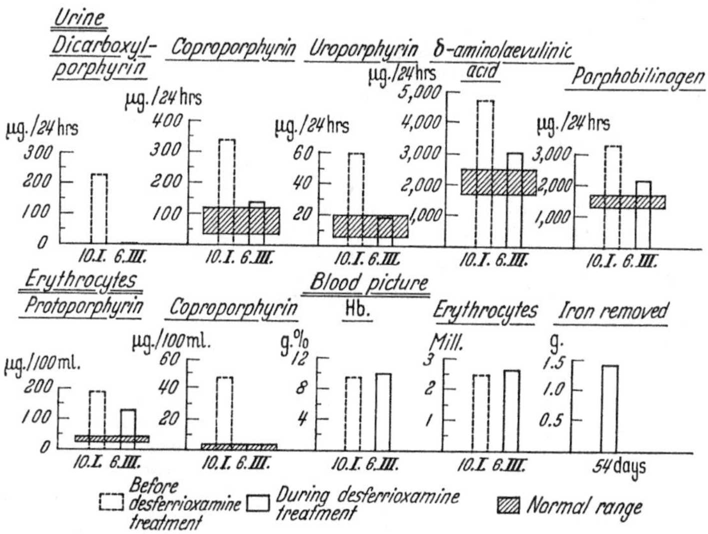

Fig. 2. Behaviour of the porphyrins in the erythrocytes and urine during treatment with desferrioxamine in another case of sideroblastic anaemia

So much for some of the hypotheses that have been advanced to explain the toxic effects of an iron overload in the erythroblasts and the action of desferrioxamine in patients with sideroachrestic anaemia. A great deal of work will still have to be done if the action of this drug is to be analysed exactly.

BEUTLER: About 8 months ago, when we first became aware of the availability of desferrioxamine, Dr. FAIRBANKS, Dr. WARSON, and I[6] undertook a study to compare the effectiveness of desferrioxamine and D.T.P.A. Initially, desferrioxamine was not available to us, so that most of our

[1] BISHOP, R. C., and F. H. BETHELL: N. England J. Med. **261**, 486 (1959).
[2] BROWN, E. G.: Nature (G.B.) **182**, 313 (1958).
[3] HEILMEYER, L.: Disturbances in Blood Heme Synthesis. C. Thomas, Springfield, Ill. (in press).
[4] GIBSON, K. D., W. G. LAVER, and A. NEUBERGER: Biochem. J. (G.B.) **70**, 71 (1958).
[5] BESSIS, M., and J. BRETON-GORIUS: Blood (U.S.A.) **19**, 635 (1962).
[6] FAIRBANKS, V. F., M. D. WARSON, and E. BEUTLER: Brit. Med. J. **1963**/I, 1414.

studies were carried out with D.T.P.A. They revealed some possibly toxic effects of this agent that had not been described hitherto. I have not found any previous references to the toxicity of this agent, except in a very recent paper by HEILMEYER and WÖHLER[1], in which they state concerning D.T.P.A.: "*Auch wir selbst benutzten diese Substanz. Sie bewährt sich jedoch wegen toxischer Nebenerscheinungen bei der Dauertherapie nicht.*" In the course of this Symposium, Dr. HEILMEYER mentioned the occurrence of painful symptoms in his patients, and I assume that these are the toxic reactions to which he referred.

We have treated three patients with D.T.P.A. One patient had red-cell aplasia with many transfusions, and in response to D.T.P.A. she showed a very excellent iron excretion, comparable to the iron excretion which Dr. BRICK has described in his paper. This woman, the first patient we studied, was very ill at the time D.T.P.A. was started. During the course of the study she grew increasingly somnolent; finally she became comatose and died. The second patient was one with myelofibrosis who had had many blood transfusions. In this case we were able to mobilise less iron. This patient, too, was very ill; at the end of the study she became comatose and died. The third patient treated with D.T.P.A. was suffering from auto-immune haemolytic disease. She excreted small amounts of iron in response to D.T.P.A. However, towards the end of the D.T.P.A. administration, she developed thrombocytopenia and reticulocytopenia, became anaemic, and suffered from ulcerations and alopecia. The therapy was stopped and all these symptoms gradually disappeared.

Although we could not at the end of these three experiences state with certainty that the results were due to D.T.P.A., this type of clinical response with a new agent is certainly alarming for any clinical investigator, and we have published a warning about these possible side effects in the form of a letter to the British Medical Journal. Since then, two other patients, also in Los Angeles, who had been treated with D.T.P.A. have come to our attention. They were studied at the University of Southern California by REDEKER and REYNOLDS, who have given me permission to present data from these two cases to you today. The first patient had possible haemochromatosis with very severe liver disease. She was given 4 g. D.T.P.A. daily i.m. Twenty-four hours after starting treatment the patient became nauseated and vomited. She continued to feel unwell for the next two days and complained of generalised pains. On the fourth day she vomited again and during that day became stuporous. D.T.P.A. treatment was discontinued after a total of 14 g. had been given. The patient then started to bleed, lapsed into hepatic coma, and died. The second patient received only 10 g. at the same dosage rate and deveopled nausea, vomiting, and severe pain in the limbs with numbness and weakness. He felt generally unwell and developed an eczematous eruption on the face. When treatment was stopped the symptoms subsided, and the rash took ten days to clear. REYNOLDS and REDEKER did some urinary excretion studies on the second patient. This patient did mobilise iron; however, he also mobilised zinc to a very marked extent, as well as manganese and calcium. The same patient showed no increase in his urinary excretion of nickel, aluminium, silver, lead, copper, and cobalt or of chromium, cadmium, barium, vanadium, tin, and titanium. Similar results were obtained in the first patient.

---

[1] HEILMEYER, L., and F. WÖHLER: Dtsch. med. Wschr. 87, 2661 (1962).

We have heard about one other patient who also developed a skin rash and thrombocytopenia, which disappeared when D.T.P.A. was stopped, and which recurred when D.T.P.A. was again given.

For these reasons we are inclined to feel that for long-term therapy D.T.P.A. may be a much more toxic agent than one might suspect from the short-term studies which Dr. Brick has carried out. I should be very interested to learn about other experiences investigators may have had with long-term D.T.P.A. therapy.

Boye Nielsen: I have been interested in the question as to whether there is a correlation between the amount of desferrioxamine infused and the urinary excretion of iron.

In order to investigate whether there is an upper limit to the amount of iron which can be excreted through the kidney per unit time under the influence of intravenous desferrioxamine, a patient with an untreated primary

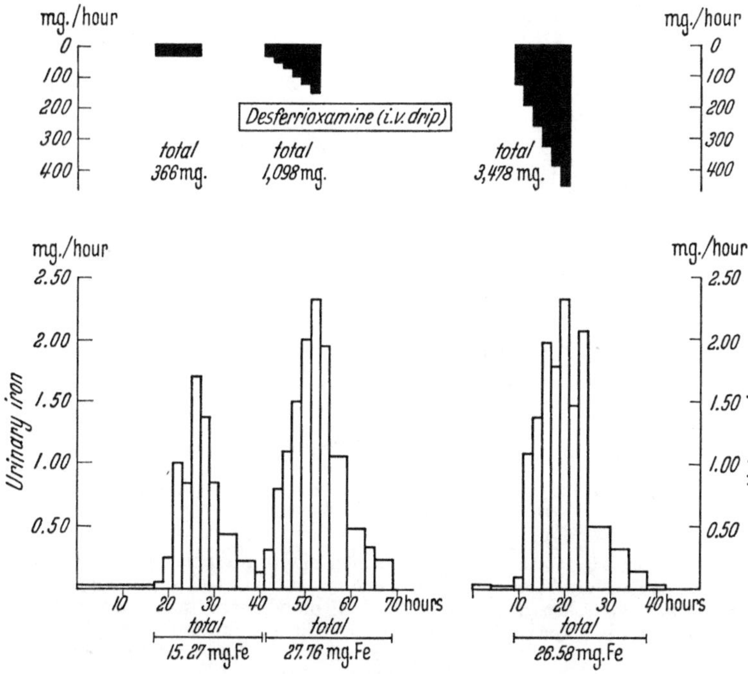

Fig. 3. Urinary iron excretion in a patient with untreated primary haemochromatosis after intravenous infusion of desferrioxamine

haemochromatosis was given a continuous intravenous infusion of increasing doses of desferrioxamine. As may be seen from Fig. 3, it was not possible to increase the urinary iron excretion beyond 2.5 mg./hour in this patient, despite further administration of considerable quantities of desferrioxamine. To exclude the possibility that this upper limit depends on the renal excretion capacity, the same patient received a continuous intravenous infusion of increasing quantities of ferrioxamine — which is desferrioxamine saturated with trivalent iron — in doses corresponding to those used in the desferrioxamine infusion. As Fig. 4 shows, the urinary excretion of iron now increased considerably, reaching about 30 mg./hour. In other words, the limit does not appear to be a question of renal capacity, and it seems reasonable to assume that the upper limit for urinary iron excretion of 2.5 mg./hour

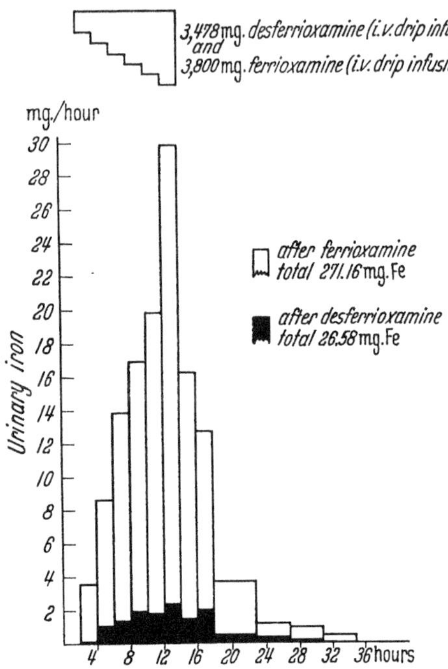

Fig. 4. Same patient as in Fig. 3. Urinary iron excretion after intravenous infusion of ferrioxamine as compared with desferrioxamine

in this patient indicates the rate at which his iron depots can be mobilised. After this test had been carried out, the patient was treated by venesection. It was not possible to withdraw 500 ml. of blood more often than every 5th day without a decrease in haemoglobin. The production of an additional 500 ml. of blood in 5 days requires an amount of iron corresponding to 2.5 mg./hour, so one might speculate that the rate at which the iron depots are mobilised may be a factor limiting haemoglobin production in the bone marrow.

Hallberg: It has been suggested that desferrioxamine takes the iron primarily from transferrin and that possibly the amount of iron excreted is related to the size of the iron stores.

I should like to mention the results that Dr. Hedenberg and I have obtained, because to some extent they conflict with what we have heard

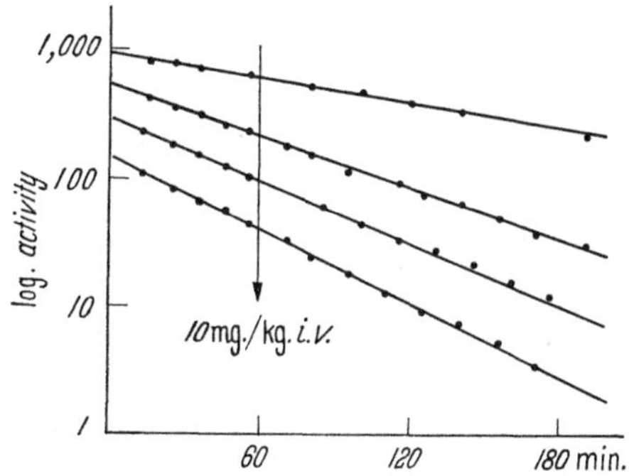

Fig. 5. Plasma iron turnover rate in 4 normal subjects in response to desferrioxamine (10 mg./kg. i.v.). Desferrioxamine has no effect on the turnover rate

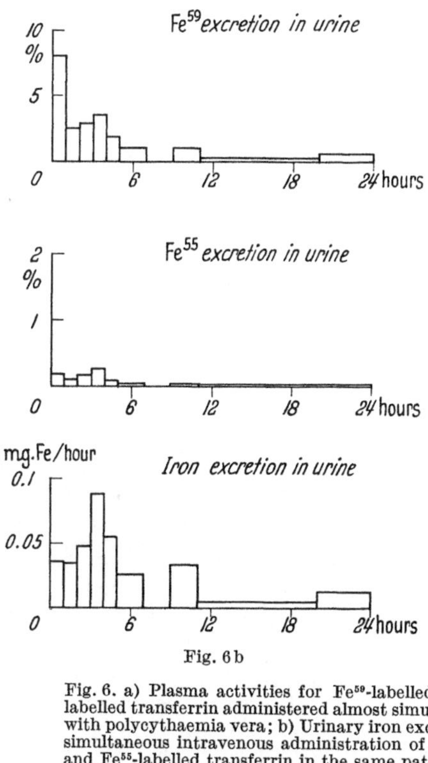

Fig. 6b

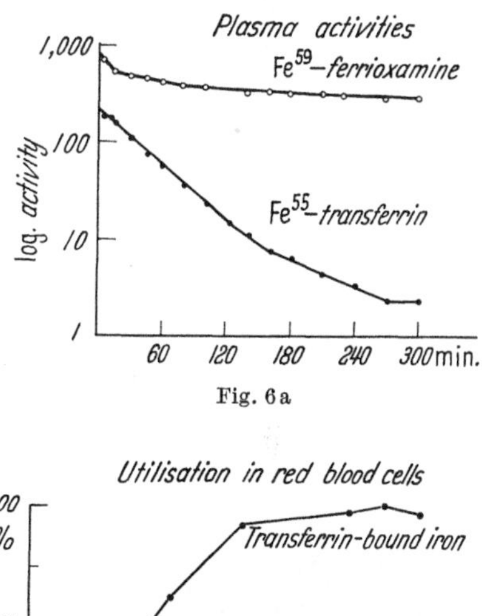

Fig. 6a

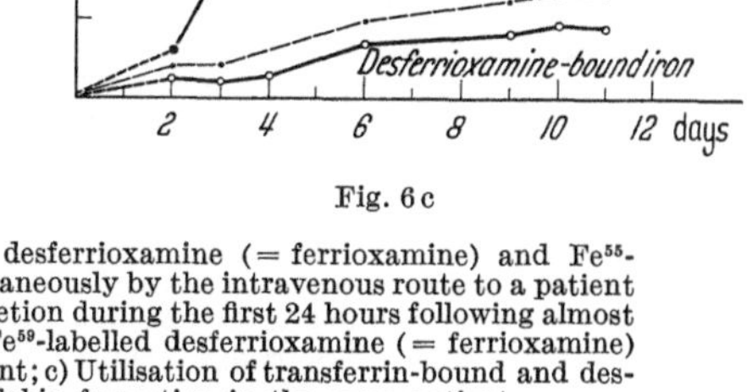

Fig. 6c

Fig. 6. a) Plasma activities for Fe^{59}-labelled desferrioxamine (= ferrioxamine) and Fe^{55}-labelled transferrin administered almost simultaneously by the intravenous route to a patient with polycythaemia vera; b) Urinary iron excretion during the first 24 hours following almost simultaneous intravenous administration of Fe^{59}-labelled desferrioxamine (= ferrioxamine) and Fe^{55}-labelled transferrin in the same patient; c) Utilisation of transferrin-bound and desferrioxamine-bound iron for haemoglobin formation in the same patient here. Firstly, we have found that in normal subjects desferrioxamine has no effect at all on the plasma iron turnover rate, and since the plasma iron level is also constant, our conclusion has been that the plasma iron turnover in normal subjects is unaffected by desferrioxamine (Fig. 5).

Another study has also shown that desferrioxamine does not take iron from transferrin. Fe^{55}-labelled transferrin and Fe^{59}-labelled ferrioxamine were given almost simultaneously by the intravenous route. About 30% of the ferrioxamine-bound tracer was excreted in the urine during the first 24 hours but only 1% of the transferrin-bound tracer — which is no more than we usually obtain when desferrioxamine is not given (Fig. 6a and b).

When comparing the utilisation of the tracers for haemoglobin formation, it was evident in this case of polycythaemia vera that about 100% of the transferrin-bound tracer was present in the red cells, but only 22.6% of the ferrioxamine-bound tracer (Fig. 6c). These results indicate that the excreted iron does not come from transferrin.

Where, then, is the iron taken from? At this point, I would like to mention briefly certain further studies we have made, which may shed some light on this problem. We administered desferrioxamine as a single intravenous injection (10 mg./kg. body-weight) to various subjects. In normal men about 0.5—1 mg. iron was then excreted in the 24-hour urine, and in normal menstruating women about 0.35—0.5 mg. (Fig. 7). These figures were higher than the normal iron excretion level as determined during the preceding 24 hours, which was usually about 0.1 mg.

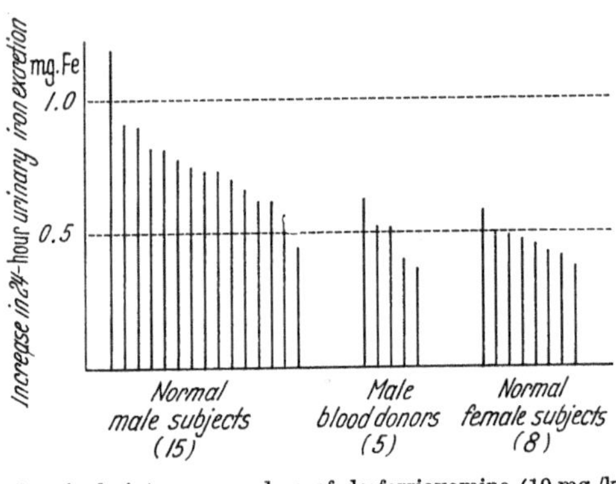

Fig. 7. Effect of a single intravenous dose of desferrioxamine (10 mg./kg.) on the urinary excretion of iron in normal men, in male blood donors, and in normal menstruating women

However, if the amount excreted were directly related to the size of the iron stores, a very low iron excretion should be expected in male blood donors who have given considerable quantities of blood without receiving any supplementary iron. The five blood donors — who had given more than 50 pints of blood, and not less than 6 pints during the last 12 months — each excreted about 0.5 mg. iron, despite the fact that their iron stores were depleted of iron. The results suggest that the iron excreted by these 5 subjects originated from iron released from newly catabolised red cells; moreover, they also suggest that such iron is more easily taken up by desferrioxamine than the iron in the so-called stores, because in normal men the amount of iron in these stores is many times greater than the pool of iron from newly catabolised red cells. If this hypothesis is correct, more iron should be excreted with desferrioxamine in haemolytic states. To test this hypothesis, desferrioxamine was administered to a male subject with pernicious anaemia before, and at weekly intervals during, treatment with vitamin B_{12} (Fig. 8). Before treatment, a large iron excretion was obtained, but already after one week of treatment, when the signs of increased destruction of red cells had disappeared, the iron excretion had dropped to normal levels. During this first week, no appreciable increase in the red-cell mass took place, which also implies that the iron stores were of roughly the same size on both occasions. (When normal subjects are given two doses of desferrioxamine with an interval of one week between each dose, the difference in the resultant urinary iron is very small.)

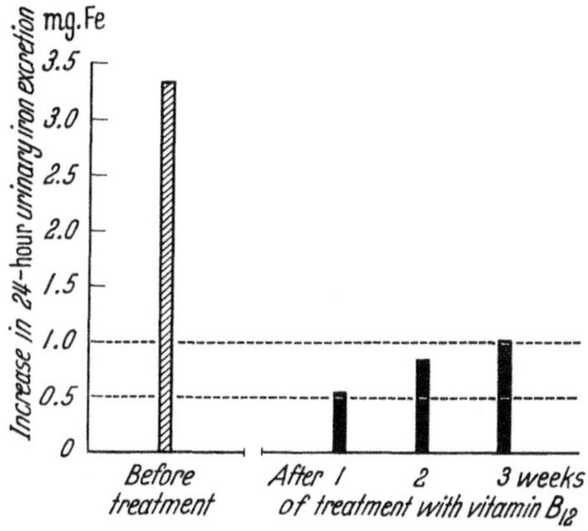

Fig. 8. Effect of single intravenous doses of desferrioxamine (10 mg./kg.) on the urinary excretion of iron in a 61-year-old male patient with pernicious anaemia before treatment and after 1, 2, and 3 weeks of treatment with vitamin B_{12}

The stored non-haem iron in the body is probably present in different forms and/or under different circumstances, leading to wide differences in its affinity for desferrioxamine and thus probably also to wide differences in its affinity for transferrin. Iron from newly catabolised red cells is probably more readily available than iron in the ordinary stores.

Katz: I think Dr. Hallberg has already partially answered the question I was going to ask, but do any of the speakers have any information on the effect of desferrioxamine infusion on red-cell utilisation or radioactive iron bound to plasma? I believe Cleton, Turnbull, and Finch[1] have shown that, despite the fact that the stability constants for certain other chelating agents are apparently higher than for transferrin, there was no evidence that iron could be removed from transferrin *in vivo*. As a corollary to this, I should like to ask if there is any evidence that human cells can utilise iron bound to ferrioxamine.

Callender: Dr. Wöhler raised the question of blocking iron absorption with oral desferrioxamine. We have some observations on rats and

[1] Cleton, F. J., A. Turnbull, and C. A. Finch: J. Clin. Invest. (U.S.A.) **42**, 327 (1963).

humans which have confirmed that you can reduce the absorption of inorganic iron, but oral desferrioxamine showed no effect on the absorption of labelled haemoglobin.

We have been giving desferrioxamine to iron-laden subjects, but have been unable to maintain a high iron excretion on continued dosage. The excretion falls quite markedly as treatment continues. I wonder if there is any possibility of there being variability between batches of desferrioxamine, some being more effective than others?

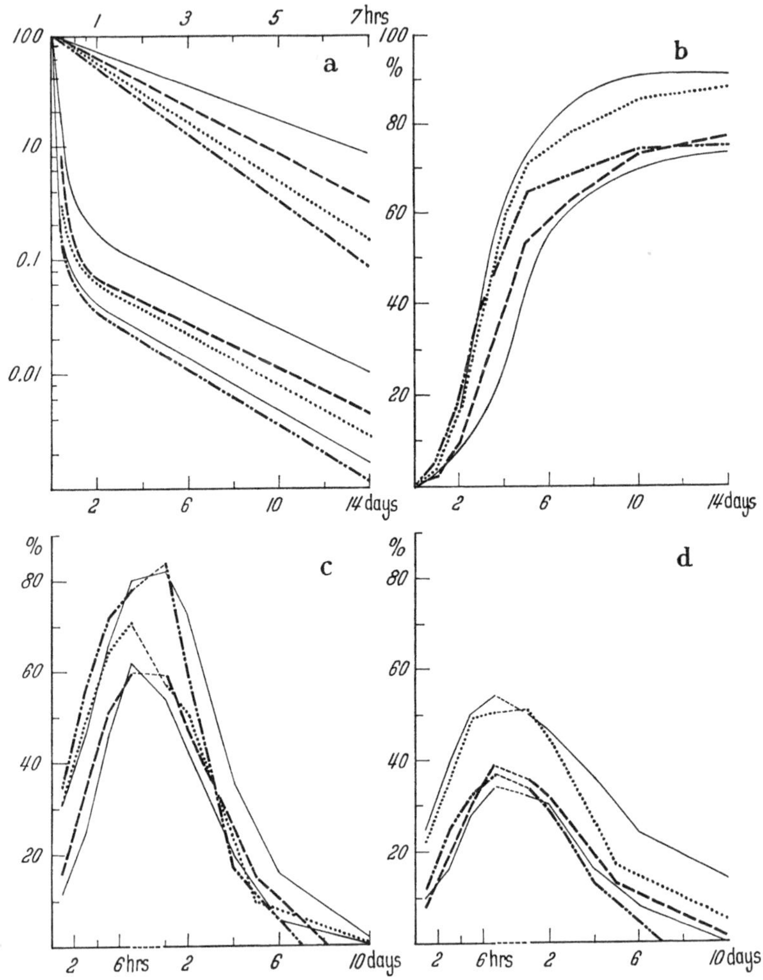

Fig. 9. Radio-iron in the plasma (a) and erythrocytes (b) and surface radioactivity of sacral marrow (c) and liver (d) after intravenous injection of Fe^{59}-transferrin in the presence of desferrioxamine. The thick lines represent the findings in 3 patients; the area within the thin lines represents the normal range

VENTURA: Like Dr. HALLBERG, we found that, when we gave intravenous injections of Fe^{59} bound to transferrin, desferrioxamine did not cause a removal of Fe^{59} from the transferrin. Regardless of the concentration of plasma desferrioxamine, Fe^{59}-transferrin, as shown in Fig. 9, follows its normal kinetic pattern. On the other hand, intravenous injection of Fe^{59} bound to desferrioxamine is followed by a change in the normal behaviour. Fig. 10 shows that the Fe^{59} leaves the plasma more slowly, and about 40% is eliminated from the body in the urine. Consequently, a smaller quantity

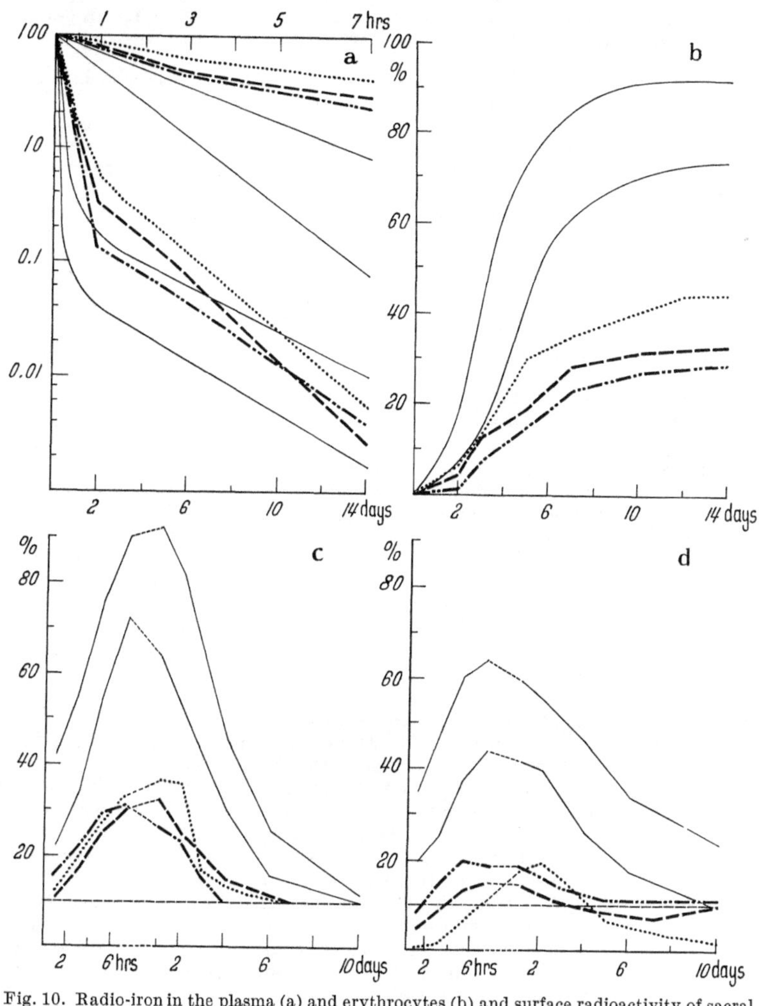

Fig. 10. Radio-iron in the plasma (a) and erythrocytes (b) and surface radioactivity of sacral marrow (c) and liver (d) after intravenous injection of Fe^{59}-desferrioxamine. The thick lines represent the findings in 3 patients; the area within the thin lines represents the normal range

of Fe^{59} is found in the bone marrow and liver, and is utilised for haemoglobin synthesis. If we now administer $Fe^{59}Cl_2$ by intramuscular injection to patients suffering from iron-deficiency anaemia and with a high quantity of transferrin and desferrioxamine in their plasma (the desferrioxamine being given intravenously before the experiment starts, and its concentration being maintained by intravenous infusion), we find that almost all of the Fe^{59} is taken up by the desferrioxamine and that it shows a ferrokinetic behaviour as illustrated in Fig. 10.

Therefore, depending on the duration of the experiment, desferrioxamine is shown to possess a higher capacity than transferrin for taking up Fe ions, but it is not capable of breaking the link between Fe and transferrin.

FIGUEROA: We have a patient with haemochromatosis who had been treated by venesection. The serum iron was elevated, and his transferrin was still saturated. He still had an excess of iron in the body. The patient was subjected to iron-balance studies. We gave him 200 mg. desferrioxamine by mouth with each meal, and later 400 mg. for the last 5 days. We were unable to demonstrate that these doses of desferrioxamine, given for 15 days, were capable of preventing the absorption of food iron at the rate of approximately 18—19 mg. per day. The urinary iron excretion rose from 0.3 to 1.5 mg. daily. Throughout the 15 days there was no effect on the urinary calcium excretion rate. There was some evidence that the calcium balance was more positive during the administration of the drug, but the period of observation is too short for any definite conclusion to be drawn. With reference to the toxicity of Ca-D.T.P.A., we have used a lot of this substance in our particular studies, simply in order to find out how much iron we could get out with it. We have also used it intermittently, instead of every single day as in the cases referred to by Dr. BEUTLER. We did this for two reasons. About 10 years ago, when we first used E.D.T.A., we found that the urinary iron excretion decreased when the drug was given daily and that the treatment was more effective if administered intermittently. Secondly, if one studies the literature, one finds that all the toxic manifestations reported in response to E.D.T.A. occurred with dosages given every single day for 5 days or more. We have also used some E.D.D.H.A. on a limited number of patients, and the amount we have given is 400 to 500 mg. With these doses as much iron could be removed as with 600 mg. desferrioxamine B.

The urinary iron excretion in the two patients shown in Fig. 11a and b was fairly closely related to the amount of Ca-D.T.P.A. administered; in the first patient with transfusion haemosiderosis, for example, urinary iron excretion was approximately 10, 20, 35, and 45 mg. in response to intravenous doses of 1, 2, 3, and 4 g. Ca-D.T.P.A. The second patient had primary haemochromatosis and excreted much larger quantities of iron in the urine than the normal controls after intravenous Ca-D.T.P.A. infusion.

If we compare the urinary iron excretion in a patient with primary haemochromatosis during 5 days of continuous Ca-D.T.P.A. therapy and 5 days of continuous Desferal infusion, it will be seen that, when the same amount of 2 g. Ca-D.T.P.A. is given each day, the urinary iron excretion progressively diminishes from 10.6 mg. on the first day to 5.6 mg. on the fifth day (Table 1). The same did not apply to desferrioxamine, at least not during the short 5-day observation period, since 0.6 g. of this drug caused approximately the same amount of iron (8—9 mg.) to be excreted in the urine on each day, making a total of 46 mg. iron for the 5 days. This is one of the reasons why I have been particularly interested in this drug.

Now with reference to your work on Ca-D.T.P.A., I noticed, Dr. WÖHLER, that you did not obtain any increase in urinary iron excretion with Ca-D.T.P.A. I do not know how to reconcile our different findings. We have used Ca-D.T.P.A. and infused it intravenously for 2 or 3 hours. I note that

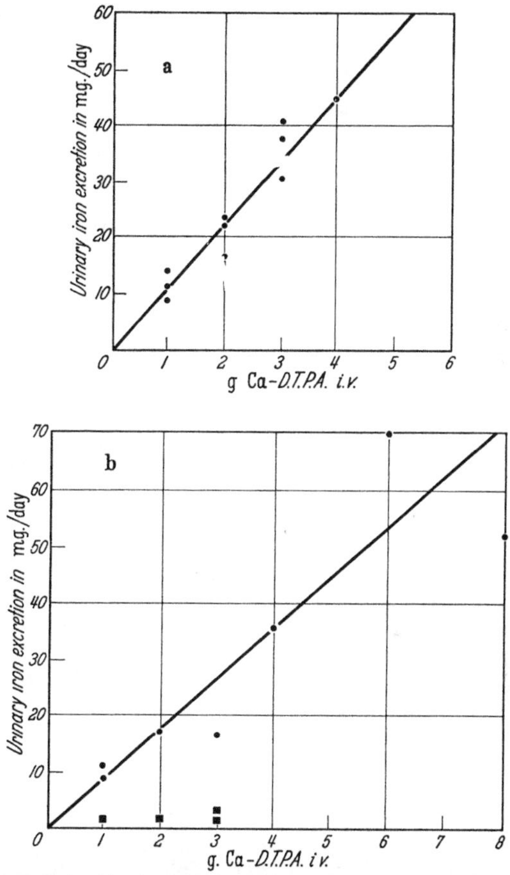

Fig. 11 a and b. Relationship of urinary iron excretion to amount of Ca-D.T.P.A. given intravenously in a patient with transfusion haemosiderosis (a) and in a patient with primary haemochromatosis (b). In (b) the iron excretion levels in several normal and cirrhotic subjects (■) are shown for comparison

you apparently injected it right away. I should like to know what method you used for the determination of urinary iron, since I wonder whether the method has something to do with it. Intramuscular injection of Ca-D.T.P.A. is, incidentally, also painful in Los Angeles! I have never given it by this route and have never recommended that it should be injected in this way. I remember giving an ampoule of Ca-D.T.P.A. to one of the doctors who wanted to use it in a patient intramuscularly. The patient developed severe pain at the site of injection. The second injection was mixed with procaine and did not produce pain. I know it is not painful in Washington, but it certainly is in Los Angeles!

Table 1. *Comparison of urinary iron excretion in a patient with primary haemochromatosis following a 5-day course of intravenous treatment with 600 mg. desferrioxamine B and with 2 g. Ca-D.T.P.A.*

Day	Desferrioxamine B 600 mg./day *	Ca-D.T.P.A. 2 g./day
1	7.5 mg.	10.58 mg.
2	11.8	8.96
3	8.8	6.43
4	8.7	6.38
5	9.3	5.61
Total:	46.1	37.96

* 800 mg. on 5th day.

I wonder whether anybody noticed any toxicity with desferrioxamine B. I have experience of one particular patient who was given 800 mg. by intravenous infusion. He developed moderate abdominal pain which disappeared 4 hours later after antacid therapy. Can anybody perhaps shed some light on the mechanism involved here?

BEARN: May I ask a brief question concerning the experiments that we have heard described on the acute toxicity induced by ferrous sulphate ingestion? Do we have any information about the physico-chemical nature of the iron in the serum when the iron-binding capacity is exceeded? Is it bound to other proteins? Do we know in what form the excess iron is excreted in the urine?

KEBERLE: In connection with the papers by Dr. MOESCHLIN and Dr. BRICK I should like to describe the results of our studies (carried out together with Dr. FITZGERALD) on the question of whether desferrioxamine can be used as a means of detecting increased iron deposition in the human organism.

First of all, tests were undertaken in 20 healthy men with normal serum iron levels, iron-binding capacity, and R.B.C., in order to find out what amounts of iron the normal subject excretes in the urine within a given space of time. Then the increase in iron excretion following a single intramuscular injection of 500 mg. desferrioxamine methane sulphonate was measured. In the case of all the subjects the urine was collected every 3 hours for a total period of 12 hours following the injection, and each specimen was assayed for iron and desferrioxamine. The results are summarised in Table 2. The figures represent the average values for the 20 subjects. The first column shows the iron excretion prior to the treatment; normally, between 29 and 45 μg. iron is excreted in the urine over a period of 3 hours. The second column indicates the iron excretion of the same subjects following the injection of desferrioxamine. In all cases, iron excretion was increased after the desferrioxamine treatment, the maximum level being attained usually between the third and the sixth hour, but quite often also within the first 4 hours. Hence, in normal subjects, the above-mentioned dose of desferrioxamine increases the iron levels in the 6-hour urine by 4.7 times on the average, the individual values varying from 2.5 times to 7.5 times. The third column shows the iron

Table 2. *Urinary iron excretion in response to a single dose of 500 mg. Desferal i.m. in 20 healthy men and in one patient with haemochromatosis*

	Iron excretion in μg.		
Time in hours	Normal untreated male subjects	Normal male subjects treated with 500 mg. Desferal*	Haemochromatosis patient treated with 500 mg. Desferal
— 3 to 0	29	29	18
0 — 3	29	110 (3.8×)	2,570 (88×)
3 — 6	33	180 (5.5×)	2,420 (74×)
6 — 9	41	175 (4.3×)	1,210 (30×)
9 —12	45	126 (2.8×)	830 (19×)
0 — 6	62	290 (4.7×)	4,990 (80×)
0 —12	148	591 (4×)	7,030 (48×)

* Average values for 20 persons.

excretion levels in a patient with haemochromatosis. This patient excreted 8 mg. iron in 24 hours following an intramuscular injection of 500 mg. desferrioxamine methane sulphonate. The 6-hour urine already contained 5 mg., i.e. 80 times more than that eliminated by normal, untreated subjects in the same period of time. Measurement of iron excretion levels in the 6-hour urine following the injection of desferrioxamine thus seems to provide a suitable method of detecting elevated iron deposits.

Table 3 shows the excretion of desferrioxamine in the urine in % of the dose administered. On the average, 33% of the desferrioxamine injected was recovered unchanged in the urine of normal subjects within 12 hours, the major portion of this amount being excreted in the first 3 hours. The remainder of the desferrioxamine is broken down in the organism and excreted in the form of metabolites.

Table 3. *Urinary excretion of Desferal, in the form of desferrioxamine and ferrioxamine, expressed as a percentage of the dose of Desferal administered to 20 healthy men and to one patient with haemochromatosis*

	Desferal excretion, in the form of desferrioxamine + ferrioxamine, in % of dose administered	
Time in hours	Normal*	Haemochromatosis
0 — 3	20.4	40.8
3 — 6	9.7	10.5
6 — 9	3.0	5.9
9 —12	1.0	3.3
0 —12	33.1	60.5

* Average values for 20 persons.

It is known from experiments performed in nephrectomised dogs by Brunner and Peters that desferrioxamine is rapidly broken down in the organism, but that ferrioxamine is not. This would explain why, as a rule, a higher percentage of the desferrioxamine administered is traced in the urine in the case of patients with iron-storage diseases. In such patients, a large proportion of the desferrioxamine is converted into ferrioxamine in the body and thus protected from degradation.

IMHOF: The question has been raised as to the nature and frequency of the side effects of desferrioxamine. Experience of several hundred cases, treated continuously for up to one year or even longer, has shown that side effects are very rare. Vague and unspecific side effects have occasionally been reported, but it is difficult to attribute them to the drug. Abdominal pains, as observed by Dr. FIGUEROA, have been reported by a few other investigators. One wonders whether these pains are related to the liberation of ferritin or to the drug itself. It is known that in some cases of primary haemochromatosis abdominal spasm may occur spontaneously, and this is thought to be due to a release of ferritin in the blood. One side effect which possibly can occur with rapid intravenous injection of doses above 600 mg. is a fall in blood pressure. Investigations in this direction have been carried out in normal persons by Dr. KELLER[1]. He found that, immediately after the rapid intravenous injection (1—2 min.) of 1,200 mg., a considerable fall in blood pressure lasting around 10 minutes occurred, together with nausea, headache, and flushing of the face. There is some evidence that this side effect may be due to a release of histamine.

PETERS: The question as to whether desferrioxamine has any renal toxicity was raised by Dr. ALBAHARY and other speakers. In this connection it is interesting to note that intravenous injections of up to 100 mg./kg. in dogs, and up to 200 mg./kg. in rats, have no influence on renal function other than that which could be explained as a direct consequence of the circulatory effect. In rats, daily intraperitoneal injections of 150 mg./kg., continued for 3 weeks, had no influence on the clearances of inulin or of P.A.H., on renal sodium and water excretion, or on the ability of the kidneys to elaborate a maximally concentrated or maximally diluted urine.

The circulatory effect of *rapid* intravenous injections of medium to large doses of desferrioxamine in cats, dogs, and rabbits takes the form of a fall in blood pressure due to a decrease in peripheral resistance (Fig. 12a and b). When repeated injections are given, the depressor response becomes less and less evident and finally sometimes disappears completely. Since we could also demonstrate a conspicuous liberation of histamine from body tissues, the circulatory response may be mediated by the release of histamine (Dr. JAQUES). The depressor response cannot, however, be prevented by antihistamines or glucocorticoids. On the other hand, when the blood pressure is lowered by desferrioxamine, it can easily be restored to normal levels by administering noradrenaline or angiotensin.

UNDRITZ: With regard to the paper by Dr. MOESCHLIN, it is alarming to hear that in England approximately 10% of all fatal cases of poisoning among children are caused by the ingestion of iron sulphate tablets. It is usually the same story in every case: the doctor prescribes iron sulphate tablets for the mother because she is expecting a child and has become anaemic as a result of previous pregnancies. A child finds the sugar-coated tablets, swallows them, and may die of acute iron sulphate poisoning.

[1] KELLER, H. M.: Personal communication.

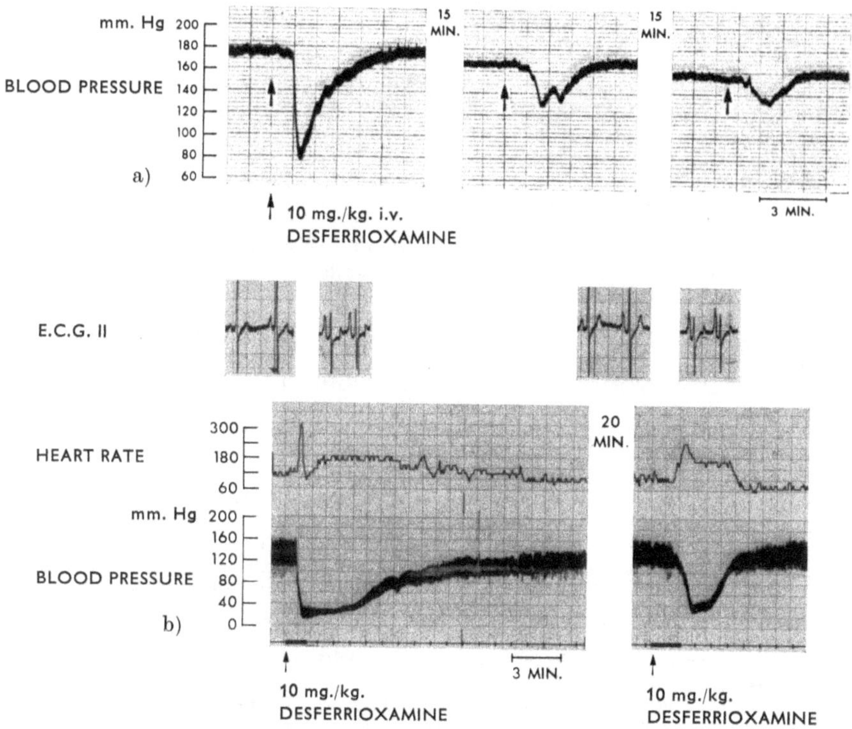

Fig. 12. Circulatory effects of repeated single intravenous doses of desferrioxamine methane sulphonate in a) the cat, anaesthetised with allobarbitone and urethane, and b) the dog, anaesthetised with pentobarbitone

Bivalent *organic* iron preparations are equally effective for combating anaemia, but are considerably less toxic than inorganic ferrous sulphate. It is incomprehensible to me why such a compound, which retains its bivalency, is not prescribed instead. Ferrous gluconate is an example of such a compound and has been in use for decades. So far as I know, this preparation has never yet caused fatal poisoning, even though large quantities of it are occasionally swallowed by children. Even the baby gorilla, Goma, at the Basle Zoo, managed to get hold of a box of ferrous gluconate tablets for children and swallowed the contents without ill-effect. It is true that ferrous gluconate is more expensive than ferrous sulphate, but a pack sufficient for one course of treatment lasts for several weeks and does not cost more than a beef-steak. It should be possible, by means of a joint effort on the part of physicians and health authorities, to replace the relatively toxic ferrous sulphate by less toxic organic iron preparations with a sufficiently long shelf-life.

Moeschlin: I am afraid I cannot answer all the questions that have been raised, and I will leave some of them — especially those relating to studies with radioactive iron — to Dr. Wöhler.

To answer Dr. ALBAHARY's first question, you will see from Figs 2—6 of my paper that the optimum dose of desferrioxamine is 500—600 mg. twice daily by the intramuscular route, i.e. 1,000—1,200 mg. daily, dissolved in distilled water. You cannot increase the excretion of iron by raising the dosage to 2,000 or 3,000 mg. daily. You have practically no side effects when giving the drug intramuscularly; the intravenous route has no advantage at all and may lead to certain side reactions as already mentioned by several speakers. The water-soluble methane sulphonate, which has now been available for about one year, causes little or no pain when administered by the intramuscular route.

Dr. ALBAHARY also asked about the possibilities of oral treatment with desferrioxamine. By giving desferrioxamine orally we can inhibit the absorption only of the inorganic iron, but not of the organic form, i.e. we cannot block the uptake of the nutritional haemoglobin iron, which is one of the main sources of food iron. Incidentally, the clinical indications for desferrioxamine are listed in paragraph 5 of my summary.

Dr. ALBAHARY asked if one could obtain a better effect by administering desferrioxamine intermittently rather than continuously. In our cases we have only omitted the injections on Sundays. The patients either injected the drug themselves or arranged for parents or relatives to give them the injections intramuscularly. As you will have seen from the figures, there was no decrease in urinary iron excretion in our patients once a steady correlation had been established between mobilisation of the iron stores and urinary excretion of iron. On the contrary, it was quite impressive to see how the iron excretion remained at an almost stable level throughout the period of treatment lasting continuously for $1^3/_4$ years. We don't think the iron excretion could be increased by giving intermittent courses of desferrioxamine, and we prefer to administer a smaller dose as continuous treatment; for psychological reasons, however, it might conceivably be desirable to give intermittent treatment, particularly in less severe cases.

The question has been raised as to whether pancreatic and hepatic functions improve in response to treatment with desferrioxamine. We have not seen this in our patients with primary or secondary haemochromatosis, but I know that Dr. HEILMEYER, Dr. WÖHLER, and Dr. FREY[1] have seen an improvement in diabetes in one patient with primary haemochromatosis. The patient finally no longer required any further treatment with insulin. Also, as you have seen from the impressive data of Dr. WÖHLER, the liver may improve histologically. Of course, one has to be careful about interpreting the histological findings, because two biopsies never show the same part of the liver. We have also found that liver function tests (Bromsulphalein) may improve in some cases, especially in secondary haemochromatosis.

I have been asked by Dr. ALBAHARY if resistance or tolerance to desferrioxamine may develop. No, we have never seen any resistance developing in our cases, and the iron excretion levels, as I have just mentioned, have remained almost stable in the patients whom we have now been treating for nearly two years.

Should we also give desferrioxamine orally in cases of primary haemochromatosis? I think desferrioxamine is an expensive drug, which should therefore be reserved for injections. We do not believe that oral administration will have any real practical value, because — as I have already pointed out — only the uptake of the non-haemoglobin bound nutritional iron can be blocked. One

---

[1] FREY, F., L. HEILMEYER, and F. WÖHLER: Schweiz. med. Wschr. **92**, 1295 (1962).

very interesting thing is (and this has also been observed by Dr. KELLER, Dr. WÖHLER, and Dr. VERLOOP) that, if you give a patient who has severe anaemia an oral dose of desferrioxamine which would be sufficient to inhibit iron absorption (Fe^{59}) in a normal subject, the anaemic patient will still absorb an impressive amount of iron. This probably means that, if there is a real need for iron, the cells of the intestinal mucosa are still able to increase their iron uptake despite the effect of the orally administered desferrioxamine. This suggests that the whole mechanism of iron absorption may possibly be different from what we have hitherto imagined it to be.

Dr. FIGUEROA has asked about the possible side effects of desferrioxamine. We have not seen any side effects in our cases. We did see some undesirable reactions when we gave it intravenously in the beginning, but since we have been administering the drug intramuscularly we have not seen any side effects. MAIER[1] has reported a shock reaction in one case, but here the preparation had also been given intravenously, and I think this was probably an allergic reaction. But any drug may give rise to allergic reactions, and this is the only case that has so far been encountered in the course of many thousands of desferrioxamine injections.

Regarding the other questions, I only want to mention again the problem of ferritin and haemosiderin mobilisation by desferrioxamine. MAIER has incubated human bone marrow containing haemosiderin, and he was unable to demonstrate that desferrioxamine took up iron from the haemosiderin. This contrasts to some extent with the data of Dr. WÖHLER, and I suggest that the problem should be studied in further experiments. Clinically, there seems to be less iron excretion in patients in whom the overload consists mainly of haemosiderin iron, as borne out by the results obtained in the cases that have already been described.

Dr. BEARN asked where the iron is bound in cases of iron poisoning in children. From the case Dr. VANNOTTI reported to us (p. 293) I think it is evident that, in the child who had no ferritin at all in her plasma, there was still some iron bound to other fractions of the gamma-globulins. In these cases with very high, toxic levels, the iron is probably bound to different fractions of the plasma-globulins, but this question is still open to further investigation.

WÖHLER: I want to say a few words about our studies on the serum electrolytes. We have found no change in any of the patients whom we have kept under observation for two years. The calcium, potassium, and other electrolytes all remained normal, and no change occurred in the thrombocyte count either. Finally, I should just like to say something about the results we obtained when we treated several cases of porphyria cutanea tarda. In the four patients to whom we administered desferrioxamine, we observed very impressive responses.

The first case (patient S.) was a 55-year-old man who had been suffering from typical symptoms and skin changes since 1960. When he was admitted to hospital, we found very high uroporphyrin values of 7,800 μg./24 hours. The delta-aminolaevulinic acid, porphobilinogen, coproporphyrin, and 5, 6, and 7-carboxylporphyrin levels were also markedly elevated. The results obtained with desferrioxamine are shown in Fig. 13. The most pronounced decrease occurred in the uroporphyrin levels, which eventually dropped to around 1,000 μg./24 hours. All the other fractions indicated in the figure also showed a significant improvement. I should perhaps add that now, after

[1] MAIER, C.: Schweiz. med. Wschr. **92**, 1295 (1962).

treatment has been in progress for several months, the patient's skin is no longer sensitive to light and his general condition is much better.

In the second case (patient B.), in which the disease had not assumed such a severe form, the uroporphyrin and coproporphyrin values reverted to

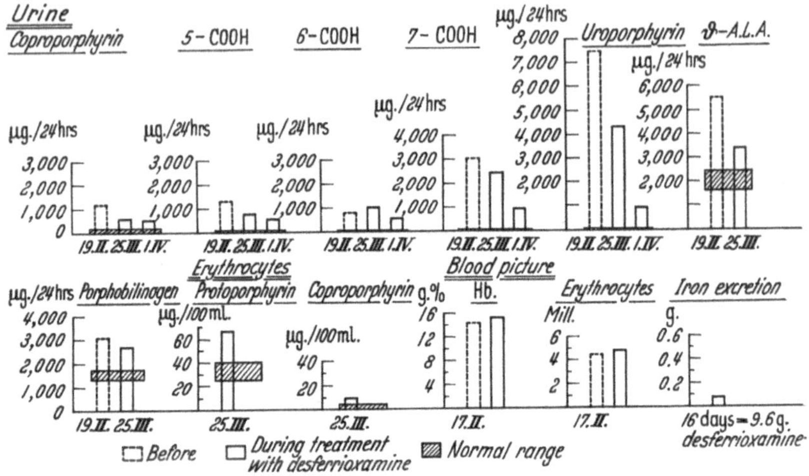

Fig. 13. Behaviour of the porphyrins in the urine and erythrocytes in a case of porphyria cutanea tarda (patient S.) under treatment with desferrioxamine. COOH = carboxylporphyrins; δ-A.L.A. = delta-aminolaevulinic acid

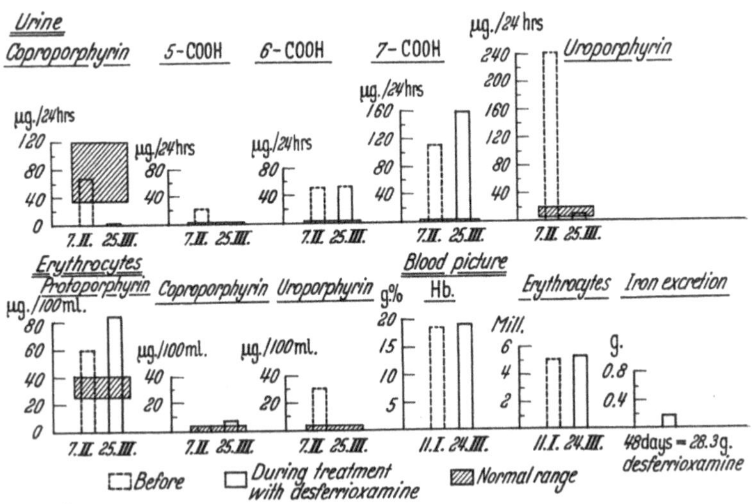

Fig. 14. Behaviour of the porphyrins in the urine and erythrocytes in a case of porphyria cutanea tarda (patient B.) under treatment with desferrioxamine

normal, as can clearly be seen from Fig. 14. Here again, a very satisfactory clinical improvement was noted during the course of treatment. In the third case, the uroporphyrin level, which had originally been around 1,200 μg./24 hours, once again fell to normal values (Fig. 15). The coproporphyrin, which

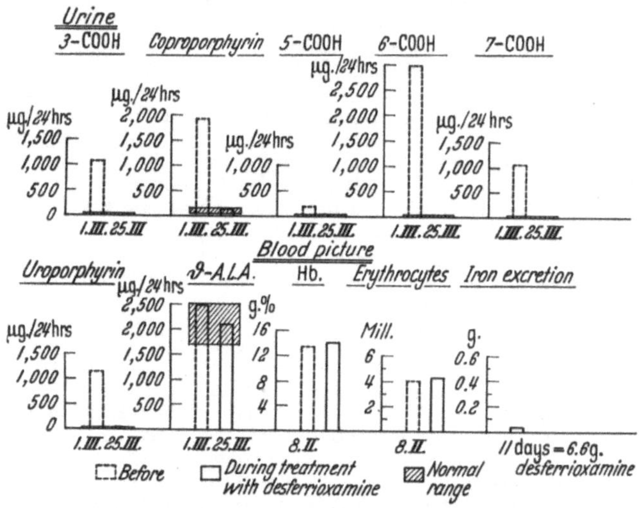

Fig. 15. Behaviour of the porphyrins in the urine and erythrocytes in a case of porphyria cutanea tarda under treatment with desferrioxamine

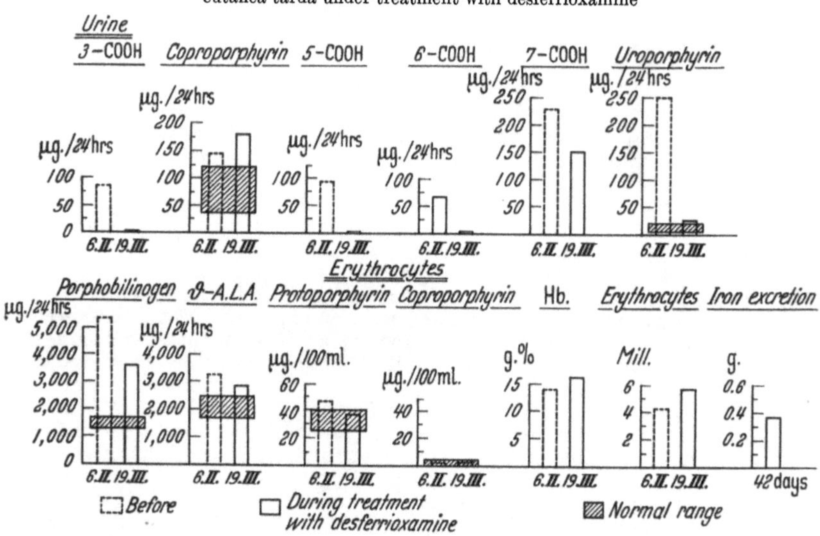

Fig. 16. Behaviour of the porphyrins in the urine and erythrocytes in a case of porphyria cutanea tarda (patient H.) under treatment with desferrioxamine

had been at 2,000 μg./24 hours, and the carboxylporphyrins likewise dropped to normal levels. In the last case of porphyria cutanea tarda (patient H.), similar results were again obtained (Fig. 16). The initially elevated uroporphyrin and 3, 5, and 6-carboxylporphyrin values became almost normal, while a marked decrease was also recorded in the values for delta-aminolaevulinic acid, porphobilinogen, and 7-carboxylporphyrin. The coproporphyrin level, however, was slightly higher than prior to treatment.

Thus, all four of these patients with porphyria cutanea tarda showed roughly the same response to desferrioxamine. A decrease occurs in the uroporphyrin, coproporphyrin, carboxylporphyrin, and porphobilinogen levels, as well as in the urinary excretion of delta-aminolaevulinic acid. This is accompanied by an improvement in the clinical picture. One striking feature of these cases is the fact that the amount of iron removed is not as great as, for example, in patients with primary haemochromatosis. In no case was more than 15 mg. iron excreted in the urine per 24 hours; indeed, in two of the patients the average urinary iron excretion worked out at only about 6 mg. daily. The blood picture invariably showed an increase in haemoglobin and in the erythrocyte count.

Although desferrioxamine produces an obvious improvement in these cases in which there is a disturbance affecting the synthesis of haem in the liver, we do not yet know where the drug's site of attack lies. One of the most likely explanations is that the iron blocks the enzymes responsible for haem synthesis, which contain SH groups, and that these enzymes become reactivated when the iron is eliminated. If this is so, then perhaps one might consider resorting to venesection in patients suffering from porphyria cutanea tarda — because venesection, of course, also removes iron and thus, in the last analysis, it has the same effect as desferrioxamine. On the other hand, treatment with desferrioxamine has the advantage of imposing less strain on the patient. At all events, I think the results I have just described demonstrate that desferrioxamine offers a new possibility for the treatment of porphyria cutanea tarda.

BRICK: I just want to answer Dr. ALBAHARY's question about the difficulty he had with D.T.P.A. in some of his patients in getting an increased iron excretion in the urine. He gave his patients immediate intravenous doses, whereas in all the patients that we have treated with intravenous infusions we administered the drug over a 3-hour period. This may explain that particular point. I think I have already emphasised that at the present time we cannot make any comment about whether this form of treatment is likely to replace venesection in haemochromatosis. I have great doubts about that. I also have great doubts about whether this is a practical proposition, since if you have to give intramuscular injections of desferrioxamine every day, it is going to prove costly, because this is an expensive drug. I think weekly venesection, which enables one to remove an exact quantity of iron, is still a convenient and satisfactory method of therapy; at least, it has proved to be so in our clinic.

I was disturbed by Dr. BEUTLER's report, since we have not had these distressing comatose episodes. However, it should be noted that his patients were very, very sick. I don't know what to attribute these episodes to, but the fact remains that they did occur. We, like Dr. FIGUEROA, have been using interrupted therapy, i.e. in most cases treatment for not more than 2 or 3 days at a time, followed by an interval of 2 or 3 weeks or longer. We have done this because of the possibility of renal damage as demonstrated in animal studies.

VISCHER: Dr. ALBAHARY asked whether there is any hope of finding orally effective preparations. We have, of course, prepared quite a number of derivatives of desferrioxamine, but unfortunately none of them has been found to be effective in animal experiments when given by mouth.

Dr. CALLENDER raised the question whether the variable results she has observed in her experiments with desferrioxamine could be attributed to differences in the preparations of desferrioxamine she was using. I think this possibility can be ruled out. However, desferrioxamine is not very stable in solution, and for this reason we recommend that the solutions should be used within 24 hours. If by any chance, in one or another of Dr. CALLENDER's experiments, solutions were used which had been standing for longer periods, this might explain the differences observed.

EICHHORN: I should like to make a brief comment on a matter that has cropped up several times, but I think the point needs some emphasis in order to correct impressions from an earlier discussion. During the discussion on the biochemistry of iron, the point was made that iron needed to be reduced to the +2 oxidation state in order to get it into, and out of, the ferritin molecule. If I understand Dr. WÖHLER's experiments correctly, he has placed ferritin inside a dialysis sac and desferrioxamine outside it, and he was able to remove the iron from the ferritin in this way without the use of reducing agents. Perhaps the conclusion that iron must be reduced to remove it from ferritin needs to be modified to the extent that if one employs a complexing agent like desferrioxamine, which binds iron(III) strongly enough, the iron can be removed in the +3 oxidation stage.

WÖHLER: That's right; the desferrioxamine takes the 3 iron ions directly from the ferritin.

SCHUBERT: A great deal of work has been done on the toxicity of D.T.P.A. The drug has been administered for long periods to people having deposits of radioactive plutonium in the body. Results relating to the toxicity of D.T.P.A. in humans, following administration over long periods, have been given in a publication by NORWOOD[1]. In any case, D.T.P.A. cannot be given daily; it is always administered intermittently. There may exist another factor which affects the toxicity of D.T.P.A. *in vivo* in cases where a large excretion of iron occurs. It may be that dissociation of the iron-D.T.P.A. produces high local concentrations of iron which result in damage to the tissues.

Desferrioxamine is an unusual chelating agent in the sense that it is highly specific for iron and remarkably unreactive with other metals under biological conditions (pH 7). This is not true of E.D.T.A. and the other polyaminocarboxylic acids. In addition, the very low degree to which desferrioxamine binds calcium improves its effectiveness *in vivo*. If one were to modify its structure so that less hydrogen binding occurred, the effectiveness of desferrioxamine at pH 7 might conceivably be enhanced, because the concentration of the chelating species would be higher. Another possibility might be esterification to increase the intracellular permeability. This has been done with polyamino acids, in which the carboxylic groups were esterified[2].

Dr. CALLENDER has referred to the diminishing effectiveness of desferrioxamine; this is something that happens with every chelating agent. In the case of heavy metals, the chelating agents remove the more labile stores from

[1] NORWOOD, W. D.: J. Occup. Med. (U.S.A.) **2**, 371 (1960).
[2] CATSCH, A.: Fed. Proc. (U.S.A.) **20**, 206 (1961).

the tissues and the blood; and then, after a certain point, the more refractory chemical forms which still remain are removed at a much slower rate. There is not much one can do about this, except to hope that with repeated treatment one may eventually manage to remove an appreciable fraction.

Finally, I should just like to make a suggestion: I think it might be worthwhile to try administering an appropriate solution of desferrioxamine by mouth, while at the same time partially neutralising the gastric acidity to about pH 5. Under these conditions, one might expect that the binding of desferrioxamine to iron would be increased several hundredfold, thus minimising dissociation of the iron chelate and hence improving absorption.

Hallberg: Just a brief remark about the side effects of desferrioxamine. When we gave desferrioxamine intravenously, we also observed flushing in some cases. The duration of this flushing and the subjective symptoms which occurred were of the same kind as those we encountered in certain cases in which iron-free transferrin was given intravenously; and they were also of the same kind as those we observed when ionised iron was given intravenously. I therefore think that the side effects of desferrioxamine are in some way related to a release of free iron ions.

J.-C. Dreyfus: Before I call upon Dr. Witts to sum up, I should like to make a few general remarks, and first to thank you all, on behalf of Dr. Schapira and myself, for participating in the Symposium. This has been a symposium of hope, since recent advances in therapy have now made it possible to provide effective treatment for certain types of patient with iron overload who could not have been satisfactorily treated before; for this reason, a great deal of time has been devoted to this question. Comparatively less emphasis has been placed on the more fundamental problems of iron metabolism, and it is to some of these that I should like to refer briefly here.

The chemistry of iron compounds has made great progress, but there is much that is still unknown; for example, it is still impossible to compare the binding of iron to protein in haem and non-haem compounds. When this has been achieved, it will perhaps become possible to synthesise simplified molecules, containing only the iron — or haem — attached to a few amino acids, and yet retaining the properties of the complete molecules.

Another important problem is the relationship between the synthesis of iron proteins and the actual presence of iron. It seems to me quite obvious that, if there is no iron, then no haemoglobin will be produced; on the other hand, it is not obvious why, under such conditions, globin should not be synthesised and should not accumulate in the erythroblats. If we consider for a moment the two non-haem iron proteins that have been well studied, we find two diametrically opposite situations: whereas transferrin is easily synthesised in the absence of iron, iron is necessary for the biosynthesis of ferritin — or at least it is a potent inducer of this protein. This phenomenon strikes me as being very interesting, since it is almost unique in the higher animals, and I suggest that the underlying mechanism would be well worth investigating at the cellular and subcellular level.

From the physiological standpoint, I would only remark that, though much has been said about the exchange of iron between the compartments of the body, very little has been added to our meagre knowledge about the way in which iron enters the organism. Granick's theory has been severely criticised, but no coherent alternative has been put forward to replace it.

In pathological states in which iron is involved, very little is known about the role played by the iron itself. The iron may accumulate in the form of an iron overload because it cannot be utilised; this would be the case where there is an absence of haem-synthesising enzyme. On the other hand, the accumulation of iron is often purely passive, i.e. because some step of porphyrin biosynthesis is impaired, because globin cannot be produced, or because the erythroblast itself cannot be made. Despite the efforts of Dr. HEILMEYER and his colleagues, much remains to be done to locate the biochemical lesion involved in the various syndromes we have been discussing, as well as to understand the way in which iron overloading damages the tissues, including particularly those of the endocrine system.

Finally, there remains the gap between the observations of physiologists and biochemists on the metabolism of iron and what has recently been described in the bone marrow by morphologists. Only a full understanding of all these findings can be expected to provide us with a clear picture of erythropoiesis.

These are only a few of the problems which remain to be solved—problems which I feel sure will provide ample scope for future symposia on iron metabolism.

Summing up

By

L. J. Witts

In a recent monograph by Dr. BEUTLER and his colleagues (*1*), I was referred to as one of the early workers in this field, and I therefore have the feeling that I have been brought forward like a Rip Van Winkle to comment on the advances of the last 35 years; but first I should like to say a word about Dr. DREYFUS and Dr. SCHAPIRA. Whereas the iron in the tissues occurs in tetrads, haematologists interested in iron seem to work in pairs, as for example, ROBSCHEIT-ROBBINS and WHIPPLE, or McCANCE and WIDDOWSON. We have been privileged this week to work under another famous pair, Dr. DREYFUS and Dr. SCHAPIRA. We were grateful to them before for their monograph on iron (*2*), and now we are grateful to them again for the way they have conducted this Symposium. Those of us who were born in English-speaking countries are indebted to the many members of the Symposium who were not and who have nevertheless all spoken in English. The one exception was the brilliant exposition by Dr. CAROLI which was given in French, and this very exception shows the sacrifices many of you made in having to translate your thoughts into English.

I have not the intention of talking about everything that has been mentioned. I am glad that we had an element of geographical pathology, and it was most interesting to hear Dr. CHATTERJEA on iron deficiency in India and Dr. BOTHWELL on iron excess in the Bantu. It was right that we should have begun with Dr. EICHHORN's paper on the function of iron in biochemistry, for much of our other research work on absorption and transfer of iron, partition between erythron, tissues, and stores, and the method of storage, is only a preliminary to this central problem. This theme was continued in the papers and discussions on hyposiderosis by Dr. MORGAN, Dr. BEUTLER, Dr. HALLBERG, and others.

Over the years I have continued to be interested in the epithelial lesions we see in iron deficiency — glossitis, Plummer-Vinson syndrome, achlorhydria, etc. We have worked on the hypothesis of WALDENSTRÖM (*3*) that the lesions are due to lack of iron for tissue enzymes in these rapidly proliferating cells, but we have stumbled on many contradictions. There are no obvious changes in the small intestine. It has not yet been possible to reproduce the changes in animals. There are considerable racial differences in the incidence of these lesions in man, and there seems to be a genetic factor which is evidenced by the occurrence of achlorhydria, iron deficiency, and pernicious anaemia in members of the same family. The position has been further complicated recently by the discovery of auto-immune reactions to gastric mucosa in patients with iron deficiency. Dr. UNDRITZ emphasised that this is not a matter of iron alone, but that other trace elements such as copper and cobalt are important. There seems to be agreement that there may be a difference between the symptoms of iron-deficiency anaemia when it is due to a deficient intake of iron (and therefore presumably of other principles) and when it is due to an increased iron loss.

We often get into semantic difficulties in talking about iron deficiency, because there are three ideas which we need to keep clear. The first is "normal", the second is "iron-sufficient", and the third is "physiological". By "normal" we mean the figures or range of values obtained from a statistically selected normal sample of a given population. By "iron-sufficient" we mean the figures obtained from animals or people on diets which cannot be improved by further supplementation with iron. For "physiological" we have no simple definition, but we mean the levels of red cells and haemoglobin which provide the optimum in terms of growth and development, freedom from illness, reproductive ability, and longevity. Confusion between these terms is most evident in discussions about the anaemias of pregnancy and of infancy, but it also underlies the controversy about *sideropenia sine anaemia*. Sideropenic symptoms such as glossitis may occur in patients whose haemoglobin is within the normal range, though they are obviously not in a state of iron sufficiency.

I wish we had had more time to talk about the problems of iron deficiency in pregnancy and infancy, because some physiologists are perturbed that we should need to give iron so frequently in these conditions. It is a puzzle to me that 20–25% of women in the reproductive epoch in Great Britain should be anaemic despite the rise in the standard of living. It seems as if Nature has managed badly. We had been led to believe that all species of animals are adapted to a particular sort of diet and that, provided the appropriate foods are available, every animal will choose the foods it eats in such a way as to satisfy its nutritional needs. It has been suggested that when *homo sapiens* first evolved he was a hunter and his diet contained much more iron than today, rather like the Eskimo, whose diet has been calculated to contain between 20 and 40 mg. of iron a day. With the discovery of cereals some 10,000 years ago, man for the first time became a food producer and ceased to rely only on gathering and hunting his foods. His diet contained less protein and less iron, and 10,000 years has been too short a time for him to adapt to the change. It is rather doubtful whether primitive man did in fact eat anything like so much meat as the Eskimo, and a more important factor may have been the contamination of food with earth, whose importance Dr. UNDRITZ has already emphasised in the nutrition of animals. When I was a child and fussed about my food, my mother used to say: "You've got to eat a peck of dirt before you die." I once calculated that a peck of dirt would just about double my intake of iron over my lifetime. Anyone who has seen the milling of wheat will have been surprised by the amount of dirt which is removed from the grain in the preliminary cleaning. There has undoubtedly been a great increase in the cleanliness of food in recent years, and this may well have meant a substantial decrease in our intake of iron. I confess I am not nearly as happy as Dr. MOORE about the level of iron in our modern diets. We need to provide a surplus, we need to discover how this can best be done, and we need to discourage foods which appeal to the palate but are poor in iron.

Had we had time we could have spent much longer discussing the absorption of iron. It seems doubtful whether the results obtained with radioisotopically labelled iron in the rat can be applied directly to the absorption of iron from the ordinary foods in man. The effects of pancreatic and hepatic disease on the absorption of iron are obviously still controversial. A relatively new subject is the occurrence of inborn errors in iron metabolism. The absence of transferrin in Dr. HEILMEYER's famous case, the hereditary differences in transferrins in man, the hereditary factor in haemochromatosis and sideroachrestic anaemia — all these are Nature's experiments which can be used to advance knowledge greatly. One wonders whether we are not missing other examples of genetic faults and whether we should not go back and look again at some of our cases which are resistant to iron therapy.

I came here with a mild prejudice against ferrokinetics, which seems to me not to have lived up to its early promise. A model is after all only an hypothesis, a curve or curves fitted to data are only an hypothesis, and a formula is merely the expression of an hypothesis in mathematical language. Models and formulae like those of Dr. POLLYCOVE must therefore be judged on a heuristic basis — in other words, by their results. It would appear from our discussions that workers are finding the study of ferrokinetics useful not only in the diagnosis of anaemia, but also in the study of conditions like haemochromatosis, in which iron metabolism is disturbed.

Scientists are like the unicellular organism paramoecium: they must conjugate from time to time if they are to remain fertile. We shall all go away from this Symposium with fresh ideas and enthusiasm for our research work. There is another way in which this Symposium has been of tremendous value. I believe we are now entering the twilight of the printed word, by which I mean that books and papers have become so numerous that it is impossible to read them all even by title. We are returning to the state of the medieval scholar who found that the best way to acquire knowledge was to travel and meet people who were learned in his subject. We have had the opportunity to meet many knowledgeable as well as delightful people, and it has been a great privilege for me to sum up this Symposium and to say how much I personally have learnt.

References

1. Beutler, E., V. F. Fairbanks, and J. L. Fahey: Clinical Disorders of Iron Metabolism. Grune & Stratton, New York/London, 1963. — 2. Dreyfus, J.-C., and G. Schapira: Le Fer. Biochimie, physiologie, pathologie. Expansion Scient. Franç., Paris, 1958. — 3. Waldenström, J.: Upsala läk.fören. förh. **46**, 215 (1941).

List of authors

Subject index

Kolibri 360 GmbH
Ferdinand-Jühlke-Straße 7
99095 Erfurt, Deutschland
produktsicherheit@kolibri360.de